J. M. Schröder
Pathology of Peripheral Nerves

Springer-Verlag Berlin Heidelberg GmbH

J. M. Schröder

Pathology
of Peripheral Nerves

An Atlas of Structural
and Molecular Pathological Changes

With 1052 Figures, partly in colour

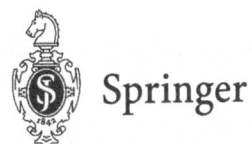 Springer

Dr. J. M. Schröder

Director
Institute of Neuropathology
University Clinic RWTH
Pauwelsstr. 30
52074 Aachen

(e-mail: jmschroder@post.klinikum.rwth-aachen.de,
Tel.: +49-241-8 08 94 28, Fax: +49-241-88 8 84 16,
homepage: http://www.klinikum.rwth-aachen.de/
webpages/neuropath/index.html)

ISBN 978-3-540-67718-5

Library of Congress Cataloging-in-Publication Data
Schröder, J. M. (J. Michael)
[Pathologie peripherer Nerven. English]
Pathology of peripheral nerves : an atlas of structural and molecular pathological changes / J. Michael
Schröder.
Includes bibliographical references and index.
ISBN 978-3-540-67718-5   ISBN 978-3-642-56808-4 (eBook)
DOI 10.1007/978-3-642-56808-4
1. Nerves, Peripheral–Diseases–Atlases. I. Title.
[DNLM: 1. Peripheral Nerves–pathology–Atlases. 2. Peripheral Nervous System Diseases–pathology–
Atlases. WL 17 S381p 2001]
RC409 .S37 2001 616.8'7–dc21

http://www.springer.de

© Springer-Verlag Berlin Heidelberg 2001
Originally published by Springer-Verlag Berlin Heidelberg New York in 2001

Typesetting: Fotosatz-Service Köhler GmbH, Würzburg
Cover design: E. Kirchner, Heidelberg
Printed on acid-free paper SPIN 10749151 24/3130/as 5 4 3 2 1 0

Preface

This atlas is based on a German textbook on the pathology of peripheral nerves, published in October 1999 [969], comprising 2,276 references and 1,052 figures compiled in 282 plates. All figures, but not all references, are included in the present atlas. Nevertheless, numerous key references from this text book are presented, which, in addition to the terms designating diseases and disorders or pathological and other alterations, may provide access to modern databases such as Medline (e. g., http://www.ncbi.nlm.nih.gov/PubMed) and Current Contents (locally available under http:\isi.digibib-www.de). One major advantage of an atlas over a literature database is the number and quality of illustrations, which are permanent, whereas textbooks may be outdated by the time they appear on the market. The figures in the present atlas are based on more than 6,000 nerve biopsies and a variety of experimental studies collected over more than 35 years. My interest in the pathology of peripheral nerves began during a research fellowship at the Harvard Medical School, Boston, Massachusetts, USA, in 1965, and continued during my time as Scientific Assistant at the Max Planck Institut für Hirnforschung, Abteilung für Neuropathologie, Frankfurt am Main, from 1966 to 1974, as Associate Professor of Neuropathology, Mainz, from 1974 to 1981, and as Full Professor of Neuropathology in Aachen, Germany, from 1981 to date. Presently, there are about 350–400 nerve biopsies, with or without muscle biopsies, submitted each year to this Department of Neuropathology for consultation from more than 100 hospitals in Germany, Luxembourg, and occasionally Austria (i. e., approximately 1–10 per hospital every year). Thus, nerve biopsy is a rare procedure usually not performed until all other diagnostic means have been applied without success (*cryptogenic neuropathies*). The tumor section, however, is based on surgical specimens which, although submitted for diagnostic purposes, were excised for therapeutic reasons.

In the textbook on which this atlas is based, the illustrations had to be reduced in size in order to fit the format of the series ("Spezielle pathologische Anatomie", edited by W. Doerr, G. Seifert, and E. Uehlinger). Its distribution is largely limited to German-speaking countries because it is written in German. Thus there are two reasons for producing the present atlas: (1) to increase the format of the illustrations from 63 % to 81.3 % of their original size, which was chosen to show details large enough to be detectable in print, and (2) to increase availability to those who are not able to read the German text.

The text between the images is kept to a minimum, whereas the descriptive legends to the figures are detailed, indicating the disorder or disease and describing the changes depicted. Many new and additional aspects may be found in the limited number of references (1,304) quoted. The index is kept as detailed as possible so that the diseases, disorders, and terms of pathological alterations can be found easily. Nowadays more information is readily accessible in all of these at the continuously updated literature databases mentioned or in other sources such as Online Mendelian Inheritance in Man (http://www.ncbi.nlm.nih.gov/omim), the Human Gene Mutation Database Cardiff (http://www.uwcm.ac.uk/uwcm/mg/hgmdo.html), and Mutation Data Base of Inherited Peripheral Neuropathies (http://molgenwww.uia.ac.be/CMTMutations).

It is a pleasure to acknowledge the secretarial help of Ms. Ingrid Schmitt and the editorial staff at Springer, Heidelberg, who effectively supported the timely appearance of this atlas. Clinical colleagues who provided biopsies for diagnostic purposes and the technicians preparing the specimens and photographs have already been mentioned in the preceding textbook version of this atlas. Again, their help and work are gratefully acknowledged. I would also like to thank my wife Monika for her patience and understanding during our vacations when I prepared the text for this book.

Aachen, September 2000   J. MICHAEL SCHRÖDER

Contents

CHAPTER 1

Introduction

Nerve fibers are prone to numerous artifacts if not properly excised, oriented, fixed or frozen, or embedded, cut, and stained (Figs. 1–3). Information about selection of nerves for biopsy and techniques of excision and preparation is provided by several authors [257, 669, 968, 969, 1085]. *Semithin sections* of plastic (epoxy resin)-embedded nerves are most informative. *Paraffin sections* of formalin-fixed nerve segments are still needed for identification of inflammatory changes, measurements of fascicular diameters or areas, and immunohistochemical determination of cellular infiltrates and macrophages. Glutaraldehyde fixation is essential for semithin sections but not for paraffin sections; it usually abolishes antigenicity for immune reactions and paraffin blocks become too hard and difficult to cut. *Teased fiber preparations* are time-consuming; they may be less essential for identification of primary than for secondary demyelination [255, 260, 483, 1127]. *Electron microscopic examination* is essential for identifying lamellar and other abnormalities of the myelin sheath (e.g., loose myelin, granular inclusions, axoglial dysjunction), and accumulation of abnormal organelles and structures in axons (e.g., in neuroaxonal dystrophy), Schwann cells (e.g., in adrenoleukodystophy), endothelial cells (e.g., in generalized gangliosidosis or ceroid lipofuscinosis), smooth muscle cells of blood vessels (e.g., CADASIL), macrophages (e.g., Niemann-Pick's disease type II), fibroblasts (e.g., mucopolysaccharidoses), extracellular precipitates (e.g., in dysproteinemias), and perineurial cells (e.g., dysplastic and degenerative changes). *Deep-frozen* nerve specimens are essential for immunohistochemical identification of cytokines and other components with low tissue concentration. To identify gene mutations in inherited neuropathies, *DNA extraction* from fresh, frozen, or paraffin-embedded sural nerve biopsies and further molecular genetic analysis may be essential [68, 208, 967, 997–999, 1015, 1017, 1018, 1121].

The most frequently and best studied human nerve is the *sural nerve*, which usually contains only sensory and autonomous components. It includes 9–21 fascicles and comprises 4,600–9,600 myelinated nerve fibers and 19,000–45,000 unmyelinated axons [978], or according to other authors 3,360–7,950 myelinated and 10,500–45,500 unmyelinated nerve fibers [459], depending on the age of the individual studied. The cross-sectional area ranges between 0.2 and 1.20 mm². Hence the density of the myelinated nerve fibers ranges between 4,080 and 25,890 per mm² and that of the unmyelinated axons between 17,300 and 193,200 per mm² [459]. The axon/myelin ratio (Figs. 4–7, 11) [975], the width of the paranodal attachment zone of the myelin sheath loops (Figs. 8, 9) [75], and the total fiber diameter (Fig. 11) have also been studied in relation to age.

Indications for a nerve biopsy are nowadays well delineated [926, 968, 1125], as are the *complications* [27, 739, 1064, 1119].

Skin nerves or other sites may also be informative [147, 149, 501, 653]. Mixed sensory and motor nerves (N. musculocutaneus or N. peroneus profundus) cannot be investigated without the risk of disturbing the motor function in the corresponding area [384]. Spinal ganglia have only rarely been studied by biopsy [361].

The *development, normal structure, and aging changes* of peripheral nerves [73–75, 260, 459, 541, 630, 826, 966, 1190, 1216] are illustrated in Figs. 4–11, and tissue culture studies in Figs. 12 and 83. The *blood–nerve barrier* [784, 785] and the *perineurial barrier* [521] are important for maintaining an adequate endoneurial milieu [827]. The *blood vessels* are of particular importance for nourishing Schwann cells, axons, and other components of peripheral nerves [50, 51]. Their number and structure are altered in the large number of inflammatory processes and the other processes involving peripheral nerves [327, 1006] (see below).

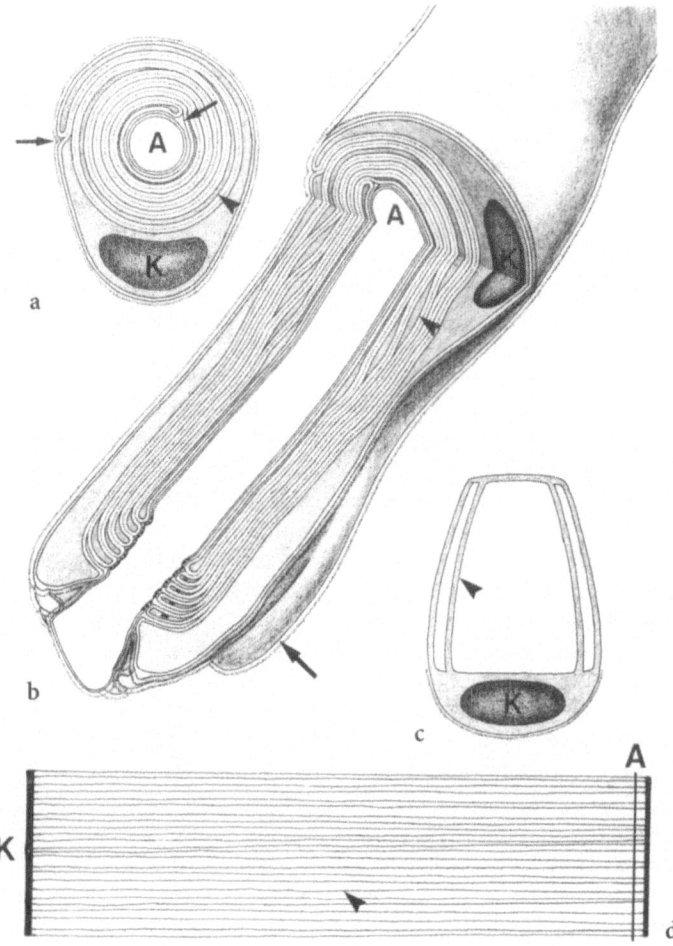

Fig. 1a–d. Four different schematic views of a Schwann cell. **a** Cross section with outer and inner mesaxon (*arrows*), intermediate lines (*dotted*), major dense lines (*continuous line*), the spirally arranged myelin lamellae, cytoplasmic extension of a Schmidt-Lanterman incisure (*arrowhead*), the nucleus (*K*) and the axon (*A*). **b** Combined cross- and longitudinal view of an internode with a node of Ranvier and a nucleus (*K*), a Schmidt-Lanterman incisure (*arrowhead*) and the outer aspect of a paranodal myelin loop (*thick arrow*). **c** Unrolled myelin lamella of a Schwann cell with paranodal cytoplasmic extensions and two Schmidt-Lanterman incisures (*arrowhead*). **d** Dimensions of an unrolled myelin sheath drawn to proportion. The thickness of the axon (*A*), the length of the internode, the length of the unrolled myelin lamella, the size of the nucleus (*K*), the decreased width of the myelin sheath at the inner mesaxon, and the number of the Schmidt-Lanterman incisures (*arrowhead*) correspond approximately to the real proportions of a nerve fiber 10 µm in thickness with 100 myelin lamellae and an internode, 1 mm in length. (From [951])

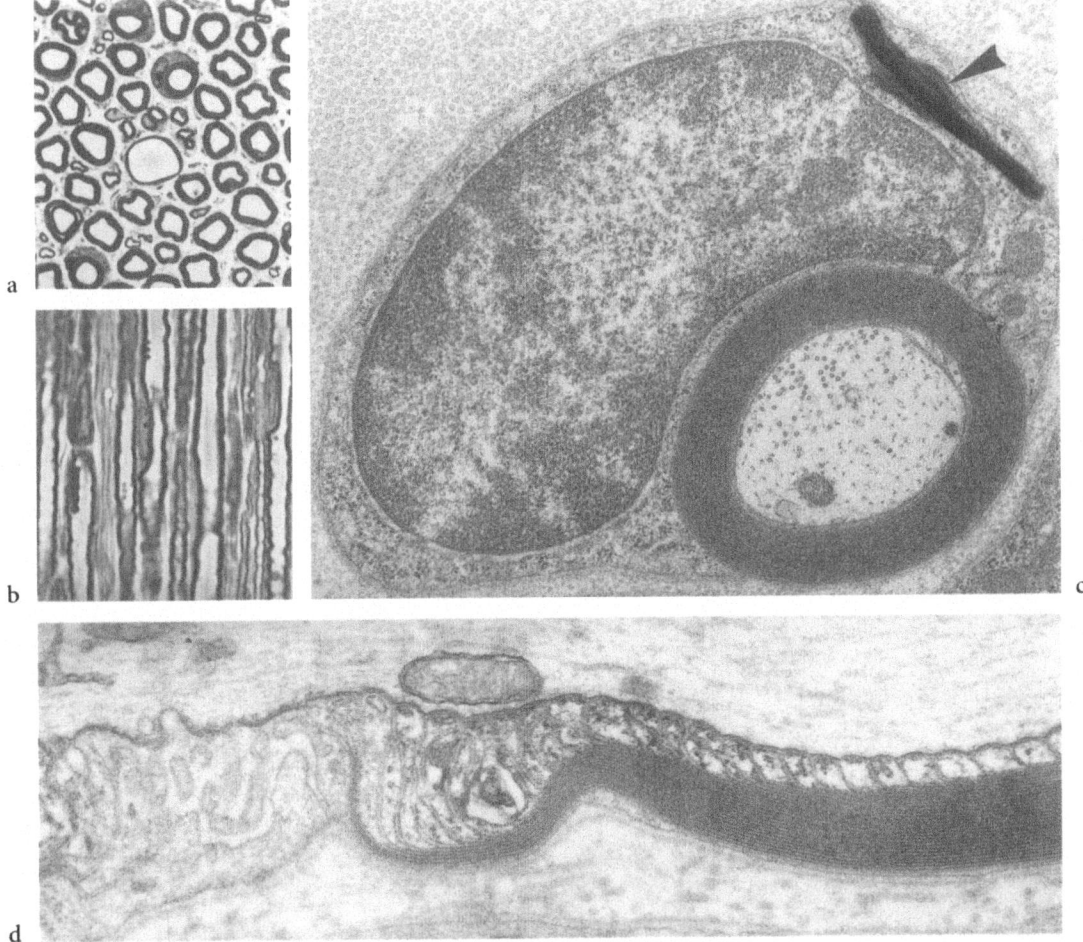

Fig. 2a–d. Optimal fixation of myelinated nerve fibers **a** in a cross section, **b** in a longitudinal section, **c** electron microscopically in a cross section, and **d** in a longitudinal section at the level of a node of Ranvier. The *arrowhead* indicates a π-granule. If not indicated otherwise, semithin sections of sural nerve biopsies were used stained with paraphenylenediamine or toluidine blue for light microscopy, and ultrathin sections following contrast enhancement with lead citrate and uranyl acetate for electron microscopy. **a** × 370; **b** × 640; **c, d** × 27,500

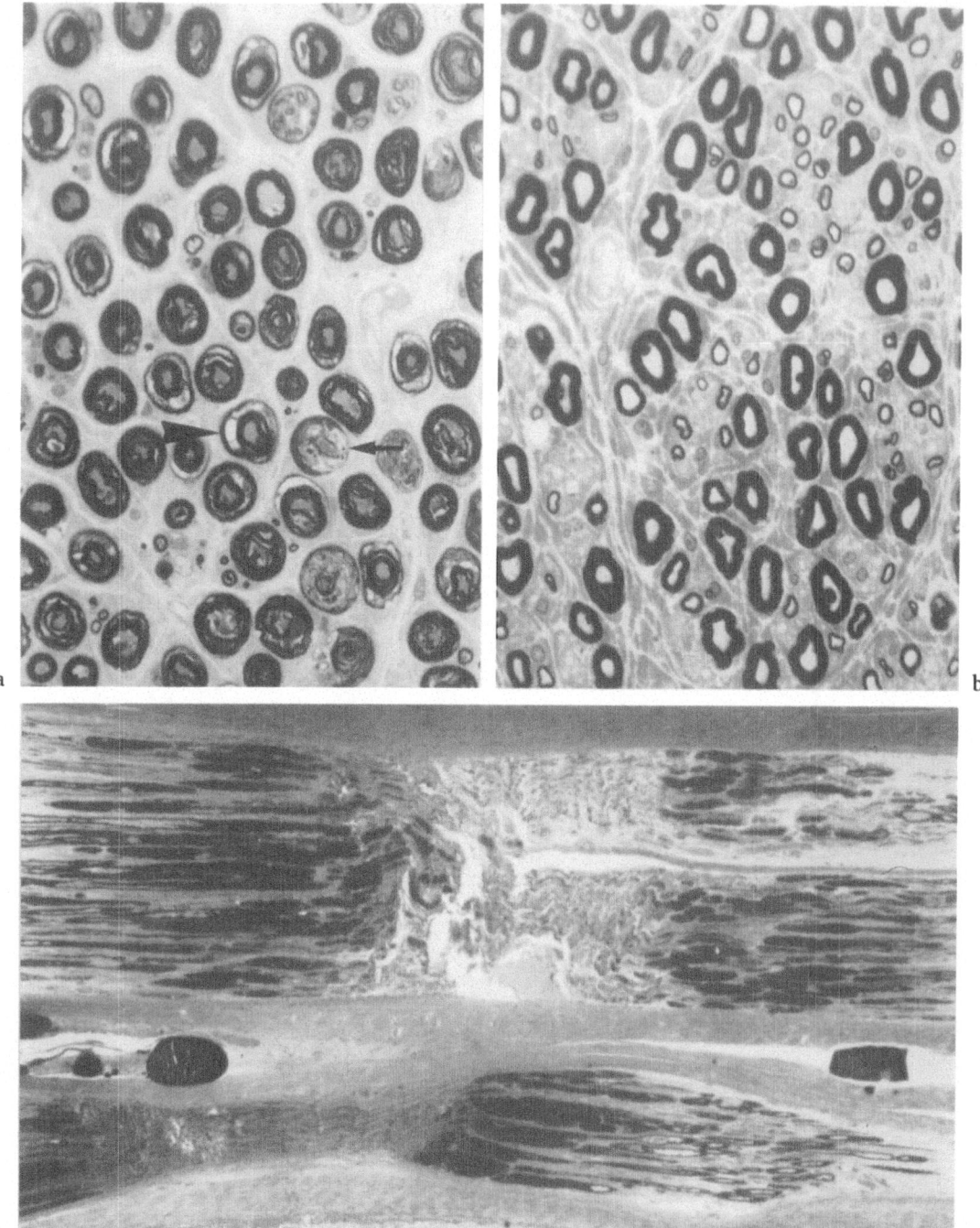

Fig. 3. **a** Typical formalin fixation artifacts with swelling of the myelin sheaths, especially of the Schmidt-Lanterman incisures (*arrowhead*), and paranodal myelin sheaths (*arrow*). **b** Following fixation of the sural nerve in a solution of 3.9% glutaraldehyde with 0.4 m phosphate buffer there are no such swelling artifacts. **a, b** Semithin sections of a nerve taken at autopsy; paraphenylenediamine. ×588. **c** Crush lesion of the sural nerve during excision for biopsy. The myelin sheaths have been squeezed out of the compressed area by the branches of the forceps used. The continuity of the more resistant connective tissue is preserved. Semithin section, toluidine blue, ×94

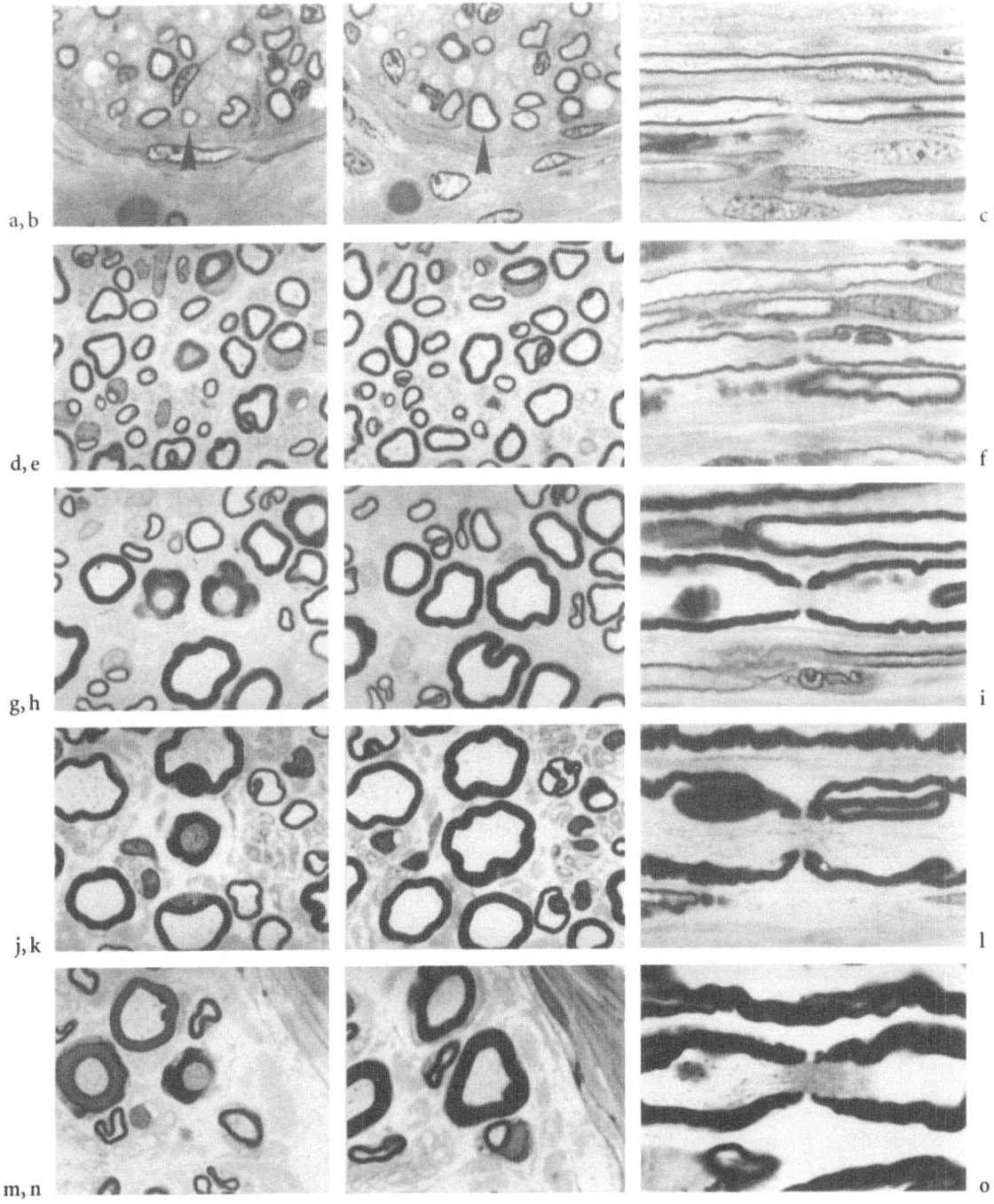

Fig. 4a–o. Light microscopic comparison of paranodal (**a, d, g, j, m**) and internodal axonal segments (**b, e, h, k, n**) of corresponding cross and longitudinally oriented (**c, f, i, l, o**) nerve fibers in sural nerves of patients at different ages. The caliber increases in both axonal segments (*arrowheads* in **a, b**) especially during the first months of life (**a–c**: 0.01 months; **d–f**: 2 months; **g–i**: 19.5 months; **j–l**: 62 months; **m–o**: 540 months). × 1,500. (Modified from [75] and [966])

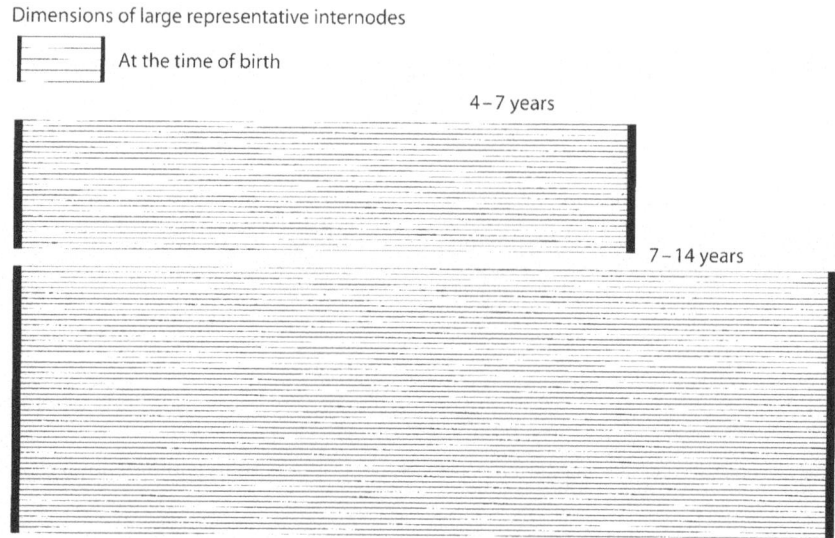

Dimensions of large representative internodes

At the time of birth

4–7 years

7–14 years

Fig. 5. Development of myelin lamellae thought to be unrolled of large, representative internodes drawn to proportion. The dimensions are based on measurements on the length of the internodes (*left vertical line*), the number of the Schmidt-Lanterman incisures (*middle horizontal lines*), the number of the myelin lamellae, and the circumference of the myelin sheaths as well as of the axons (*right vertical line*: adaxonal cytoplasm of the Schwann cells). The largest internode at the time of birth measures about 250 μm (*upper figure: left margin*). (From [958])

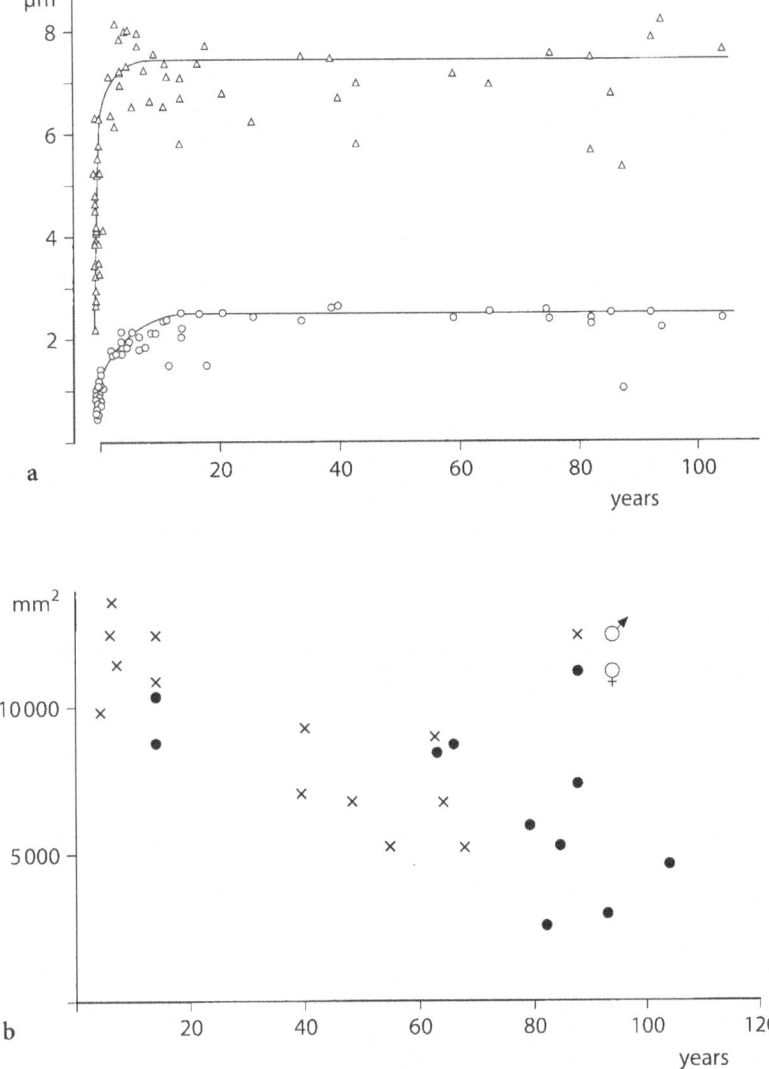

Fig. 6. a Development of axonal diameter and myelin sheath thickness in the sural nerve of man (biopsy and autopsy cases; the latter may include clinically unidentified neuropathies). The ten largest nerve fibers were measured in each nerve at the age of 4 months before term until the age of 104 years with the help of an ocular micrometer using maximal light microscopic magnification. **b** Number of myelinated nerve fibers per mm² (nerve fiber density) in sural nerves of men and women. The nerve fiber density decreases during life which is partly due to an increase of the endoneurial collagen. (From [958])

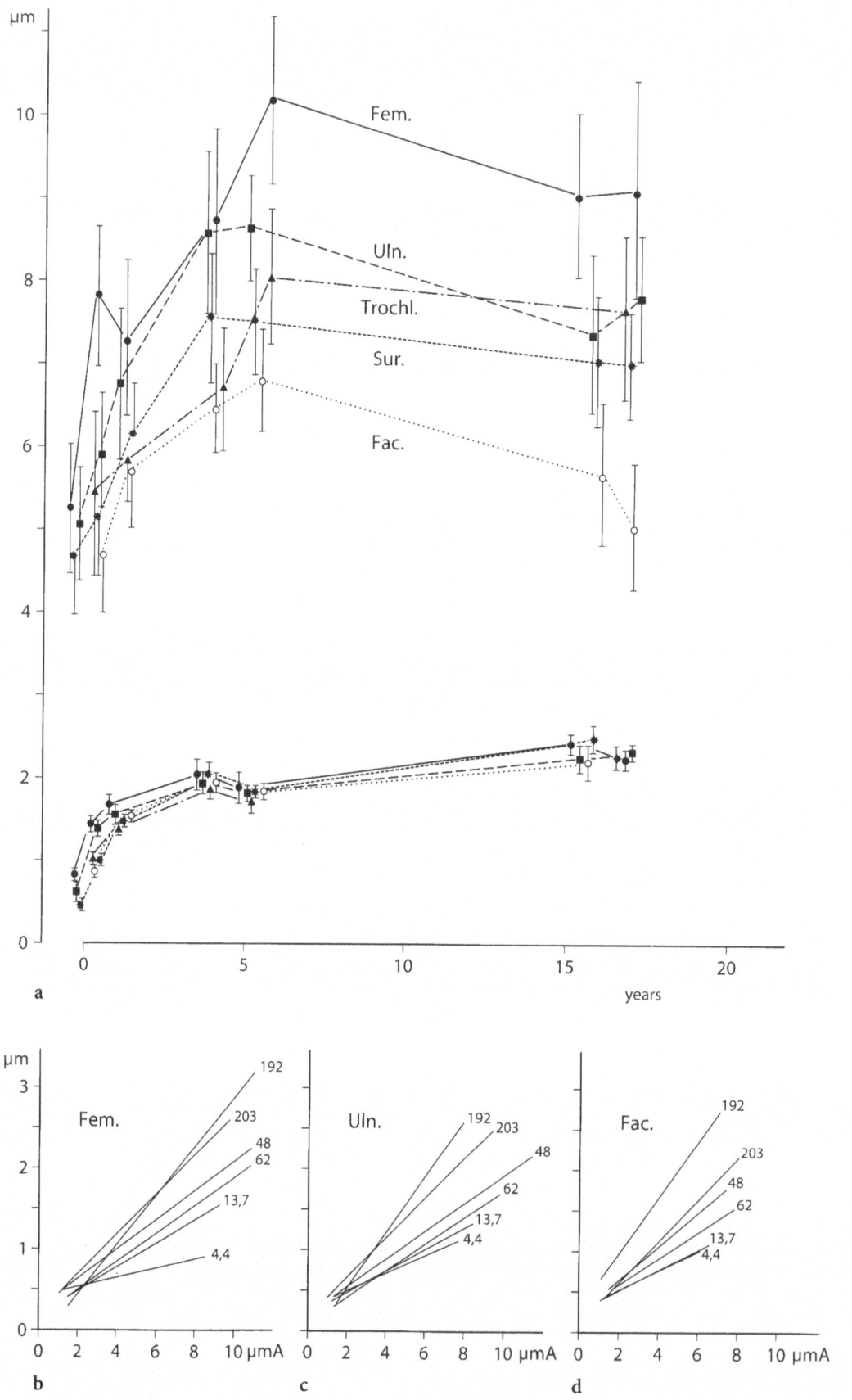

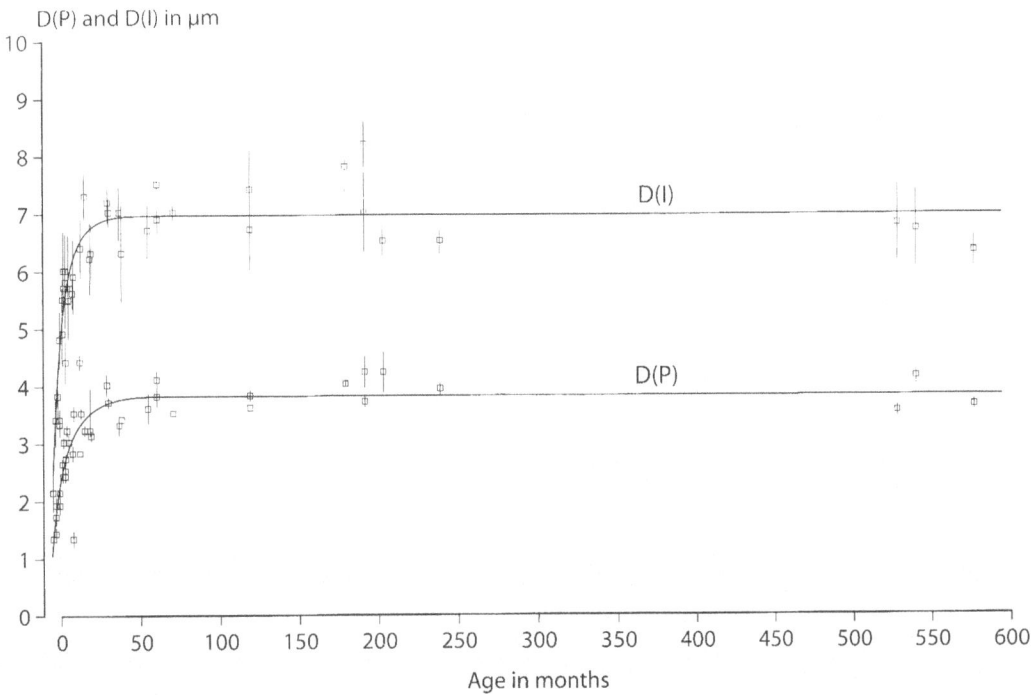

Fig. 8. Light microscopic measurements of the internodal [D(I)] and paranodal [D(P)] axon diameter (*ordinate*) of the largest sural nerve fibers in relation to the age of the individuals studied (*abscissa*). In both axonal segments there is a nearly continuous increase of the caliber with increasing age. Regression analysis reveals a nonlinear, exponential caliber growth during the life period studied corresponding to the formula $y = a\,[1 - \exp(-lx)] + b$. (From [75])

Fig. 7. **a** Mean values with standard deviations (*vertical lines*) of ocular micrometer measurements of the 20 largest myelinated nerve fibers in femoral, ulnar, trochlear, sural, and facial nerves at seven different stages of age. In the *upper part* of the diagram, the axons of the different nerves are indicated by various *symbols* which are connected by different *lines* delineating corresponding nerves. In the *lower part* of the figure, *analogue symbols* and *lines* were used to indicate the mean values for the myelin sheath thickness of the same nerve fibers. Maximal values for the axons are already reached at the age of 5 years or before, whereas the maximal myelin sheath thickness is not reached before the age of 15 years. **b–d** Simplified (linear) regression lines for the ratio between axon diameter (*abscissa*) and myelin sheath thickness (*ordinate*) for a large number of nerve fibers, measured and calculated with the help of a TGZ3-Automatik (Zeiss, Oberkochen, Germany) for femoral, ulnar, and facial nerves at the age of 4.4–203 months. The age is indicated in months at the *right upper end* of each line. In general, the regression lines are shorter and increase less steeply in younger children than in older children. (From [975])

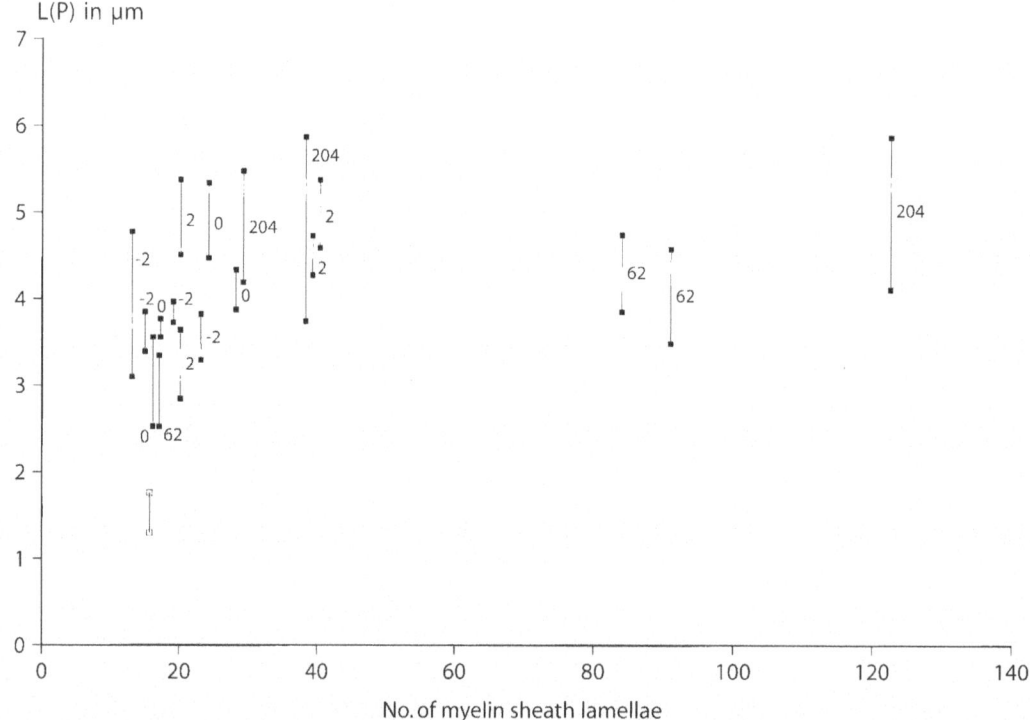

Fig. 9. Relation between the length of the paranodal myelin sheath attachment zone at the axon [L(P); *ordinate*] and the number of the lamellae (*abscissa*) of the myelin sheath in corresponding nerve fibers. The *connecting lines* indicate the lowest and the highest value, measured on both sides of an individual node of Ranvier. The *numbers* at the connecting lines indicate the age in months of the individuals studied. In contrast to the considerable increase of the number of the lamellae during development, there is no corresponding change in the length of the paranode when fibers of the same caliber group are compared with each other. The paranodes of small fibers in a single sural nerve tend to be shorter than those of large fibers. (From [75])

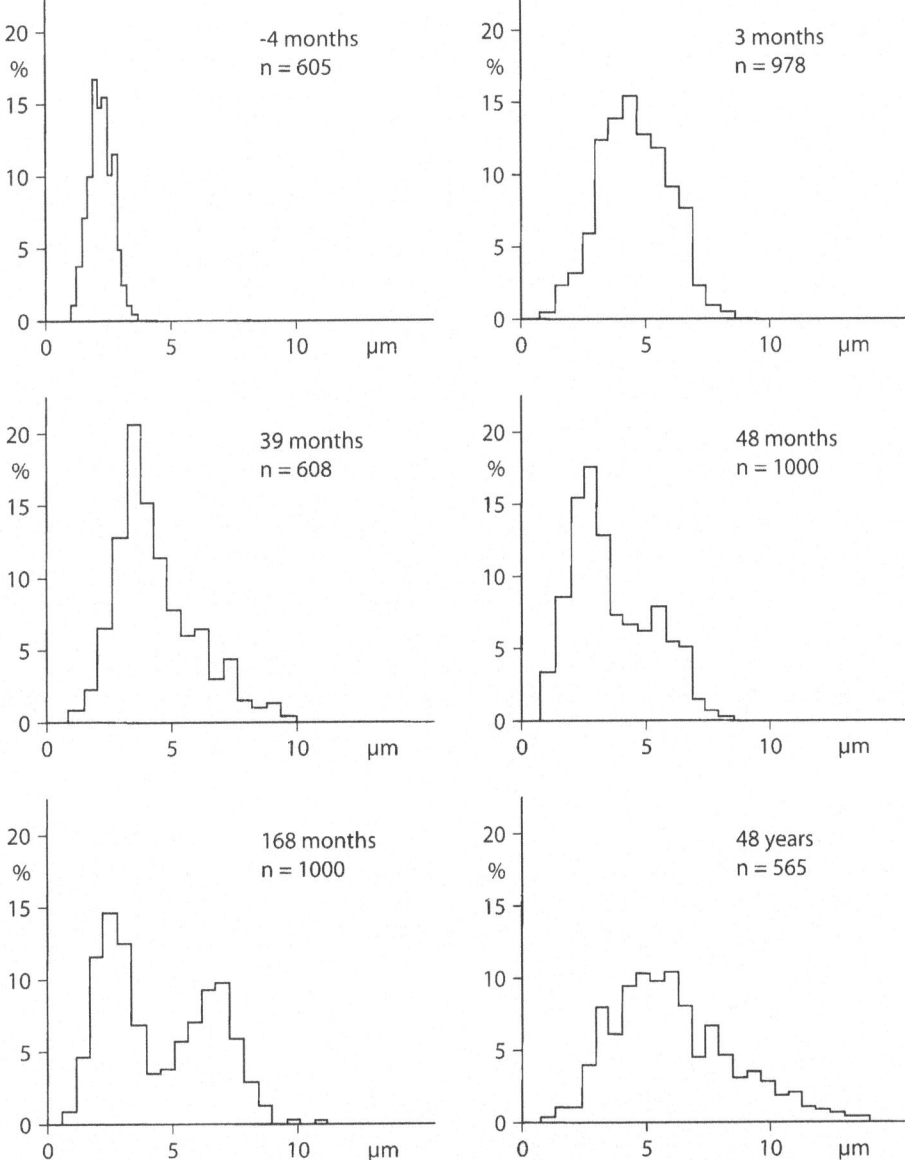

Fig. 10. Development of myelinated nerve fibers at the age of 4 months before term (–4 months) to 92 years. *n* = number of evaluated nerve fibers

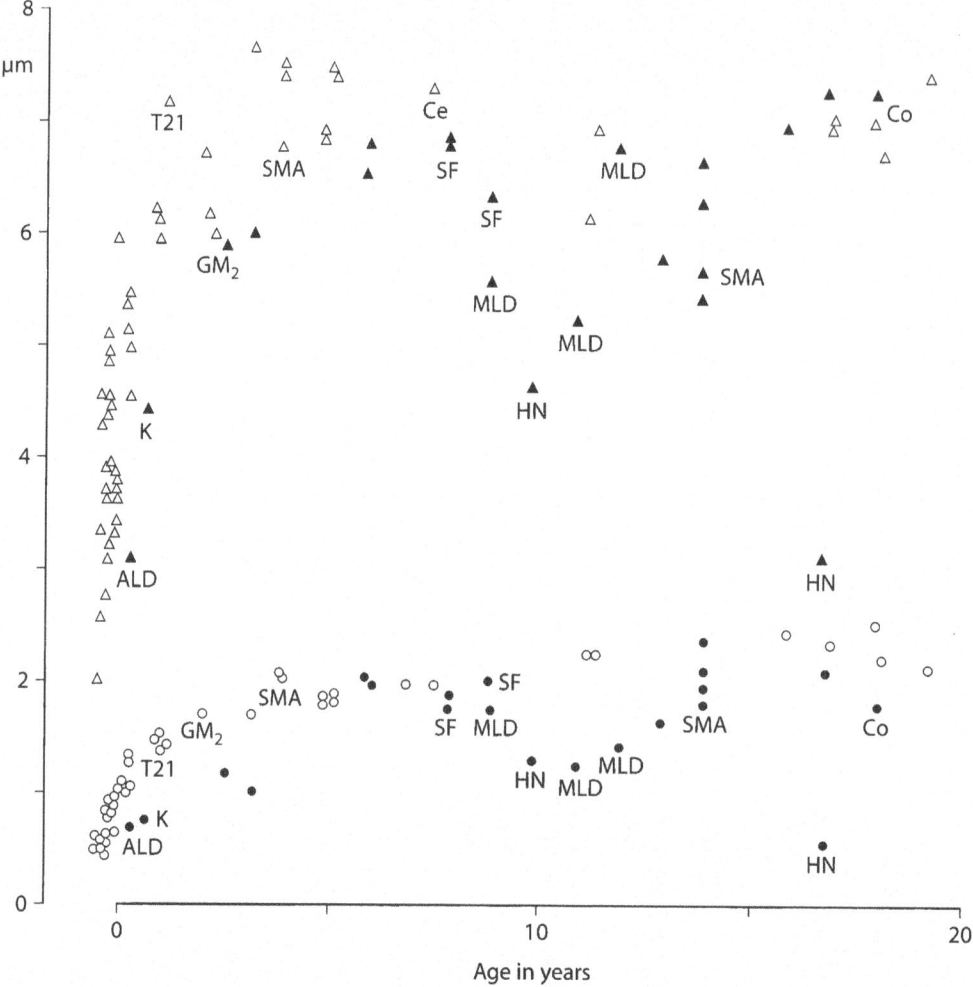

Fig. 11. Sural nerves: axon caliber (△) and myelin sheath thickness (○) in the 20 largest myelinated nerve fibers of control cases (*open triangles and circles*) and of various polyneuropathies (*filled triangles and circles*) some of which are unidentified (not labelled). *ALD*, adrenoleukodystrophy; *Ce*, ceroid lipofuscinosis; *Co*, Cockayne's syndrome; *GM2*, GM$_2$-gangliosidosis; *HN*, hypertrophic neuropathy (Dejerine Sottas); *K*, Krabbe's leukodystrophy; *MLD*, metachromatic leukodystrophy; *SF*, Sanfilippo's disease; *SMA*, spinal muscular atrophy; *T21*, trisomy 21. (Figs. 10 and 11 from [960])

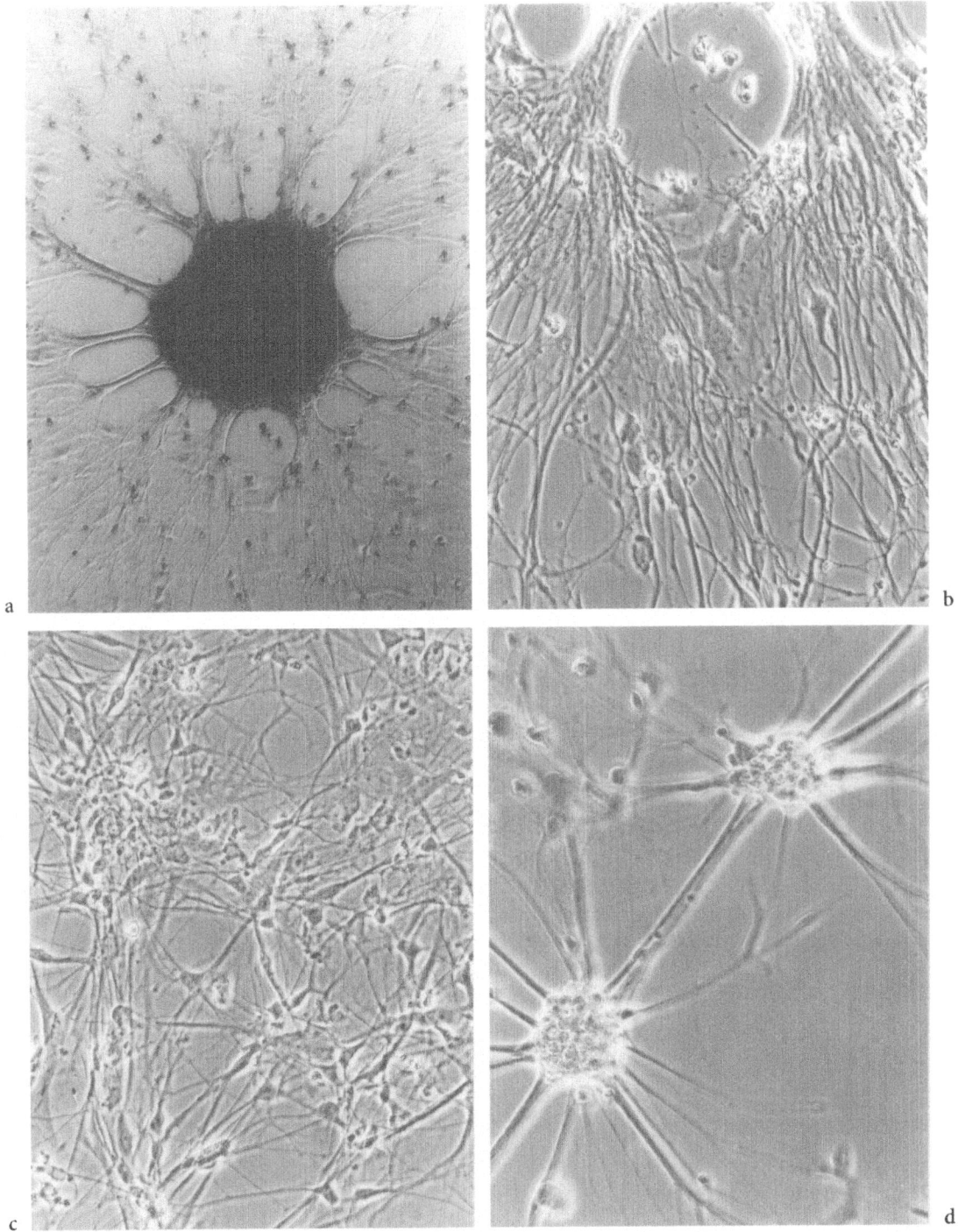

Fig. 12. Organotypic cultures of spinal ganglia showing centrifugal growth of neurites which may vary considerably in different explants with no addition of neurotrophic factors. Such variations need to be considered in experimental studies of pharmacological actions. (From Weber; Inauguraldissertation, Aachen 1988)

CHAPTER 2

Epidemiology and Classification of Peripheral Nerve Disorders

The *annual incidence* of mononeuropathies as well as polyneuropathies has been estimated as 40 per 100,000 persons [551]. Analysis of health care data in the United States revealed that 17.6% of ambulant neurological patients showed disorders of the musculoskeletal and connective tissue system [663]. The *etiology* of peripheral neuropathies remained unsettled in 13% of these patients after 1 year of follow-up [656]. It will always be difficult to determine the exact borderline between a normal state and a minimal manifestation of motor, sensory, and autonomic disturbances caused by peripheral nerve lesions. A field study in northern Italy [439] revealed a possible polyneuropathy in 7% (8.1%), and probable polyneuropathy in 3.7% (3.4%) of a population of 4,191 patients aged over 55 years and examined by general practitioners in the regions of Varese and San Givanni Rotondo, respectively. Rates per 100,000 persons per annum are available for diabetic neuropathy (54), compressive neuropathies (49), and all types of peripheral neuropathies (15) [622].

In an international *classification* of neuromuscular disorders made by the Research Group on Neuromuscular Disorders of the World Federation of Neurology [1204], 809 items were enumerated; 347 comprised primary disorders of skeletal muscles, 271 were forms and causes of peripheral neuropathies. Yet these are only rough and preliminary data on the number and frequency of disorders of the peripheral nervous system.

CHAPTER 3

General Lesions and Reactions of Peripheral Nerves

The most frequent lesions of peripheral nerves are schematically illustrated in Fig. 13a–f'', the sequence of changes during and following *Wallerian degeneration* in Figs. 14a–h and 37a–f. Fine structural alterations of *axons* are shown in Fig. 15a–f (and other Figs.; see Subject index!), at the *node of Ranvier* in Fig. 16a–c, at *Schmidt-Lanterman incisures* in Fig. 17a–i, and in *adaxonal compartments* in Figs. 18–21. The *abaxonal cytoplasm of Schwann cells* may include different shapes of π-granules of Reich (Figs. 22, 23), nuclei (Figs. 24–27, 60, 234), mitochondria (Fig. 28a, b, 164–168), and lysosomes (Figs. 28d, 33d), or unidentified structures (Figs. 28c, 29d) and μ-granules of Elzholz (Fig. 29a, b). Presumptive *transnodal remyelination* is shown in Fig. 29b and severe *siderosis* in Fig. 30a–d.

Degenerating endoneurial fibroblasts (Figs. 31a–d, 32a–c) occur as a nonspecific phenomenon, but are particularly frequent in inflammatory disorders [360]. A *defective nuclear membrane* (Fig. 31e) is of special interest since this change was noted as a characteristic nuclear alteration of nuclei in skeletal muscle fibers of a patient with emerin deficiency [289]. We noted a similar change in Schwann cell nuclei of myelinated and unmyelinated fibers as well as endoneurial fibroblasts in this disease [1092]. The presence of *melanin-like pigment granules* in endoneurial fibroblasts (Fig. 31f) is a unique, unexplained finding.

The number of *endoneurial mast cells* (Fig. 33a–c) is increased in inflammatory neuropathies [407, 523].

The *endoneurial connective tissue*, especially the *collagen*, increases in a large number of conditions representing a nonspecific reaction. Collagen is the main component causing the pseudohypertrophy in hypertrophic neuropathy [1217] (Figs. 99, 100, 209). A combined increase of *oxytalan fibrils* (as one component of elastic fibers) and collagen in association with perineurial cells is seen in *Renaut bodies* (Figs. 34–36), which occur at sites of compression [1221], especially in association with *carpal tunnel syndrome*, *meralgia paraesthetica* (Fig. 35), and *Morton's metatarsalgia* (Fig. 36). Lectin binding to

Renaut bodies indicates the presence of mannose, glNAc, and sialinic acid [719]. There is a correlation between body mass and carpal tunnel syndrome [1229]. Other compression syndromes include *lotus neuropathy* [651], cervical or other *radiculopathies*, thoracic outlet syndrome, brachial neuropathy, *mononeuropathy* of the ulnar or the common peroneal nerve, and disturbances of *pelvic floor innervation* in association with chronic obstipation and perineal descensus causing anorectal incontinence [1056].

Experimental models and surgical procedures have largely clarified the pathomechanisms underlying *compression syndromes* and *nerve constriction* [317, 535, 583, 608, 612, 623, 761, 883, 917, 931, 982].

Transection of nerves causes Wallerian degeneration and changes in the endoneurial, perineurial, and epineurial connective tissue with subsequent *neuroma* formation if the connection to the peripheral nerve stump is lost [72, 125, 160, 295, 305, 342, 350, 375, 416, 614, 824, 909, 993, 1051, 1090, 1109, 1110, 1226, 1237].

Nerve grafting [279, 668, 673, 924, 993, 994, 1013, 1031, 1095, 1250] may then be necessary (Figs. 38–50). Tubulization experiments offer interesting insights for nerve grafting [611, 989]. Tubules seeded with Schwann cells grown in tissue culture to be used instead of nerve grafts are still at an experimental stage [19]. The same holds true for experiments with end-to-side anastomosis [613]. Any experimental effort to bridge gaps in peripheral nerves should focus on investigating gaps larger than approximately 1–3 cm because distances below this limit will spontaneously be overcome by the regenerative power of the peripheral nervous system with no aid [114]. The crucial point is vascularization and supply with nutrients in grafts longer than roughly 3 cm and thicker than approximately 2–3 mm [994].

Following any nerve lesion, especially transection and grafting, *terminal reinnervation* of end organs is crucial. This concerns *motor end plates* and *muscle spindles* (Figs. 51, 52) [227, 231], *Pacini corpuscles*, and other end organs including sweat glands. Definite statements regarding the final outcome following interruption of nerve fibers (not simply segmental demyelination) should not be made before approximately 2 years. Thereafter complications such as *fibrosis* of muscle tissue, *retrograde atrophy*, and finally *retrograde degeneration* of nerve fibers (Figs. 53, 54) may influence the long-term outcome of reinnervation [106, 925, 1178]. The long-term influence of the short-living *growth factors* and other *cytokines* [21, 87, 126, 183, 184, 209, 340, 348, 401, 428, 440, 503, 590, 600, 617, 683, 729, 745, 828, 861, 887, 1043, 1074, 1161, 1171, 1208, 1243, 1281, 1285] is probably minor if not maintained by the feedback mecha-nisms from contact with adequate end organs such as muscle fibers.

Traction of spinal roots out of the spinal cord [118, 601] probably causes irreversible loss of function (Fig. 55) although there is some unconfirmed experimental evidence that neurosurgical reunion may be beneficial [419].

Tension [1174], *cold injury* [471, 502, 1134], *heating* [1253], *electric injury* [283, 1048], and *radiation* (Fig. 56) may all cause nerve lesions. A radiation dose of more than 20 Gy may cause considerable clinical symptoms [1201].

Segmental demyelination   Secondary degeneration

Neurotmesis

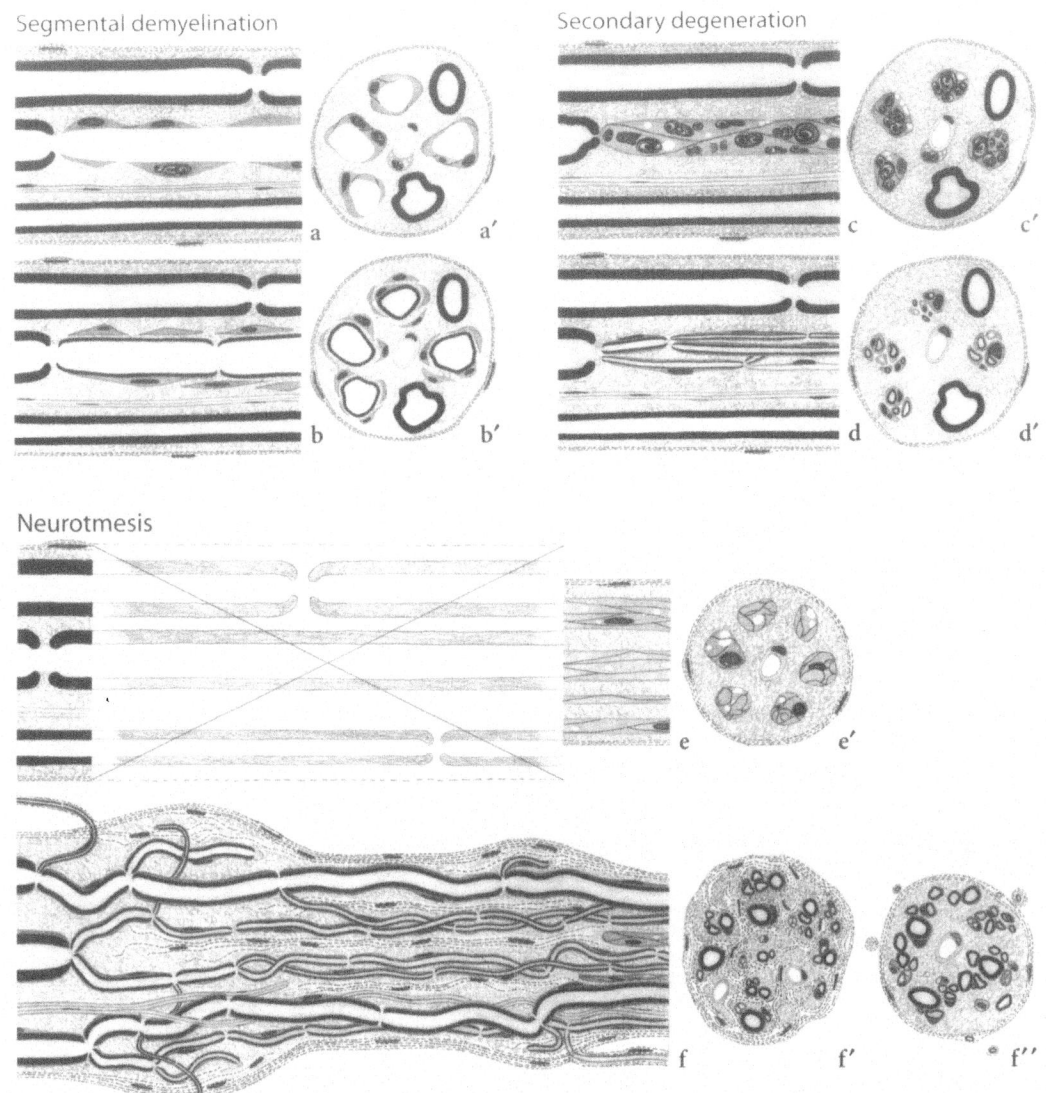

Fig. 13 a–f''. Schematic view of the three most important lesions of peripheral nerves with the corresponding patterns of repair. (From [965]). **a** and **a'** Longitudinal and cross-sectional areas of a nerve with one or more segmentally demyelinated axons, the continuity of which was not interrupted. The Schwann cells of the affected internodes are proliferated and contain still some myelin degradation products. **b** and **b'** Longitudinal and cross sections showing the corresponding pattern of repair. The demyelinated axons remain thinly remyelinated. The newly formed internodes are shortened. Some supernumerary proliferated Schwann cells lie circularly arranged around the remyelinated nerve fibers. **c** and **c'** Cross and longitudinal views of degenerating nerve fibers, the continuity of which is completely interrupted (secondary, Wallerian degeneration). The proliferating Schwann cells contain numerous myelin degradation products. **d** and **d'** Clusters of myelinated nerve fibers are seen at the site of the degenerated nerve fibers while the endoneurium is preserved. The regenerated nerve fibers are of uneven thickness and remain partially unmyelinated. **e** and **e'** Distal to a complete interruption of the whole nerve the proliferated Schwann cells remain at the site of the degenerated nerve fibers in the form of longitudinally oriented, empty bands of Büngner in the endoneurium, which may or may not become reinnervated. **f, f'** and **f''** A nerve defect or a nerve graft has been reinnervated in a neuromatous pattern by bundles of small regenerated nerve fibers surrounded by a newly formed perineurial cells (*dotted lines*) isolating the regenerated clusters from the surrounding connective tissue (minifascicles) (**f** and **f'**). Some nerve fibers may be branching laterally or recurring or ending freely in the adjacent connective tissue. Others may reach the distal nerve fascicle (**f''**) finding a band of Büngner. Here, the bundles of nerve fibers will not be surrounded by newly formed perineurial cells, but by the preexisting perineurium of the original fascicles. Isolated aberrant fascicles lie in the epineurium of the distal nerve segment surrounded by a separate perineurium

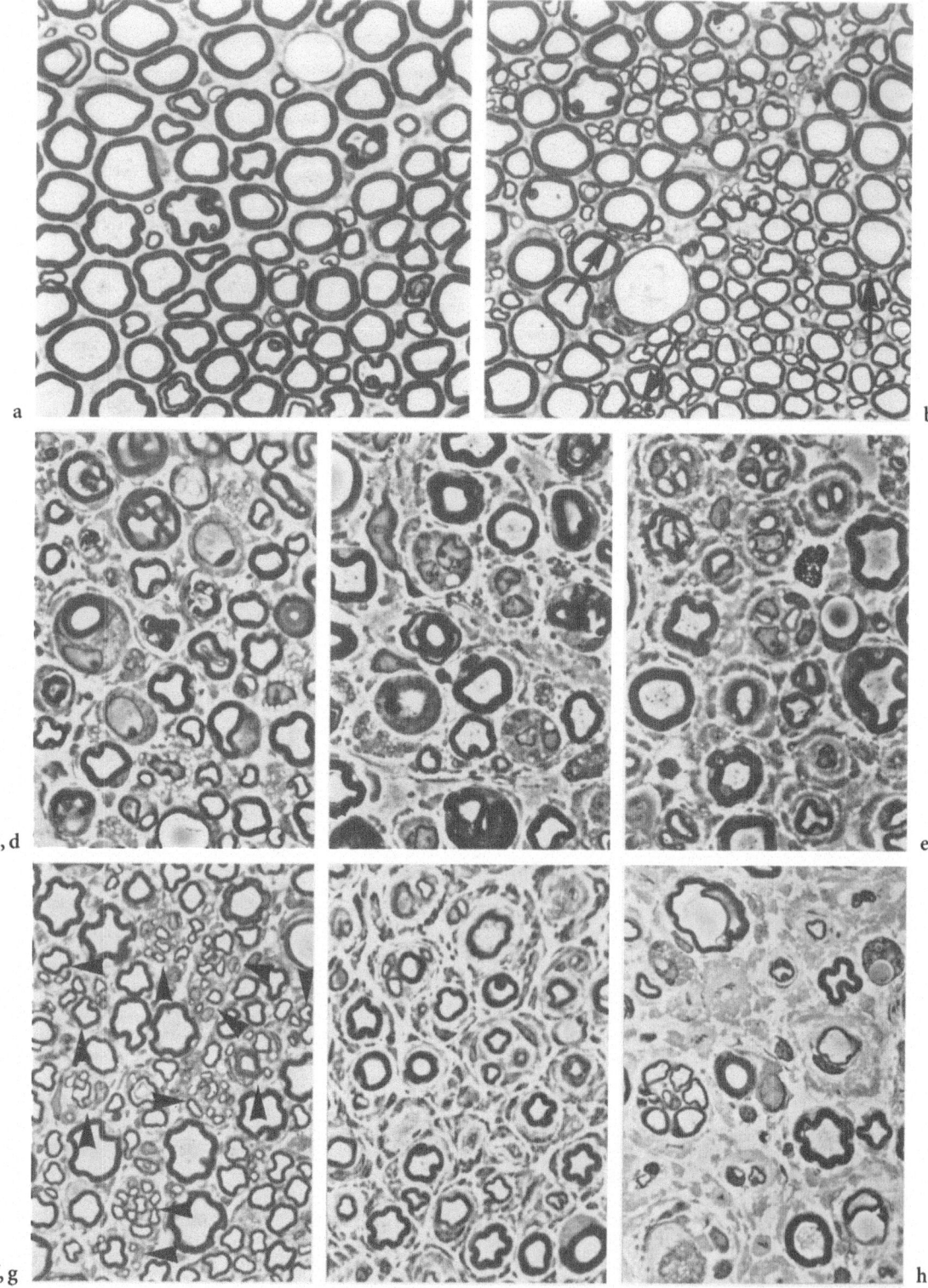

Fig. 14a–h. Legend s. p. 22

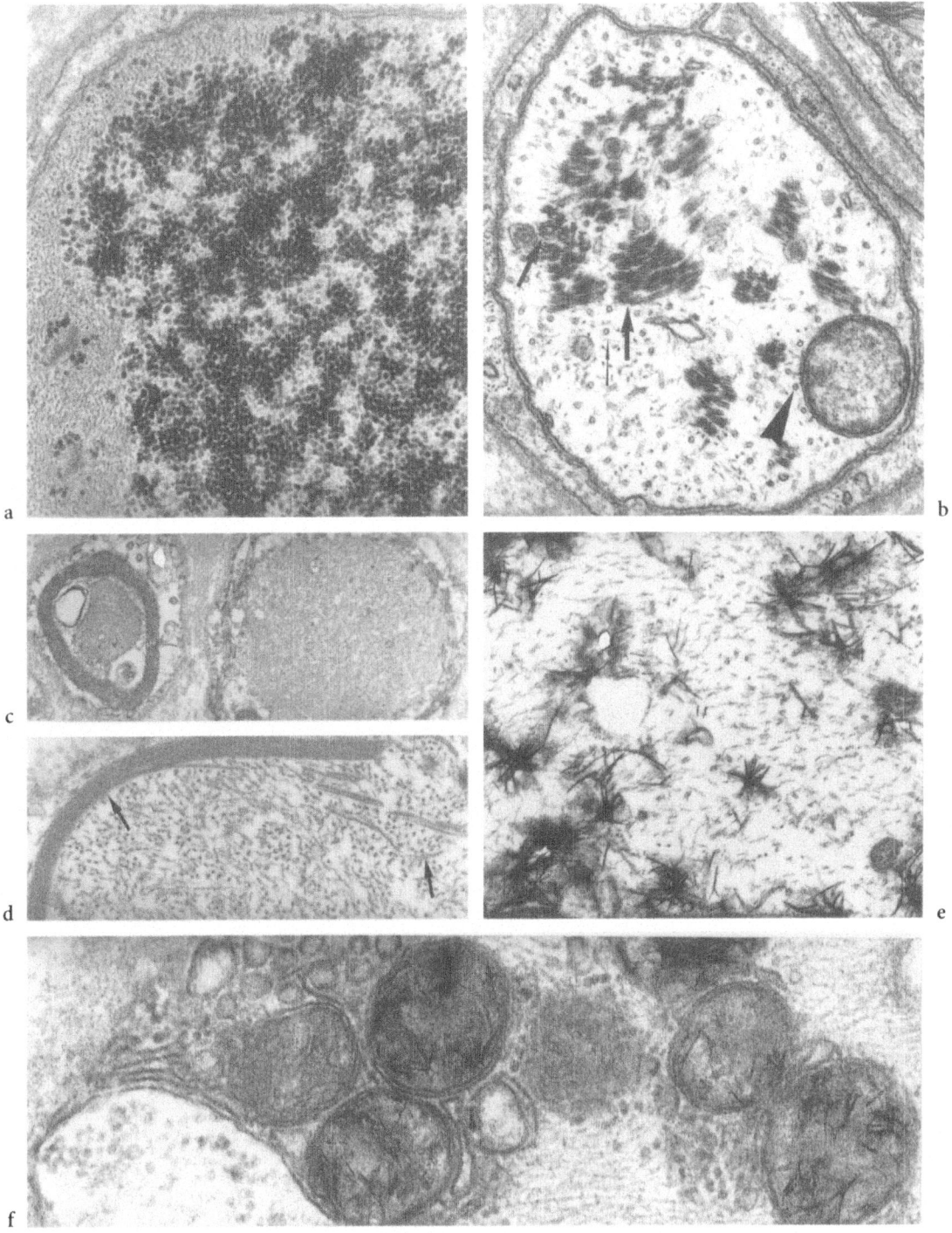

Fig. 15 a–f. Legend s. p. 22

Fig. 14a–h. Representative areas of sciatic nerves of rats (From [941, 946, 965]). **a** Control nerve. **b** Twelve months after a crush lesion (distal to the crush area). The largest regenerated nerve fibers are surrounded by (in relation to the axonal calibers) disproportionately thin myelin sheaths. The *arrows* indicate atrophic nerve fibers. **c–h** Experimental isoniazid (INH) neuropathy: sciatic nerves of different rats **c** 4 days, **d** 3 weeks, **e** 7 weeks after the beginning of INH intoxication, and **f** after 3 months and **g** after 24 months of survival time following short INH intoxication. The number of the supernumerary regenerated nerve fibers and the proliferated Schwann cells has decreased significantly after 2 years, the endoneurial connective tissue, however, is clearly increased. **h** Control rat at relatively old age of 3.5 years with a large variety of different forms of spontaneous nerve fiber changes: degeneration and regeneration, demyelination and remyelination, bands of Büngner, edema, and increase in the endoneurial connective tissue. **a, b, f, g** × 720; **c, d, e** × 1,000; **h** × 690

Fig. 15a–f. Characteristic though not specific axonal changes. **a** Accumulation of glycogen granules in a nonmyelinated axon with increased neurofilaments in the sural nerve of a 62-year-old man, who 5 months later succumbed to Creutzfeldt Jakob disease. × 53,600. **b** Intra-axonal, partly paracrystalline bundles of filaments (*thick arrows*) in a 74-year-old female with diabetes mellitus and suggested costal metastases derived from an unknown carcinoma. The filaments are with a distance and diameter of approximately 14 nm considerably thicker than the neurofilaments (8–10 nm) (*thin arrow*), but thinner than microtubules (25 nm) (*arrowhead*). × 41,400. **c** Giant axonal neuropathy in a 2-year-old girl (intramuscular nerve; autopsy case). The neurofilaments are severely increased in number despite advanced autolysis; at least some axons are enlarged up to 12 μm (instead of 6–7 μm) in this case favoring the diagnosis of giant axonal neuropathy. × 7,800. **d** Same case as in **c**. Hirano body (*arrows*) (cf. [886]) in a stage of advanced autolysis. × 32,000. **e** Needle-like arrangement of calcium crystals in the axoplasm of a patient with a neuropathy of an axonal type of unidentified pathogenesis (70-year-old female). × 36,000. **f** Needle-like calcium precipitates in axonal mitochondria in a 65-year-old patient with neuropathy of the Vizioli type (HMSN type VI, with optic atrophy). The calcium precipitates are suggestive of hypercalcemia. × 71,000 (From [958])

Fig. 16a–c. Node of Ranvier type I (according to the classification of Phillips et al. 1972 [829]) with myelin loops terminating at the axon with a narrow angle (**a**), and of type II (**b**) with myelin loops terminating at the axon in a wide angle; both types of node of Ranvier are normal variants. Components of the cytoplasm of the Schwann cell are included in the outer abaxonal part of the paranodal myelin sheath (*arrows*) which contain an increased number of glycogen granules. A small so-called axon/Schwann cell network is indicated in the lower part of the nerve fiber in **a** by *arrowheads*. Tubular and vesicular components of the axons are accumulated above the node of Ranvier in **a** and **b** thereby indicating the proximal part of the node of Ranvier in respect to the perikaryon. Glycogen-like granules are noted more frequently in the distal paranodal region of the axons. The nodal segment of the axons is unusually electron dense in **a**. **c** Remyelinated internode with a thin myelin sheath on the right side opposite a presumably preexisting thick myelin sheath segment on the left side. Myelin-like figures can be seen in the axon as well as in the myelin sheath. **a** × 8,000; **b** × 12,000; **c** × 11,000. (Modified from [966])

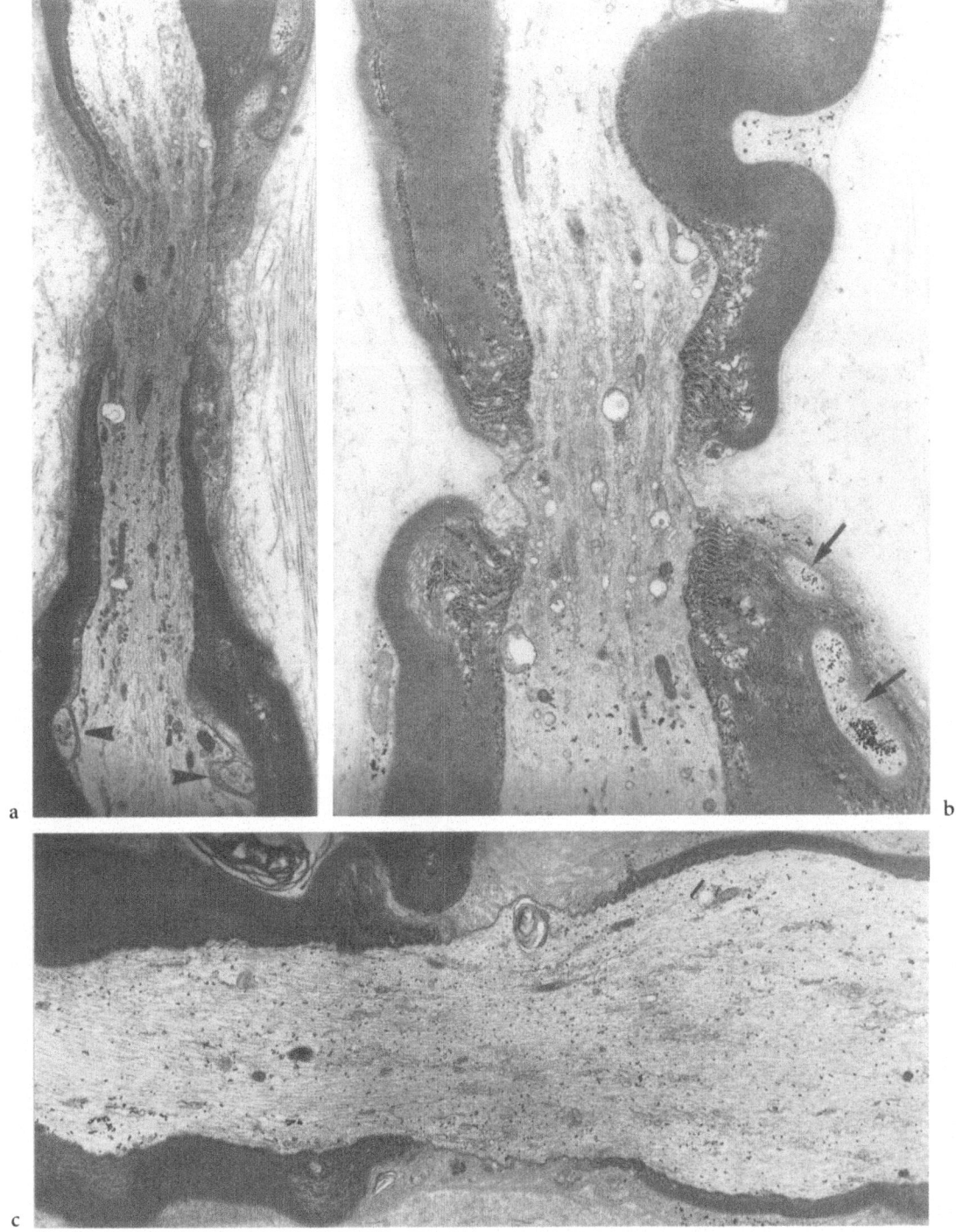

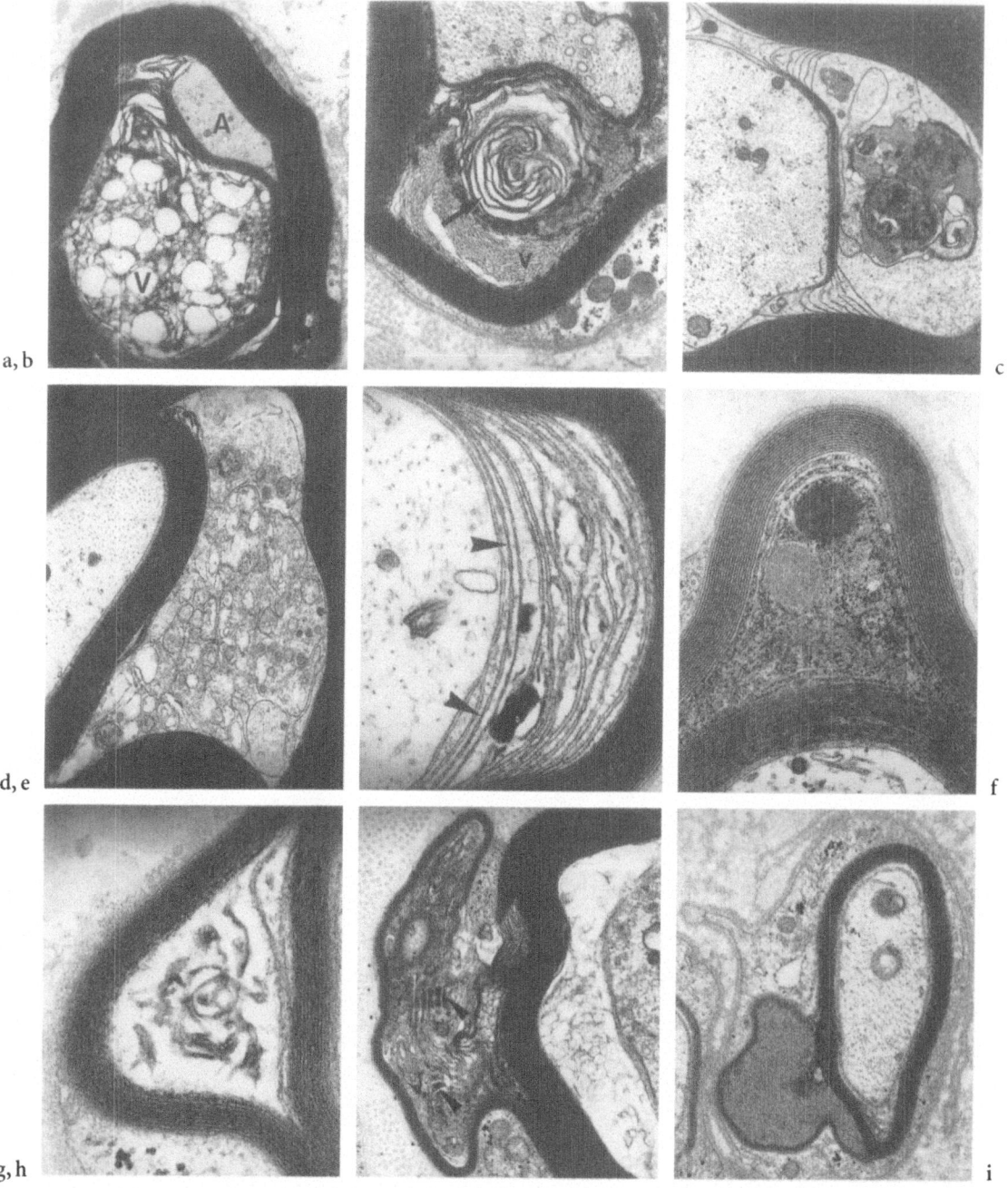

Fig. 17a–i. General reactions of Schmidt-Lanterman incisures. **a** A myelin loop is located adjacent to an atrophic axon and a Schmidt-Lanterman incisure, the center of which shows multivesicular degeneration (in a patient with plasmocytoma). × 4,600. **b** In a swollen incisure adjacent to a myelin-like, concentrically lamellated body there is fine vesicular lysis of the myelin sheath (dorsal branch of the 5th cervical nerve in a patient with spasmodic torticollis). × 16,200. **c** Pleomorphic inclusions in an incisure with membranous and granular components of different electron density (in a patient with suggested lysosomal storage disease). × 10,000. **d** Multiple processes with dense bodies, membranous and amorphic inclusions in an incisure (in a patient with autosomal dominant neuropathy). × 11,000. **e** Uncompacted myelin lamellae with osmiophilic, condensed membranous structures and circumscribed fusions between neighboring lamellae (*arrowheads*) (in a 3-year-old girl with Friedreich's ataxia). × 17,000. **f** Electron dense and finely granulated substances in a dilated major dense line of an incisure with lysosome-like bodies and different electron density of the inclusions (46-year-old man with HMSN I). × 18,700. **g** This incisure includes irregular membranous components (same case as in **e**). × 46,000. **h** Focal protrusion of a distended, complicated incisure, which contains desmosome-like structures (*arrowheads*) as well as vesicular and granular components (patient with cryoglobulinemia). × 16,500. **i** Dilatation and deformation of an incisure with finely granulated material of homogeneous, medium electron density (in a 1.5-year-old girl with demyelinating neuropathy of undetermined cause). × 18,700

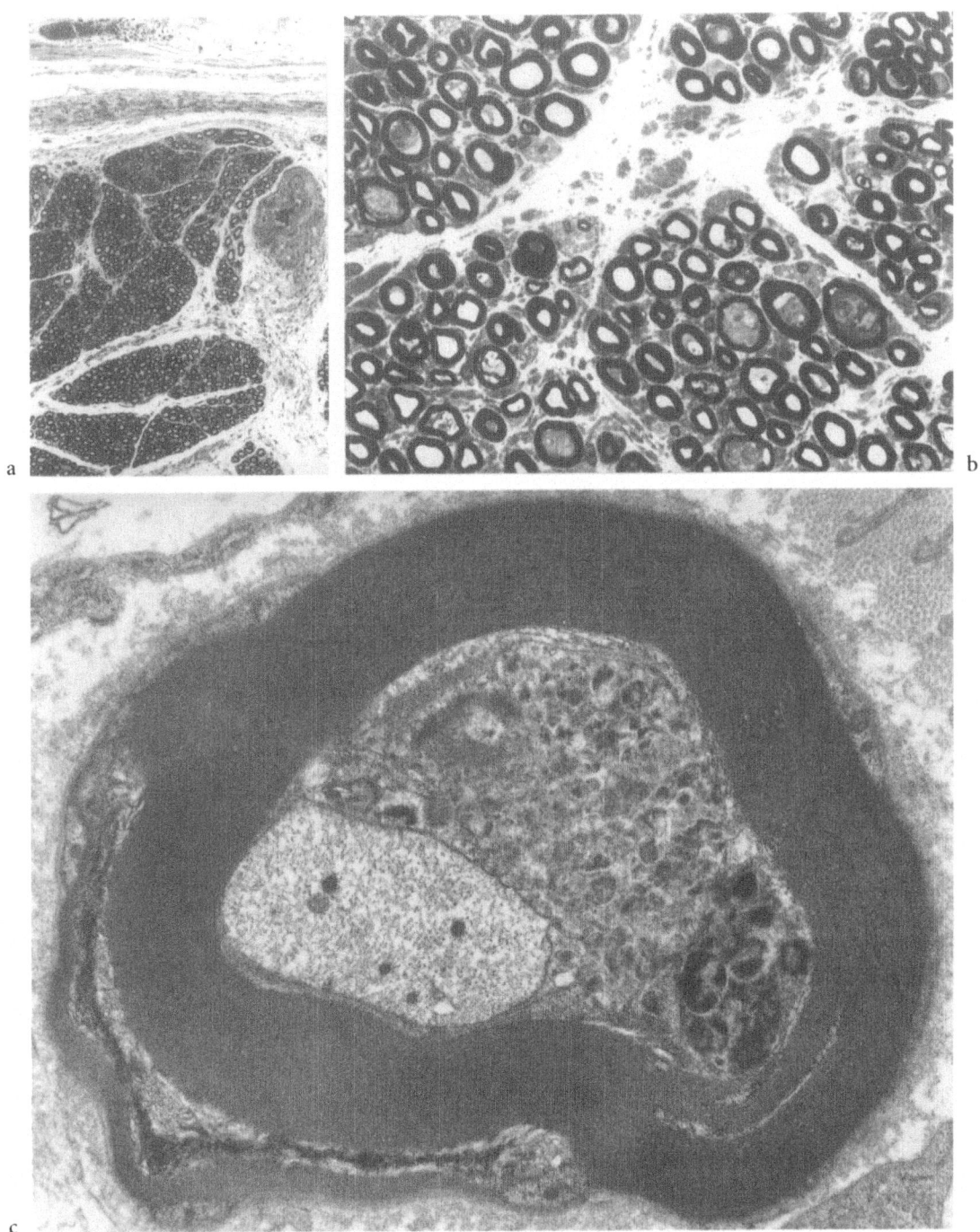

Fig. 18 a–c. Hypoglossal nerve following neck dissection after three recurrences (5 and 10 years before) of a carcinoma of the base of the tongue in a 63-year-old female. There are unusually numerous and pronounced axonal compressions by pleomorphic distensions of the adaxonal cytoplasm of the Schwann cell (partly by disintegrating macrophages) in this type of paraneoplastic neuropathy. **a** × 66; **b** × 426; **c** × 9,800. (From [958])

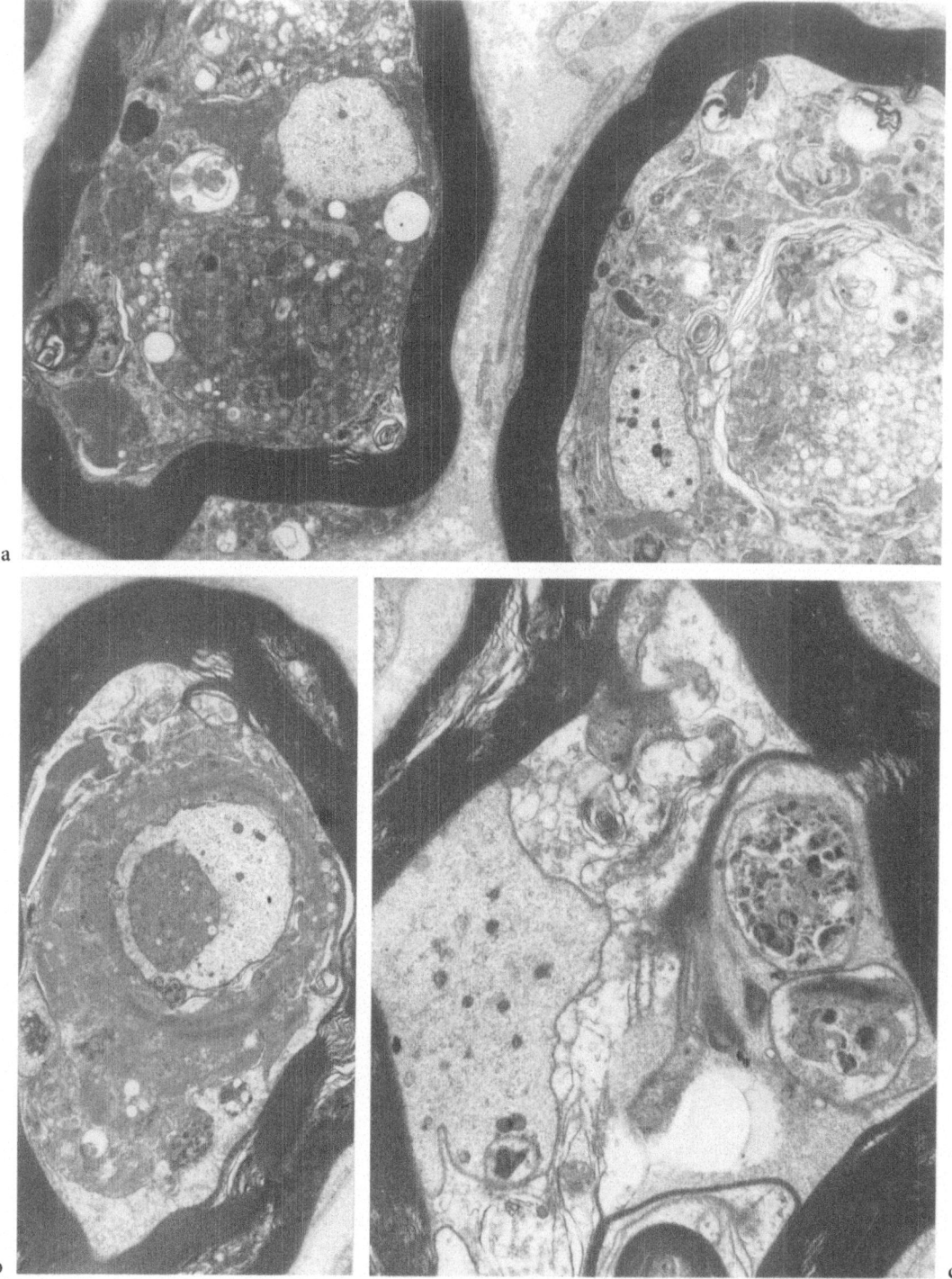

Fig. 19. Pleomorphic adaxonal inclusions in the same case as in the preceding figure. In **a**, **b**, and **c** autophagolysosomal structures with vesicular disintegration of myelin lamellae dominate, whereas in **c** deposition of amorphic material around the axon predominates, lying in the extracellular space. Adjacent pleomorphic lysosomal structures can also be seen. The adaxonal myelin lamellae are irregularly widened and altered. **a** × 7,600; **b** × 9,000; **c** × 12,000

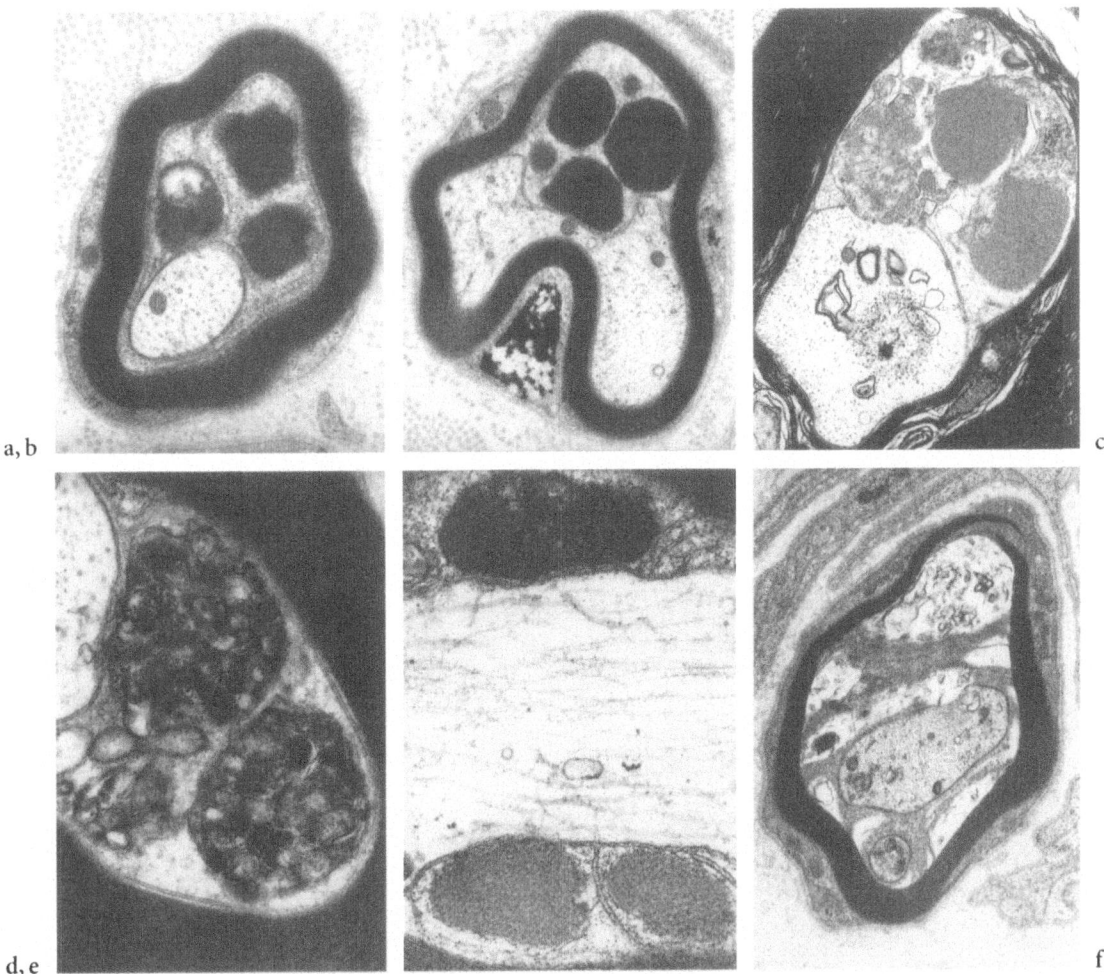

Fig. 20 a–f. Structured inclusions in the adaxonal cytoplasm of Schwann cells. There are electron dense lysosome-like structures **a** in a chronic neuropathy of the axonal type and unknown cause, and **b** in a 19-year-old man with HMSN type VI, Vizioli. **a** × 18,000; **b** × 15,000. **c** Less electron dense granular lysosome-like inclusions in the same case as in Figs. 18 and 19. × 13,000. **d** Pleomorphic autophagolysosomes in a 16-year-old boy with HMSN I. × 29,000. **e** Finely granulated lysosome-like depositions in a 44-year-old man with CIDP. × 36,000. **f** Pleomorphic adaxonal alterations with vesicular disintegration, homogeneous, or granular deposits in a paranodal area of an onion bulb formation in a 21-year-old man with suspected HMSN I. × 3,000

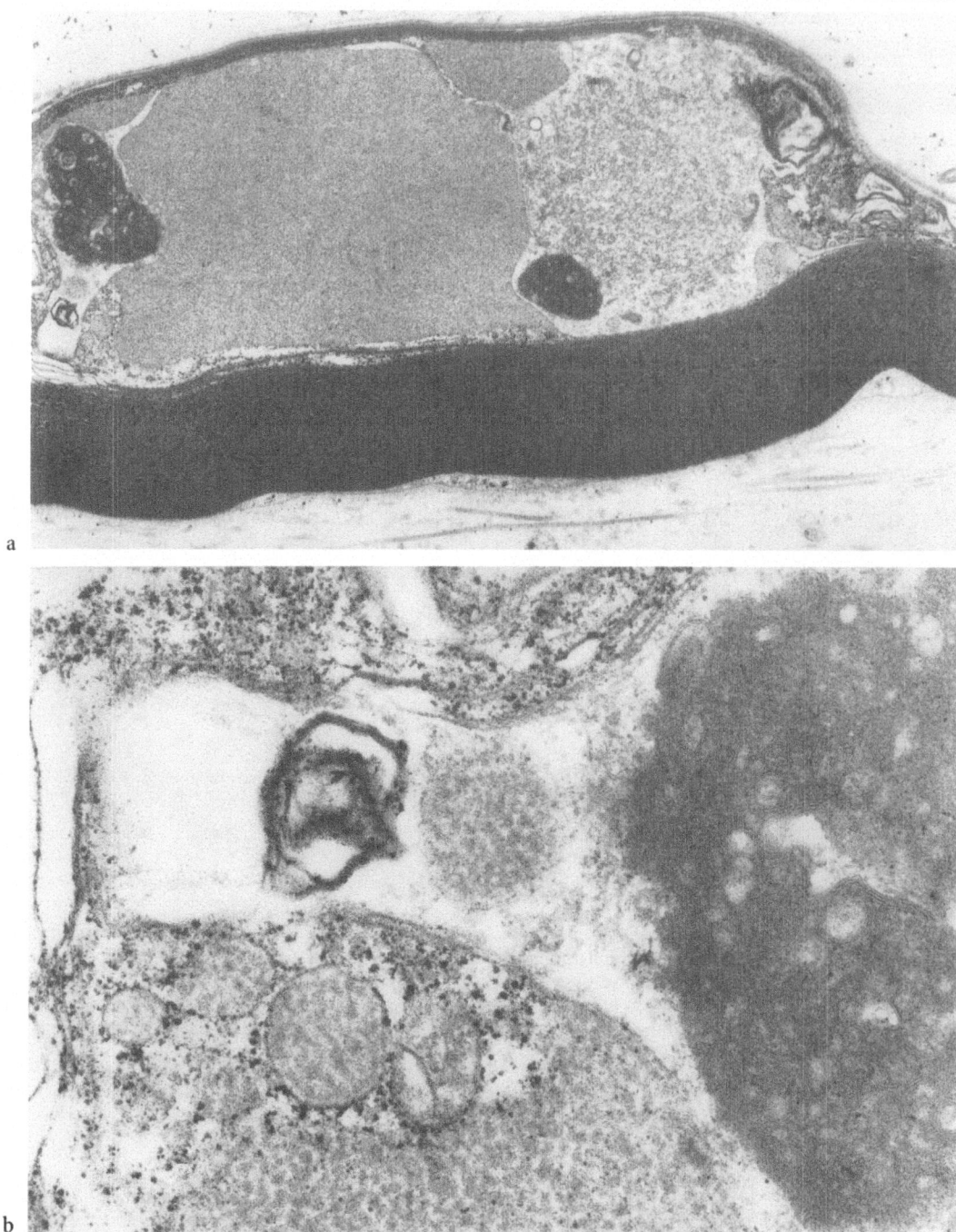

Fig. 21a, b. Unusual, extensive, granular inclusions of varying density in the inner myelin sheath of a 60-year-old man with suspected autoimmune disorder. **a** × 15,000; **b** × 93,000

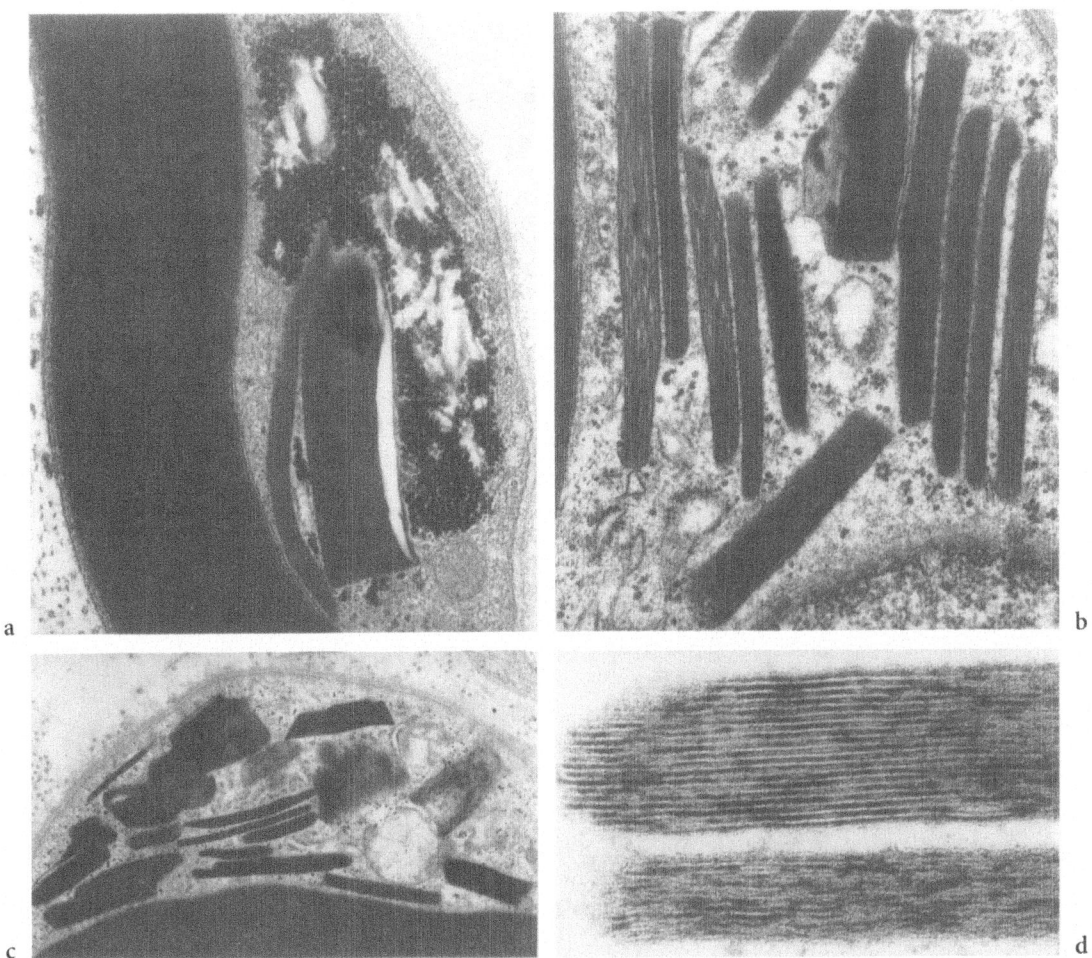

Fig. 22 a – d. Varying aspects of π-granules in different neuropathies. **a** Neuropathy of mixed, partly axonal, and partly de-myelinating type. **b** Mitochondrial myopathy in a 59-year-old female. **c, d** Chronic neuropathy in a 54-year-old man. **a** × 46,000; **b** × 39,000; **c** × 13,000; **d** × 170,000

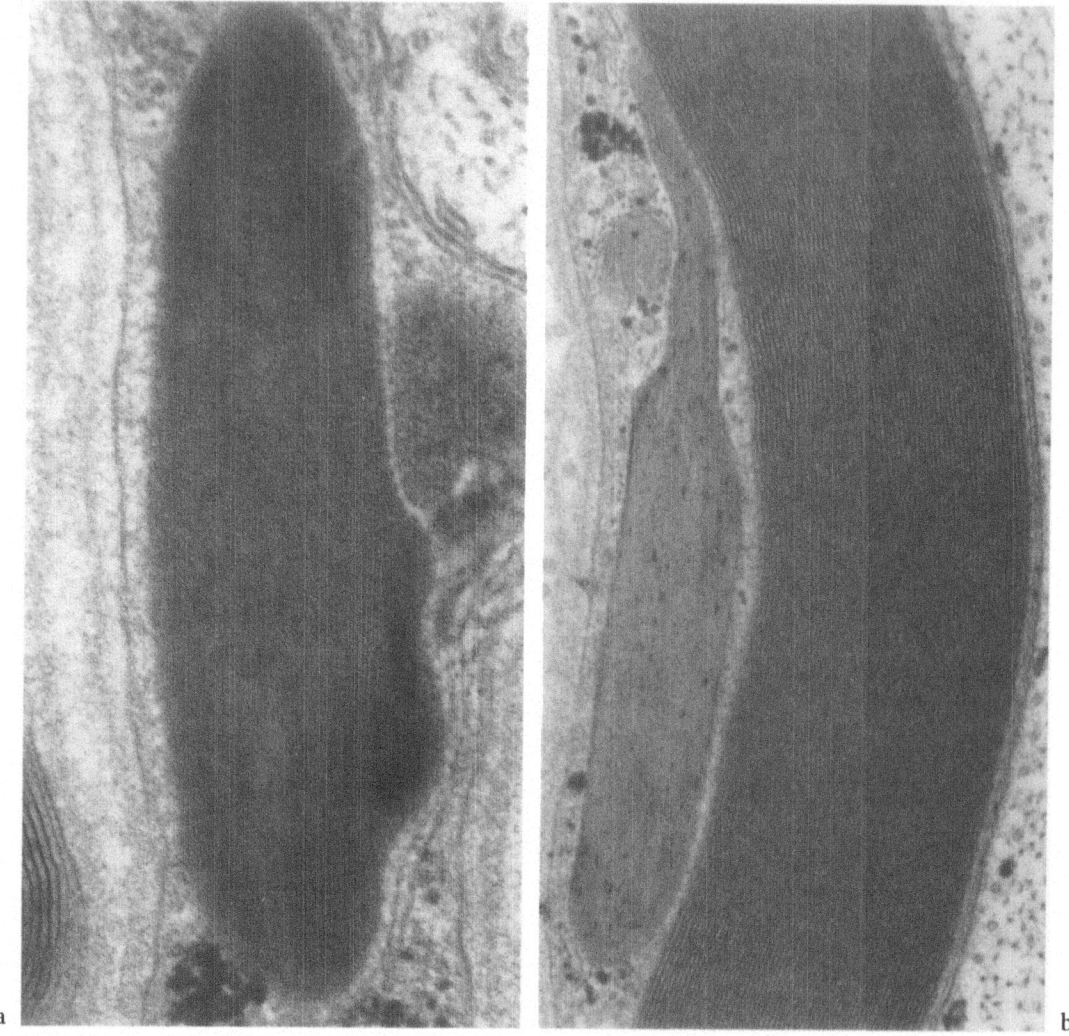

Fig. 23. Higher magnifications of π-granules in a patient with polyglucosan-body myopathy. **a** × 110,000; **b** × 64,000

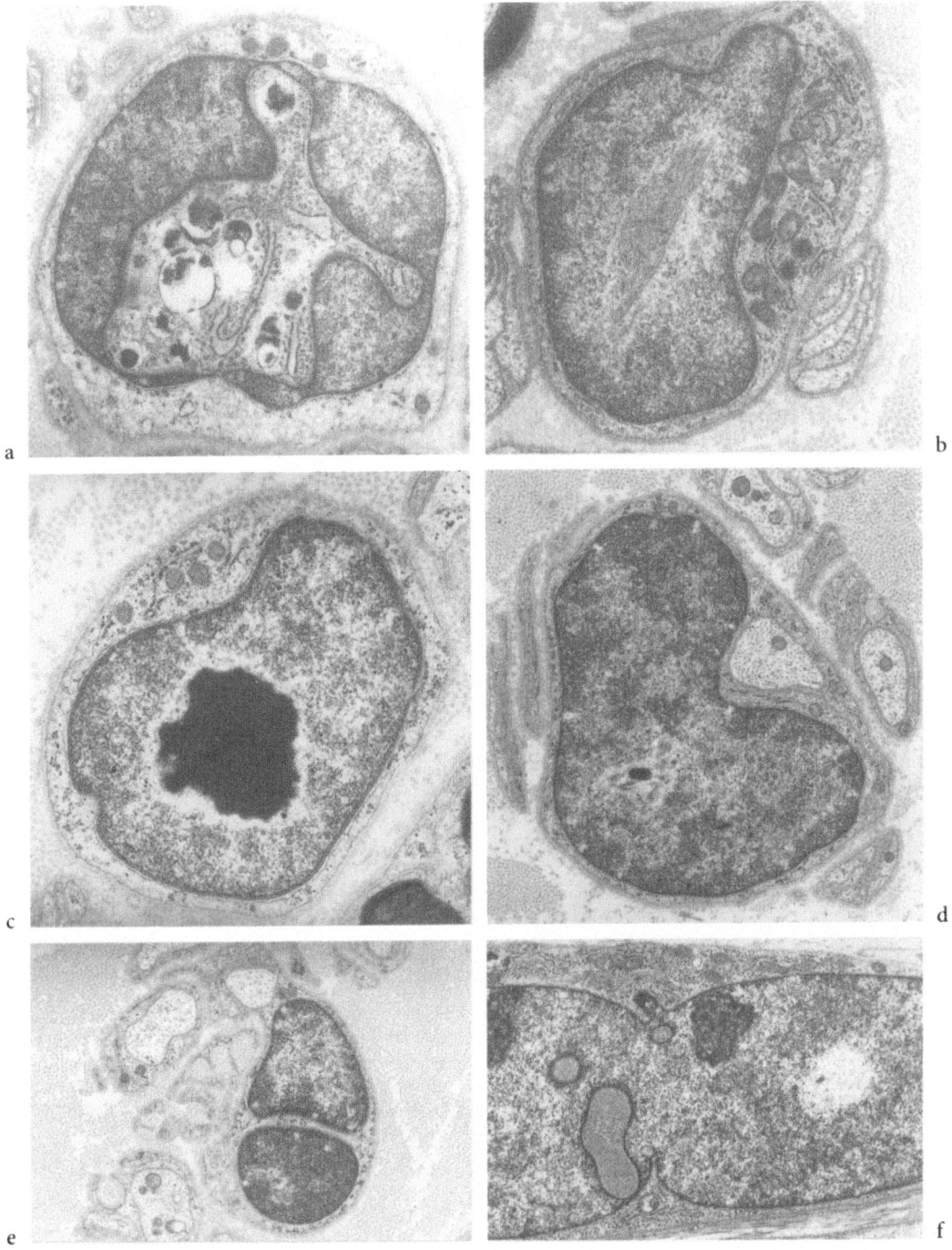

Fig. 24 a–f. Various nuclear changes in Schwann cells. **a** Prominent cytoplasmic invaginations with granular endoplasmic reticulum and several vesicles containing a variety of ill-defined osmiophilic substances (presumably of lysosomal origin) (in amyloidosis of the AL type). × 12,400. **b** Abnormal filaments in a Schwann cell nucleus of a 52-year-old female with neuropathy of the axonal/neuronal type of uncertain etiology (perhaps due to spinocerebellar atrophy). × 16,000. **c** Large homogeneous osmiophilic, non-membrane-bound nuclear inclusion in a 74-year-old female with neuropathy in MGUS. × 18,700. **d** Much smaller nuclear inclusion than in **c**, a Schwann cell with an unmyelinated axon (same case as in **c**). × 11,000. **e** Double nuclear profiles which are presumably caused by a cytoplasmic invagination in a Schwann cell with an unmyelinated axon (same case as in **c** and **d**). × 9,000. **f** Unusual, indented form of a nucleus with focal lysis and several homogeneous cytoplasmic invaginations in a 61-year-old man with advanced, chronic neuropathy in diabetes mellitus and additional inflammatory cellular infiltrates. × 7,200

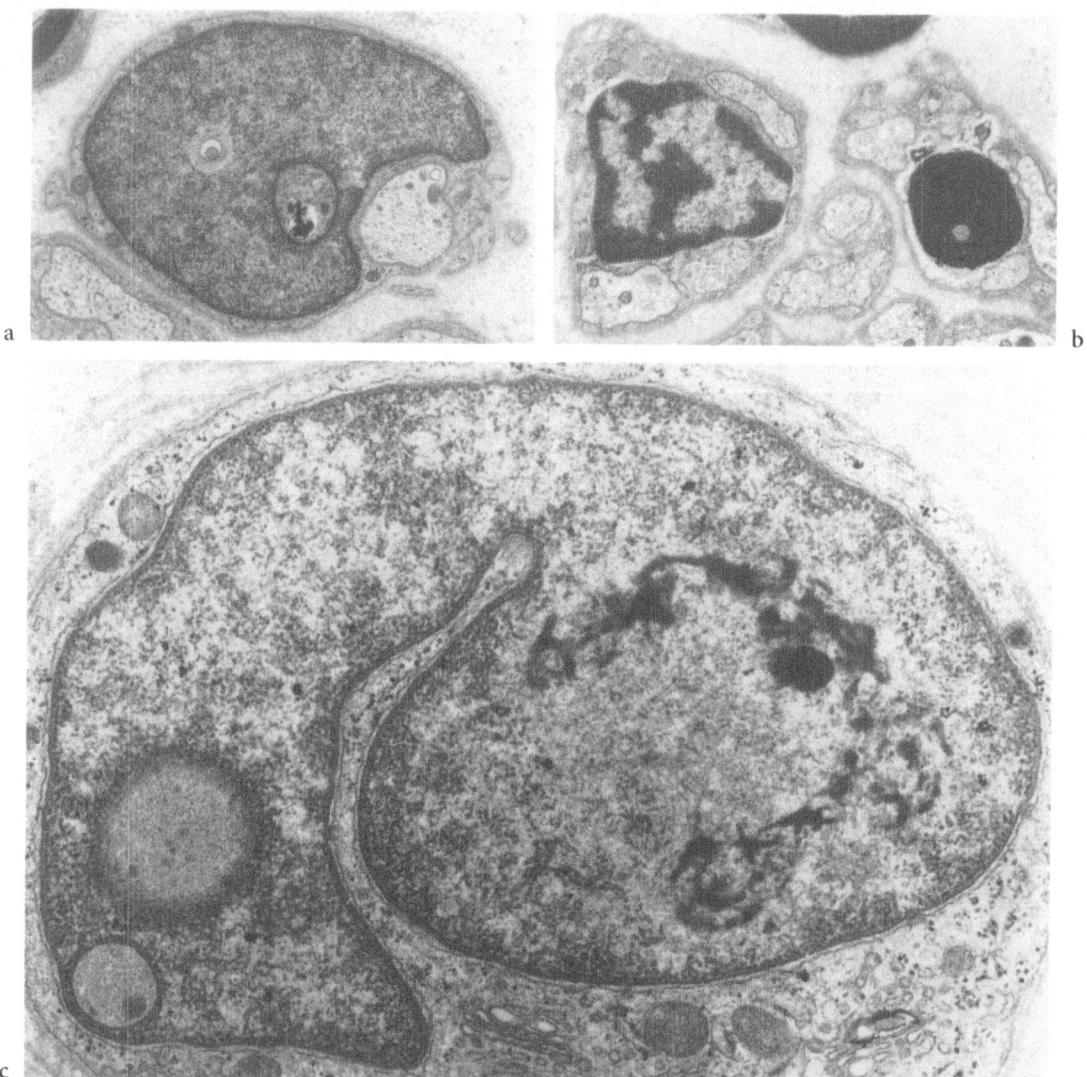

Fig. 25 a–c. Further nuclear abnormalities in Schwann cells. **a** Unusual vacuolar nuclear inclusion adjacent to a cytoplasmic invagination. The latter contains a vesicle with osmiophilic substances (in a 62-year-old man with a demyelinating neuropathy and microangiopathy). × 11,000. **b** Severely pycnotic nucleus (apoptosis) in a Schwann cell with unmyelinated axons in a 31-month-old boy with suggested adrenoleukodystrophy. × 12,000. **c** At least three different partly fuzzy, partly finely granulated nuclear inclusions in a Schwann cell nucleus indented by a cytoplasmic invagination in a 52-year-old man with polyneuritis. × 33,000

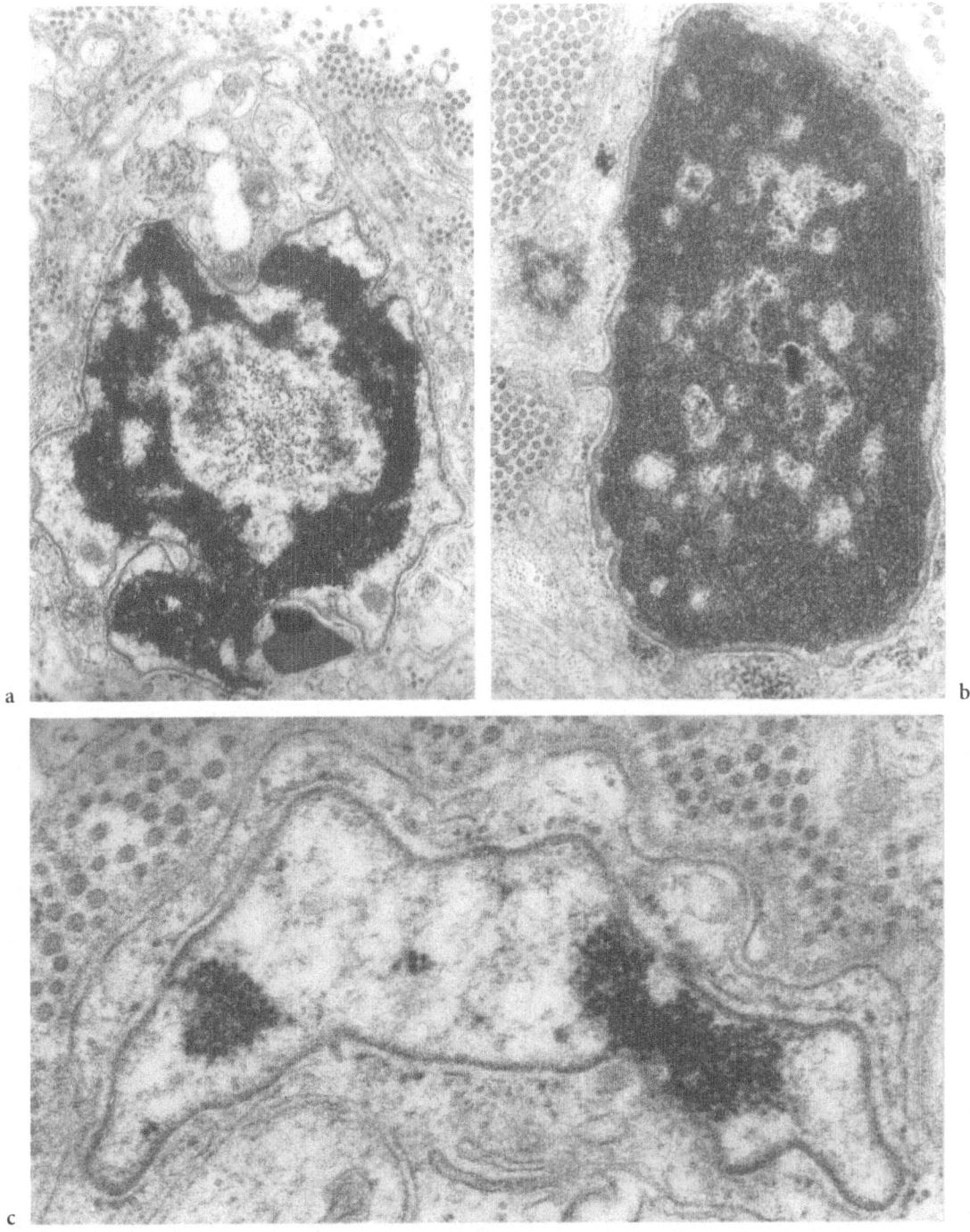

Fig. 26 a–c. Further nuclear changes in Schwann cells in a 58-year-old female with chronic neuropathy of the axonal type. **a** Separation of the heterochromatin from the inner nuclear membrane and central loosening of several granular components. × 25,000. **b** Condensed Schwann cell nucleus with abnormal superficial protrusions and multiple clear areas. × 40,000. **c** Extensive loss of chromatin in a nucleus of a Schwann (Remak) cell. × 64,000

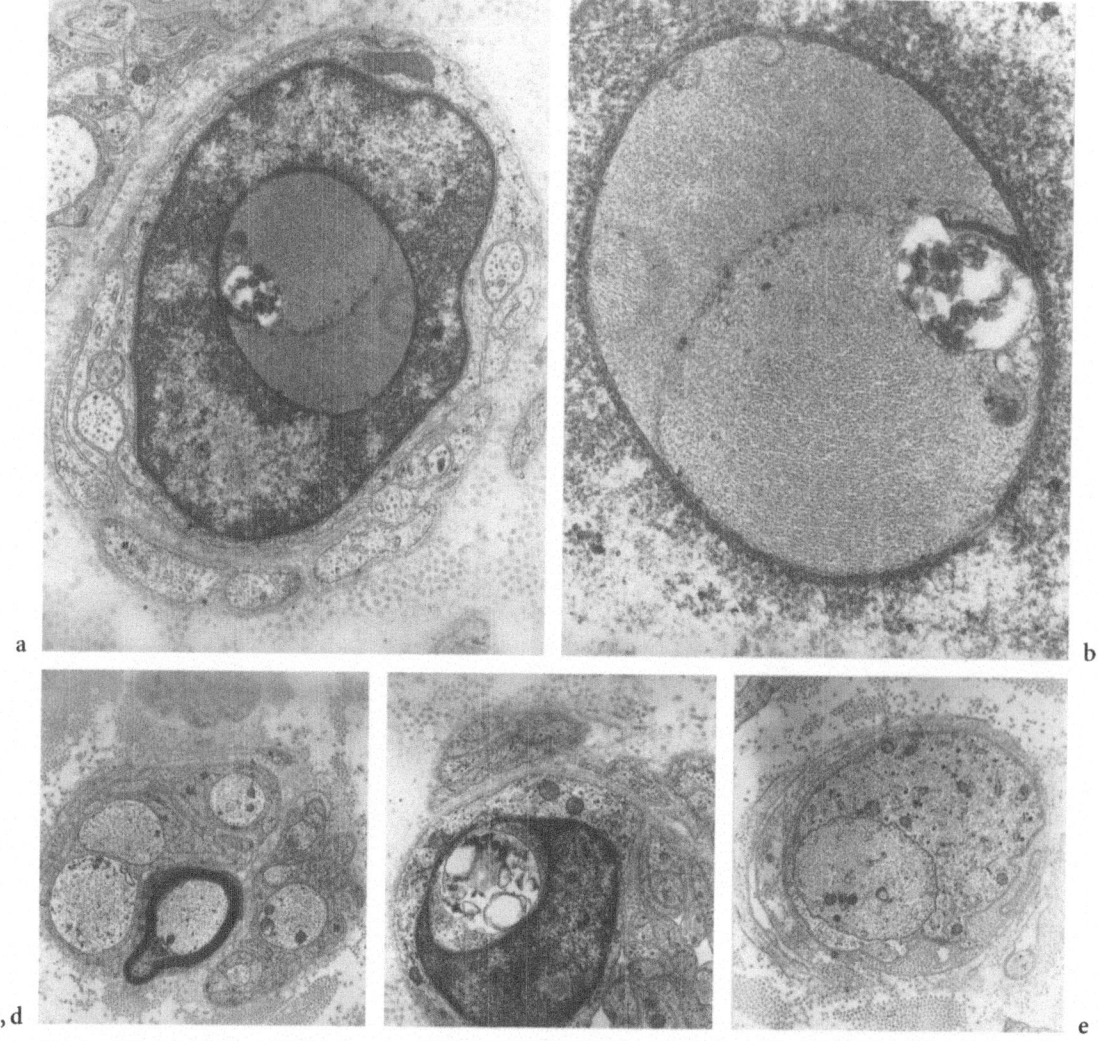

Fig. 27a–e. Abnormal cytoplasmic invaginations in a Schwann cell nucleus with accumulation of partly cross-, partly oblique, partly longitudinally oriented filamentous components in the dimension of actin filaments (in an ethanol-addicted 57-year-old man). There is also a vesicular inclusion with amorphic osmiophilic components. **a** × 20,000; **b** × 44,000. In the same case there are clusters of regenerated fibers (**c**), further nuclear invaginations with vesicular components (**d**) and a demyelinated large, previously myelinated axon (**e**). **c** × 6,700; **d** × 14,000; **e** × 7,800

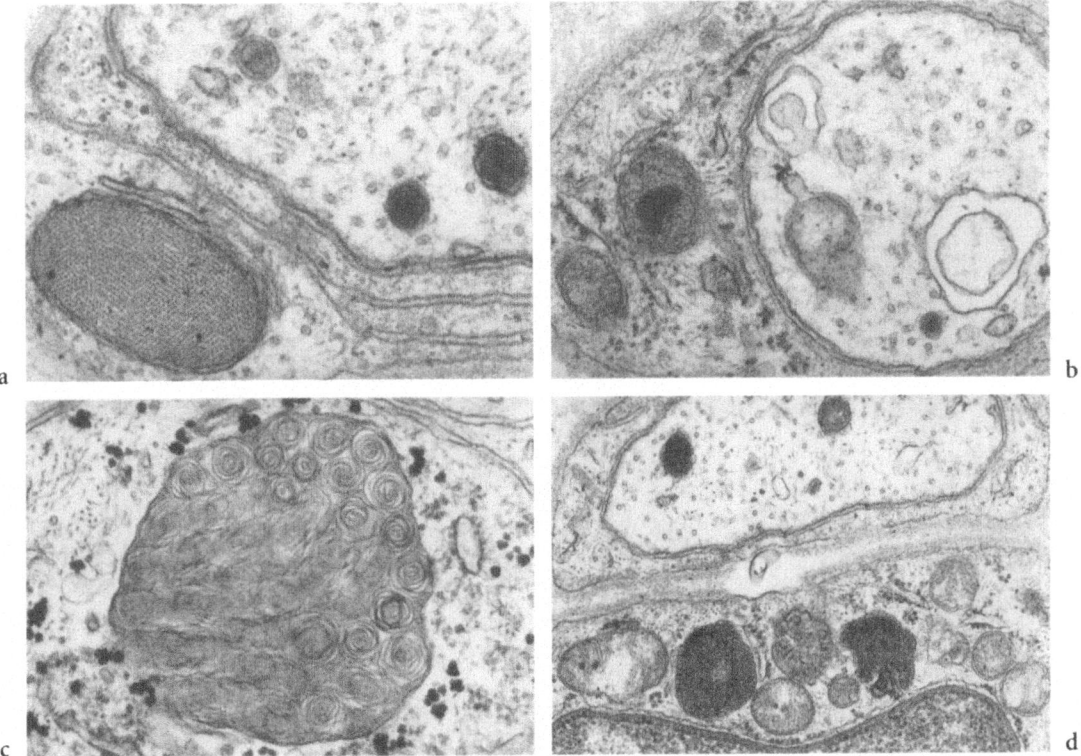

Fig. 28a–d. Different Schwann cell inclusions in a patient with demyelinating neuropathy and suspected ALS, but in fact mitochondrial myopathy. **a** Mitochondrion with paracrystalline arrangement of granular inclusions. × 59,000. **b** Mitochondrion with amorphous electron dense inclusion. × 45,000. **c** Multicentric lamellar inclusion of uncertain (myelin or mitochondrial) origin. × 58,000. **d** Variable lysosomal structures adjacent to and between several mitochondria. × 30,000

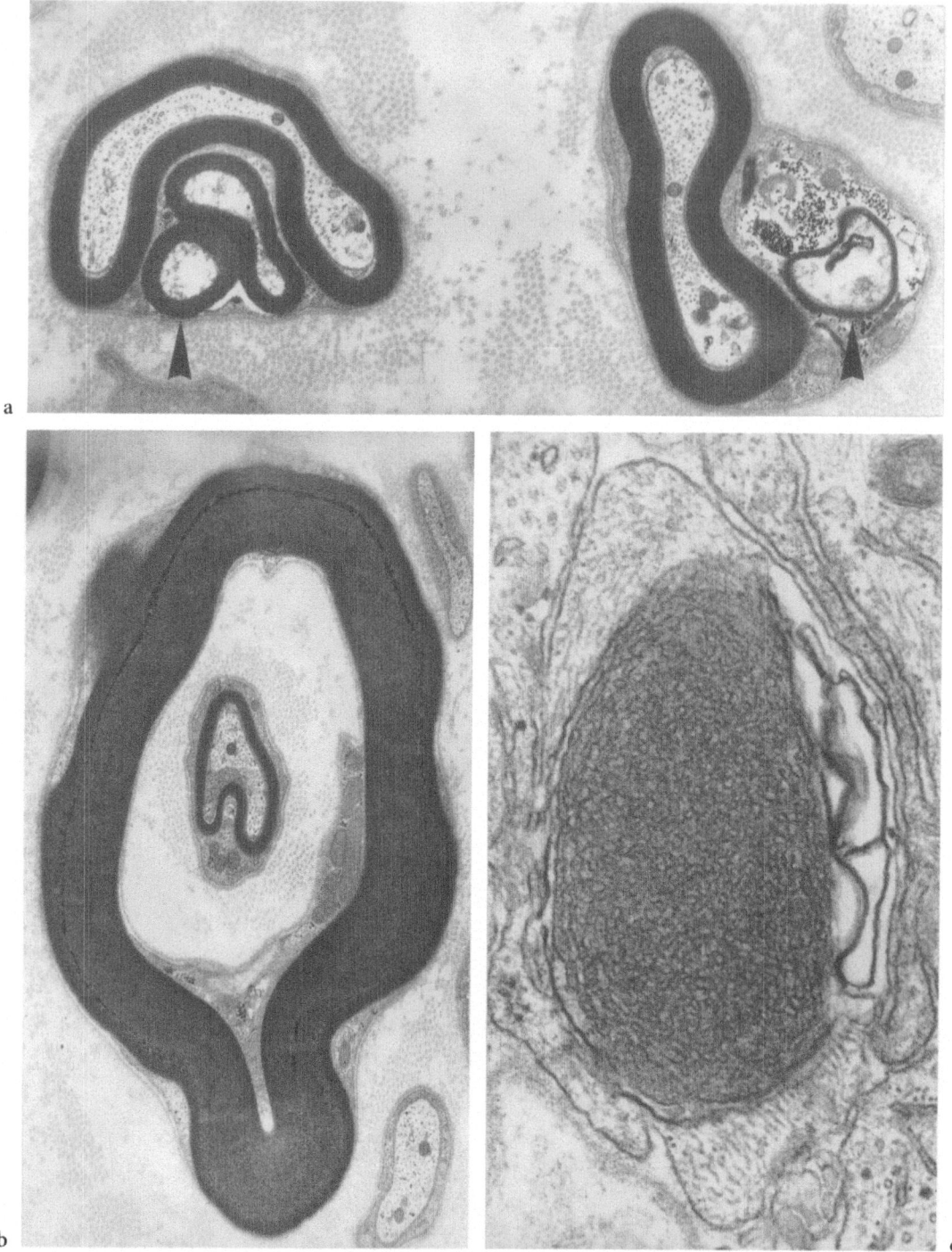

Fig. 29 a – c. Fifty two-year-old male with neuromyopathy of unidentified etiology. **a** Variable μ-granules (*arrowheads*) in the adaxonal cytoplasm of Schwann cells. × 15,000. **b** Transnodal remyelination with duplication of the myelin sheath: there is a thick myelin sheath around a very small myelinated fiber. Numerous collagen fibrils are located between the two myelin sheaths within a large extracellular space. × 13,000. **c** Tubulovesicular body in a band of Büngner (Schwann cell complex). × 77,000

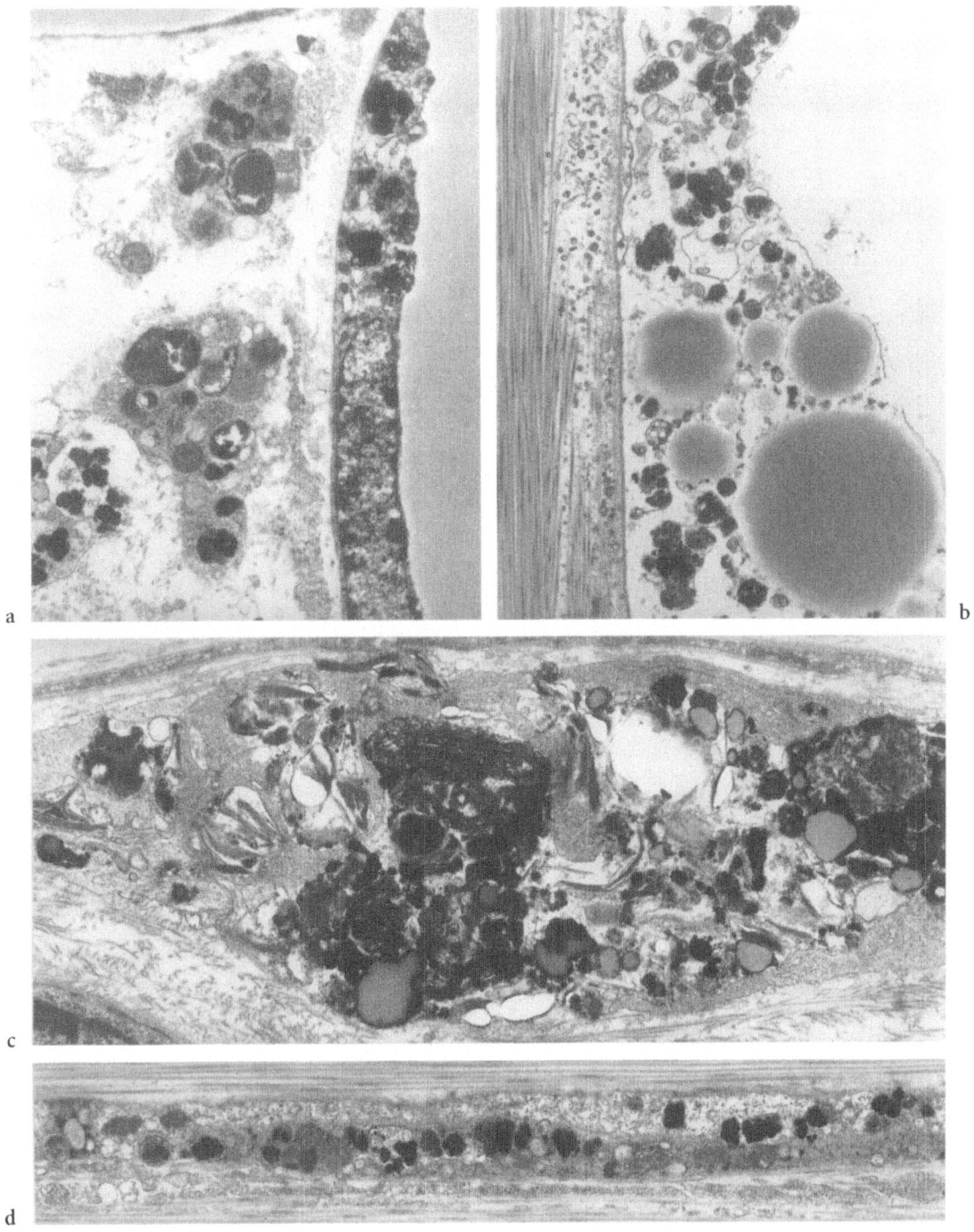

Fig. 30a–d. Epineurial siderosis presumably following a traumatic nerve lesion in a 43-year-old man with predominating demyelinating neuropathy. Numerous lysosome-like cytosomes contain predominantly finely granulated substances, **a** in the marginal cytoplasm of a fat cell with a homogeneous lipid component on the right, **b** together with large lipid droplets in an endothelial cell, **c** together with large lipofuscin bodies and membranous structures in a macrophage, and **d** in a perineurial cell. **a** × 940; **b** × 8,300; **c, d** × 10,500

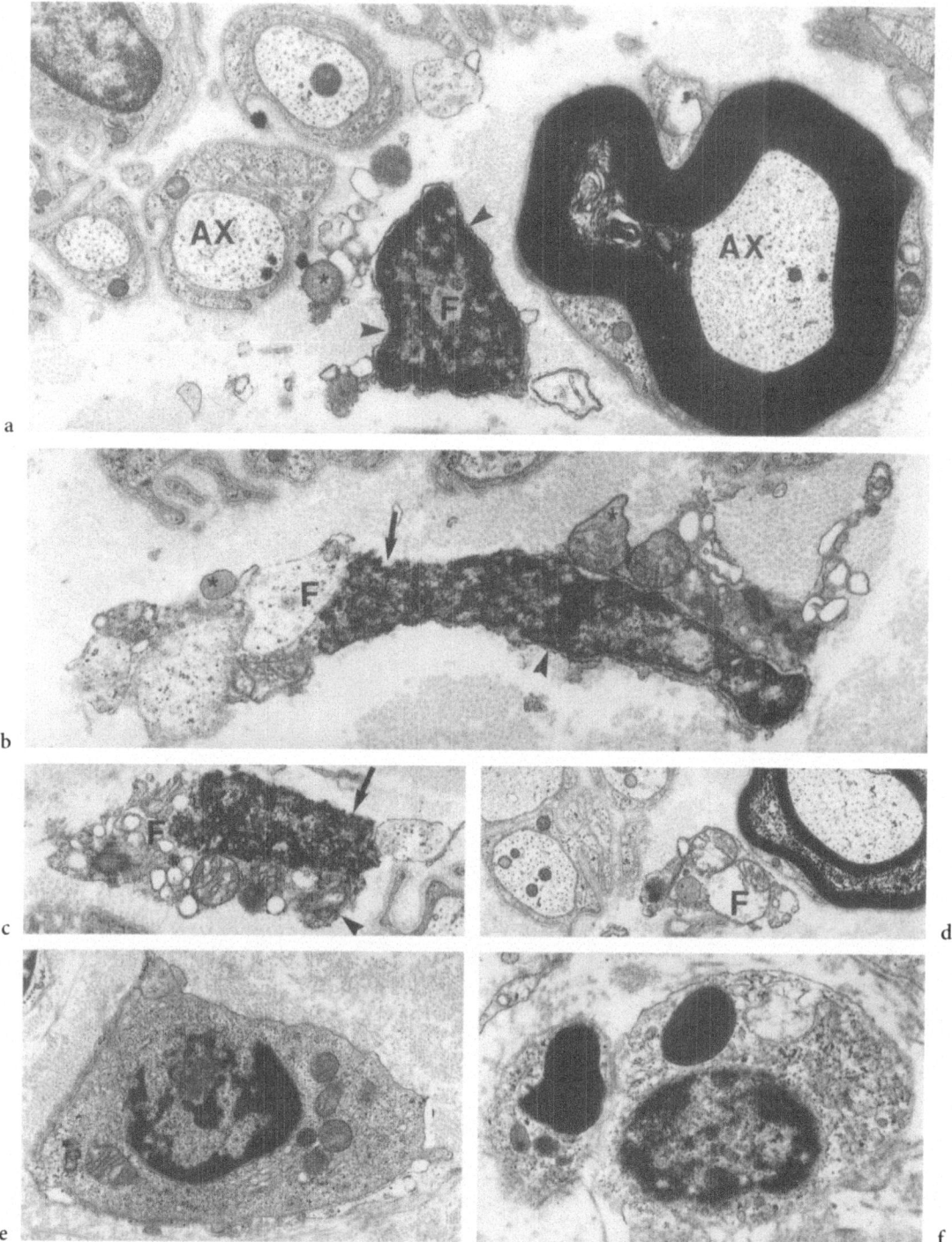

Fig. 31a–f. Degenerating endoneurial fibroblasts are indicated (*F*). The defects of the cytoplasmic membrane of the fibroblasts are indicated by *arrowheads*, those of the nuclear membranes by *arrows*. The myelinated and unmyelinated axons (*AX*) in the vicinity of the degenerating cells are well preserved. Some mitochondria (*) and other organelles of the fibroblasts are already located in the extracellular space and are no longer surrounded by a cytoplasmic membrane. The nuclear chromatin in the degenerating cells is condensed. In **e** the nuclear membrane is incompletely preserved. In **f** the intensely osmiophilic pigment granules resemble those in eosinophilic granulocytes. **a** × 13,000; **b** × 15,200; **c** × 14,300; **d** × 10,600; **e** × 12,000; **f** × 13,500

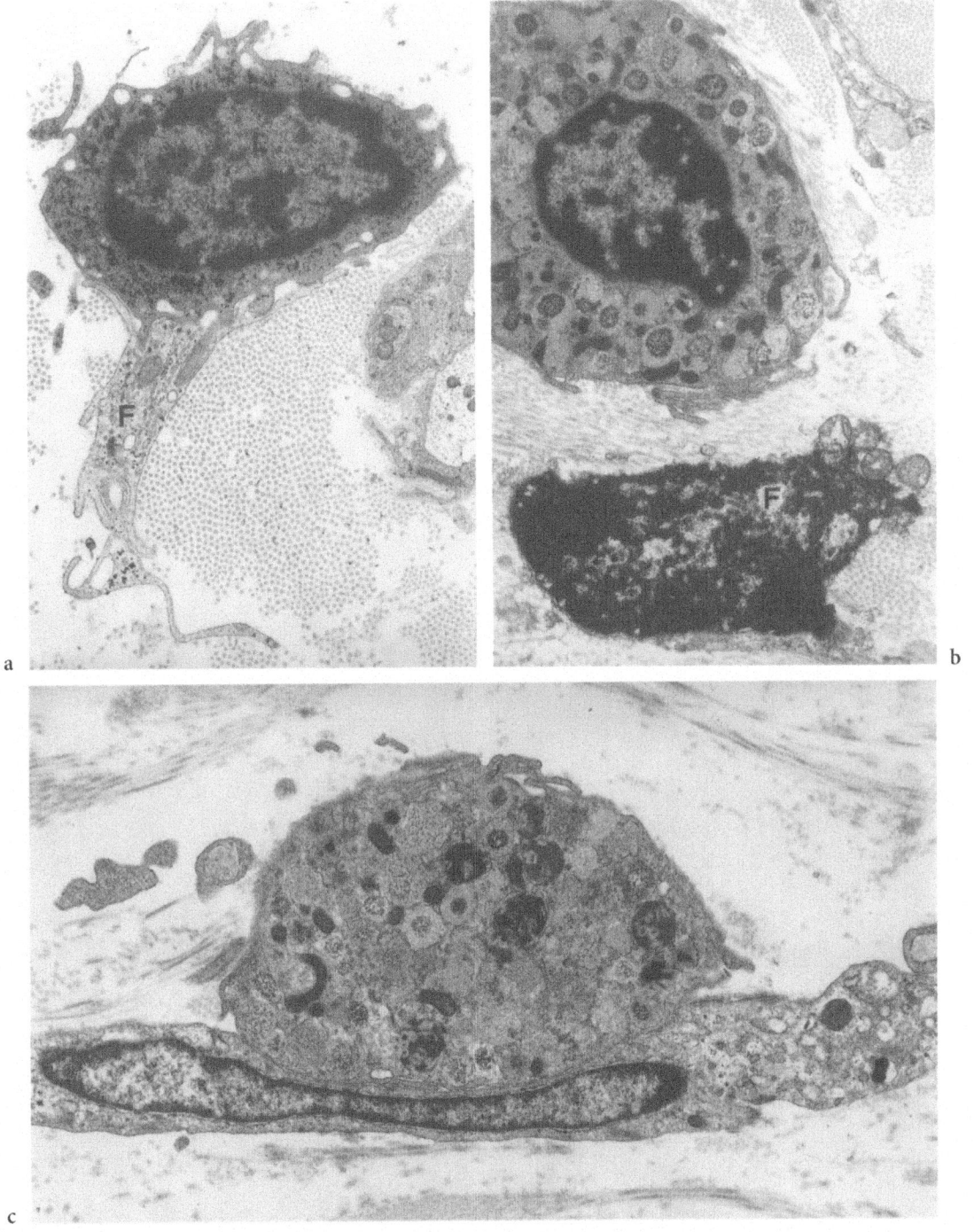

Fig. 32a–c. Close contact between a preserved endoneurial fibroblast (*F*) and a lymphocyte in a patient with severe neuropathy due to IgM cryoglobulinemia. Mast cells can be seen in the vicinity of a degenerating (**b**) and in close contact to a preserved (**c**) endoneurial fibroblast in a patient with panarteritis nodosa. **a** × 12,000; **b** × 10,400; **c** × 11,900 (Figs. 31 and 32 From [360])

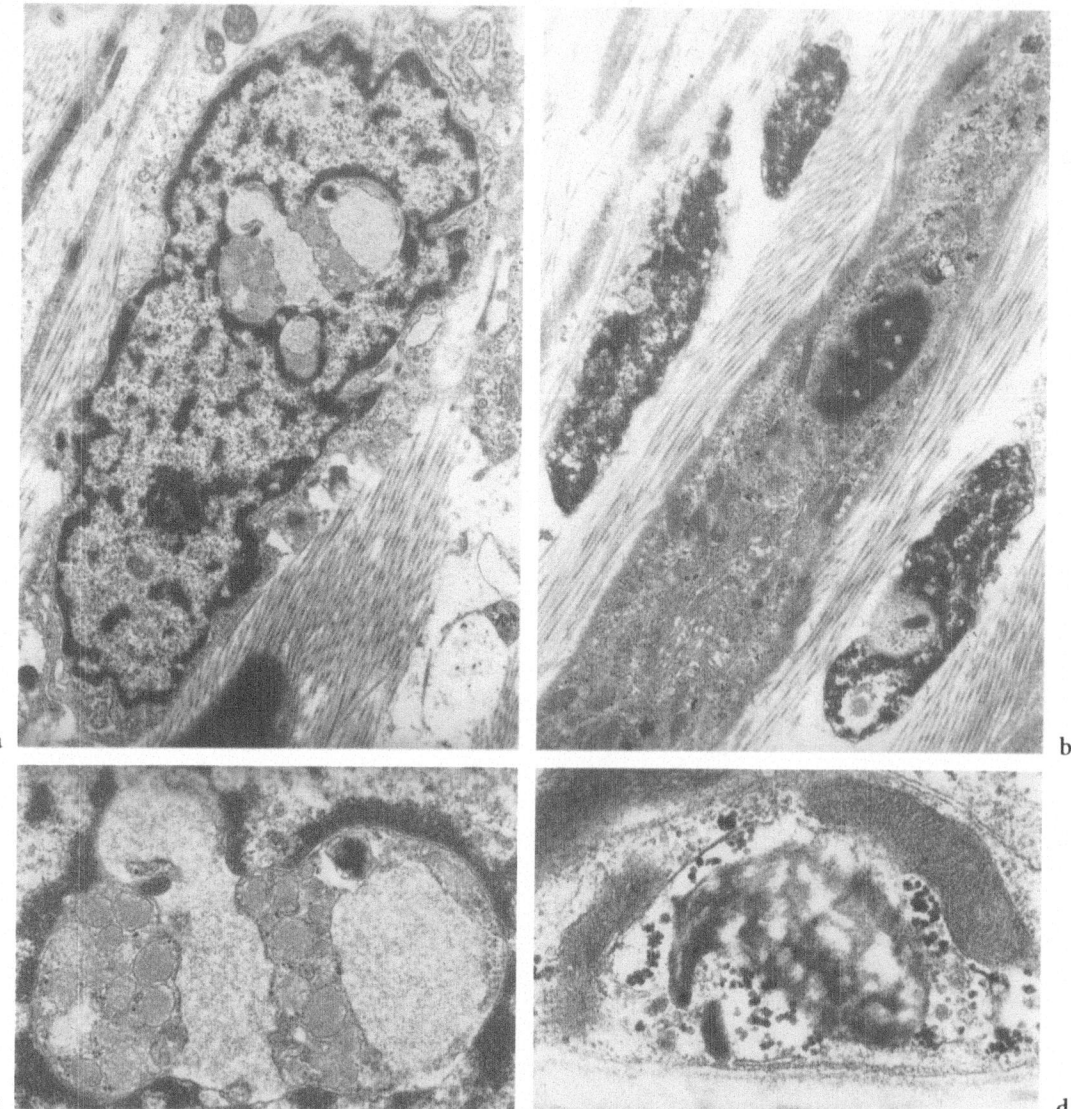

Fig. 33 a – d. Degenerating endoneurial fibroblasts in a 4-month-old boy with amnion infectious syndrome and multisystem disease as well as hydrocephalus. **a** Unusual cytoplasmic inclusions in the nucleus with several vacuoles of the endoplasmic reticulum containing amorphous substances of variable density. **a** × 9,400. Higher magnification of the fibroblast's nuclear inclusions in **c**. × 25,000. **b** Several degenerating endoneurial fibroblasts which have lost their cytoplasm completely. **d** Vacuolated lysosome-like structure in the cytoplasm of a Schwann cell. × 43,000

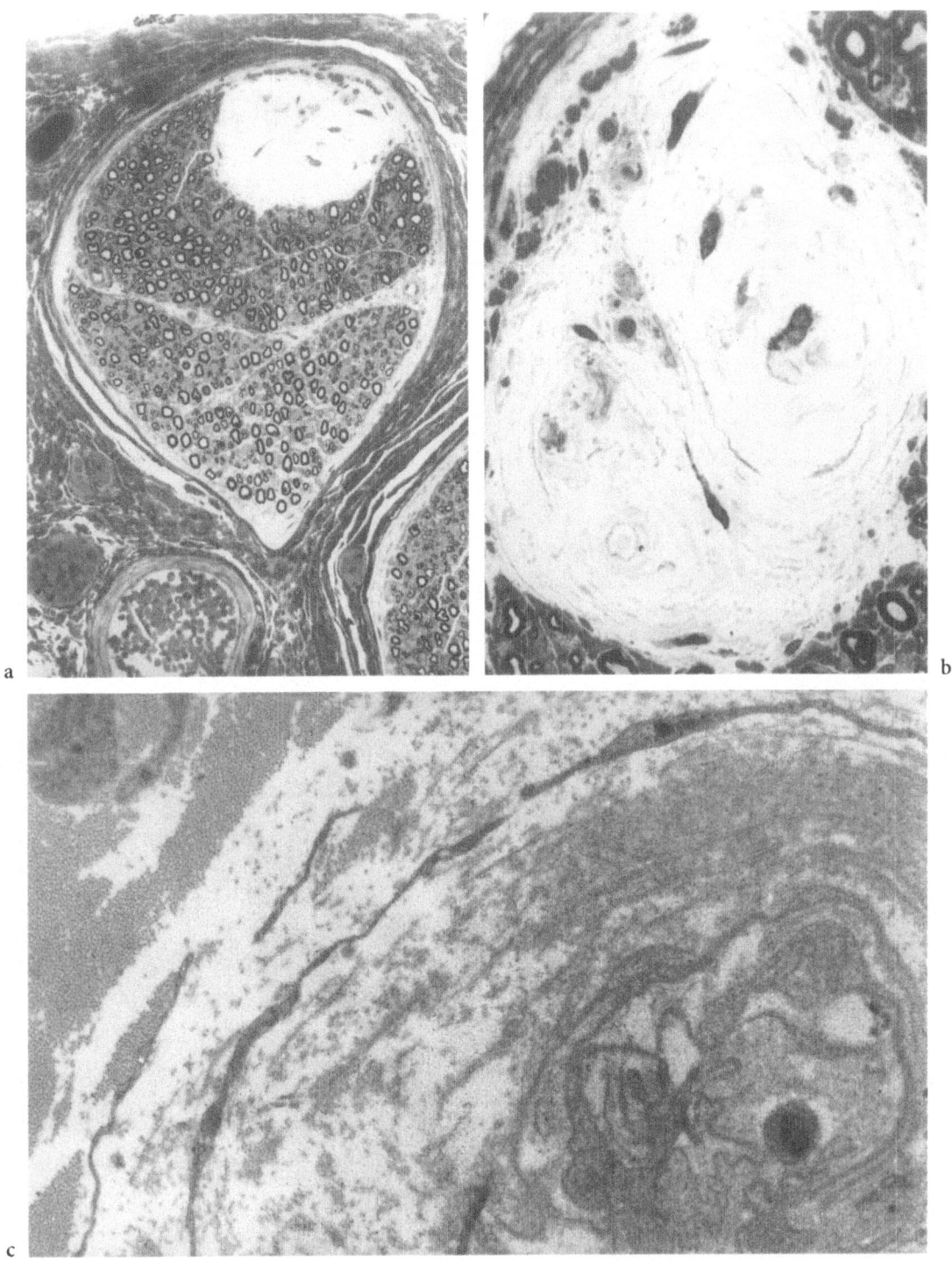

Fig. 34a – c. Renaut body in the sural nerve of a 20-year-old man with spinal muscular atrophy. The alterations in the nerve are otherwise in the normal range. **a** × 157; **b** × 526. **c** Electron microscopic magnification of the presumptive initial stage of Renaut body formation in a 55-year-old male patient with severely advanced alcoholic neuropathy. Illustrated are cellular debris, basal laminae remnants, and collagen fibrils in the *lower right*; a band of Büngner can be seen in the *upper left*. × 7,000 (From [958])

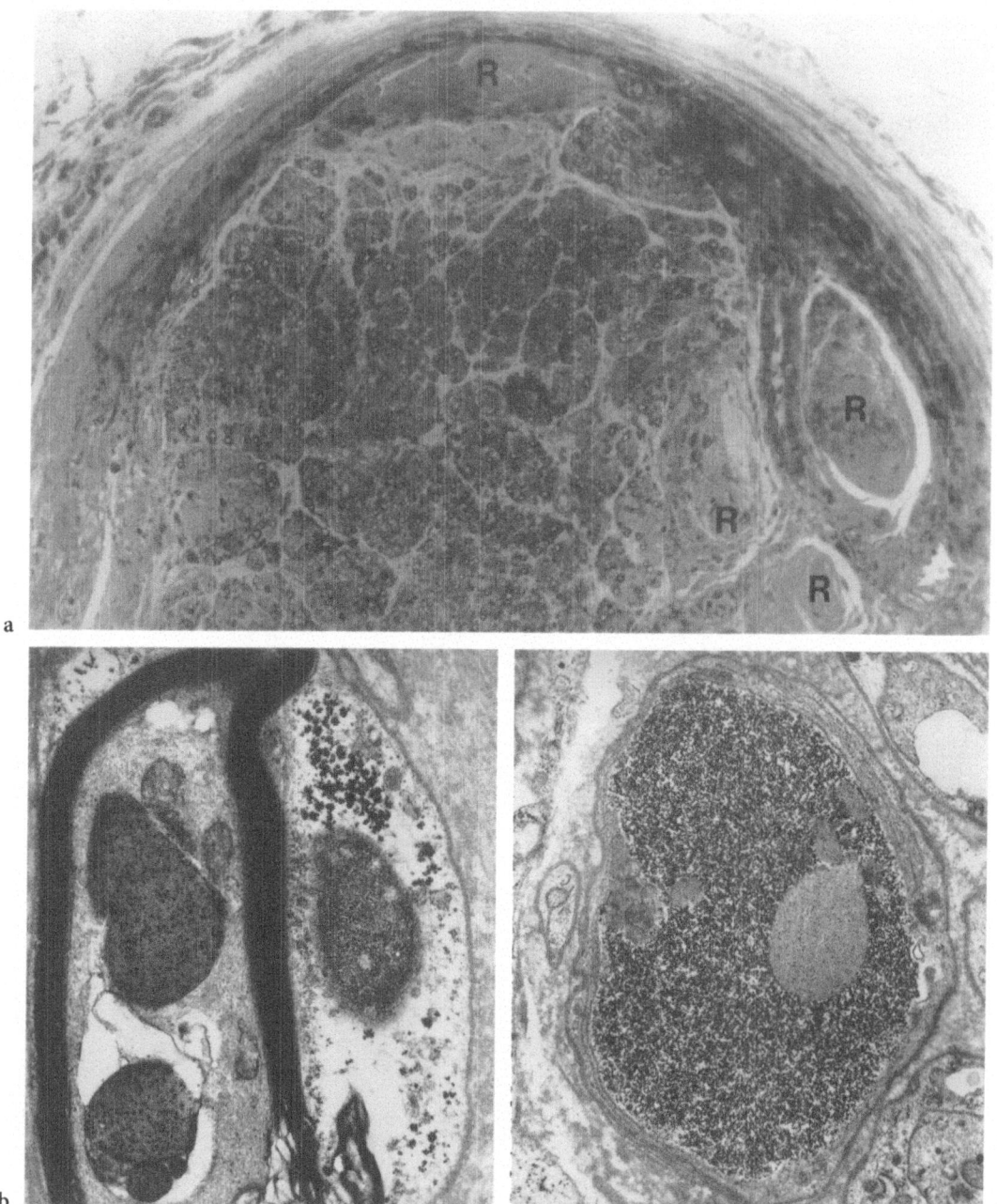

Fig. 35 a–c. N. cutaneus femoris lateralis in a case of meralgia paresthetica in a 39-year-old man. **a** The perineurium is unevenly thickened. There are Renaut bodies at several sites. The number of large myelinated nerve fibers is considerably reduced and the endoneurial connective tissue is altogether increased. × 206. **b** A myelinated nerve fiber contains unusual, partly vacuolated, enlarged lysosome-like cytosomes with glycogen granules in the axoplasm. The glycogen in the perikaryon of the corresponding Schwann cell is increased. × 16,000. **c** A presumably demyelinated axon is filled with glycogen. Therein are some mitochondria and a cytosome resembling those in **b**. × 11,000

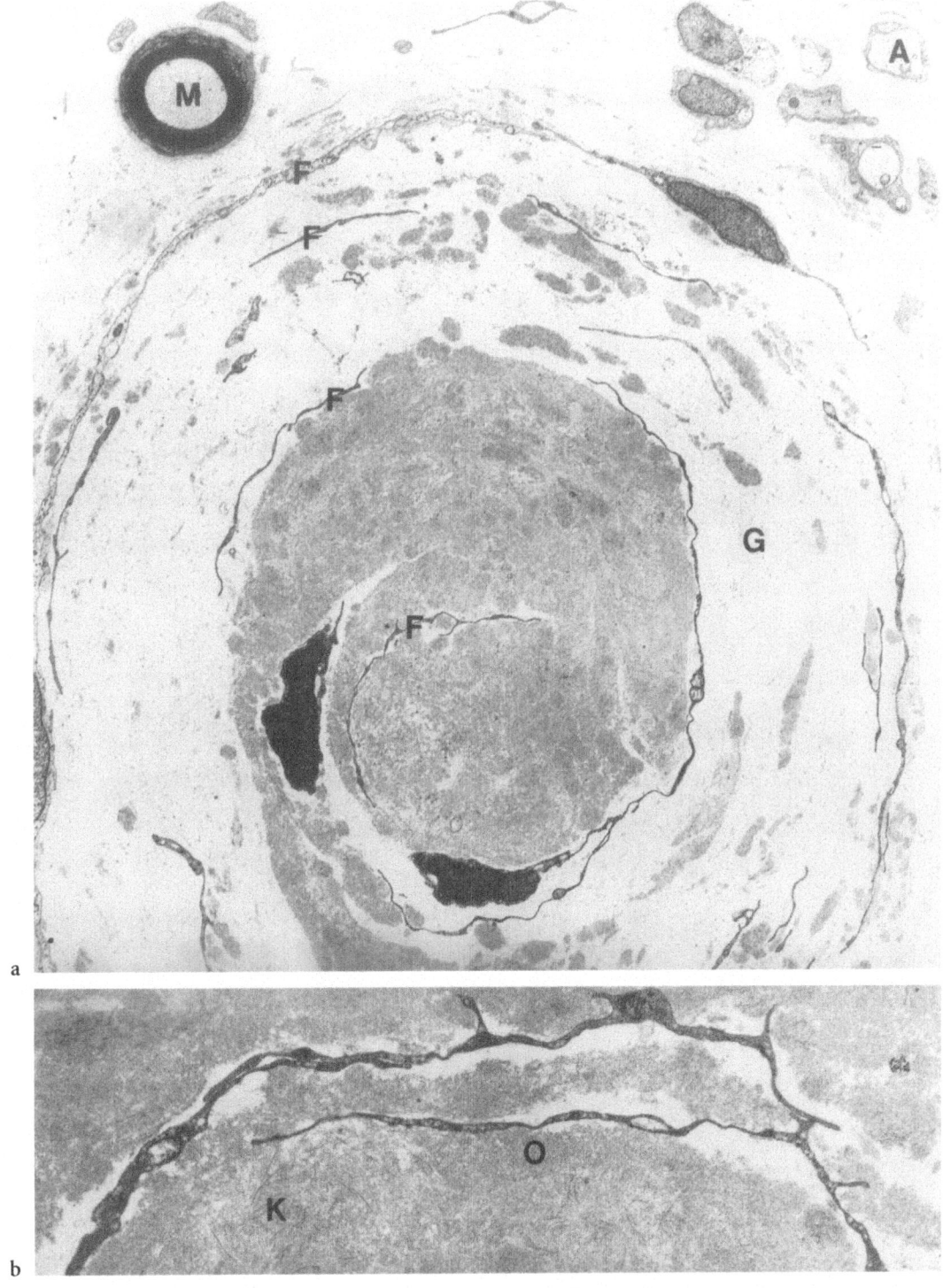

Fig. 36. a Electron microscopic area of the N. digitalis plantaris proprius between the third and fourth toe of a 51-year-old female with Morton's metatarsalgia. Only rare myelinated (*M*) and unmyelinated axons (*A*) are preserved. Instead there is a Renaut body with concentrically arranged fibroblast-like cells (*F*) (which according to EMA immune reactions were identified as perineurial cells) associated with an accumulation of oxytalan filaments in the center and surrounded by granular, mucoid substances (*G*). × 7,500. b Higher magnification of a neighboring area of a. Between and adjacent to flat cell processes there are collagen fibrils oriented in different directions (*K*) and masses of oxytalan filaments (*O*). × 10,300. (From [964])

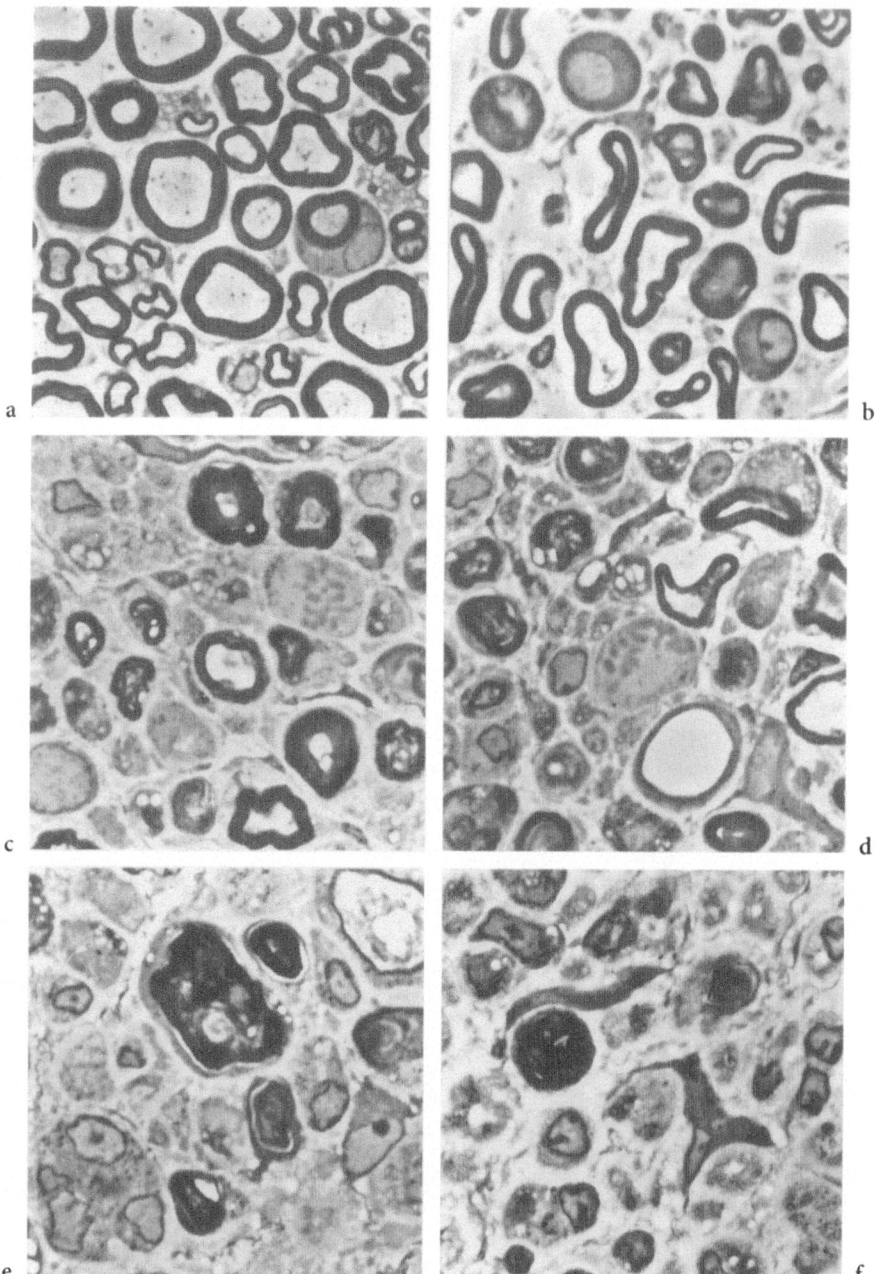

Fig. 37 a–f. Different stages of Wallerian degeneration: 24 (**a**) and 48 h (**b**), and 5 (**c**), 10 (**d**), 20 (**e**), and 31 days (**f**) after the transection of the sciatic nerve of rats. The nerve fiber degradation progresses relatively slowly including large and small myelinated nerve fibers affecting both at a different pace. A mitotic figure is seen at 5 and 10 days. The bands of Büngner contain up to 3 nuclei per cross section indicating considerable proliferation of Schwann cells (and macrophages). After 1 month regressive alterations dominate: shrinkage of the bands of Büngner including the cell nuclei. Myelin sheath remnants may persist to even later stages. × 1,120 (From [1014])

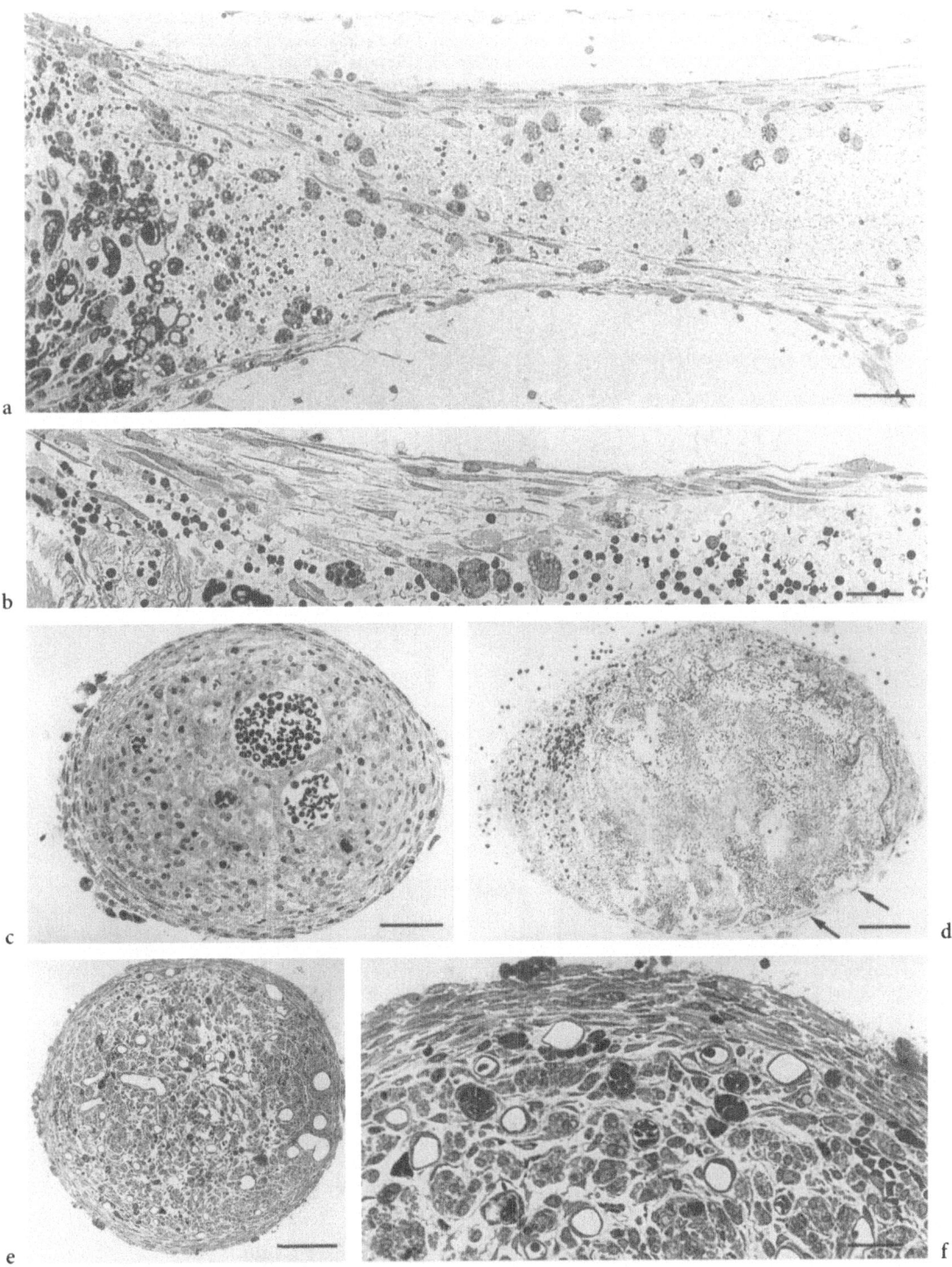

Fig. 38. Legend s. p. 46

Fig. 38. **a** Early stage of a perineurial cell tube, which connects the proximal with the distal stump of the sciatic nerve of a rat within a silicon tube, 7 days after the excision of a nerve segment about 1 cm in length. Within the tube are numerous macrophages and degenerating blood cells. (From [989]). **b** Higher magnification of the perineurial cell tube at the site of the connection between the preexisting proximal perineurium and the newly formed perineurial cell tube. **c** Cross section of the proximal segment of the regenerating cord within the silicon tube, 12 days after surgery. The cord is surrounded by concentrically arranged perineurial cells; it contains numerous fibroblasts and Schwann cells as well as surprisingly large blood vessels. **d** In the intermediate portion of the same regeneration chamber as shown in **c**, the cord is mainly composed of fibrin fibrils which are surrounded by sparse, longitudinally oriented cells that have spread along its surface (*arrows*). **e** After 18 days, this cross section of the regenerating cord shows numerous cells and blood vessels. **f** At higher magnification several layers of a well-differentiated perineurium and numerous capillaries, fibroblasts, Schwann cells, and still unmyelinated axons can be seen lying together in groups, but not surrounded by a separate perineurium (such as seen in minifascicles following a neuromatous type of reinnervation). Bar in **a, c, d** = 50 μm; **b, f** = 25 μm; **e** = 100 μm. (**b**–**f** From [1224]).

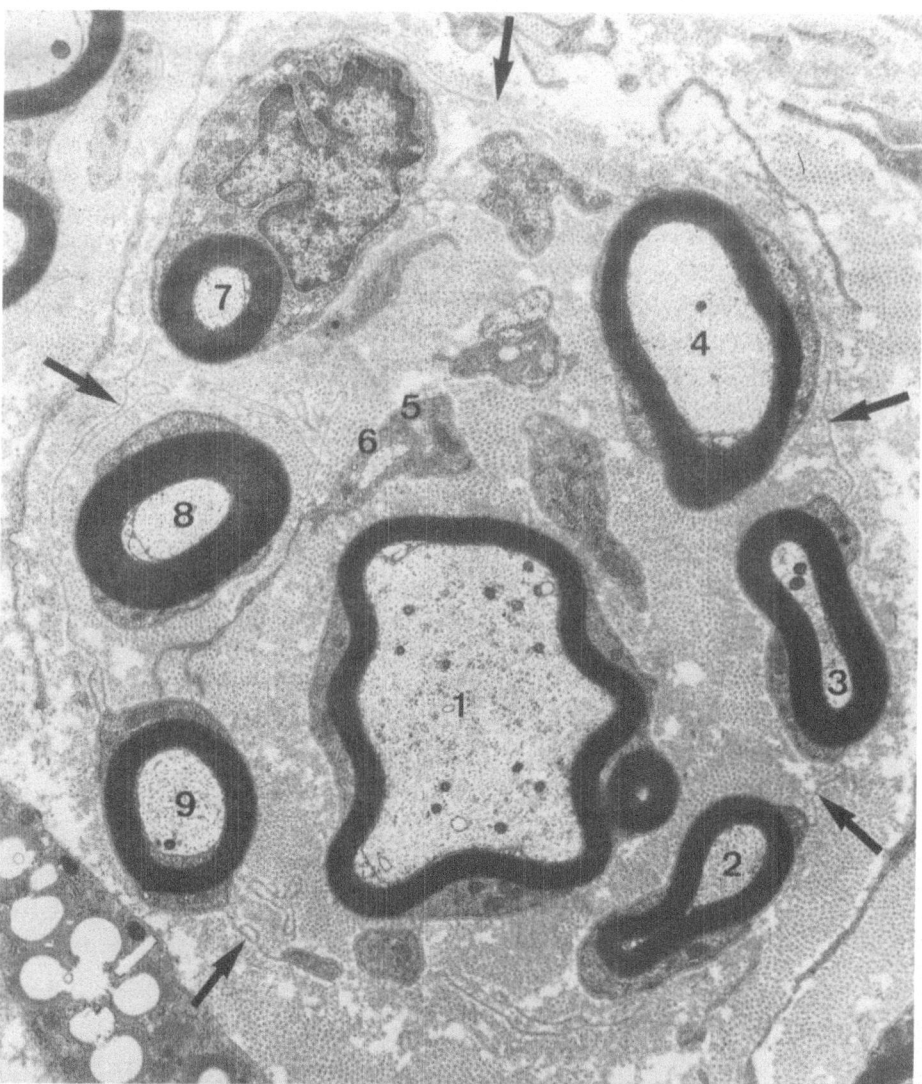

Fig. 39. Cluster of nine regenerated, partly myelinated (nos. 1–4, 7–9), partly unmyelinated (5 and 6) axons, of which only nerve fiber 1 has become rather large, whereas nerve fibers 2, 3, 7–9 have become atrophic, presumably because they have not found an adequate end contact. This group is surrounded by a completely preserved basal lamina indicating that it is derived from a single myelinated nerve fiber (*arrows*). (From [986])

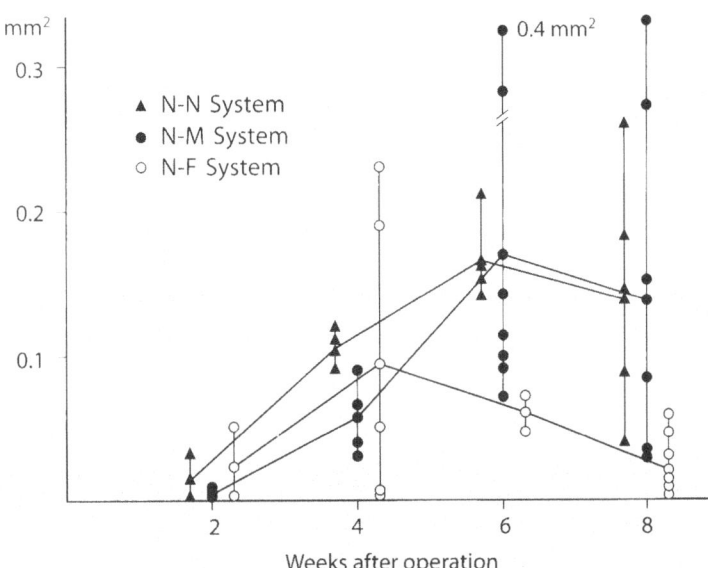

Fig. 40. Dimensions of nerve fascicles 2–8 weeks after the implantation of a silicon tube at the site where a 1-cm-long segment of the sciatic nerve of rats has been excised. The best results were obtained after connecting the silicon tubes with the peripheral nerve stump (N-N system) or with muscle tissue (N-M system). Following connection of the tubes with fat tissue, a relatively large number of nerve fibers has outgrown proximally within the first 4 weeks; after 6 and 8 weeks, however, there are regressive changes and a reduction in the diameter of the regenerating cord, presumably because of a lack of adequate peripheral end contacts and therefore an insufficient supply of neurotrophic substances, etc. (From [1225])

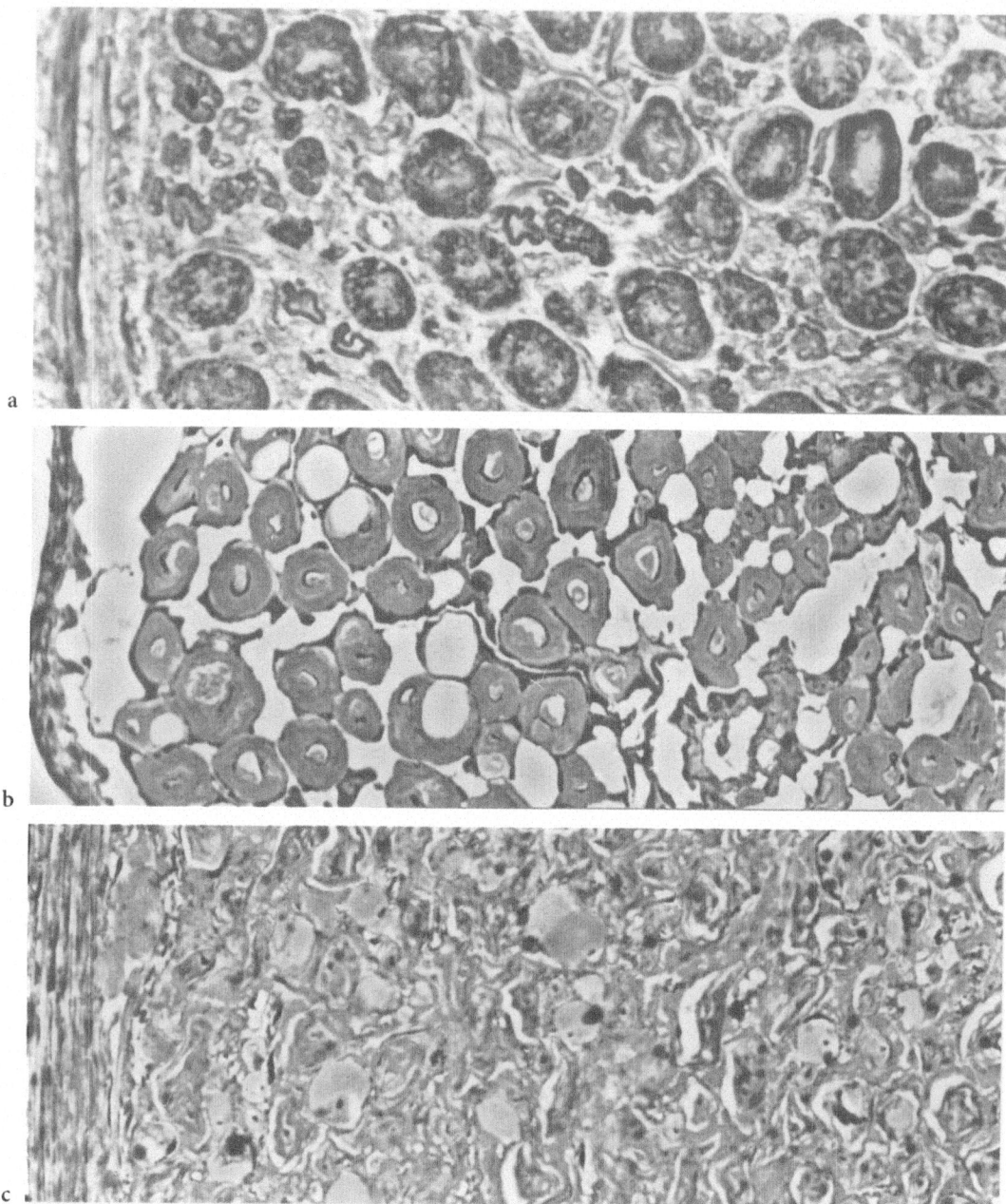

Fig. 41. a Deep-frozen, **b** freeze-dried, and **c** cialit-solution-preserved nerve specimens after standard fixation and embedding for electron microscopy (semithin sections). The freeze-dried specimen in contrast to the usual procedure for nerve grafting, was not kept in physiological NaCl solution, but fixed immediately; correspondingly, there are numerous gaps and vacuoles in the tissue. In the deep-frozen specimen the structure of the nerve and the nerve fibers appear to be better preserved, while in the cialit-specimen preservation is the worst. × 720 (From [994])

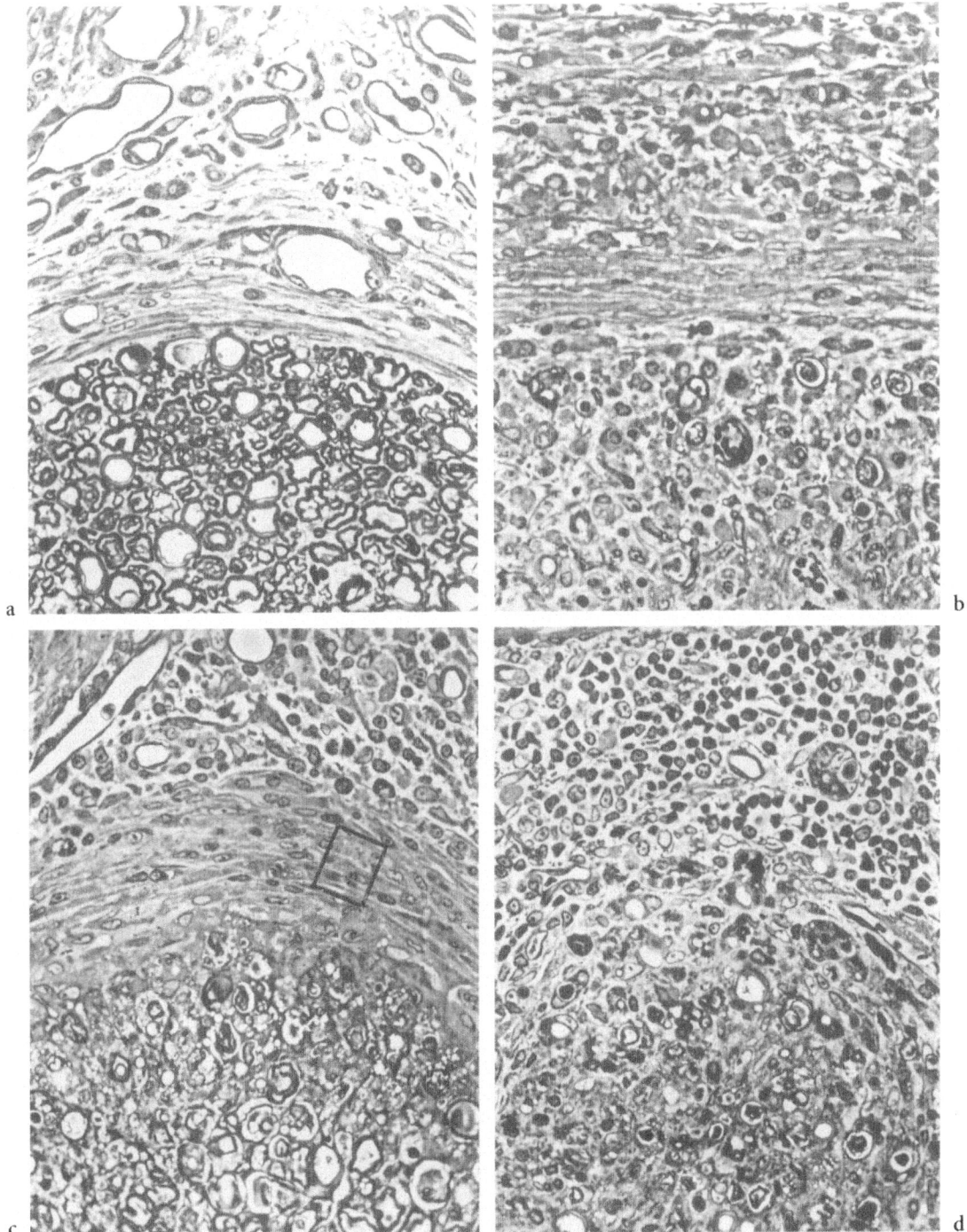

Fig. 42a–d. Heterologous, heterotopically implanted nerve grafts of rats 1 (**a**), 2 (**b**), 3 (**c**), and 4 weeks (**d**) after the implantation under the skin of the dorsum of guinea pigs. After 2–4 weeks there are increasing numbers of cellular infiltrates, mainly of mononuclear cells. The perineurium after 3 weeks has surprisingly increased in thickness. [The *boxed area* is magnified in the subsequent electron micrograph (Fig. 43)]. After 4 weeks there is massive cellular infiltration also of the perineurium (perineuritis). Degradation of myelin sheaths is delayed up to this time. × 290

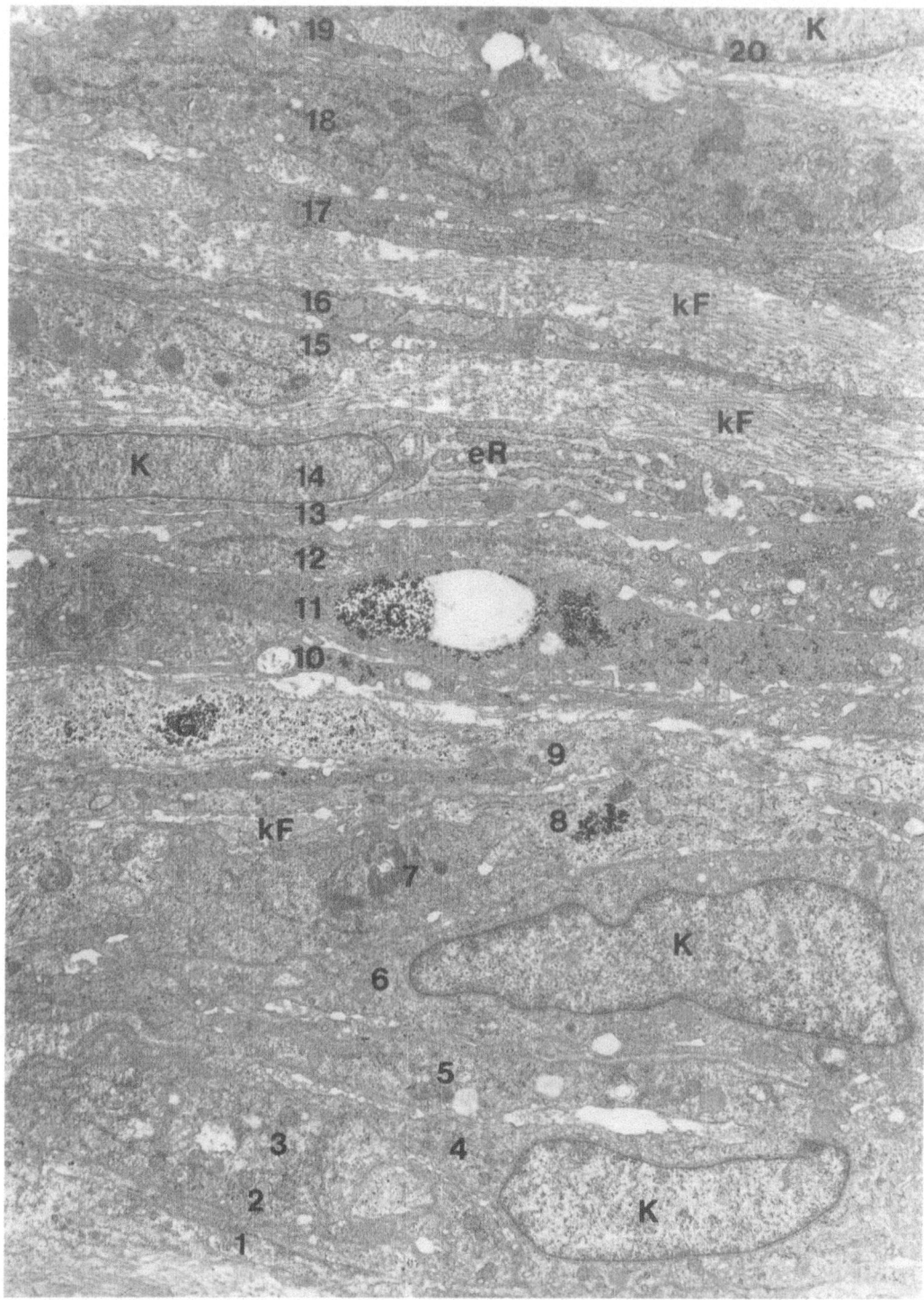

Fig. 43. Higher magnification of the extremely thickened perineurium shown in Fig. 42c. The cellular layers of the perineurium are substantially increased in number (1–20) and partly thickened. A basal lamina is not detectable at the surface of most of the cells. The endoplasmic reticulum (*eR*) is enlarged in some cells. At several sites there are numerous glycogen granules (*G*) in the cytoplasm of some cells. *K*, nucleus; *kF*, collagen fibrils. × 6,900 (Figs. 42 and 43 from [947])

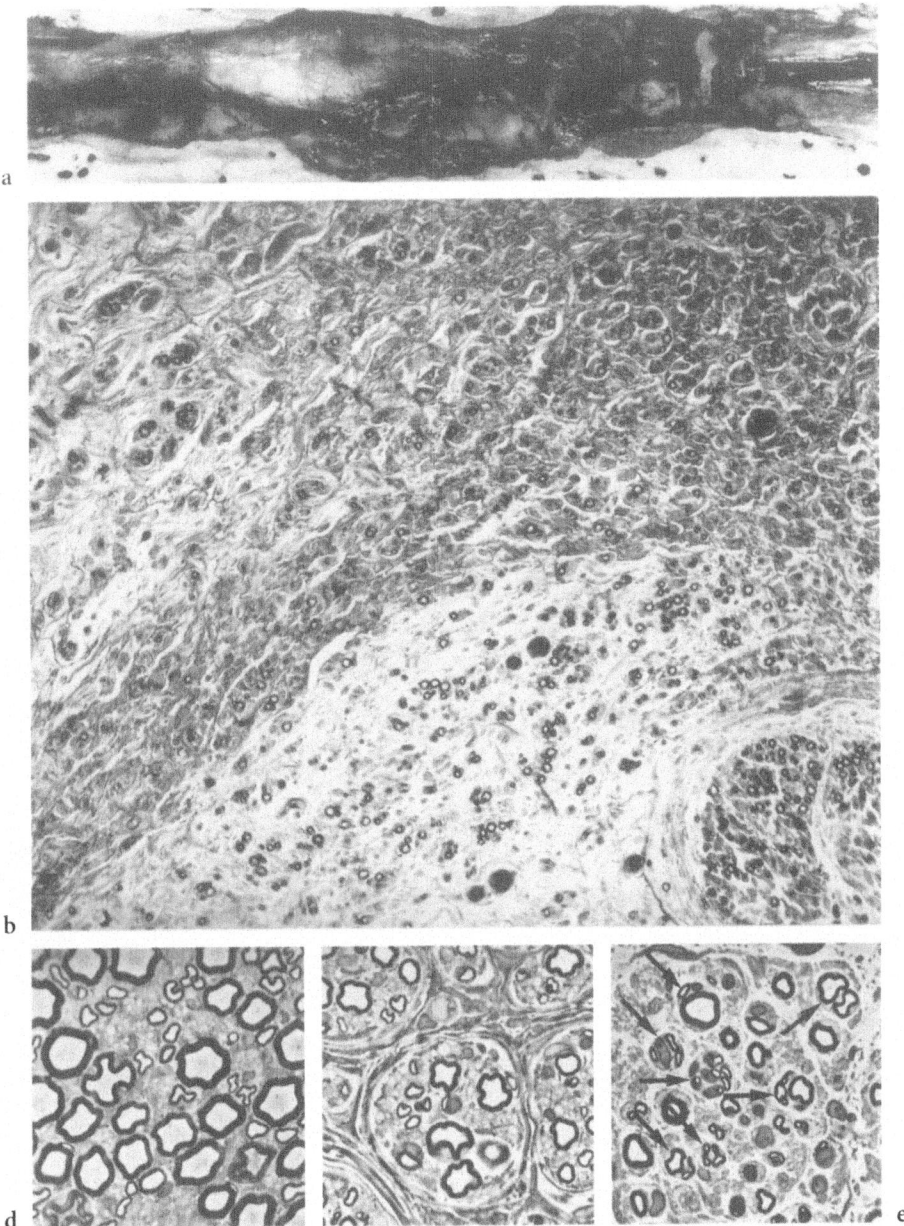

Fig. 44. a Cialit-treated, allogenic nerve graft, 3.1 cm in length, 1 year after implantation. The adhesions at the level of the graft and somewhat proximal thereof are clearly apparent. The proximal neuroma (on the *left side*) is more prominent than the distal one (on the *right side* proximal to the division of the sciatic nerve of a dog). × 2. **b** 2.5 cm-long fresh allogenic graft 1 year after the implantation. Numerous regenerated nerve fibers lie amidst the connective tissue; only in the *lower right corner* is still a larger fascicle apparent. × 40. **c** Proximal to **d**, a 3.2 cm-long deep-frozen allogenic graft; the nerve fibers and the architecture of the endoneurium appear to be completely normal in this area. In **d** there are several very small fascicles (minifascicles) closely adjacent to each other. The regenerated nerve fibers therein are thinner than proximal nerve fibers. **e** Distal to the 3.1 cm-long cialit-treated graft (in **a**), 6 months after implantation. Numerous regenerated nerve fibers of uneven size (clusters of regenerated fibers) have reinnervated the bands of Büngner (causing hyperneurotization of the bands of Büngner, *arrows*). **c, d** × 560 (From [943, 993])

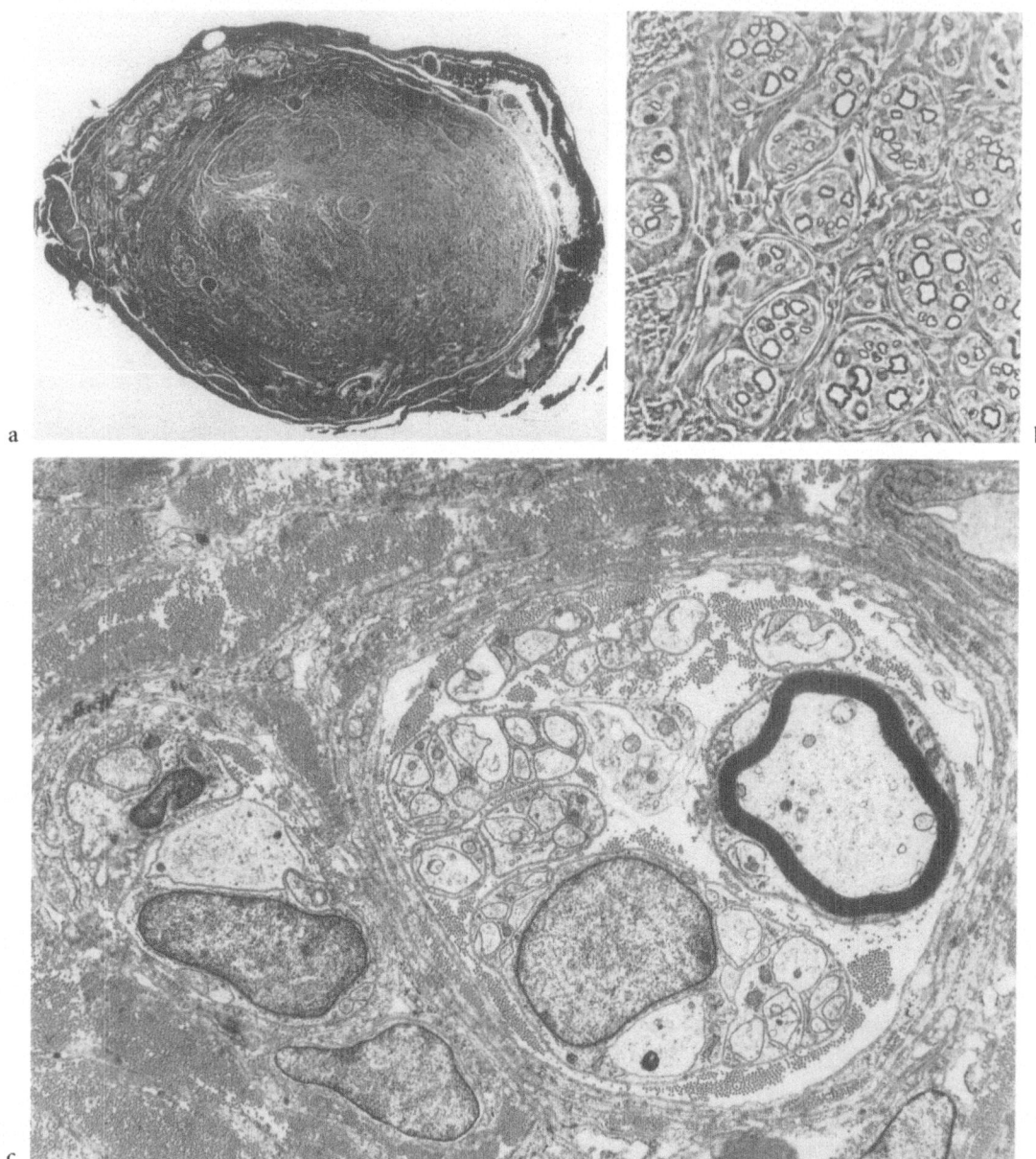

Fig. 45 a – c. Neuromatous reinnervation (neurotization) of nerve grafts. **a** Cialit-treated 3.1 cm-long homologous graft 1 year after the implantation into the sciatic nerve of a dog (same nerve as in Fig. 44 a – d). **b** Deep-frozen fresh homologous graft 1 year after the reinnervation with numerous small isomorphically arranged, newly formed nerve fascicles (minifascicles). × 487. **c** Cialit-treated homologous nerve graft 6 months after the implantation. This newly formed minifascicle is completely isolated from the surrounding connective tissue by a multilayered perineurium. The collagen fibrils in the new endoneurium are thicker than in the surrounding epineurium. The fascicles contain numerous unmyelinated axons, but only one thinly myelinated regenerated nerve fiber. × 5,220. (From [958])

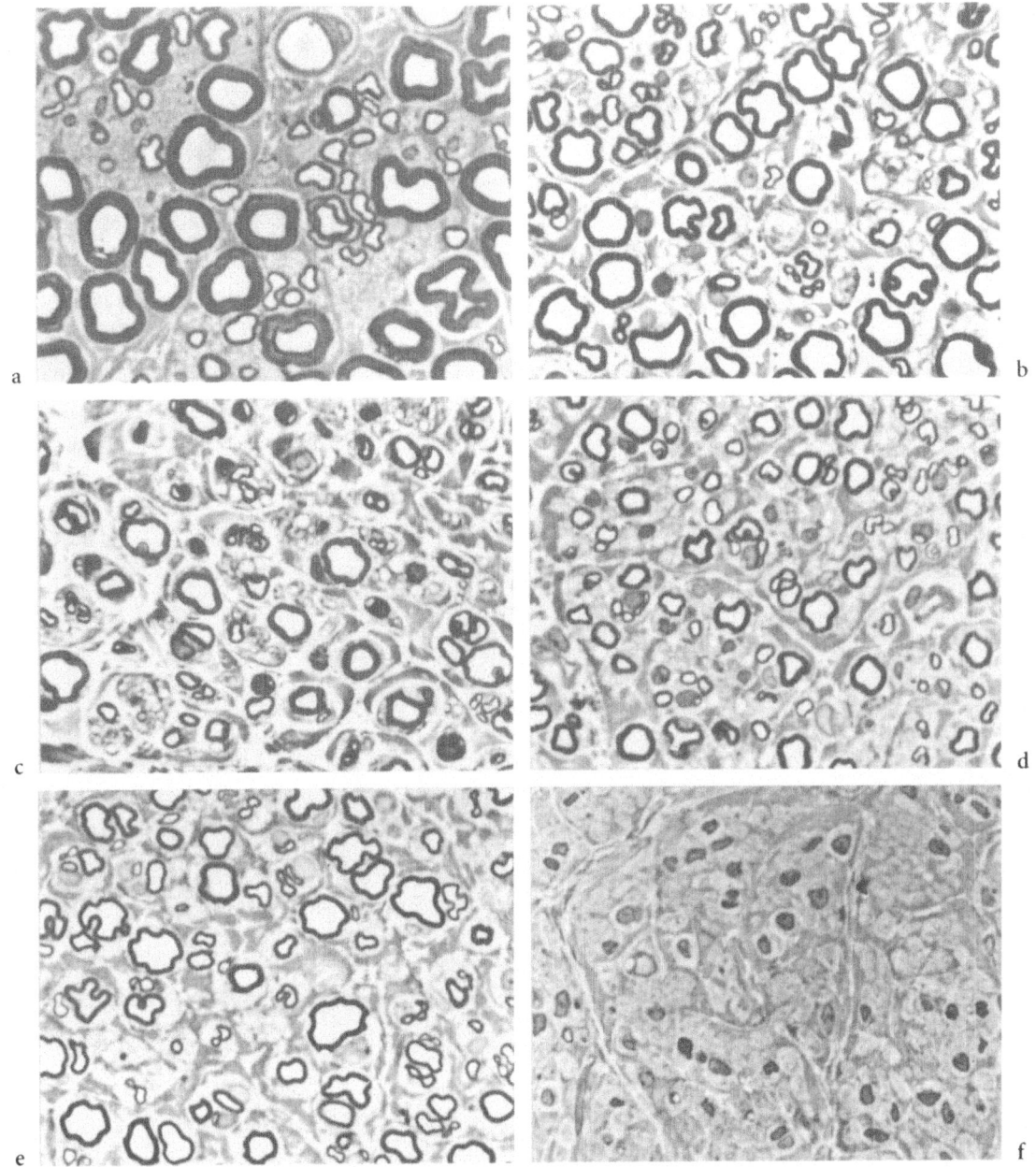

Fig. 46. a Normal nerve, **b** distal to a 2 cm-long autologous nerve graft, **c** distal to a 3.1 cm-long cialit-preserved nerve graft, **d** distal to a 3.2 cm-long deep-frozen nerve graft, **e** distal to a 3 cm-long freeze-dried nerve graft, and **f** distal to a 8 cm-long cialit-treated nerve graft. The newly formed myelin sheaths are in all cases considerably thinner than in normal nerves although axonal calibers approach normal values quite closely. The autologous graft resulted in optimal reinnervation, i. e., it contains the largest number of nerve fibers with useful calibers. No nerve fibers can be seen distal to the long graft in the area illustrated (f); there are only empty bands of Büngner. × 670. (From [994])

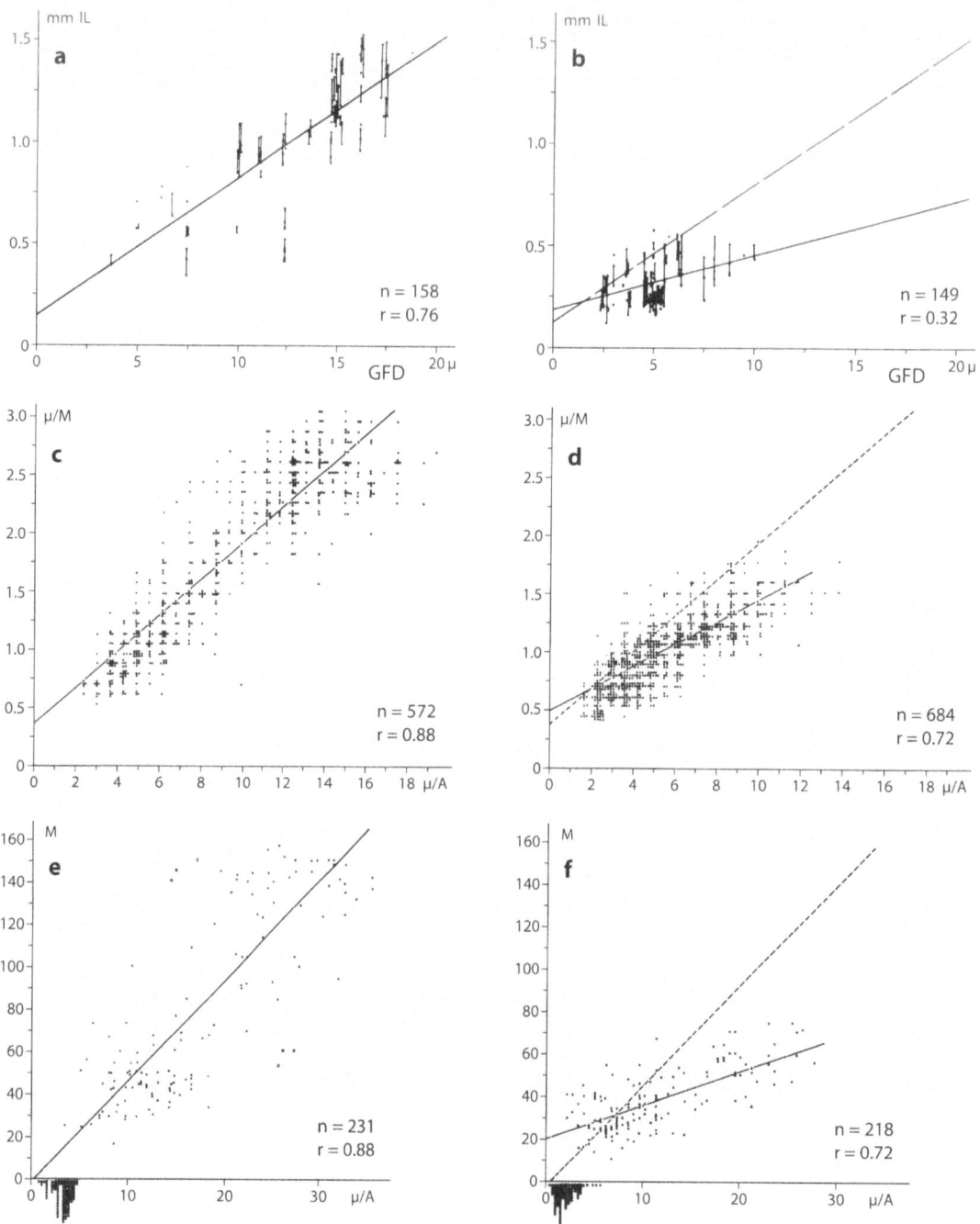

Fig. 47. **a**, **c**, and **e** normal, **b**, **d**, and **f** regenerated nerve fibers in the contralateral sciatic nerve of a dog 12 months after the implantation of a deeply frozen, 3.5 cm-long homologous nerve graft. **a** and **b** Length of the internode (*IL*) in relation to the total nerve fiber diameter (*GFD*); **c** and **d** myelin sheath thickness in μm (μ/M) in relation to the total nerve fiber diameter in μm (μ/A) according to light microscopic measurements; **e** and **f** number of the myelin sheath lamellae (*M*) in relation to the axon circumference in μm (μ/D) according to electron microscopic measurements. The unmyelinated nerve fibers measured by electron microscopy are indicated in **e** and **f** *below the abscissa*. Many regenerated unmyelinated axons are thinner than the normal ones. (From [951])

Dog: normal myelin sheath

Restored myelin sheath

Rat: normal myelin sheath

Restored myelin sheath

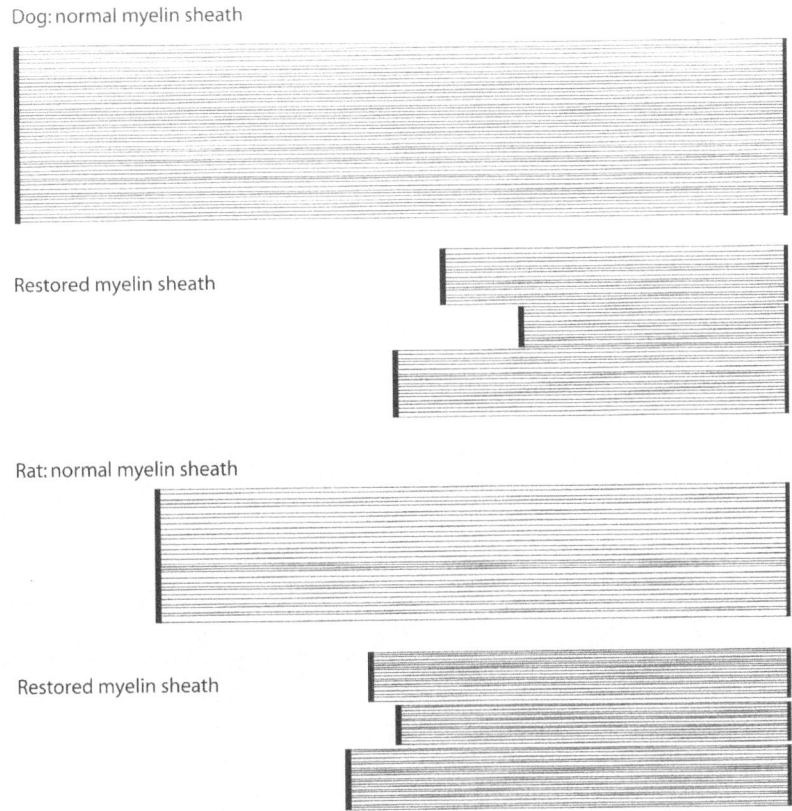

Fig. 48. Proportionate, two-dimensional reconstruction of the largest normal and three regenerated internodes, the myelin lamellae of which are thought to be unrolled in sciatic nerves of dogs and rats. The cytoplasm of the Schwann cells is drawn to scale in *black* at the outer and inner mesaxons. Both cytoplasmic sides are connected to each other by horizontal lines corresponding to the paranodal myelin loops and Schmidt-Lanterman incisures. The number of Schmidt-Lanterman incisures is considerably increased in relation to the thickness of the newly formed myelin sheaths. The internodes of the regenerated nerve fibers are uniformly shortened, and the thickness of the myelin sheaths (or the length of the myelin lamellae which are thought to be unrolled) is absolutely and relatively more reduced in the dog than in the rat. (From [951])

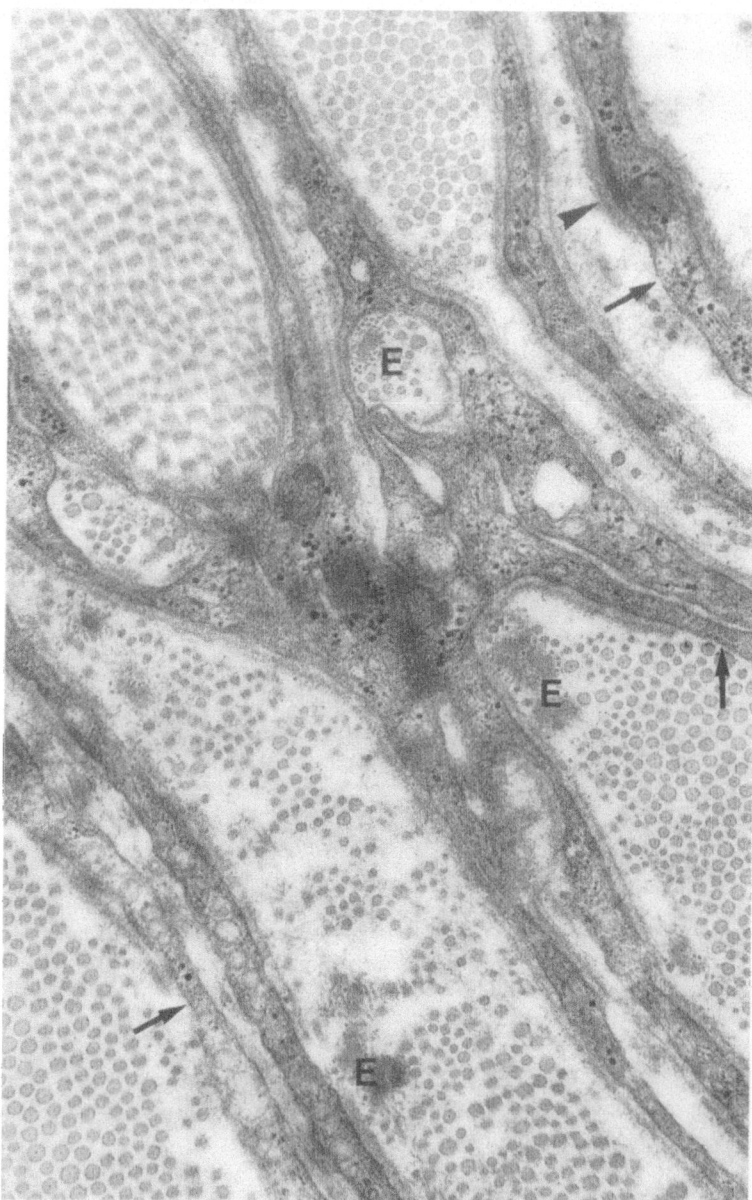

Fig. 49. The newly formed perineurial cells enclose bundles of collagen fibrils which show different calibers. Interspersed are elastic fibers (*E*). Sites where the basal laminae at the surface of the perineurial cells are lacking are indicated by *arrows*; a hemi-desmosome-like structure is indicated by an *arrowhead*. Between the processes, the perineurial cells show different forms of contacts. × 40,500 (From [993])

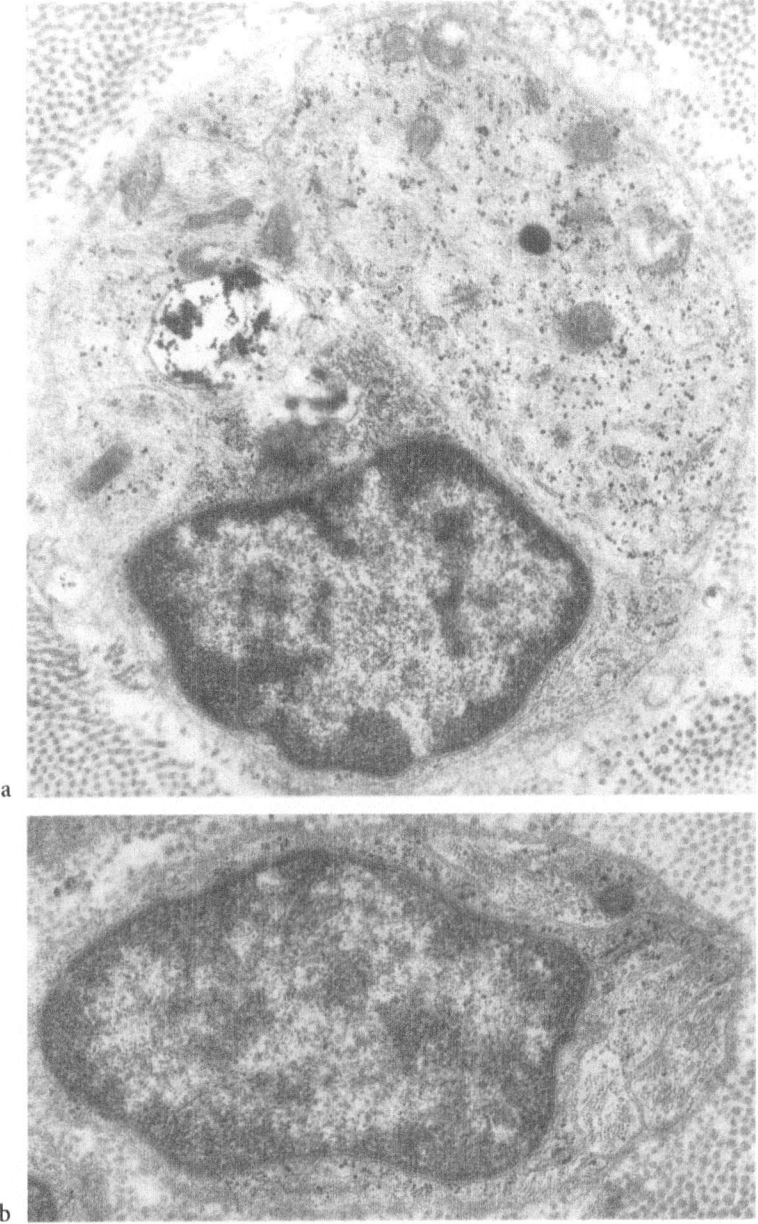

Fig. 50 a, b. Bands of Büngner distal to an inefficient long graft 8 cm in length, 6 months after implantation. In the cytoplasm of the proliferated Schwann cells or Schwann cell processes, which are surrounded by a common basal lamina, there are numerous intermediate filaments oriented in different directions, glycogen granules, tubules and ribosomes, an autophagic vacuole, mitochondria, and a nucleus which is rich in heterochromatin. **a** × 20,000; **b** × 23,500

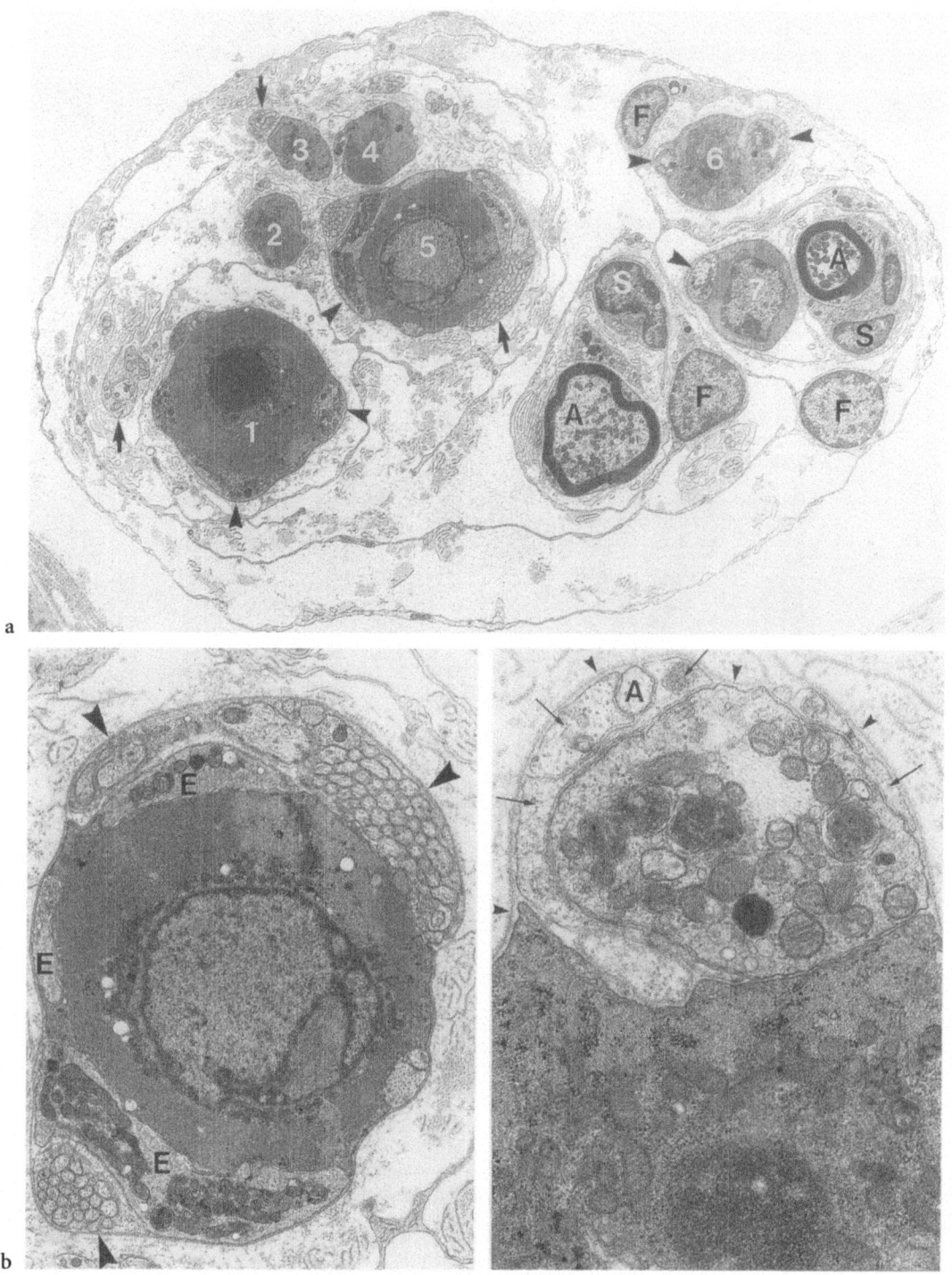

Fig. 51a–c. Legend s. p. 60

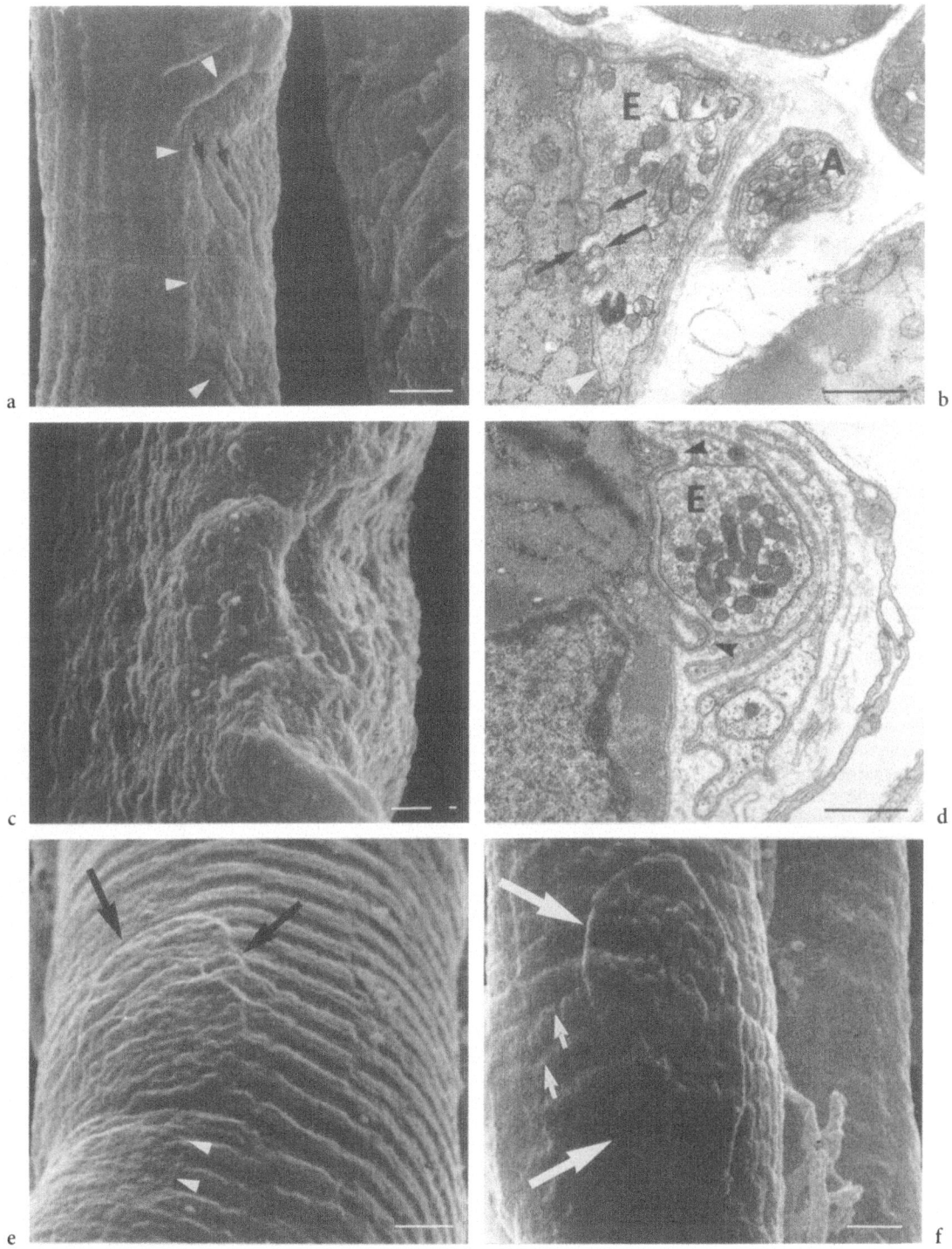

Fig. 52a–f. Legend s. p. 60

Fig. 51a-c. Equatorial area of a muscle spindle 6 months after transection and immediate suture of the sciatic nerve of a rat. **a** An increased number of intrafusal muscle fibers (*IMF*; normal: 1–4) is indicated by numbers (*1–7*), some of which are partially surrounded by regenerated sensory nerve endings (*arrowheads*). Fibroblasts (*F*) and their processes form the inner spindle capsule and subdivide the outer from the inner periaxial space; the latter contains thinly remyelinated axons (*A*) and multiple sprouts of nonmyelinated axons (*arrows*), Schwann cells (*S*), collagen fibrils, elastic fibers, and remnants of numerous basal laminae. IMF 1 contains an electron-dense body. × 3,000. **b** Higher magnification of IMF 5 in **a**. A nuclear chain fiber is partially surrounded by a regenerated sensory nerve terminal (*E*); the axolemma and the sarcolemma are closely apposed. The nerve terminal and the IMF are surrounded by a common basal lamina. Two Schwann cell processes which enclose numerous nonmyelinated axons can be seen immediately adjacent (*arrowheads*) and are in close contact with the sensory nerve terminal or the IMF. The axonal sprouts in the *lower left corner* are isolated from collagen fibrils and from the regenerated nerve terminal by a Schwann cell process. The axial space contains collagen fibrils, elastic fibers, fibroblast processes, and remnants of basal laminae. × 7,700. **c** Higher magnification of parts of IMF 6 in **a**. The regenerated sensory nerve terminal is filled with mitochondria, neurofilaments, microtubules, neurogenic vesicles, and small membranous cytoplasmic bodies. Immediately adjacent to the nerve terminal are Schwann cell processes (*arrows*), which separate the nerve terminal at least partially from the IMF lying beneath as well as from a nonmyelinated axon (*A*). The sensory nerve terminal, the Schwann cell processes, and the IMF are surrounded by a common basal lamina (*arrowheads*). × 23,000. (From [227])

Fig. 52a-f. Teased denervated and reinnervated muscle spindles. **a** Normal-looking subsynaptic folds and rims beneath a motor end plate of an intrafusal muscle fiber in the distal polar region, 6 months after crushing the sciatic nerve of a rat. The flat impression with synaptic folds is subdivided by sarcoplasmic protrusions, indicated by *arrowheads*. Bar = 2 μm. **b** Transmission electron microscopic aspect of the subneural region of an intrafusal muscle fiber with a motor nerve terminal in the polar region of a normal rat muscle spindle. The nerve terminal (*E*) is filled with small, light synaptic vesicles and mitochondria. An unmyelinated preterminal axon (*A*) can be seen close to the nerve terminal. A basal lamina separates the motor nerve terminal from the intrafusal muscle fiber (*arrowhead*). The subneural apparatus is formed by small sarcoplasmic protrusions and rims (*arrows*). Bar = 1 μm. **c** A reinnervated intrafusal muscle fiber, 12 months after crushing the sciatic nerve, shows a subsynaptic area in the middle polar region. It is surrounded by a sarcolemmal rim. Bar = 2 μm. **d** Transmission electron microscopic aspect of the subneural apparatus of an intrafusal muscle fiber. A regenerated motor nerve terminal (*E*) is illustrated in the polar region, 3 months after a crush lesion of the sciatic nerve. The muscle fiber beneath the nerve terminal shows a moderate indentation which is bordered by a sarcolemmal rim (*arrowheads*). Bar = 1 μm. **e** Three months after transection and immediate suture of the sciatic nerve, the distal polar region of a nuclear bag fiber shows a flat plate-like elevation (*arrows*). The sarcomeric pattern at the elevation close to the equator is flattened (*arrowheads*). Bar = 3 μm. **f** One month after a nerve crush lesion there is a plate-like elevation (*large arrows*) as shown in Fig. **e** in the polar region of an intrafusal muscle fiber. It shows small irregular elevations at the surface. The sarcomeric pattern of the intrafusal muscle fiber (*small arrows*) is interrupted at the elevation. Bar = 2 μm. (From [231])

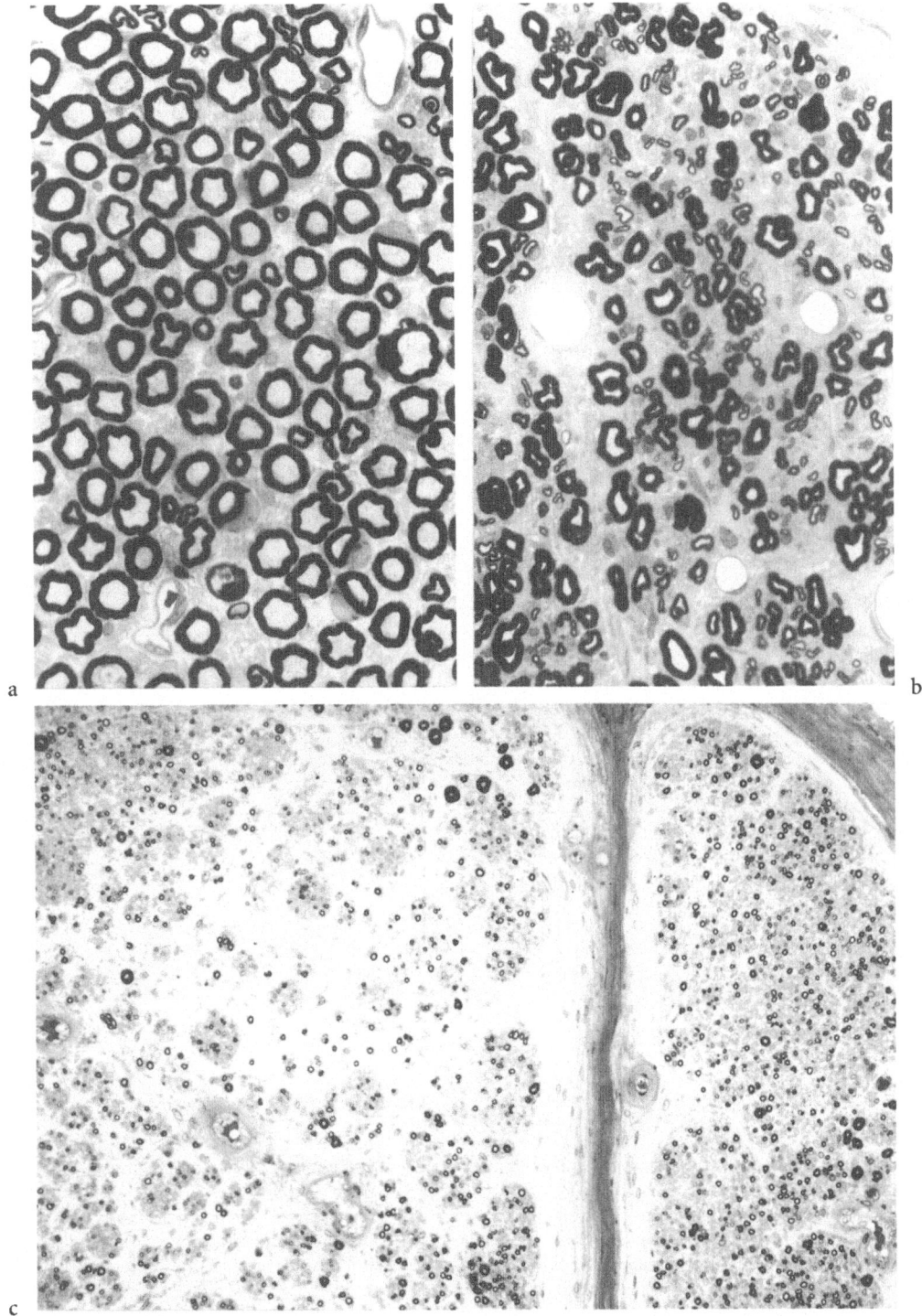

Fig. 53. a Normal and **b** retrograde-atrophic sciatic nerve of a dog 6 months after implantation of a homologous, ineffective, approximately 10 cm-long nerve graft distal to **b** is shown. The axons in **b** are shrunken, the myelin sheaths of which are more or less severely collapsed without evidence of degeneration. × 380. **c** Retrograde nerve fiber loss in a sciatic nerve of a 46-year-old man whose leg was amputated at the age of 4. Nearly all large myelinated nerve fibers are retrograde-degenerated. Remaining are mainly small regenerated, myelinated nerve fibers. × 96. (From [958])

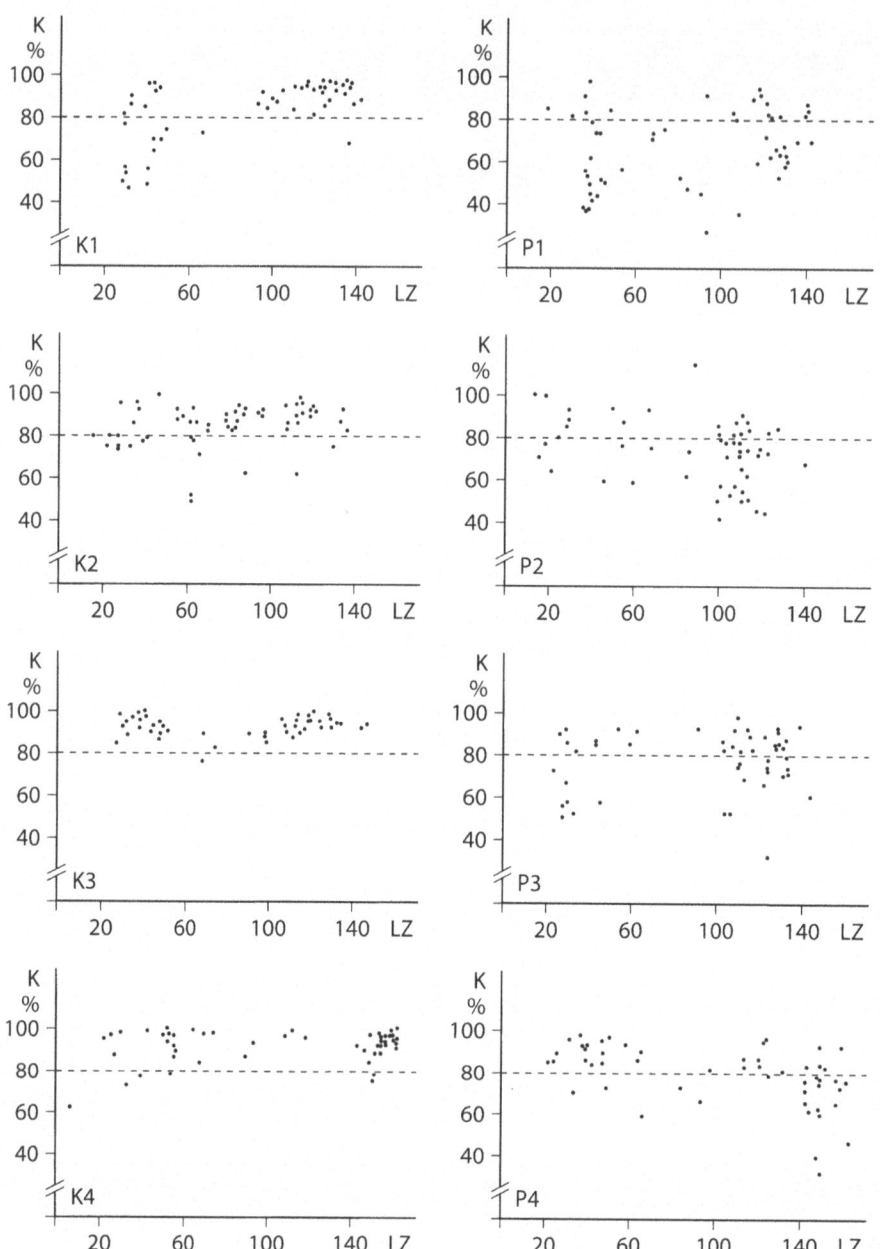

Fig. 54. Deviation of the circularity of individual myelinated nerve fibers in percentage (K value in %, ordinate) in normal (K 1–4) and retrograde-altered nerves proximal to different ineffective, approximately 10-cm-long nerve grafts (P 1–4) in sciatic nerves of dogs 6 months after implantation. There are already deviations from the ideal circularity in control nerves. In the retrograde-altered nerves (see Fig. 53b) these deformations are considerably more numerous and severe (values below the 80% line). On the *abscissa*, the number of myelin lamellae (*LZ*) of individual nerve fibers determined with the electron microscope is indicated (as a measure for the original dimensions of the nerve fibers). Thin myelinated nerve fibers in normal nerves show deviations of the circularity more frequently than large ones. (From Schröder and Müller 1982, unpublished results)

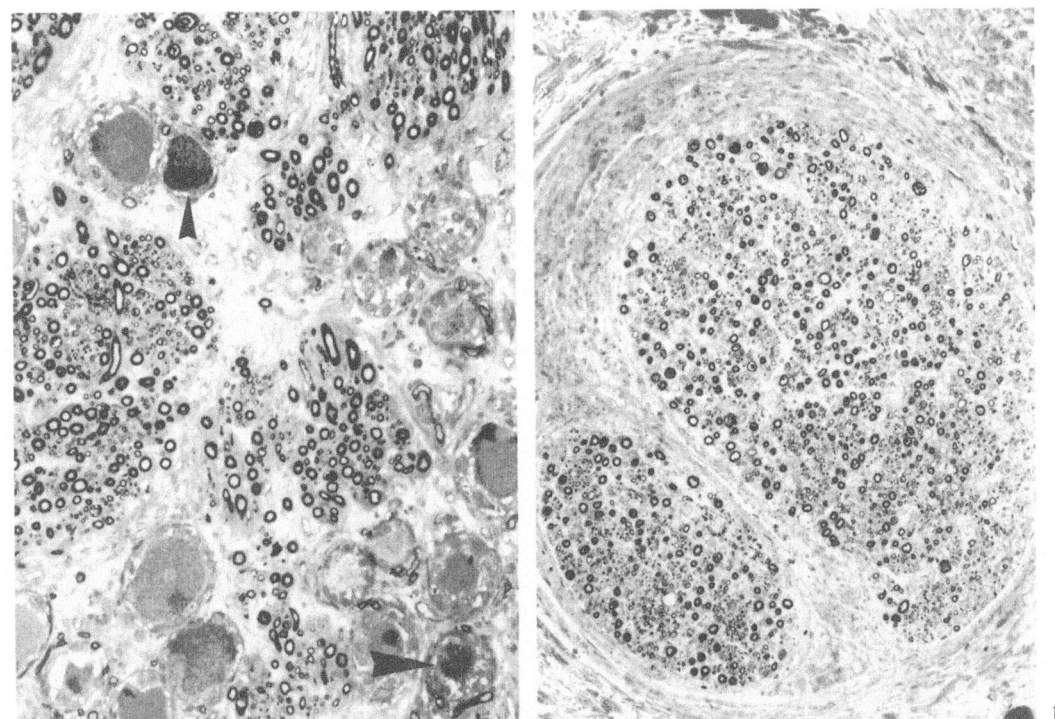

a   b

Fig. 55 a, b. Spinal nerve root avulsion at the level of C 7/Th 1 with roughly 4 – 5 cm distally dislocated, surviving spinal ganglion cells 5 months after an accident in a 17-year-old patient. Many small myelinated nerve fibers in **a** and more numerous in **b** (distal nerve fascicle) are regenerated. The severe dislocation of this spinal ganglion could have caused an interruption of the supplying blood vessels with degeneration of nerve fibers and subsequent regeneration (similar to the ischemic lesions that are seen in thick heterotopic autologous nerve grafts). Other fibers show a normal proportion of the axon/ myelin ratio and are presumably preserved. **a, b** × 156. (From [956])

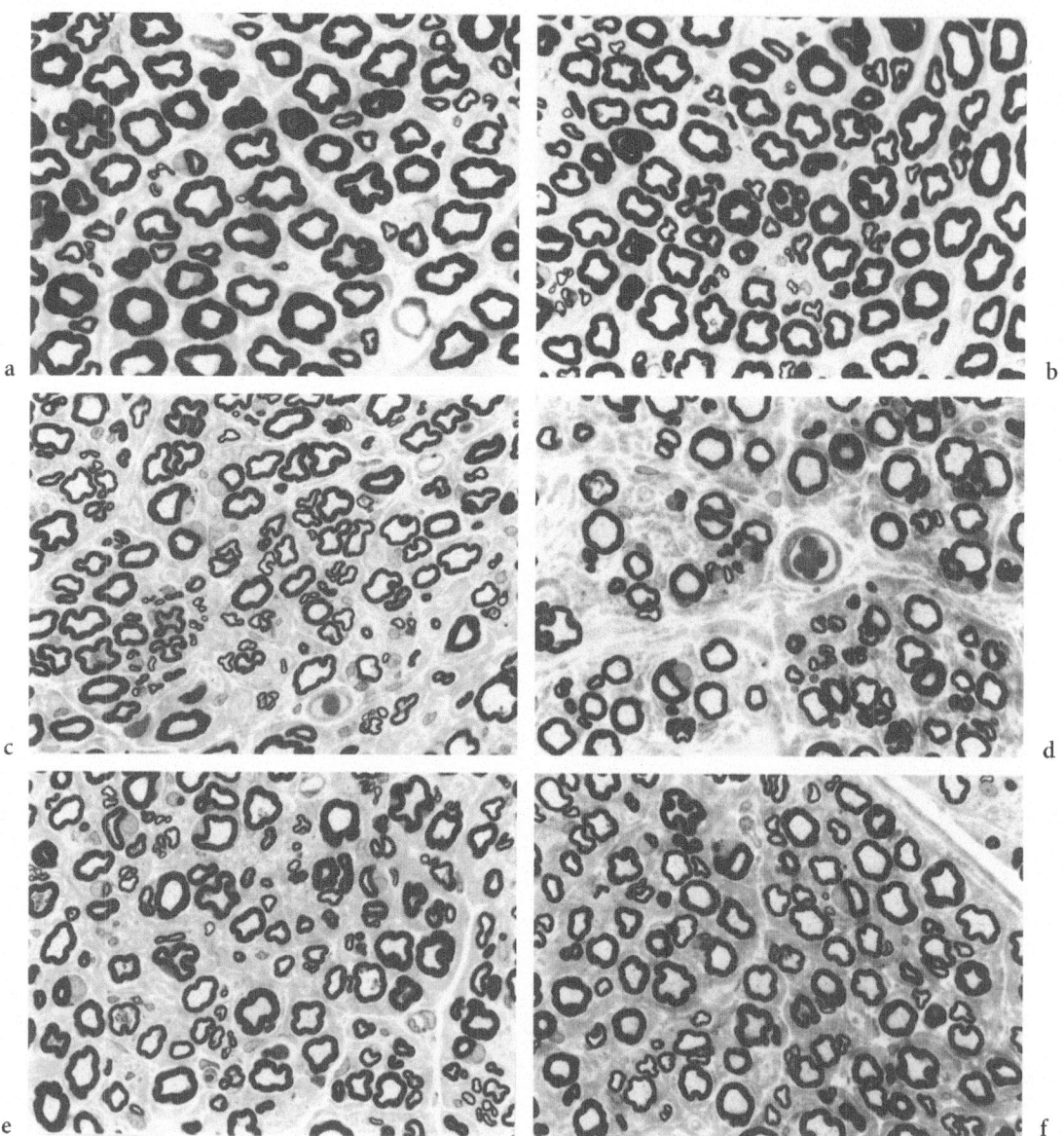

Fig. 56a–f. Sequelae of experimental radiation in cats (specimens of C. U. Fritzemeyer, Düsseldorf). **a, b** Proximal nerve segments, **c** and **d** irradiated nerve segments, **e** and **f** distal nerve segments. The endoneurial connective tissue is clearly increased in the irradiated area. In addition, there are clusters of regenerated fibers, but no onion bulb formations, similar to the distal nerve segment where the connective tissue is less severely increased. **a–e** × 1,080

CHAPTER 4

Nutrition Deficiency

In *anorexia nervosa* [657] and *vitamin deficiencies* [201, 292, 562, 738, 1075, 1093, 1264], the peripheral nervous system may be involved. Of special interest is a persistent sensory neuropathy following overdose of *pyridoxin* (vitamin B$_6$) [5, 67, 538, 695]. The symptoms remained progressive despite discontinuation of pyridoxin application (*the "coasting" phenomenon*) [67]. *Vitamin B$_{12}$* deficiency (Figs. 57, 58) results in combined system disease (funicular myelosis), atrophy of the optic nerve, and dementia [292]. Deficiency of *biotinidase* caused unique axonal inclusions (Figs. 59, 60) which I have not seen before and which have not been reported to the best of my knowledge in any other neuropathy.

Alcoholic neuropathy (Figs. 27a–d, 34c, 61–63) appears to be the most frequent neuropathy after diabetic neuropathy [533, 738, 744, 1239, 1245]. It is clearly of a neuronal type with very little evidence of paranodal demyelination after focal ethanol application (Figs. 64–65). Vitamin deficiencies are usually involved in alcoholic neuropathy. However, a direct toxic effect as a result of oral ingestion cannot be excluded [693].

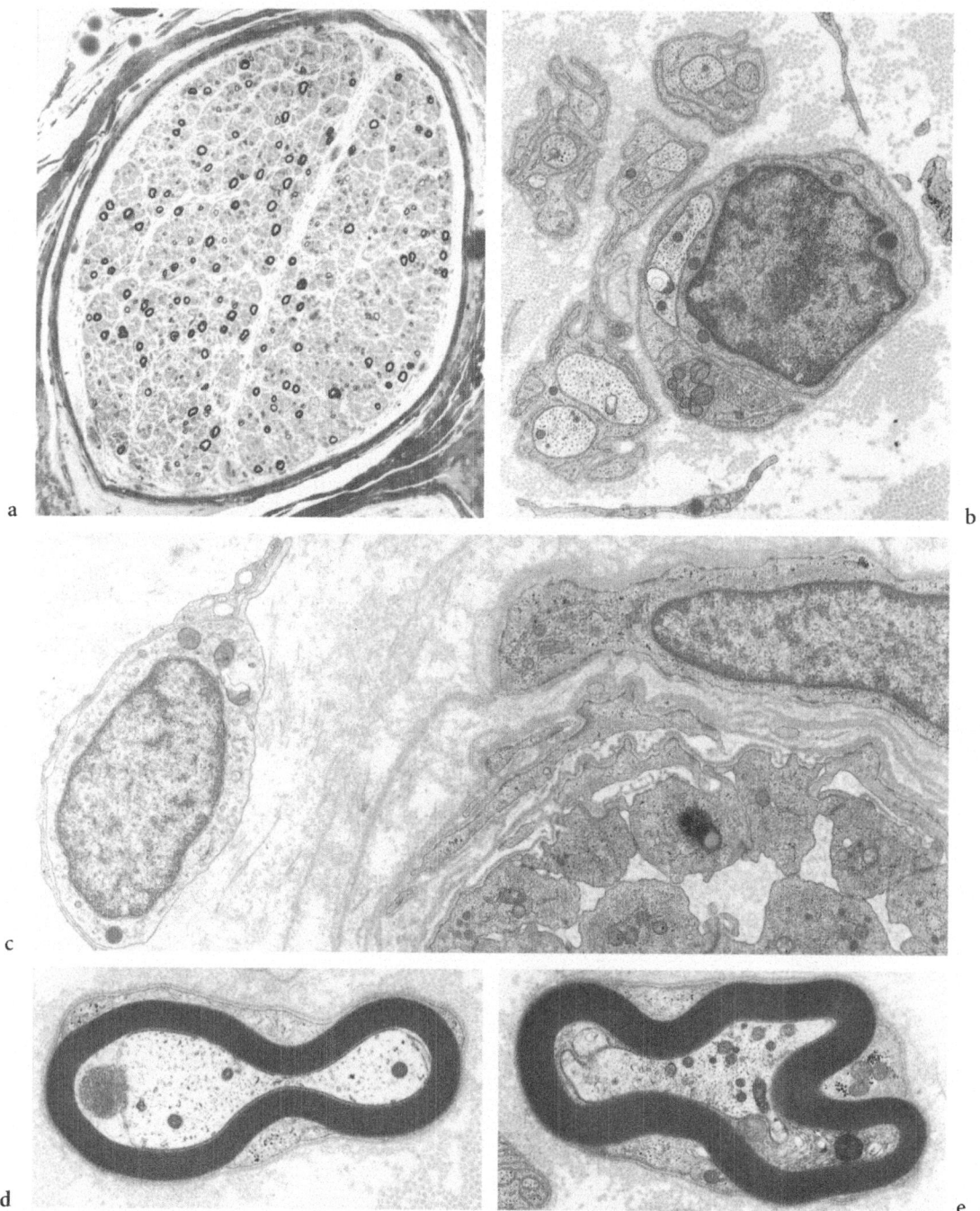

Fig. 57a – d. Disturbance of vitamin B$_{12}$ resorption in a 52-year-old man with subacute combined system degeneration of the spinal cord (funicular myelosis). **a** Prominent neuropathy with predominant loss of small myelinated nerve fibers. × 156. **b** Incomplete loss of unmyelinated nerve fibers. × 11,000. **c** Arteriole with focally separated basal lamina and neighboring inactive macrophage which is attached to a fibroblastic process. × 9,700. **d, e** Atrophic myelinated nerve fibers with several mitochondria in the axon and adaxonal Schwann cell inclusions of different kinds. **d** × 13,500; **e** × 11,500

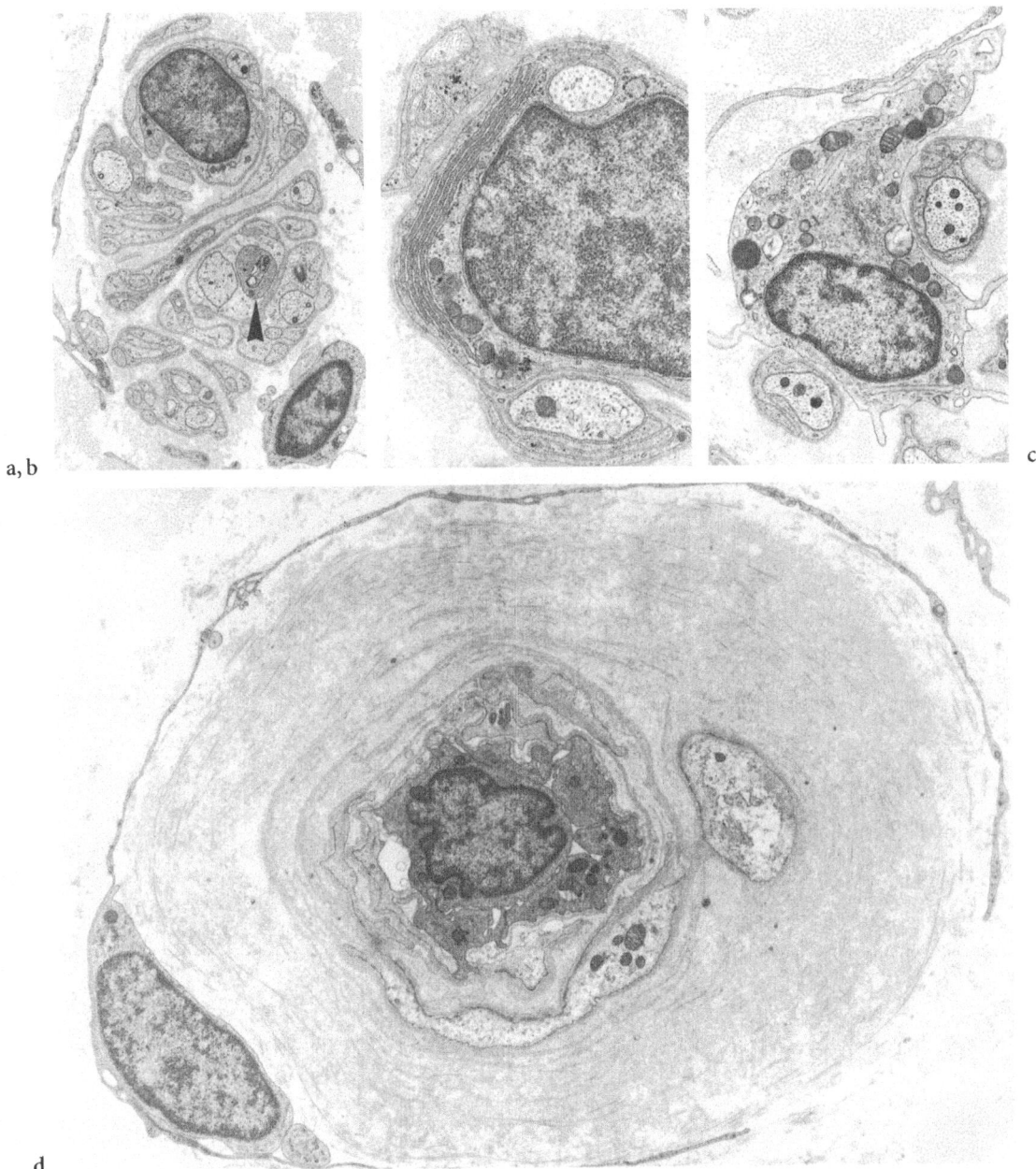

Fig. 58 a–d. Same case as in Fig. 57. **a** Group of unmyelinated axons and Schwann cell processes as well as a macrophage in the *lower right corner*. An axon appears to be condensed and contains loose membranous structures (*arrowhead*). × 6,200. **b** Confronting cisternae in a Schwann cell with unmyelinated axons. × 15,500. **c** Macrophage with numerous organelles and two prismatic inclusions between two preserved unmyelinated axons. × 8,700. **d** Endoneurial capillary which is surrounded by several layers of basal laminae and interspersed collagen fibrils. A thin fibroblastic process with an attached inactive macrophage encircles this area. × 6,000

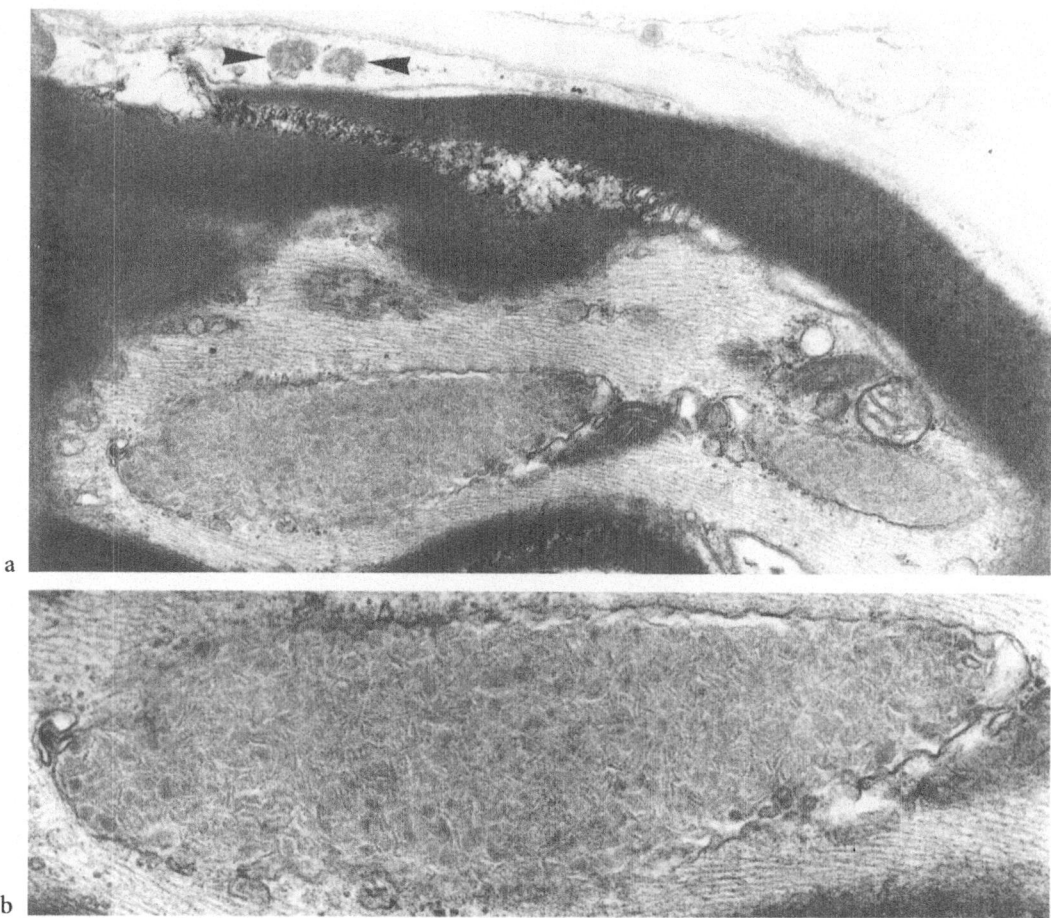

Fig. 59 a, b. Biotinidase deficiency in a 14-year-old boy. Unusual curvilinear structures, incompletely surrounded by a remarkably dense membrane in a myelinated axon. Granules of intermediate electron density are included between the curvilinear membranous structures. The membrane at the surface of theses corpuscles shows vesicular degradation. There are further remarkable cytosomes (*arrowheads*) in the cytoplasm of the Schwann cell. **a** × 27,000; **b** × 49,000

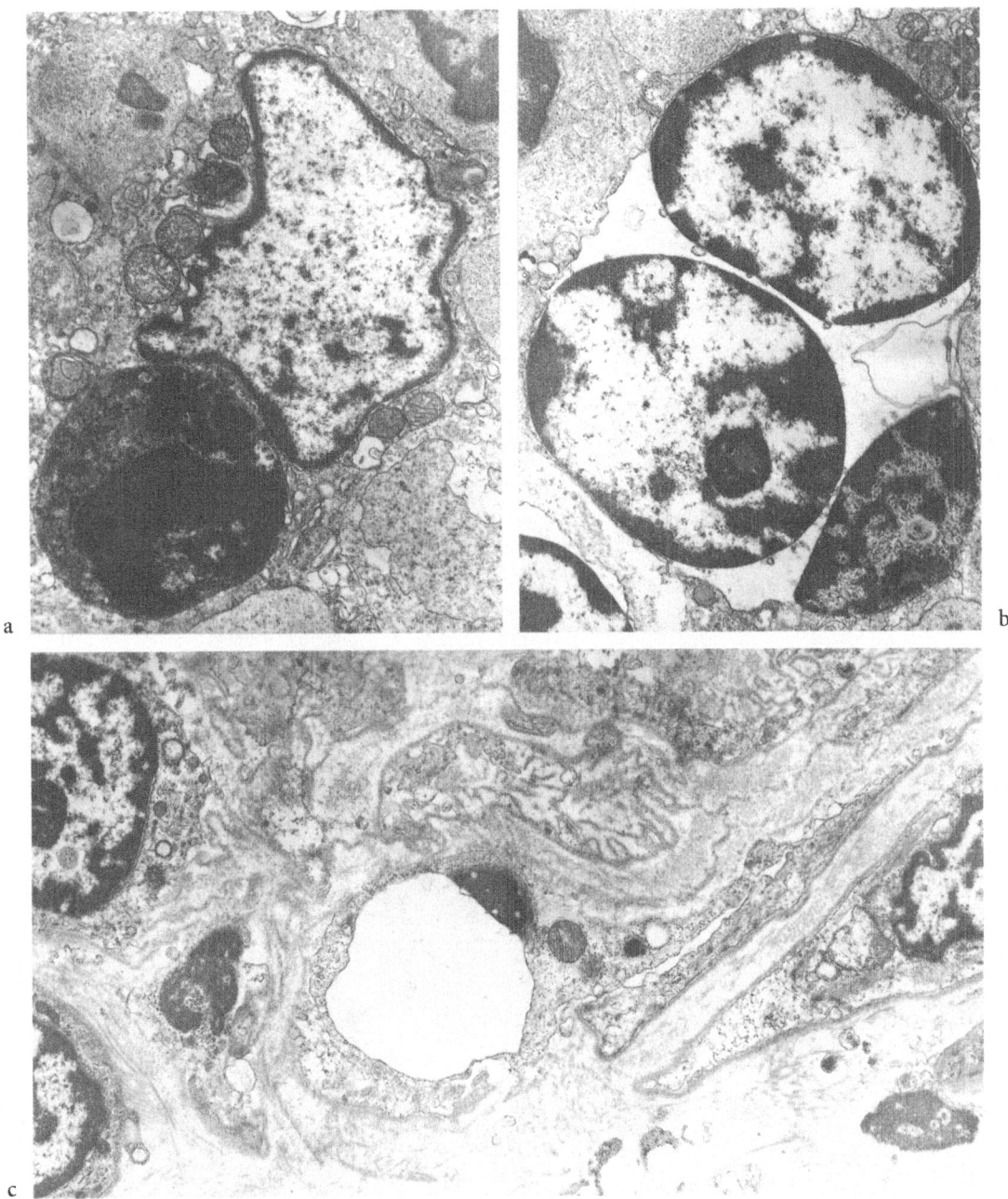

Fig. 60 a–c. Same case as in Fig. 59. Different forms of nuclear changes and cell degeneration in the sural nerve. **a** Pycnotic nucleus in a shrunken, rounded, degenerating cell (apoptotic body) which has obviously been phagocytosed by another cell, a macrophage, rich in mitochondria. × 3,400. **b** Three nuclei which are obviously surrounded by a common outer nuclear membrane within an aggregate of cells. **c** Severe distension of the outer nuclear membrane adjacent to a pycnotic remnant of a nucleus in a degenerating cell which is only incompletely covered by a basal lamina. Also, some of the neighboring cells show considerable regressive changes. **b, c** × 10,000

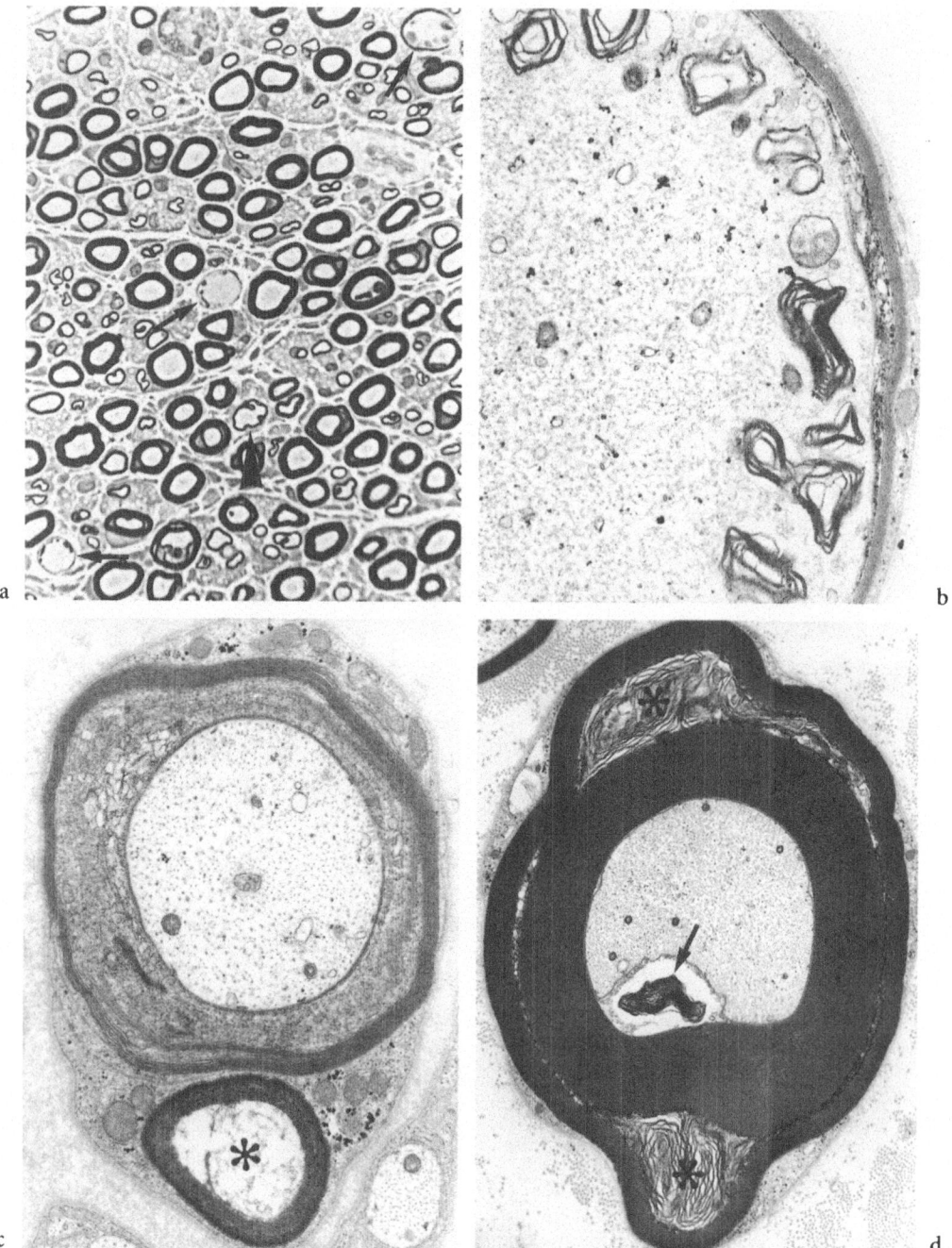

Fig. 61a–d. An unusual form of alcoholic neuropathy in a 66-year-old male with prominent cerebellar atrophy, cortical brain atrophy, and carotic calcification. **a** Three nerve fibers show retractions of paranodal myelin sheaths with subaxolemmal membranous bodies (*arrows*) which, however, may be fixation artifacts due to prolonged fixation in glutaraldehyde. Hypomyelinated large axons can also be seen at other sites (*arrowhead*). A band of Büngner is apparent at the *upper left margin.* × 3,900. **b** In addition to neurofilaments, a nerve fiber (like the ones indicated in **a** by *arrows*) shows microtubules, some mitochondria, glycogen granules, subaxolemmal membranous bodies, and amorphous substances in the axoplasm. Obvious thinning of the myelin sheath is suggestive of incipient paranodal demyelination. × 22,400. **c** The μ-granule (Elzholz body, indicated by an *asterisk*) below the paranodal myelin sheath segment differs from a paranodal myelin loop by the density of the lamellar structure (reduced periodicity) and the unstructured center. × 20,000. **d** Membranous body (*arrow*) in the adaxonal cytoplasm of a Schwann cell which can already be recognized at the light microscope level and which in normal nerve fibers occurs more frequently with increasing age. The complex membranous formations (*asterisks*) within the Schmidt-Lanterman incisure may occur in many other conditions; they presumably have a similar pathogenesis as the membranous bodies in the adaxonal cytoplasm (*arrow*). × 7,560. (From [958]).

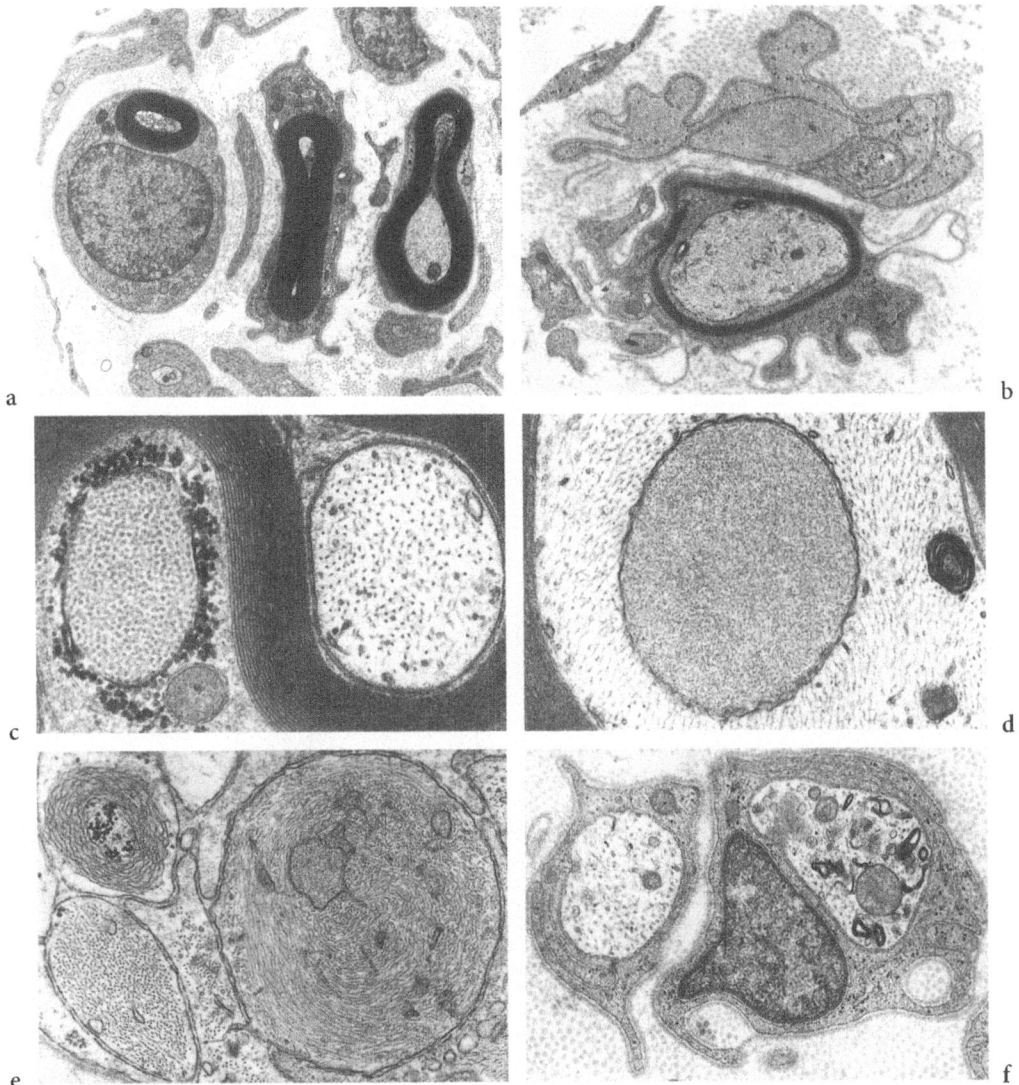

Fig. 62 a–f. Neuropathy of an axonal type in an alcoholic who was said to have also been exposed to toxic solvents. **a** Two severely atrophic myelinated nerve fibers contain axonal remnants and are surrounded by several Schwann cell processes which still contain rare unmyelinated axons. × 7,100. **b** Cluster of Schwann cell processes with an obviously regenerated and remyelinated axon. × 10,500. **c** Unusual cytosome with a granular matrix and surrounding glycogen granules in the cytoplasm of a Schwann cell of a myelinated fiber. × 43,000. **d** Unusual cytosome surrounded by an abnormal double membrane in the axon of a myelinated nerve fiber. The organelle is filled with a finely granulated substance. Two membranous cytoplasmic bodies can also be seen in the axon. × 39,000. **e** Unusual arrangement of neurofilaments in an axon, surrounded by Schwann cell processes within a band of Büngner in which there are other unmyelinated axons. In another axon the neurofilaments can all be seen in cross section. Another Schwann cell process contains loosely arranged concentric membranes with several glycogen granules in the center. × 26,000. **f** Several small membranous cytoplasmic bodies in an unmyelinated axon that is surrounded by a Schwann cell containing bundles of collagen fibrils at the site of degenerated unmyelinated axons ("collagen pockets"). × 18,800

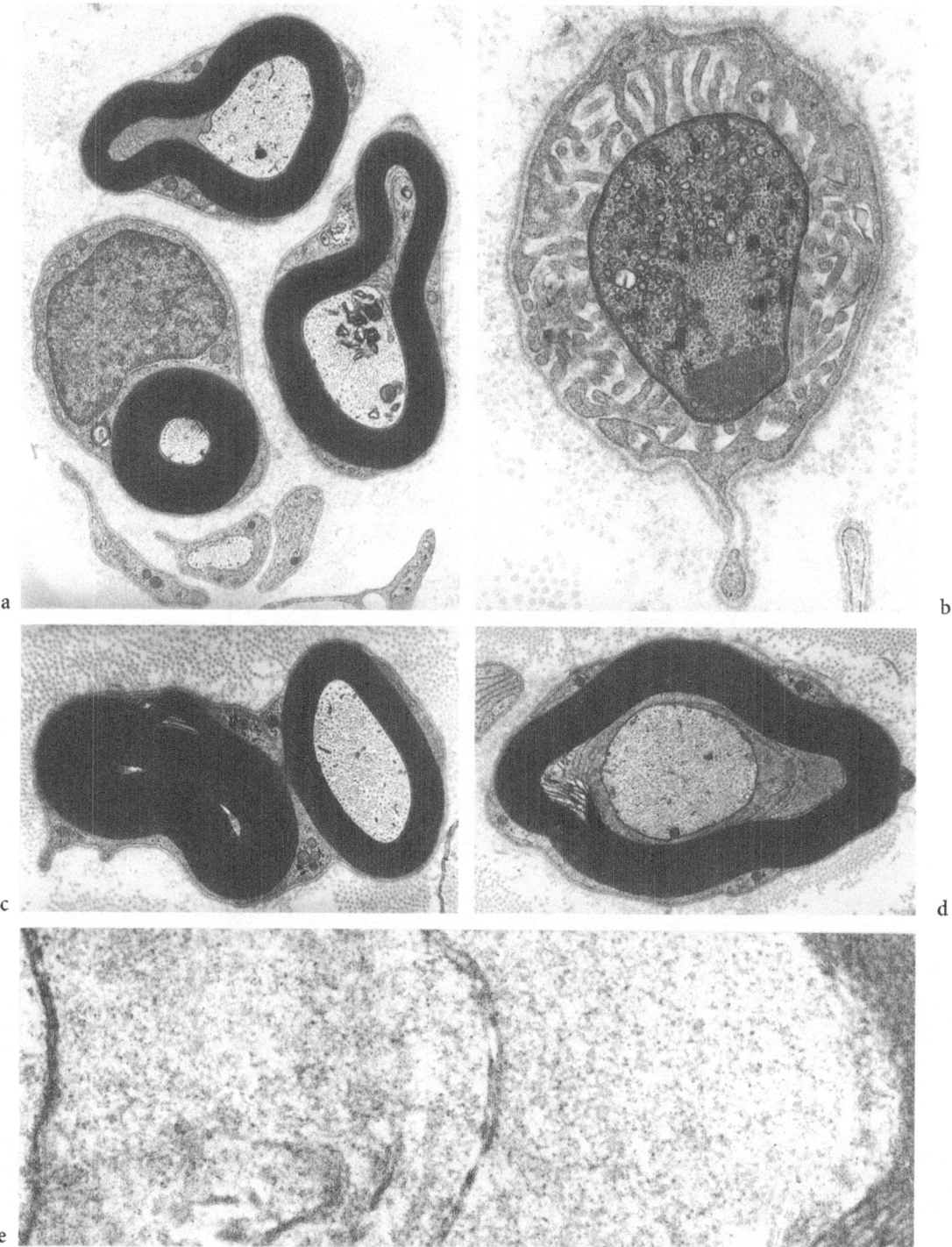

Fig. 63a–e. Same case as in Fig. 62. **a** In the adaxonal cytoplasm of a myelinated nerve fiber in a cluster of regenerated fibers, there are finely granulated inclusions in the noncompacted adaxonal myelin lamellae. A neighboring nerve fiber is cut at the level of the nucleus and is obviously atrophic. × 10,300. **b** Nodal axon segment with an unusually large and condensed mito-chondrion in the *lower right*. × 28,000. **c** Myelinated nerve fiber with an unusually thick, seemingly doubled myelin loop, which is presumably caused by intussusception. × 10,300. **d** Abnormal adaxonal homogeneous granular Schwann cell inclusions, shown in **e** at higher magnification. **d** × 9,200; **e** × 94,000

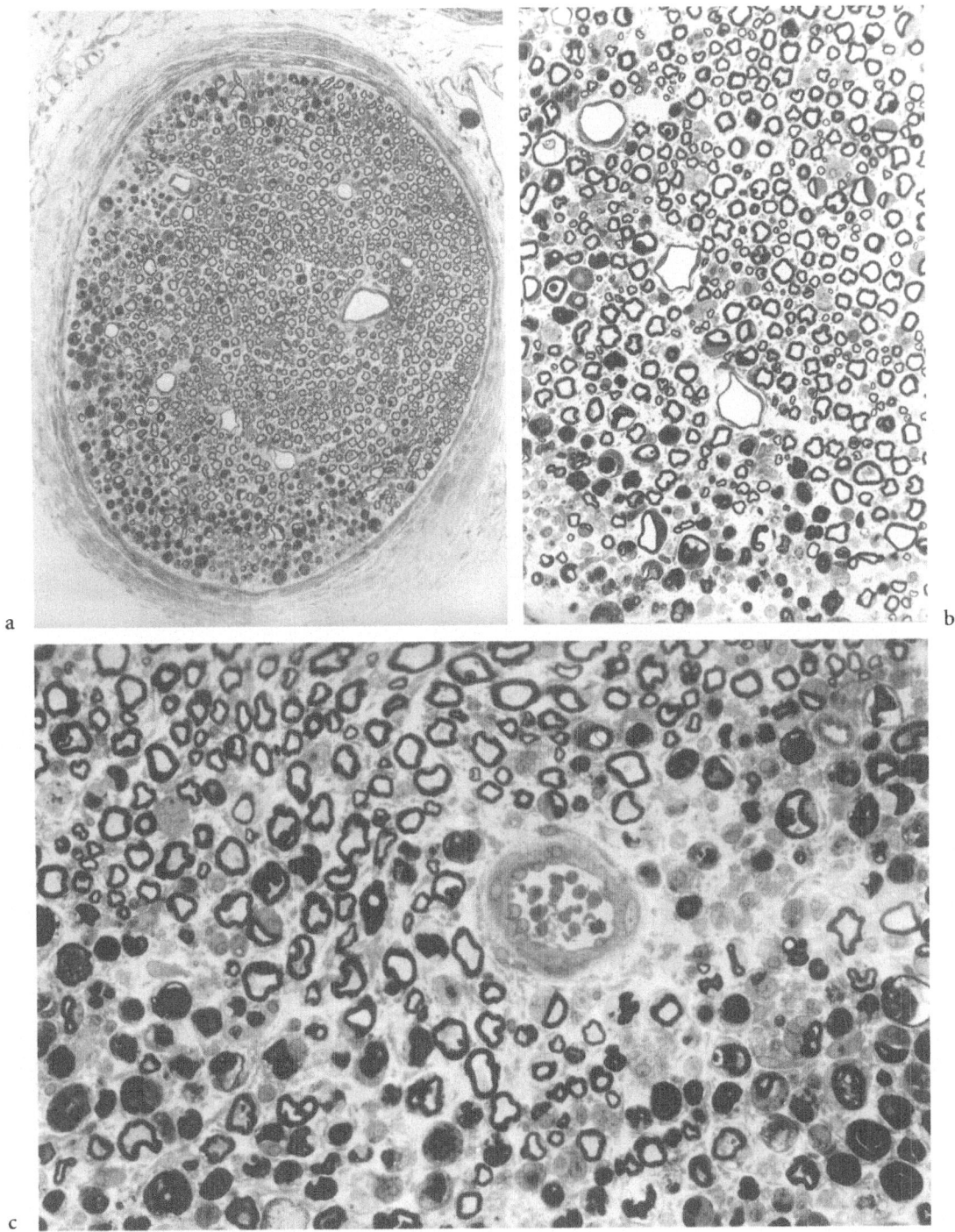

Fig. 64a–c. Six days after 3 min of immersion of the sciatic nerve in 10% ethanol. **a** Subperineurial lesional pattern with Wallerian degeneration of about ³/₄ of the circumference of this fascicle. The epineurial and perineurial connective tissue at this site shows minor thickening. × 160. **b, c** Higher magnifications of the damaged nerve fibers in **a**. Segmentally demyelinated axons are not apparent. There is a moderate endoneurial edema. The nerve fibers show different stages of disintegration. **b** × 330; **c** × 410 (Inaugural dissertation of E. Krämer, Aachen, 1992)

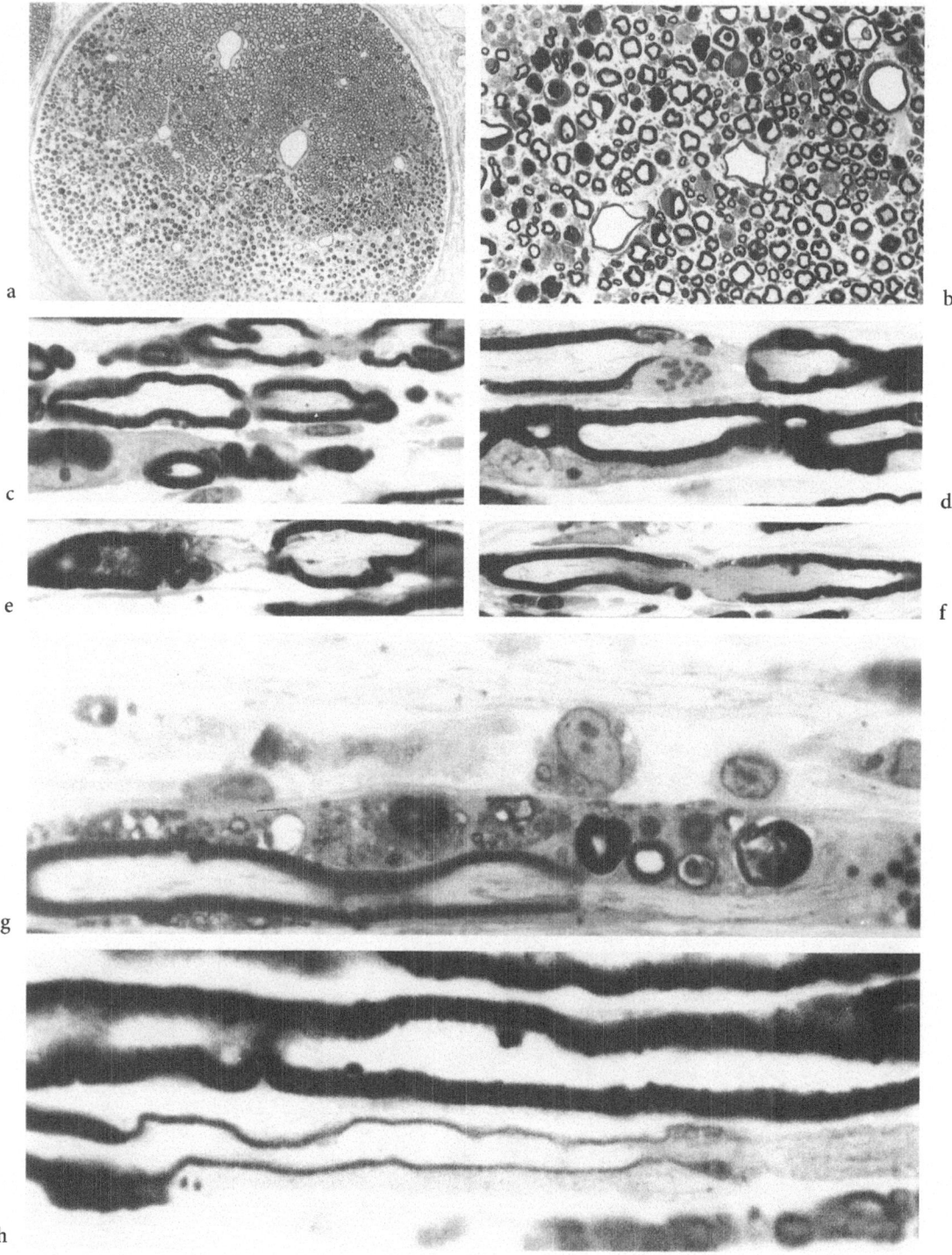

Fig. 65a–h. a Six days after 2 min of immersion of the sciatic nerve of a rat in 96% alcohol. The lesion in the uncovered sector of the nerve fascicle is considerably more prominent than in Fig. 64a. × 35. **b** Same nerve as in Fig. 64b. × 140. **c–f** Paranodal retraction of the myelin sheaths with a paranodal mitosis in **d** 6 days after 2 min of immersion in 10% ethanol. × 100. **g** Same nerve as in **b**, cut longitudinally. There is segmental demyelination with prominent paranodal myelin degradation products, whereas the left part of the nerve fiber appears to be intact. × 660. **h** Same nerve as in **g**. Incomplete paranodal demyelination with a very thin myelin segment, while the right part of the node of Ranvier shows complete segmental demyelination. × 685. (Schröder, Wendtland, Krämer, unpublished results)

CHAPTER 5

Toxic Neuropathies

Knowledge of the toxic effects of chemicals and drugs on the peripheral nervous system is of major importance in estimating and judging the vast effects of medicinal, occupational, and environmental exposure. An extensive treatise is presently available for detailed information [1076].

Extremely toxic substances such as botulinus toxin may nevertheless be beneficial when applied in proper dosage, e.g., for treating dystonic syndromes such as spasmodic torticollis [179, 358, 982] and others (see below).

Characteristic, though not absolutely specific, structural changes are seen following a considerable number of substances, although personal experience is restricted to:

- *Cadmium* resulting in numerous changes of the spinal ganglia in organotypic tissue cultures and in other findings [784, 812, 971, 1138]
- *Lead* (Fig. 66) [349, 566, 694, 801, 845]
- *Ethylenoxide* (Figs. 67, 68) [112, 132, 143, 199, 320, 556, 774, 981]
- *Trichlorethylene* (Fig. 69) [132, 143]
- *Chloroquine* (Figs. 70, 71) [980, 1116]
- *Ciliary neurotrophic factor (CNTF)* [12, 21, 44, 232, 333, 440, 543, 559, 584, 681, 791, 793, 938, 1019–1021, 1043, 1120, 1154, 1171, 1223, 1241]
- *Dextrin*-like substances (Fig. 72)
- *Adriamycin (doxorubicin)* (unpublished tissue culture experiments causing severe nuclear

changes similar to those reported by others [144, 270, 271, 354], *ergotism* (J.M. Schröder, unpublished observation)
- *Gangliosides* causing Guillain-Barré syndrome (J.M. Schröder, unpublished observation) [22, 110, 135, 138, 164, 268, 352, 430, 441, 442, 567, 578, 678, 724, 725, 747, 764, 766, 768, 840, 856, 929, 1032, 1033, 1077, 1079, 1200, 1238, 1267, 1271, 1273, 1275, 1276]
- *Thalidomide* neuropathy (Fig. 73) [30, 213, 346, 347, 373, 542, 627, 978, 987, 996, 1005]
- *Isoniazid* neuropathy (Figs. 74–82) [418, 941, 944, 945, 950, 970, 972, 1256]
- *Zidovudine* (Fig. 83a, b) [42, 89, 207, 398, 570, 586, 643, 704, 973, 983, 1228]
- *Vincristin/vinblastin* [42, 89, 207, 398, 570, 586, 643, 704, 973, 983, 1207, 1228]
- *Colchicine* (Figs. 84a–e) [413, 547]

In a large number of sural nerve biopsies submitted for identification of the suggested underlying, possibly specific structural substrate, a mixture of environmental substances was thought to be involved in causing the neuropathy. In these and other cases, only nonspecific changes were observed at the light microscopic level and frequently also at the electron microscopic level if there was not an inflammatory process (unpublished observations) or an inherited disposition [1016] detectable. For further substances and details see [969, 1076], among others.

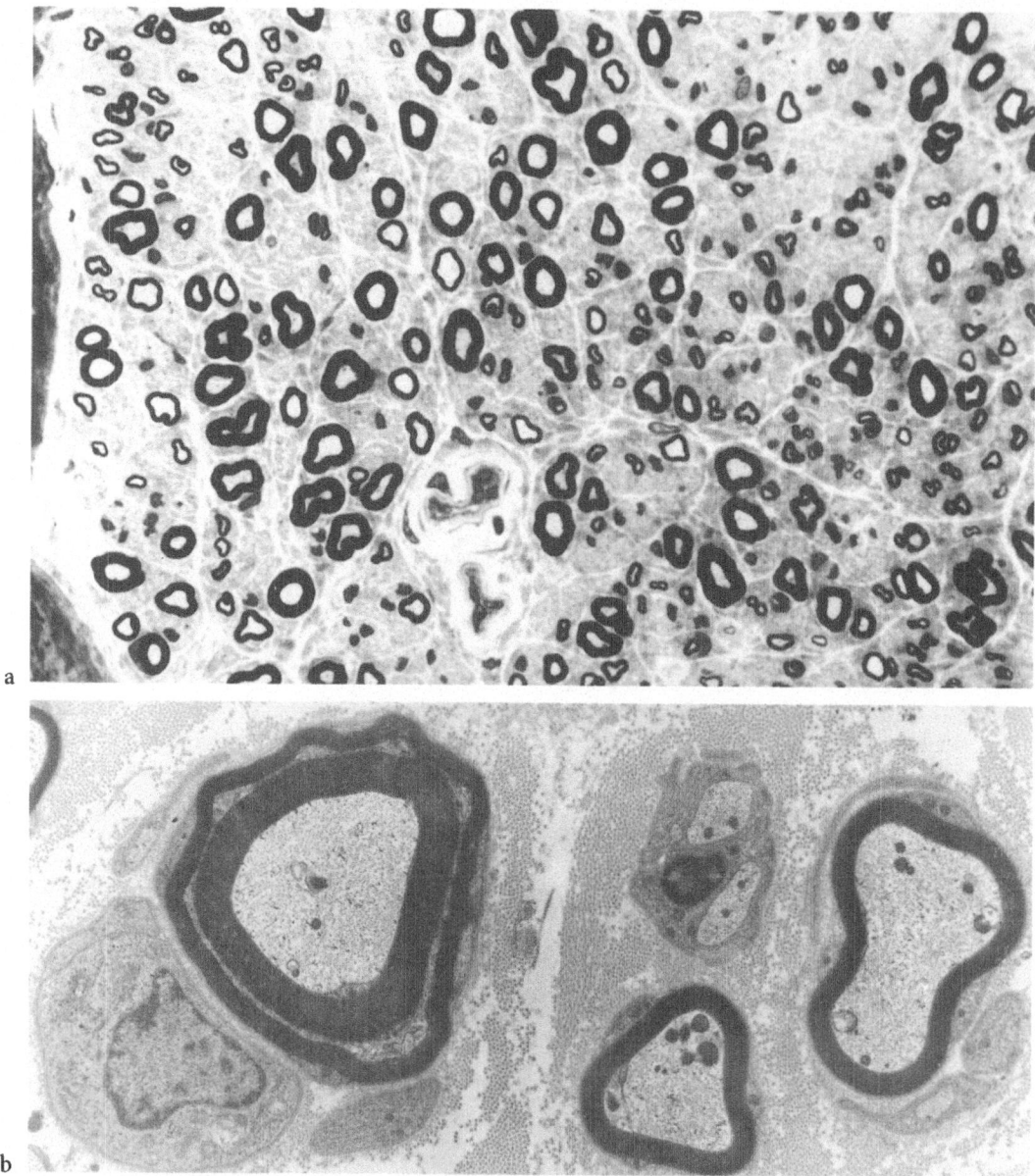

Fig. 66. a Chronic neuropathy of a demyelinating type, now in a stage of remyelination, after chronic lead exposure in a 53-year-old man. Several isolated myelinated nerve fibers show disproportionately thin remyelinated fibers. × 690. **b** Electron microscope magnification of a disproportionately thin myelin sheath around the fiber on the *right* with circumferentially arranged Schwann cell processes that enclose an unmyelinated axon. On the *left* are other empty Schwann cell processes containing no axons partially surrounding another myelinated fiber. × 7,600

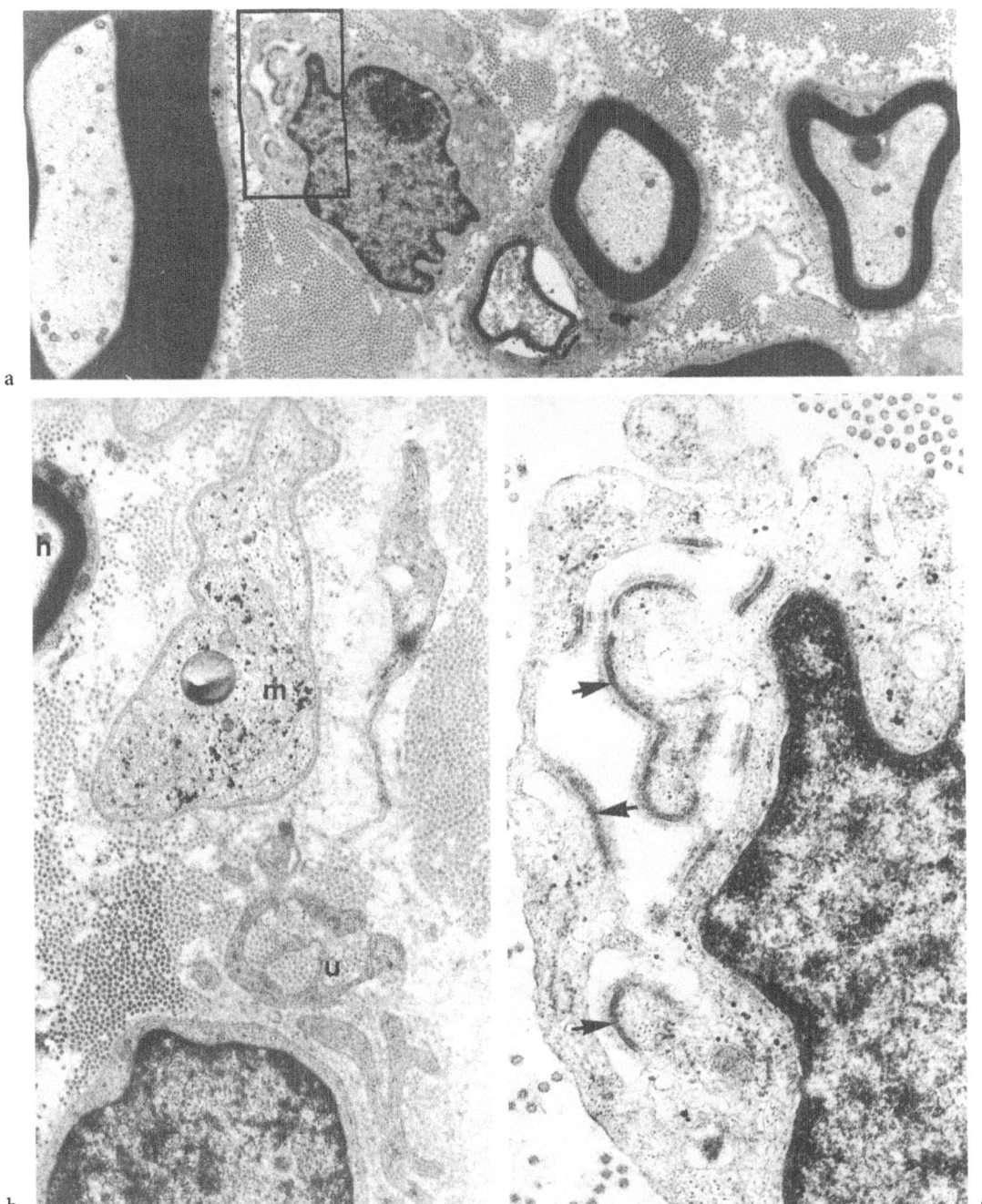

Fig. 67a–c. Ethylene oxide intoxication in a 23-year-old man. (From [981]). **a** An endoneurial fibroblast contains an unusual cistern, which is partially covered by a basal lamina (c). × 8,700. **b** Bands of Büngner of myelinated (*m*) and unmyelinated nerve fibers (*u*) adjacent to a myelinated axon with a disproportionately thin myelin sheath (*h*). × 14,000. **c** Higher magnification of the boxed area in **a**. The *arrows* indicate several introverted hemidesmosomes. × 40,000

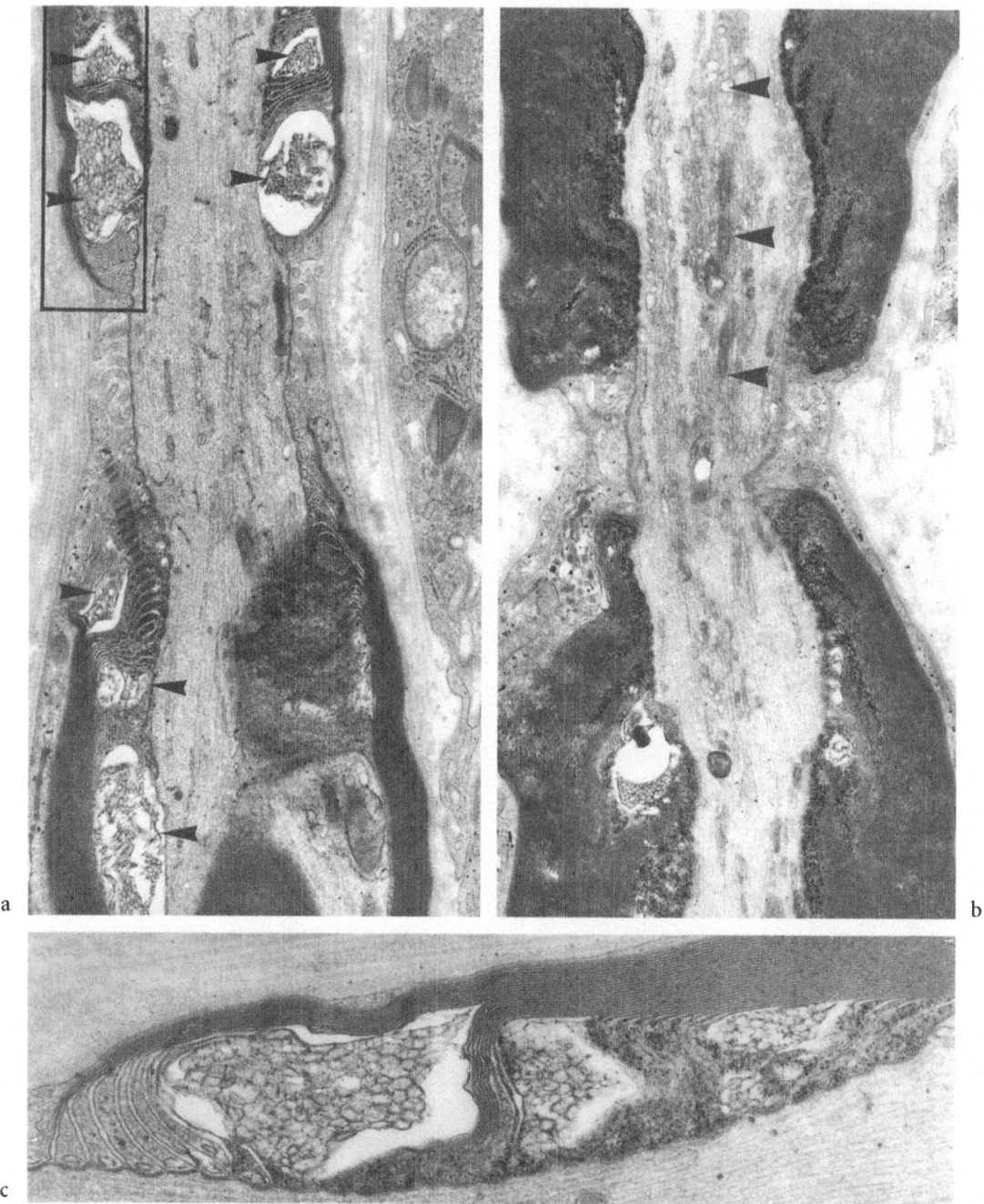

Fig. 68 a – c. Same case as in Fig. 67. Electron microscopic images of longitudinally sectioned nodes of Ranvier. **a** Several para-nodal myelin lamellae show focal fine vesicular lysis (*arrowheads*). × 16,000. **b** The axon contains vesicular and tubular mem-branous profiles with some mitochondria only on one side, presumably the proximal side of the node (*arrowheads*). × 16,000. **c** Higher magnification of the boxed area in **a** indicates focal microvesicular disintegration of some myelin lamellae at the site of paranodal myelin loops. × 7,000

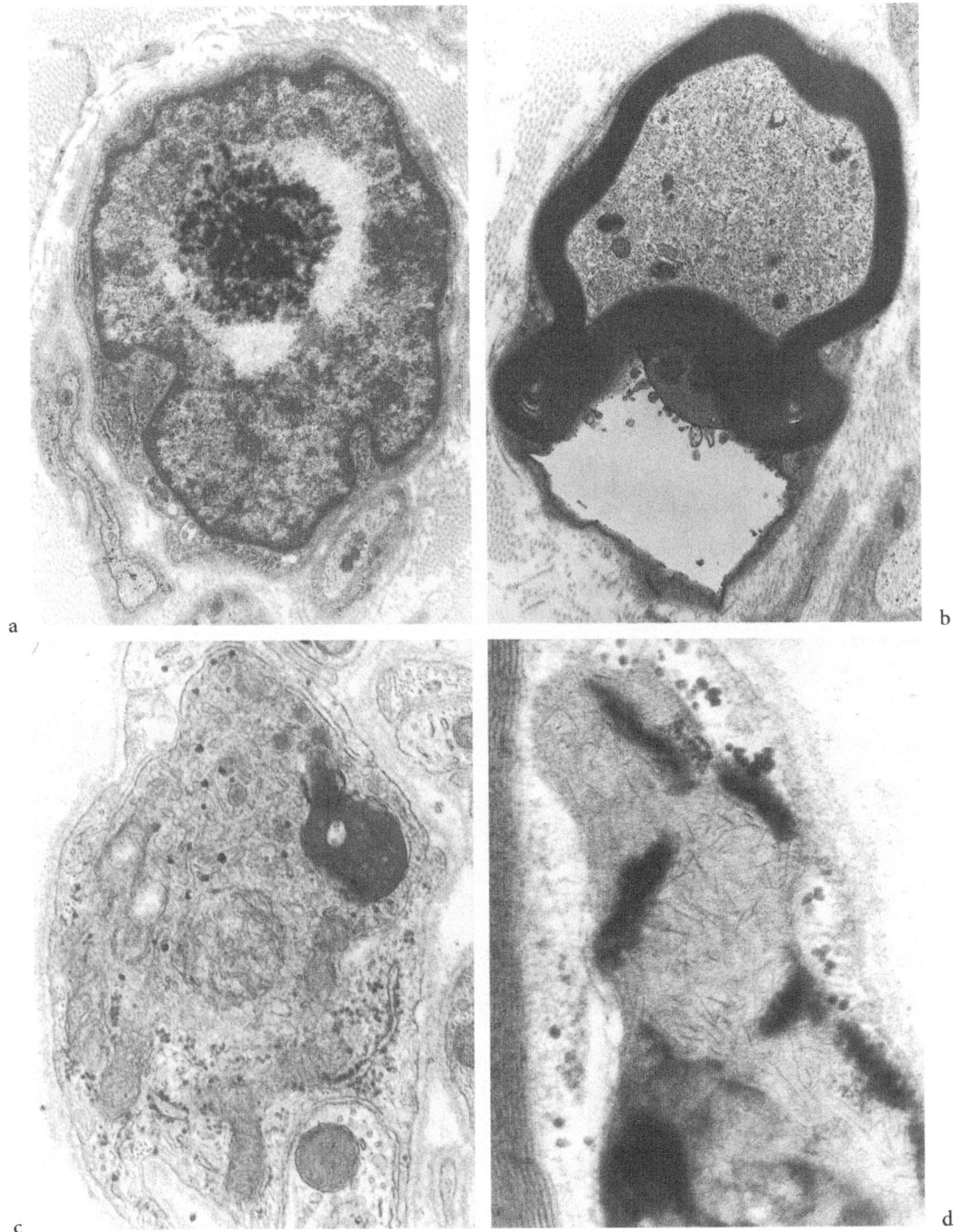

Fig. 69a–d. Trichlorethylene intoxication in a 57-year-old man with neuropathy of a neuronal type. **a** Unusual nucleolus with perinucleolar swelling in a Schwann cell without axons. × 12,000. **b** The myelinated axon shows a disproportionately thin myelin sheath with abnormal granular and other inclusions and a large vacuole in the abaxonal cytoplasm of the Schwann cell. × 11,000. **c** Abnormal, dystrophic axon within a band of Büngner with partly tubulovesicular, partly membranous cytoplasmic inclusions. × 46,000. **d** Abnormal cytoplasmic inclusion, presumably of lysosomal origin, with linear sheet-like or membranous components within an amorphous, medium osmiophilic mass, in which there are other more osmiophilic deposits located in the abaxonal cytoplasm of a Schwann cell of a myelinated fiber. × 81,000

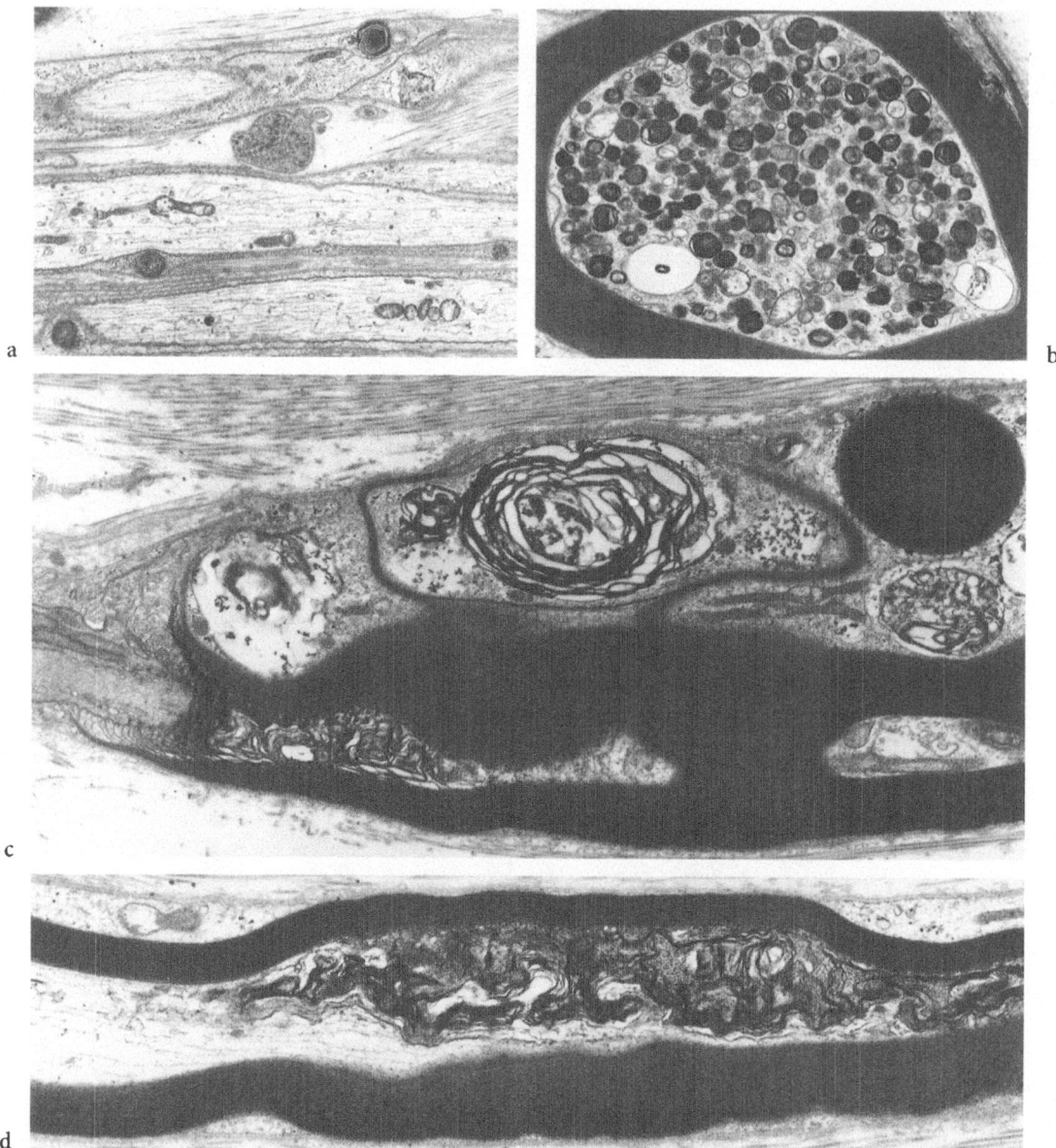

Fig. 70 a–d. Severe chloroquine neuromyopathy with membranous cytoplasmic bodies in the cytoplasm of Schwann cells of unmyelinated axons (**a**), in the axoplasm (**b**), and in the abaxonal cytoplasm of a Schwann cell of a myelinated nerve fiber and in a paranodal Schmidt-Lanterman incisure (**c**) as well as in the adaxonal cytoplasm of the Schwann cell of a myelinated nerve fiber (**d**). **a** × 6,700; **b** × 9,400; **c** × 9,500; **d** × 12,000

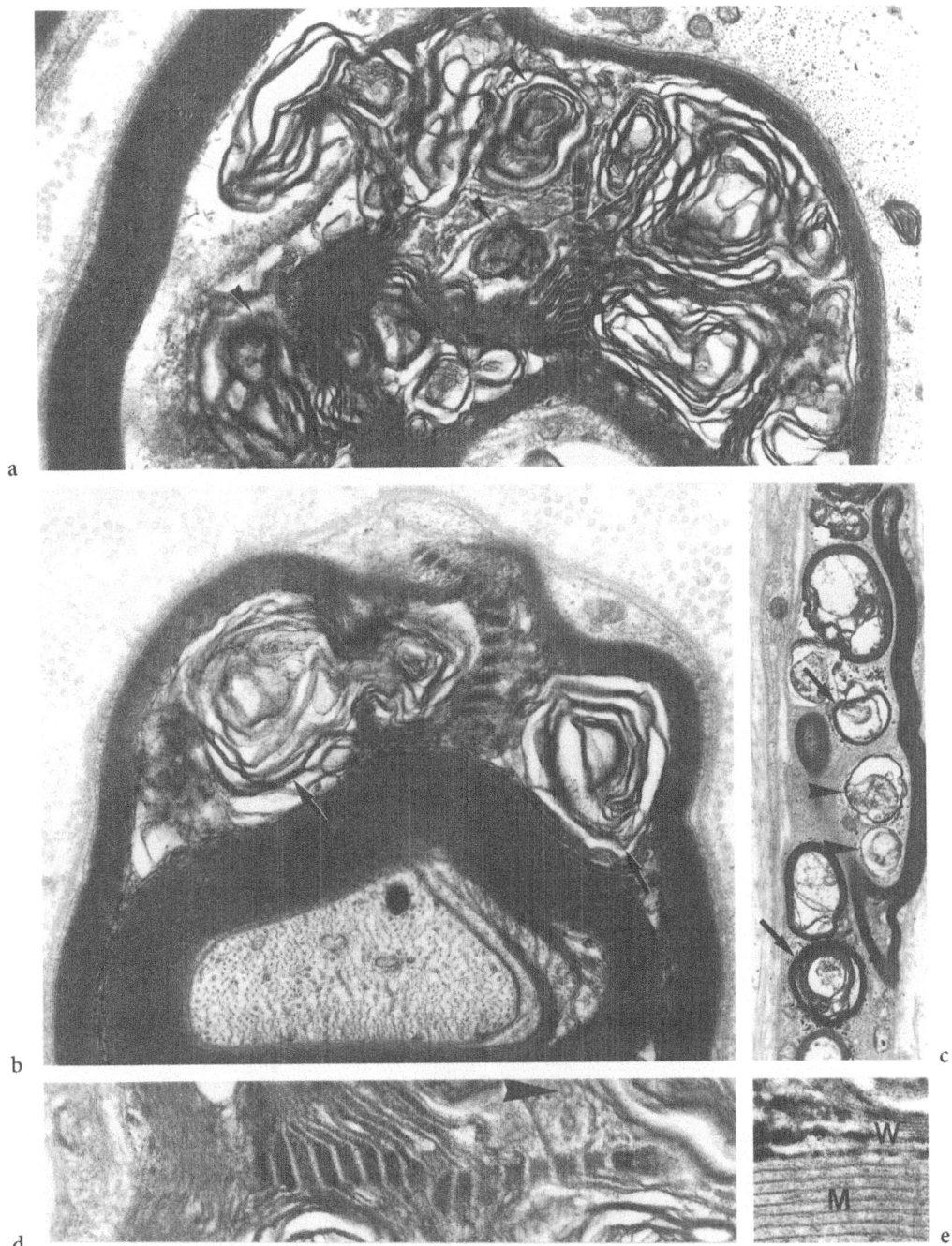

Fig. 71a–e. Same patient as in Fig. 70. Multiple extraordinarily prominent membranous cytoplasmic bodies in Schmidt-Lanterman incisures (**a, b**) and in the abaxonal cytoplasm of a degenerating myelinated nerve fiber, where the myelin ovoids, i. e., the myelin degradation products, cannot easily be distinguished from the membranous cytoplasmic bodies (MCBs) which are due to the chloroquine intoxication. Desmosome-like series of electron densities are apparent in **a, b**, and **d**. The different periodicity of the membranous cytoplasmic bodies (*W*) in contrast to the myelin lamella (*M*) are illustrated in **e**. The periodicity of the membranous cytoplasmic bodies is only about 5 nm, in contrast to those of the normal myelin lamella, which is about 15 nm. The *arrowheads* in **a, c**, and **d** indicate membranous cytoplasmic bodies, the *arrow* in **a** points to the series of desmosome-like structures, the *arrows* in **b** again to membranous cytoplasmic bodies. **a** × 23,000; **b** × 31,000; **c** × 6,000; **d** × 53,000; **e** × 136,000. (From [980])

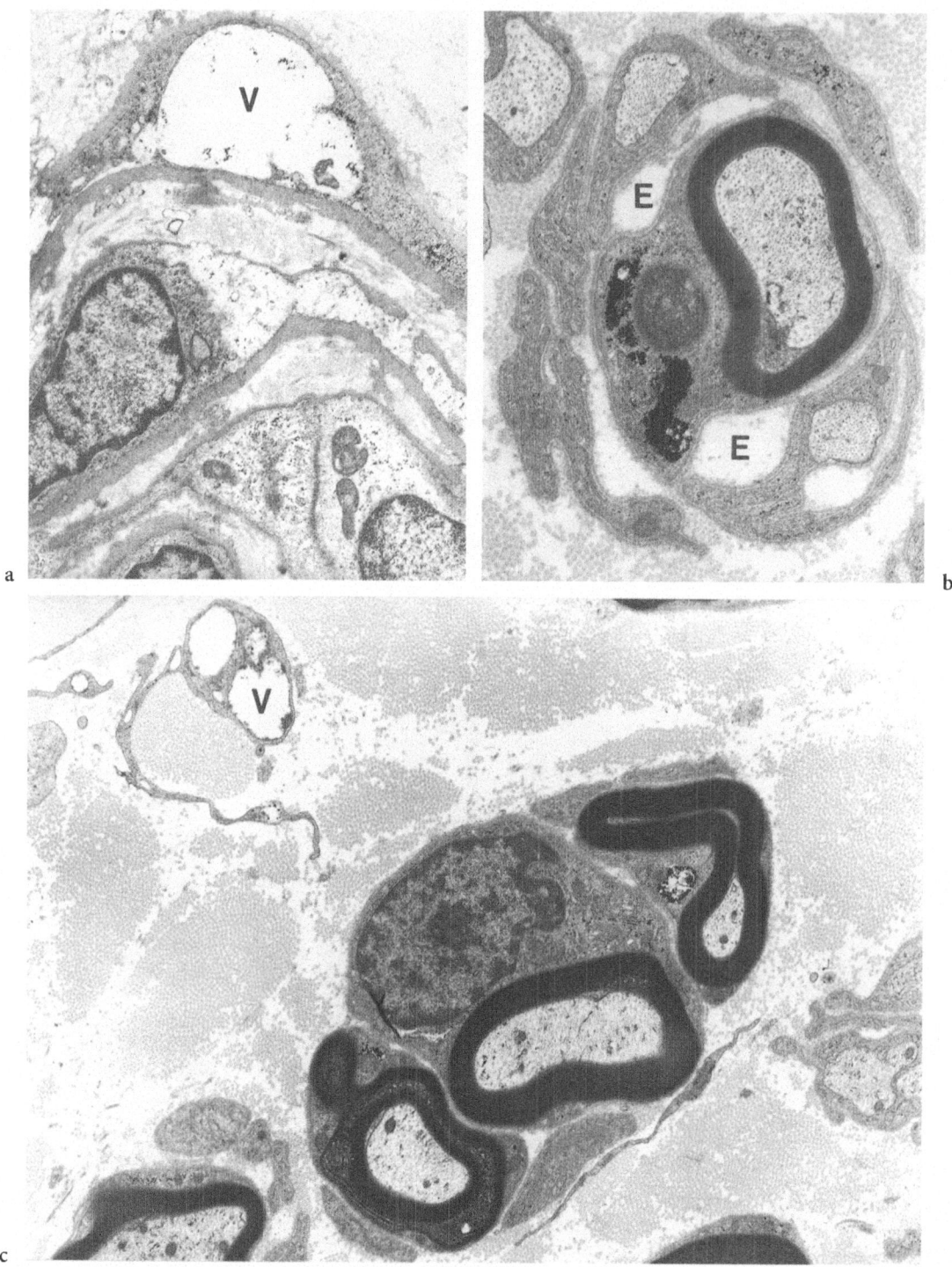

Fig. 72 a–c. Suggestive dextrin deposits in perineurial (**a**) and endoneurial, fibroblast (or macrophage)-like cells (**c**) in a case with polymyositis. The typical vacuoles in the muscle biopsy of this patient are considerably more prominent than in this nerve biopsy. The vacuoles are indicated by *V*. In **b** there are remarkable electron optically empty extracellular spaces between Schwann cell processes inside a cluster of regenerated nerve fibers (*E*), which are usually not seen in such clusters. By contrast, such collagen-free cavities are not apparent in the cluster in **c**. **a** × 11,000; **b** × 14,000; **c** × 8,300

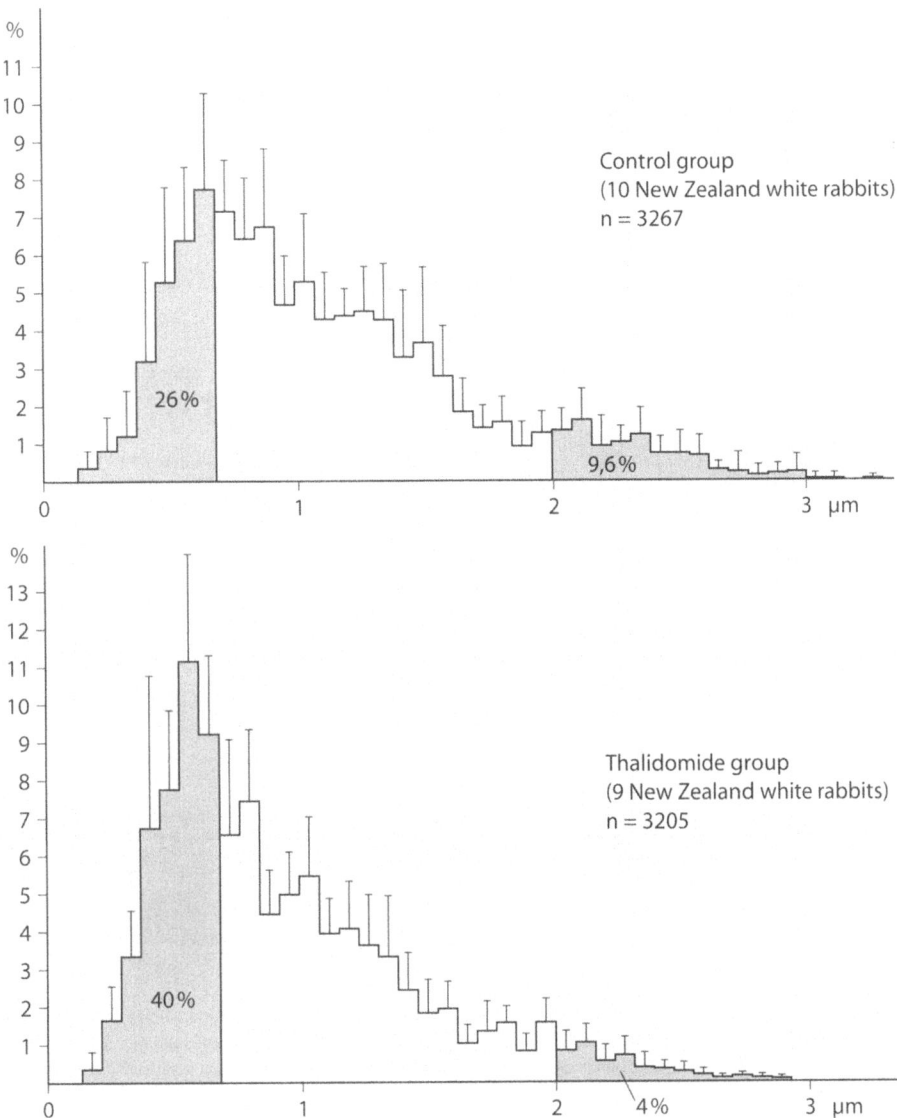

Fig. 73. Diagram showing results of the morphometric evaluation of experimental thalidomide neuropathy. The number of large myelinated nerve fibers is after 6 months of thalidomide application reduced from 9.6% to 4%; the number of small myelinated nerve fibers increased from 26% to 40%. (From [987])

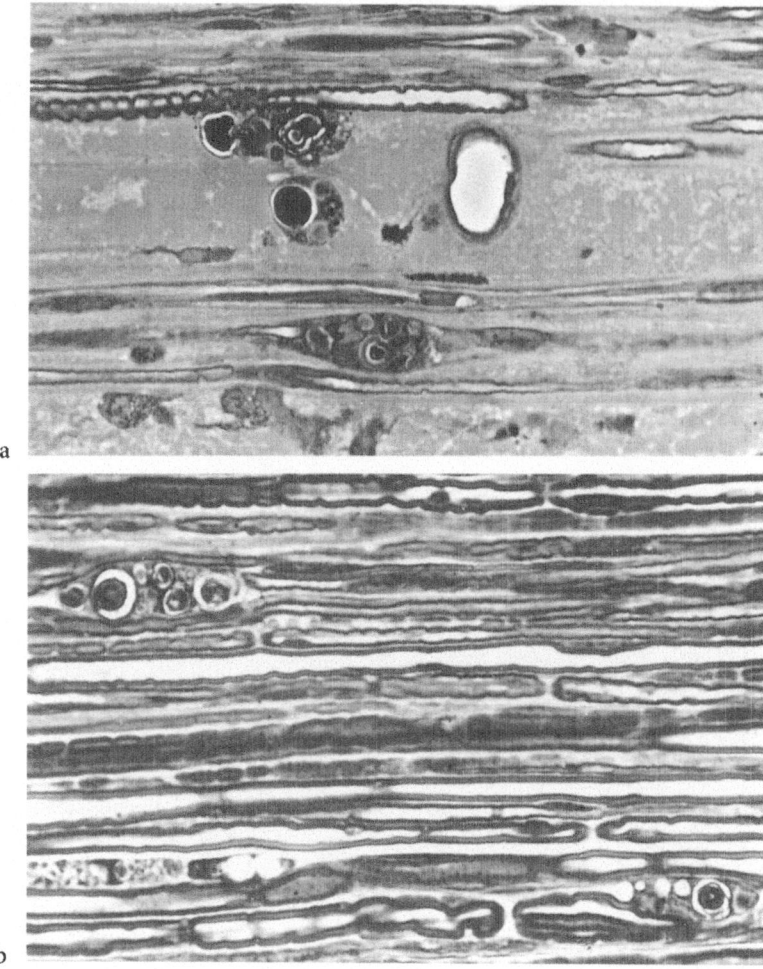

Fig. 74a, b. Experimental isoniazid (INH) neuropathy in rats. **a** Four weeks after onset of INH application (7 × 650 mg/kg per day). The rare preserved or regenerated nerve fibers are separated by extensive perivascular plasma infiltrates (endoneurial edema). Several cells contain large myelin degradation products. **b** Two months after a similar degree of INH intoxication. Myelin ovoids indicate the preceding lesion; in addition, there are numerous regenerated nerve fibers. The endoneurial edema is completely resolved. **a, b** × 450. (From [944])

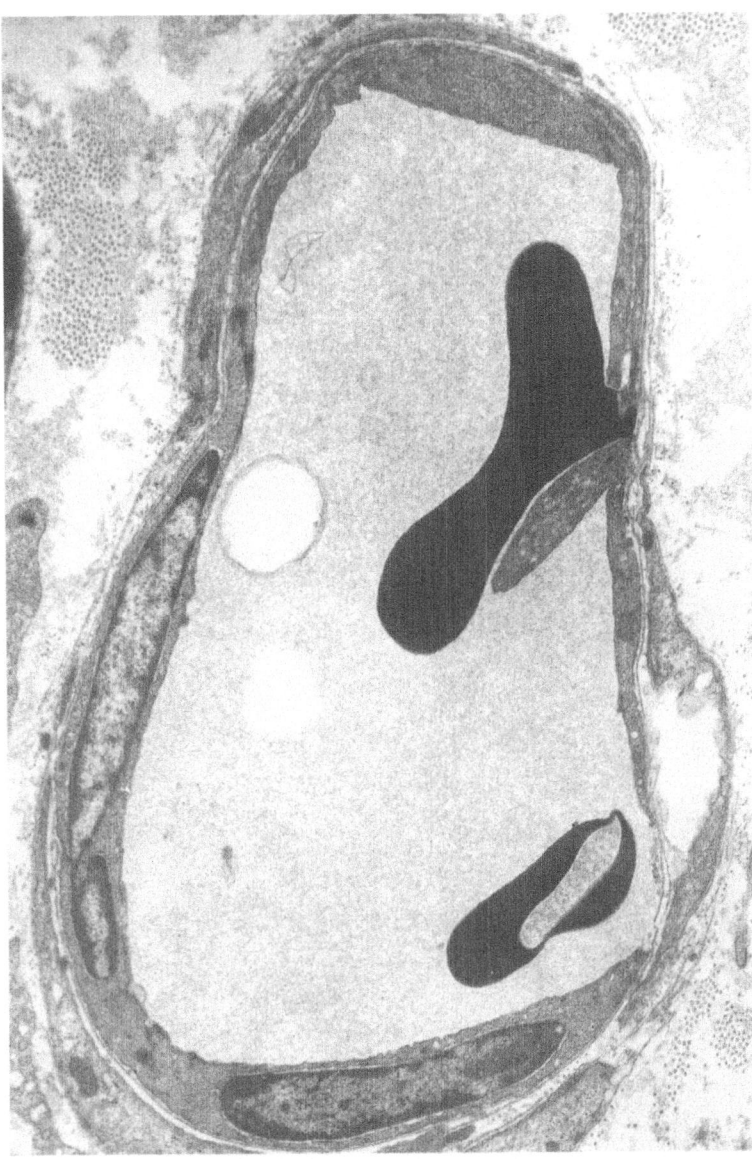

Fig. 75. Isoniazid neuropathy 9 days after beginning the INH-application (6 × 650 mg/kg). Severely altered endoneurial blood vessel showing erythrodiapedesis. (In the neighboring endoneurium there are some erythrocytes, which are not visible in this figure.) The endothelial continuity is interrupted at two sites and the connection with the perithelium is partially destroyed. The amorphous plasma-like content of the blood vessels indicates that the perfusion fixation has not been effective at this site. × 10,500. (From [944])

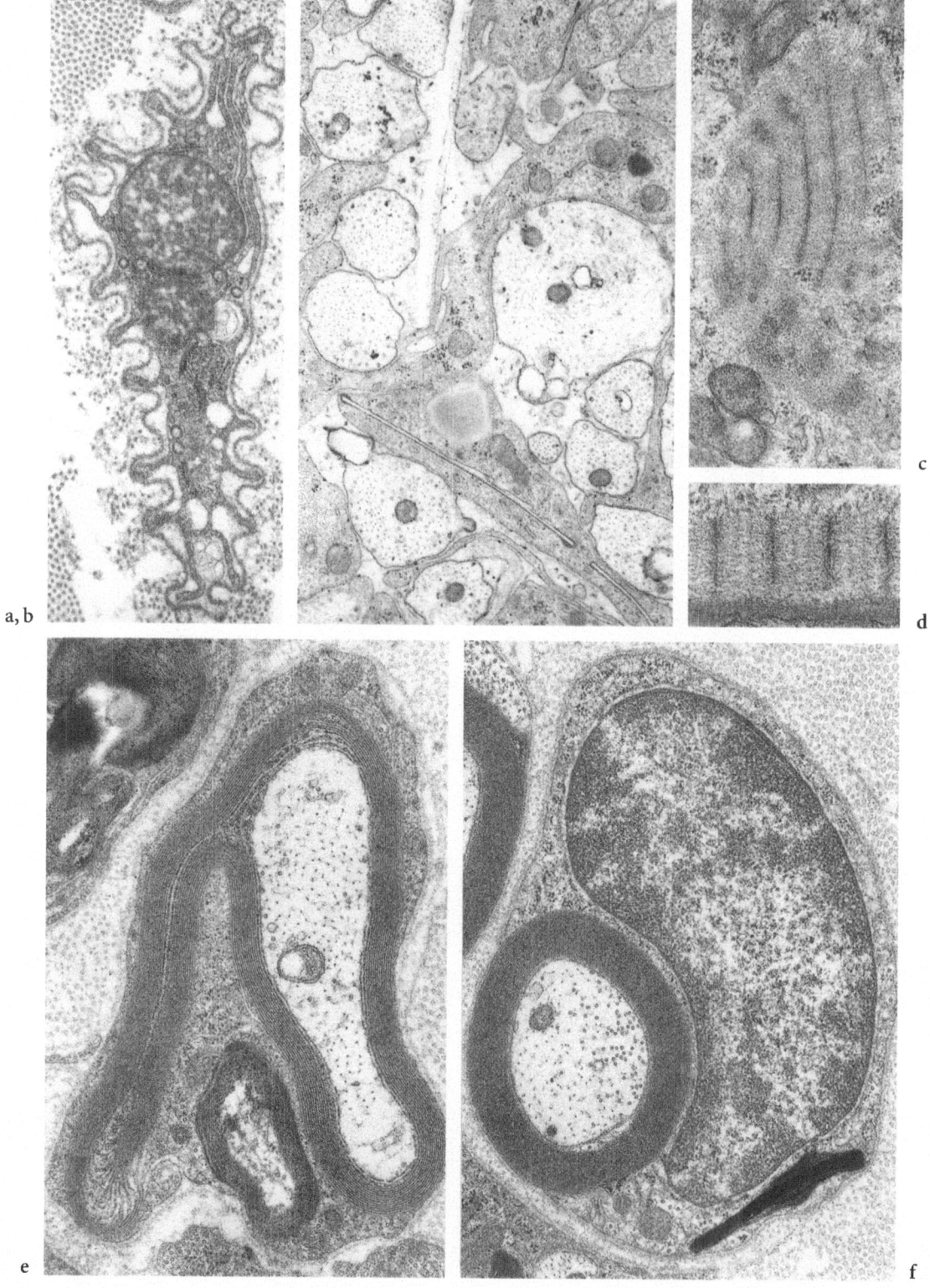

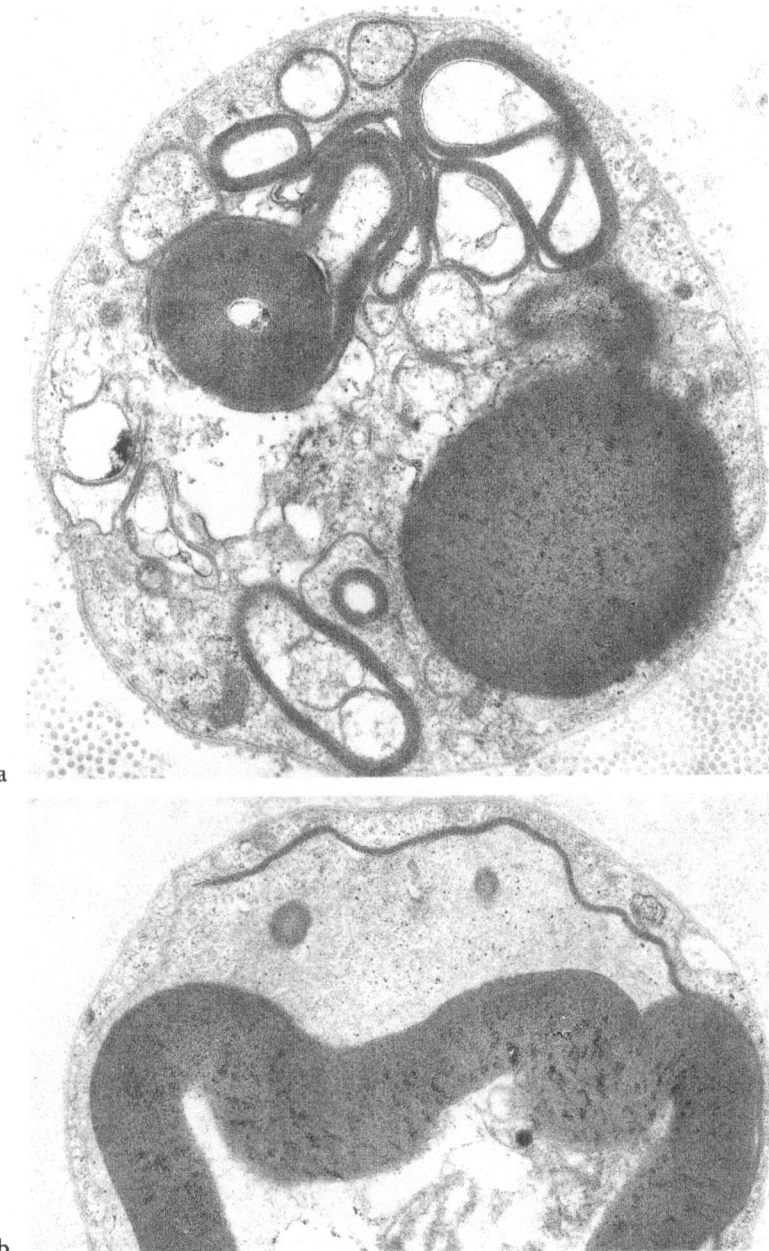

Fig. 77 a, b. Isoniazid neuropathy: tibial nerve 4 days after onset of INH-application (2 × 400 mg/kg per day). **a** Myelin degradation within its Schwann cell after interruption of the continuity of the axons showing manifold forms of lysis and fragmentation into small ovoids. Individual myelin lamellae often remain regularly layered until the last stage of lysis. × 18,500. **b** Same specimen as in **a**. Some myelin lamellae separate themselves from the otherwise still largely preserved myelin sheath and reach out freely into the cytoplasm of the Schwann cell. × 13,000. (From [944])

◄───

Fig. 76 a – f. Different Schwann cell inclusions in isoniazid neuropathy. **a** Nine days after onset of INH-application. A shrunken Schwann cell which is completely surrounded by a basal lamina contains enlarged lysosomal bodies. The finger-like processes of this cell extend partially into the folds of the basal laminae without being closely attached. × 18,000. **b** Band of Büngner 4 weeks after onset of INH-application. Between regenerated axons and proliferated Schwann cell processes a needle-like, crystalline structure can be seen lying in the extracellular space, which appears electron-optically empty without a limiting membrane. In addition, there are two further needle-like or prismatic structures in the cytoplasm of a Schwann cell which here are surrounded by an electron dense rim. × 29,400. **c, d** Leptomer fibrils in Schwann cells. × 28,000. **e** μ-granule (Elzholz body) in a regenerated nerve fiber. × 55,000. **f** π-granule (of Reich) in a regenerated myelinated nerve fiber, each in isoniazid neuropathy. × 19,000. (From [949])

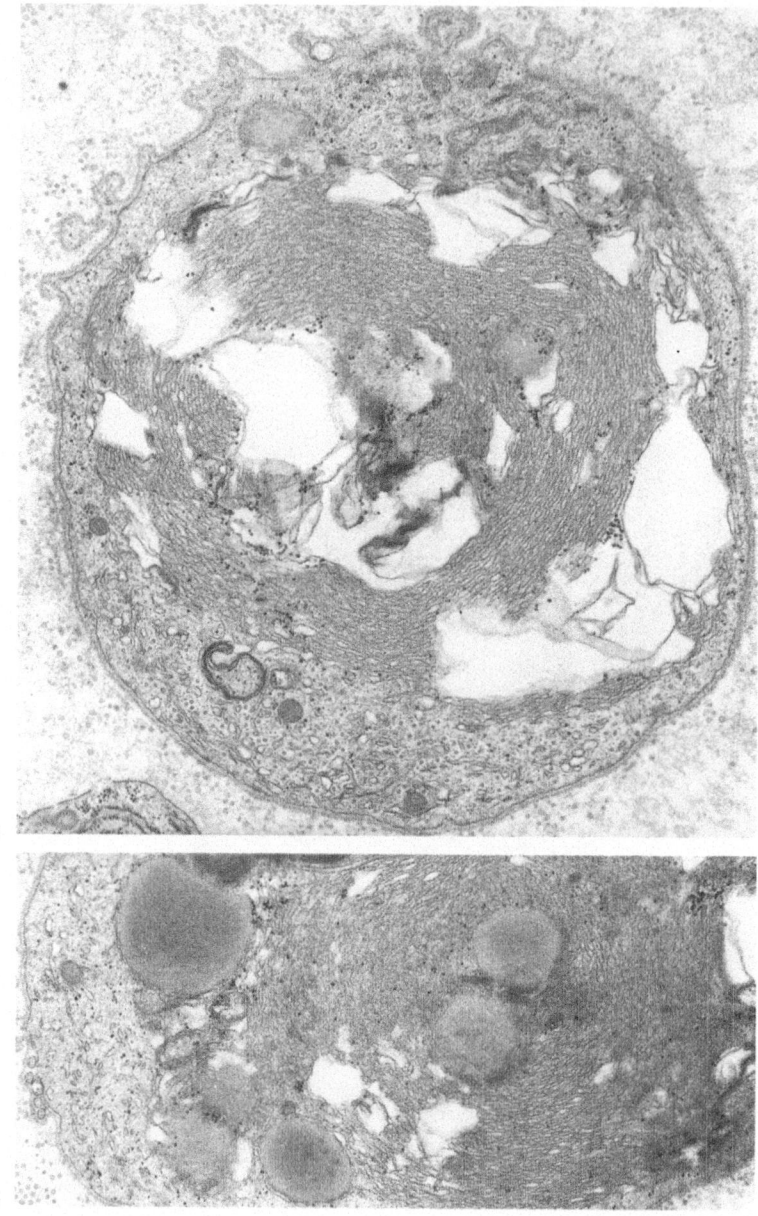

Fig. 78 a, b. Isoniazid neuropathy. Sciatic nerve, otherwise as in Fig. 77. **a** An extensive system of loosely arranged membranes fills the cross-sectional area of a Schwann cell rather completely. In between lie some vacuoles with electron-optically clear content and several glycogen granules. × 17,400. **b** Several lipid droplets are apparent between the more or less concentrically arranged membranes. A degenerating myelin sheath can be seen at the *upper margin*. × 14,500

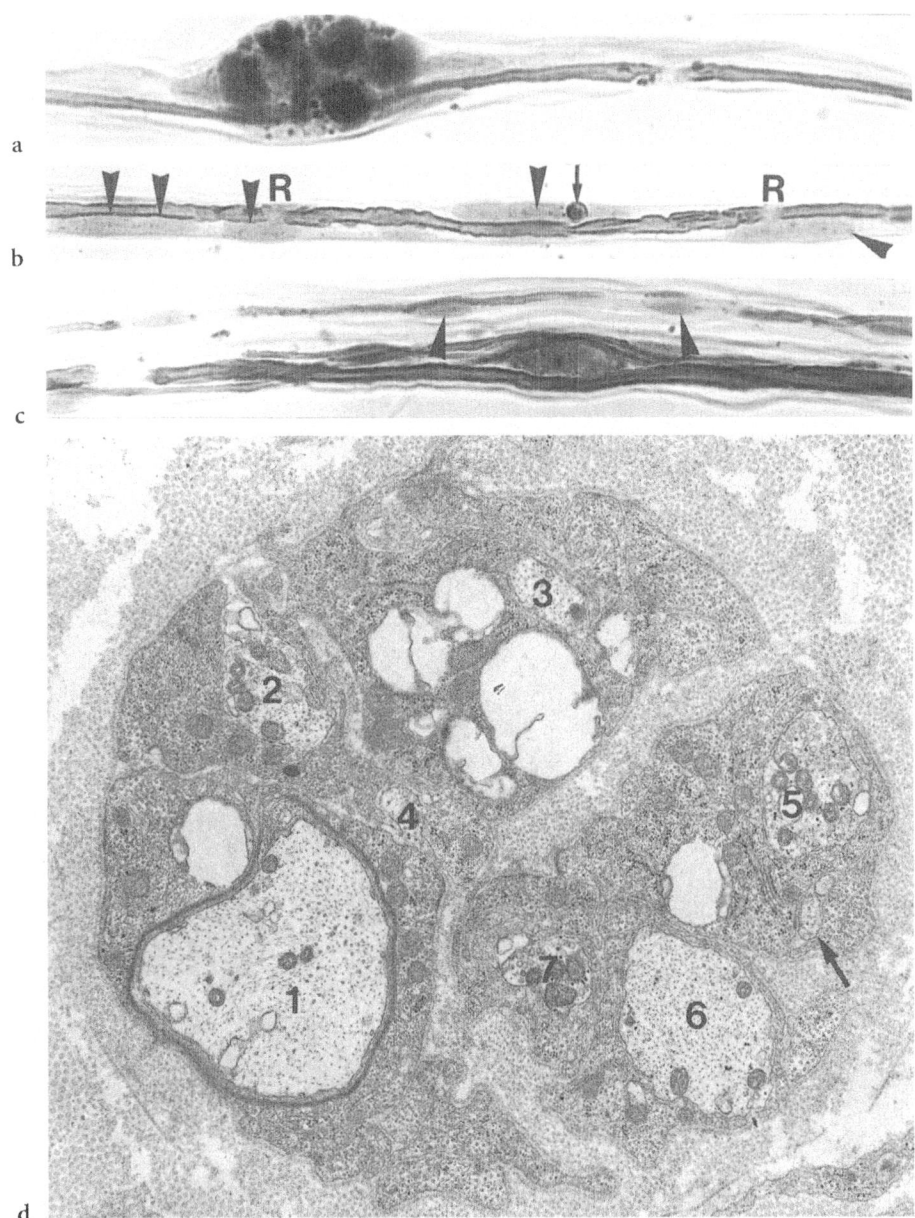

Fig. 79a–d. Regenerating nerve fibers in isoniazid neuropathy. **a–c** Teased regenerating nerve fibers 6 weeks after onset of isoniazid application. **a** Extensive myelin degradation products lie adjacent to a thinly myelinated nerve fiber. **b** Numerous Schwann cell nuclei (*arrowheads*) and a μ-granule (*arrow*) in a band of Büngner, which is reinnervated by a small myelinated nerve fiber with short internodes (*R*, nodes of Ranvier). **c** Bundle of intermingled, thin regenerated nerve fibers adjacent to a fiber with incompletely remyelinated internodes, the nuclei of which are indicated by *arrowheads*. **a–c** × 620. **d** Bundle of seven regenerating nerve fibers (labeled by numbers *1–7*) in a band of Büngner 3 months after continuous isoniazid application. The largest axon (*1*) is remyelinated by only 2 compact myelin lamellae. Two others (*5* and *7*) contain numerous vesicular structures and several mitochondria. The *arrow* indicates 2 further processes which are possibly degenerating axonal sprouts. The Schwann cell processes contain increased numbers of intermediate filaments and microtubules as well as lipid droplets which have partially been extracted during the embedding procedure. The collagen filaments between the reinnervated Schwann cells are thinner than in the surrounding endoneurium. × 16,500

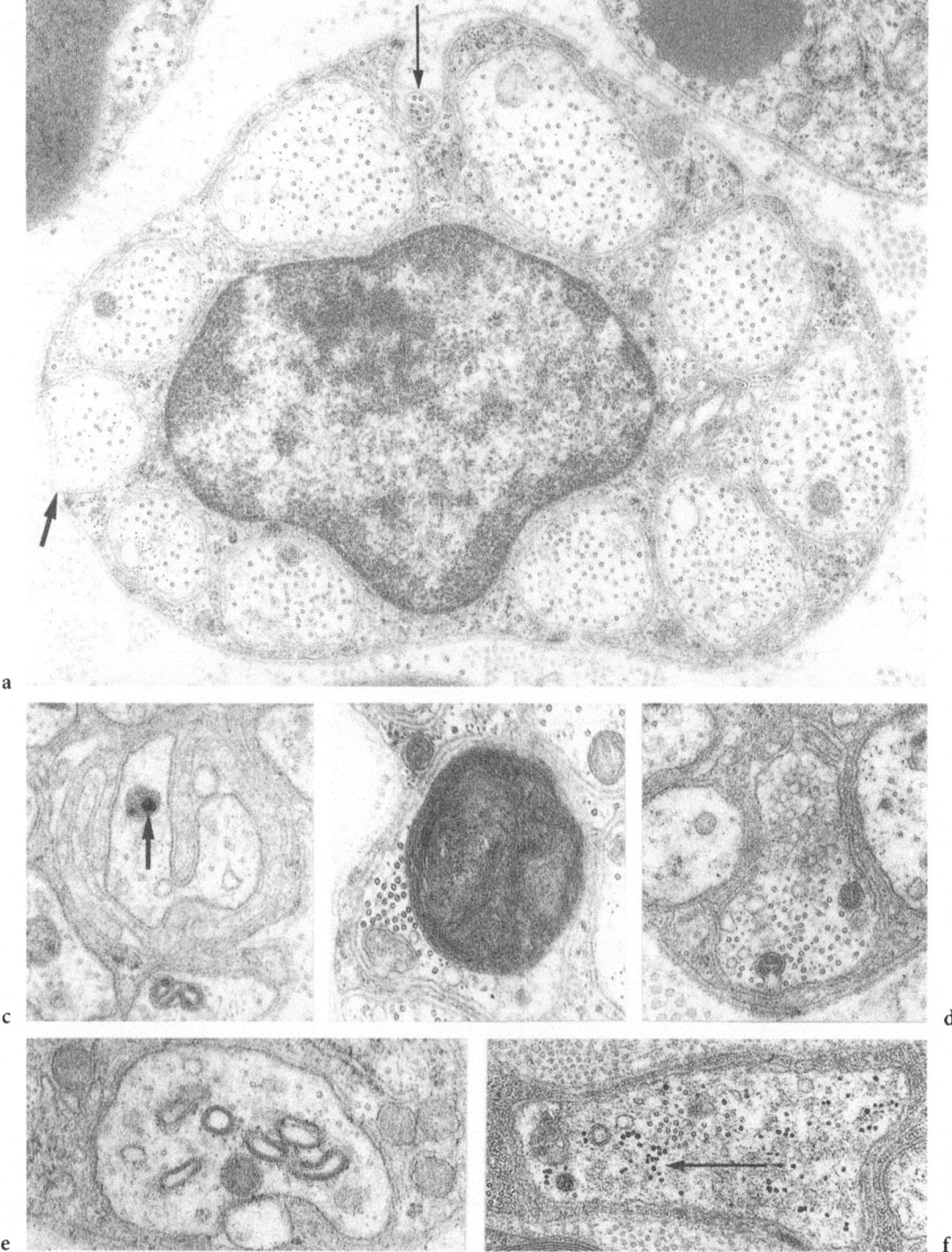

Fig. 80. a Nonspecific axonal changes (after INH-application) which occasionally may also occur in normal nerves of control animals. Eleven different axons with a normal number of tubules and filaments are here cut at the level of the Schwann cell nucleus. The *upper arrow* indicates an unusual thin axon, the *arrow on the left* an open mesaxon. × 20,500. **b** Irregular contour of an axon; the *arrow* indicates mitochondrial granules which we have only seen in INH neuropathy. × 20,500. **c** Electron-dense lamellated, presumably lysosomal body in an axon with numerous microtubules. × 31,000. **d** Aggregated vesicles in an otherwise normal appearing axon. × 24,600. **e** Suspicious vesicles with thick membranes. × 20,500. **f** Intra-axonal glycogen granules (*arrow*). × 32,400

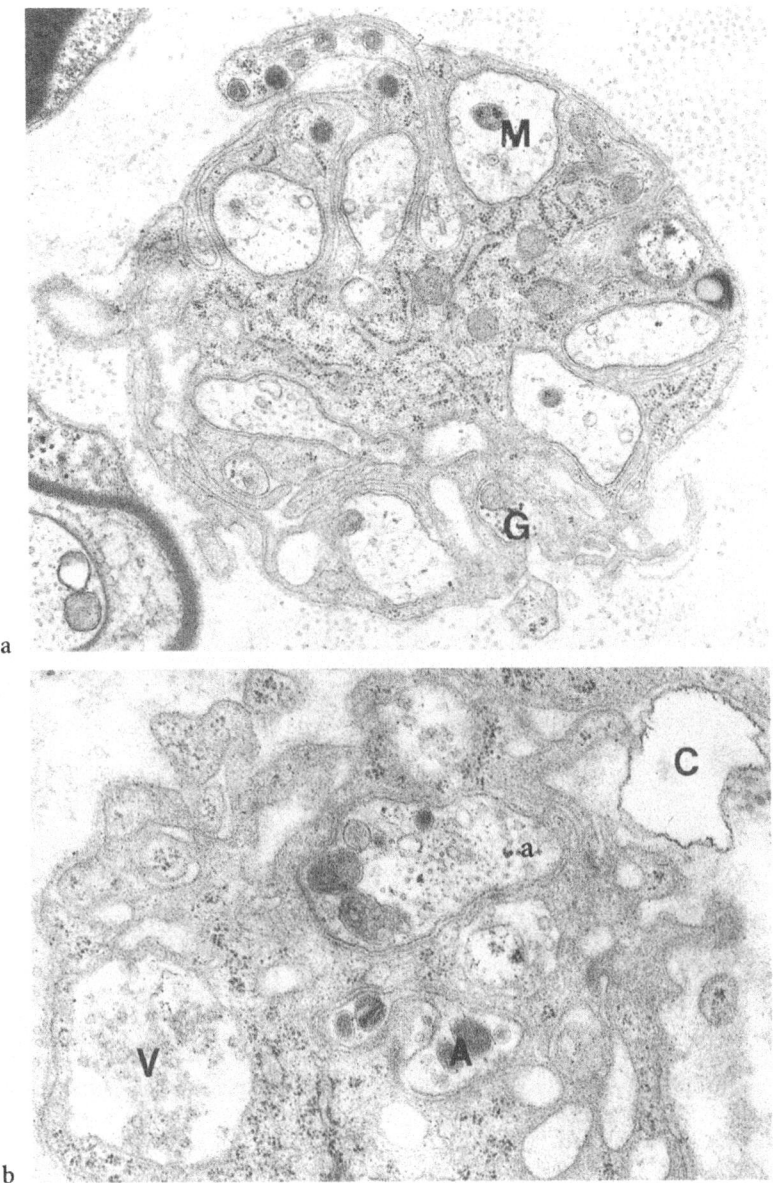

Fig. 81a, b. Isoniazid neuropathy 4 days after onset of INH-application. **a** A prolapse-like axonal deformation is partially covered by a Schwann cell process. Other axons appear normal; they may contain some glycogen granules (*G*), whereas others include only rare normal microtubules and filaments or fragmented mitochondrial matrix granules (*M*). The Schwann cell processes below are irregularly shaped, increased in length, or branched. The Schwann cell surface shows conspicuous focal indentations or protrusions. × 29,400. **b** Even more severe irregularities of the Schwann cell surface are apparent here. An intracellular autophagic vacuole (*V*), a cystic process located outside the cell (*C*), and a severely deformed axon (*A*) with four mitochondria are labeled. The basal laminae at some sites are defective or difficult to be distinguished from an endoneurial plasma exsudate. × 19,800

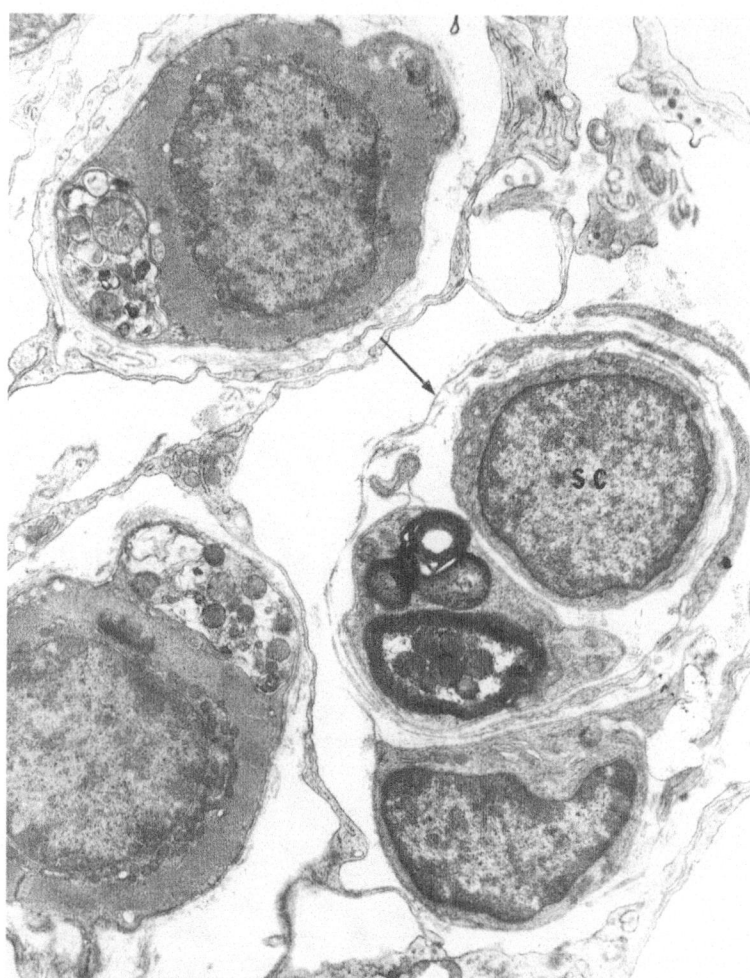

Fig. 82. Isoniazid neuropathy 7 days after onset of INH-application. The sensory nerve terminals at both intrafusal nuclear chain fibers and the preterminal nerve fiber show severe signs of degeneration. A preterminal, degenerating nerve fiber is almost completely filled with osmiophilic organelles. Adjacent is a rounded Schwann cell (*SC*) which in this plane of section contains no remnants of nerve fibers. The inner spindle sheath around this Schwann cell is completed by a basal lamina (*arrow*). The inner capsule cells appear not to be affected. × 8,000

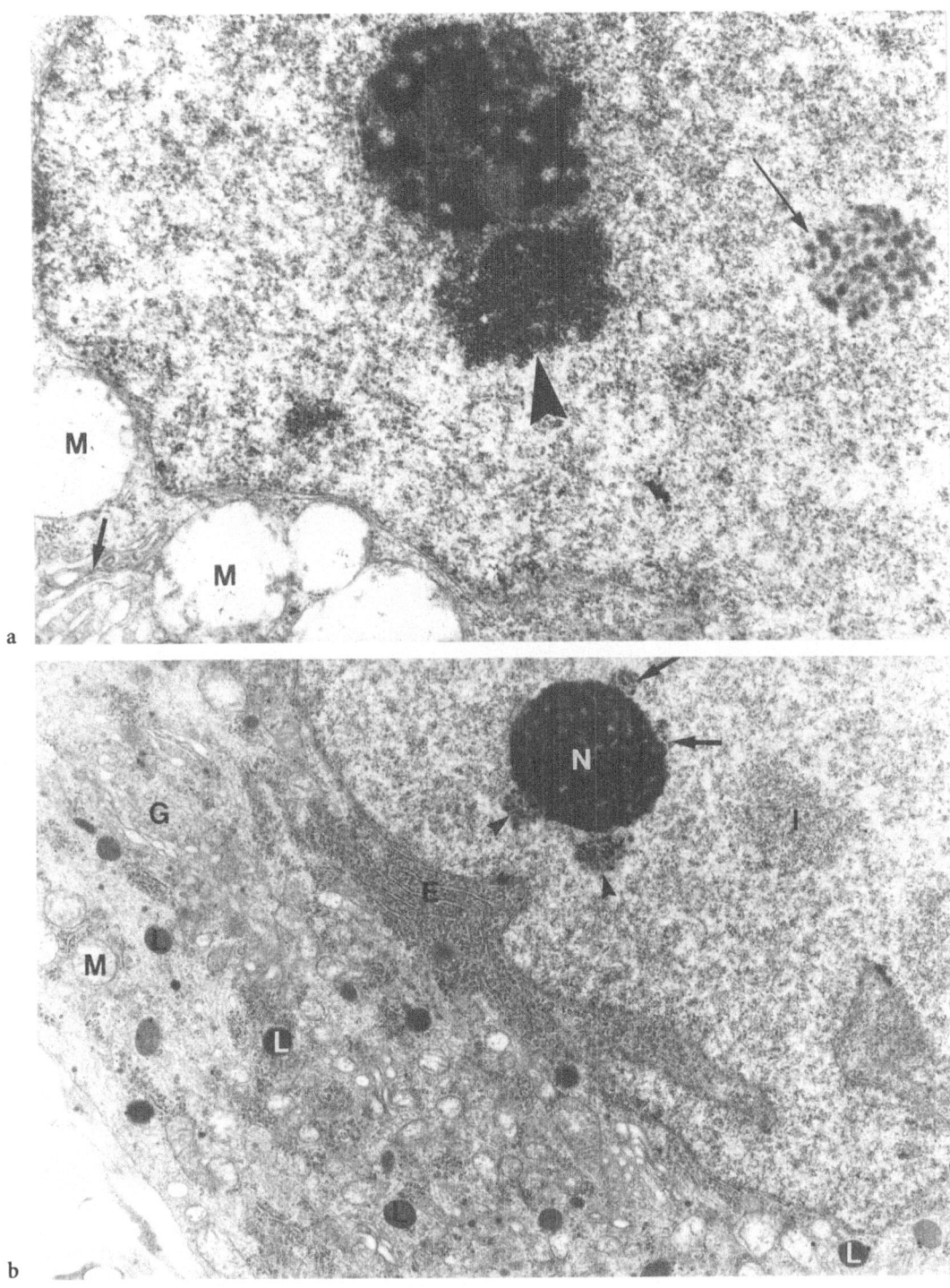

Fig. 83 a, b. Zidovudine intoxication in organotypic tissue cultures of spinal ganglia together with spinal cord cells and muscle fibers. **a** Five days after application of 1,000 μmol zidovudine (AZT), the nucleolus of a neuron in the spinal cord appears to be segregated and shows prominent cap formation (*large arrowhead*). The perichromatin granules are increased in size and number (*long arrow*), the mitochondria are swollen (*M*) and the Golgi complex slightly dilated (*small arrow*). × 32,000. **b** Spinal neuron 8 days after 1 μmol AZT. Perichromatin granules are associated with a conspicuous nucleolus (*N*) (*arrowheads*). The *arrows* indicate nucleolus associated chromatin. *I*, clusters of interchromatin-granules; *L*, lysosome; *G*, Golgi complex; *M*, swollen mitochondria; *E*, fragmented ergastoplasma. (Modified from [983])

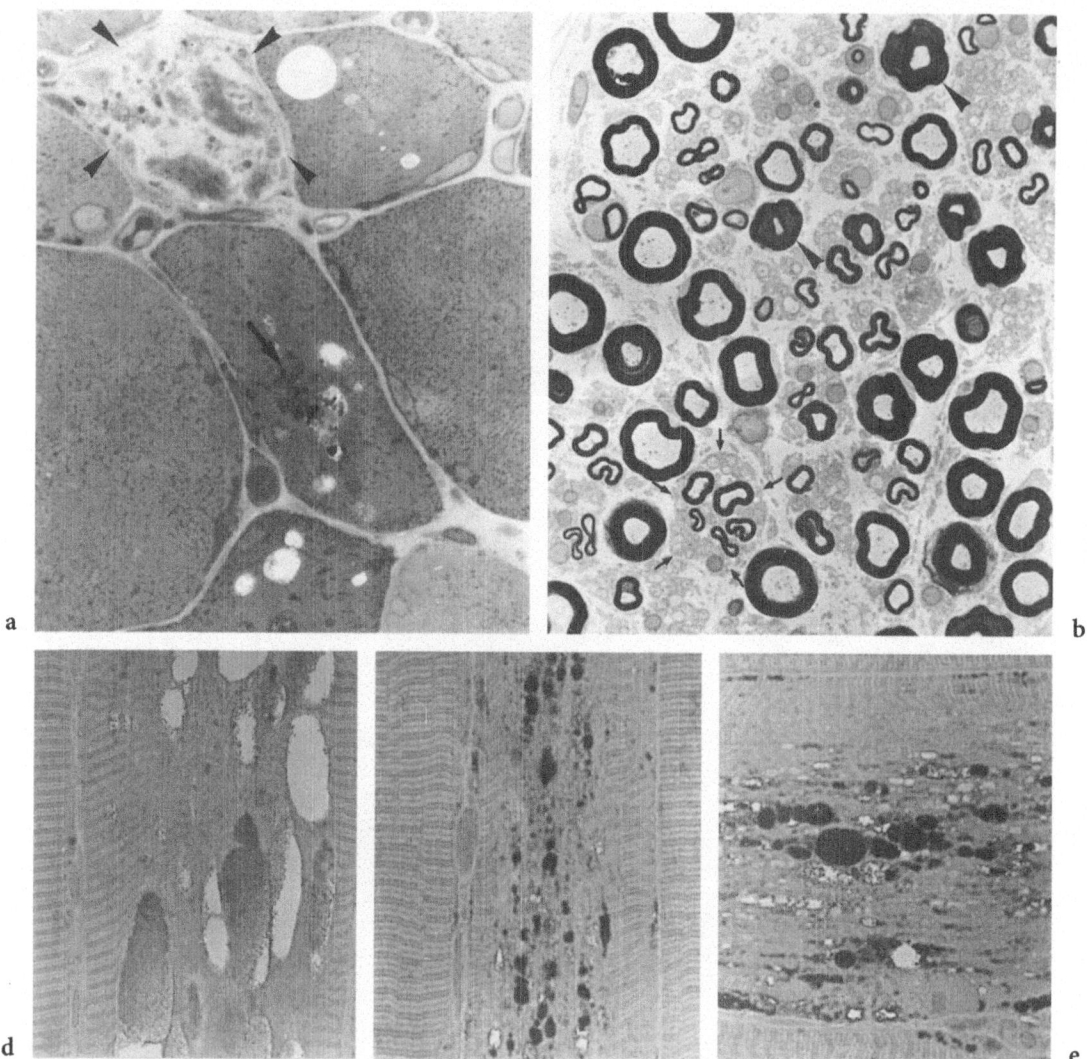

Fig. 84a–e. Colchicin neuromyopathy with prominent alterations in muscle (**a, c–e**), but relatively uncharacteristic atrophic nerve fibers (*arrowheads*) and clusters of regenerated fibers (*small arrows*) in the sural nerve biopsy (**b**) of a 24-year-old man with familial thalassemia, amyloidosis, and massive subacute myopathy in association with a viral infection. **a** × 1,200; **b** × 1,300; **c** × 750; **d** × 975; **e** × 875. (From [413])

CHAPTER 6

Neuropathies Due to Systemic Metabolic Disturbances

The most frequent peripheral neuropathy of all is probably diabetic neuropathy (above or below alcoholic neuropathy as stated already in the preceding section), which is caused by the underlying metabolic disturbances of diabetes mellitus. Three variants of *diabetic neuropathy* need to be distinguished:

- Symmetric polyneuropathy
- A predominantly sensory or autonomic form
- Focal and multifocal neuropathies

The pathomechanism leading to the different forms is complex, but the focal forms are usually attributed to a vascular component known as diabetic angiopathy [28, 54, 109, 127, 211, 250, 261, 262, 357, 473, 478, 484, 501, 508, 652, 658, 684, 726, 746, 847, 857, 862, 902, 922, 1077, 1254, 1255, 1260, 1295, 1299].

The combined effects of diabetic neuropathy, diabetic angiopathy, and diabetic arthropathy may cause ulceration of the feet (known as *diabetic foot* or *Charcot foot*).

Histopathological changes are dominated by a loss of myelinated and unmyelinated nerve fibers (Fig. 85a–d), and an increased thickness of the pericapillary basal laminae (Fig. 240a, d) [327], loss of neurons in the spinal ganglia and in the anterior horn of the spinal cord, degeneration of nerve fibers in the dorsal tracts in the spinal cord [1295], and other changes (Fig. 24f). Thickening of the basal laminae of the perineurial cells is reversible to a certain extent [52, 109]. Loss of small myelinated and unmyelinated fibers results in so-called diabetic *pseudo-syringomyelic neuropathy* [726]. There are fewer clusters of regenerated fibers than expected [108]. *Combination of diabetes with HMSN Ia* (see below) results in an unusually severe neuropathy with less distinct onion bulb formations [49, 1121, 1128]. In experimental *streptozotocin-induced diabetes*, diabetic amyotrophy may be more prominent than nerve fiber changes (Fig. 86) [1222].

Hypoglycemia [688] and *hypoxia* [862] may play a major role.

Uremic polyneuropathy [29, 547, 879] was the first neuropathy in which the concept of *secondary segmental demyelination* was introduced and statistically proven by evaluating teased nerve fiber preparations [254, 1127], later also in Friedreich's ataxia [255]. Individual atrophic axons more frequently showed demyelinated and remyelinated internodes than expected if segmental demyelination had occurred at random. Vesicular disintegration of paranodal myelin sheaths may be detected at the electron microscopic level (Figs. 87a, b, 141b). The main clinical symptoms are due to a loss of myelinated nerve fibers causing a distal sensorimotor polyneuropathy. This may develop very rapidly [879]. We were able to document a *devastating neuropathy* by examining two sural nerve biopsies at a time interval of 68 days in a *rapidly progressive glomerulonephritis* subsequent to *streptococcus type A* infection (Figs. 88a, b) [1070].

Neuropathy may also occur in *primary biliary cirrhosis* [1133], which is characterized by xanthomatous deposits, and *hepatitis* [505, 858, 903, 1117, 1152], which may be associated with panarteritis nodosa. It is also seen in *hypothyroidism* [256, 353, 835, 1045] in which the pericapillary basal laminae may be extremely thickened [952], *hyperthyroidism* [285], *akromegalia*, *pituitary insufficiency* (Figs. 89), and in *critically ill* patients [93, 94, 150, 1246, 1298].

Neuromyotonia, which may not be adequately presented at the end of this chapter is seemingly caused by antibodies directed against potassium channels at preterminal motor nerve fibers [396, 1028, 1126]. It is also seen in *mice with hereditary myelinopathies* [1290]. We have seen muscle biopsies with this disorder showing minor degrees of denervation of muscle fibers, but thus far no nerve biopsies.

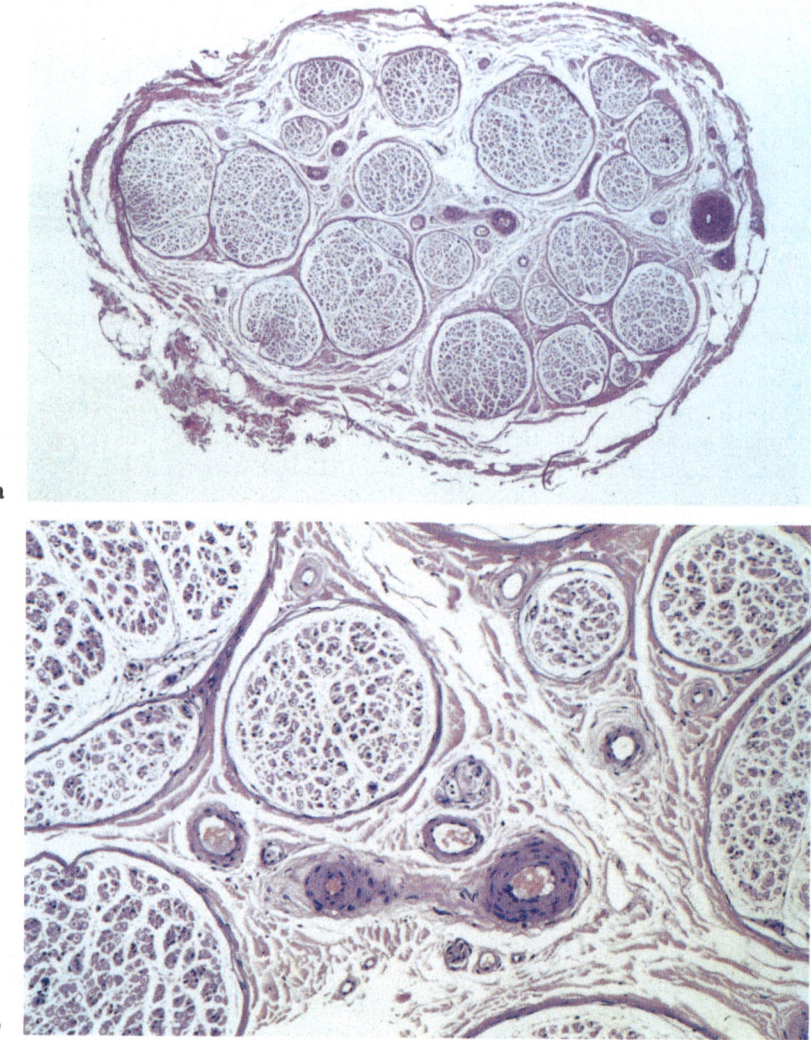

Fig. 85 a, b. Legend s. p. 97

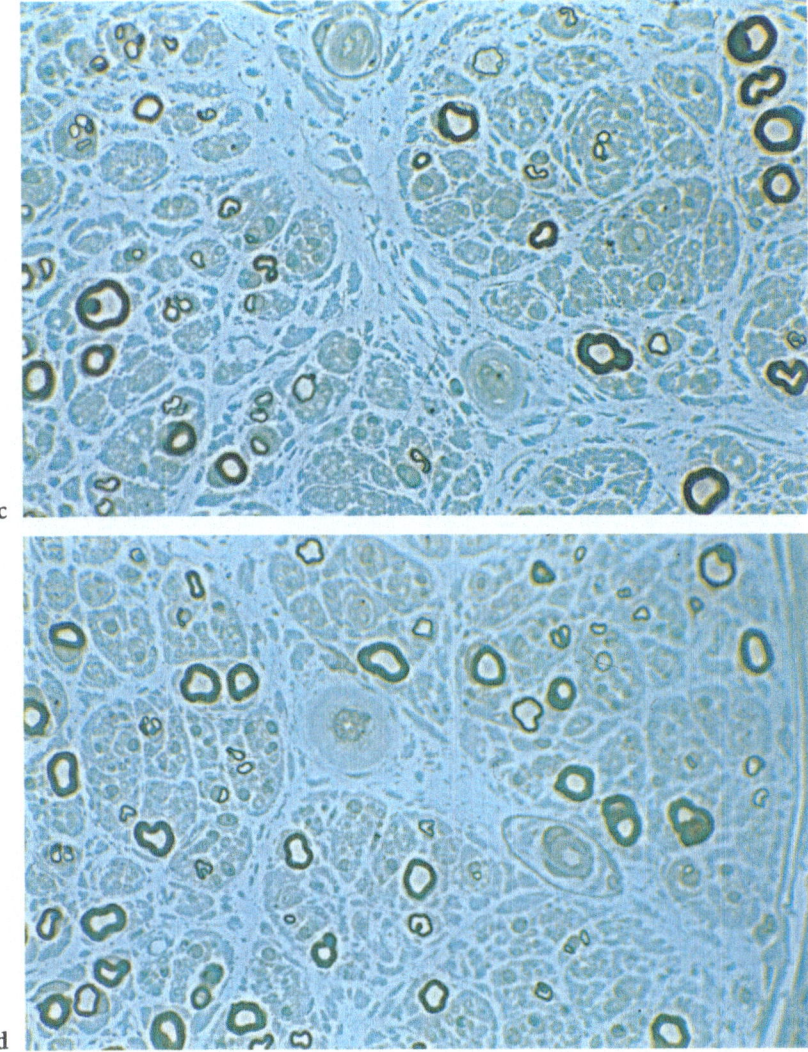

Fig. 85a–d. Prominent diabetic neuropathy in a 69-year-old man with an approximately 70%–80% loss of large and small myelinated nerve fibers. The perivascular basal laminae are thickened

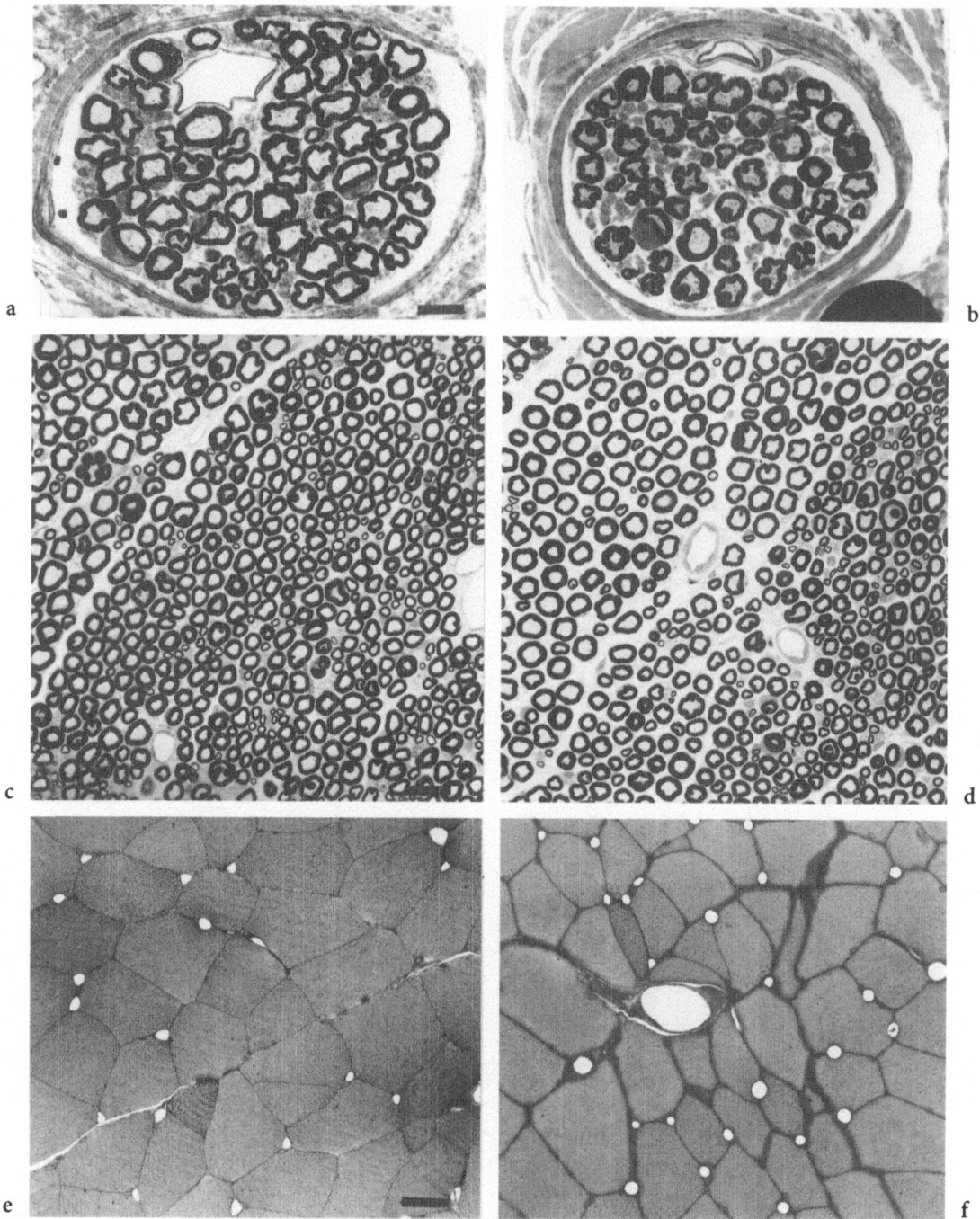

Fig. 86. Experimental diabetic neuropathy (**b**), after streptozotocin-intoxication (**d**). There is only endoneurial edema (**d**) and diabetic amyotrophy (**f**) in comparison to normal controls (**a, c, e**). Bar = 25 μm. (From [1222])

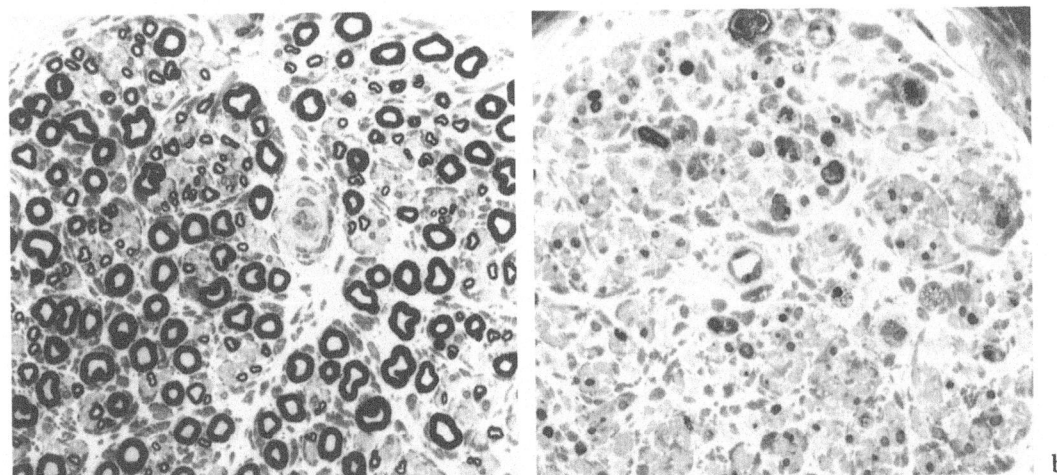

Fig. 87a, b. Uremic neuropathy in a 22-year-old man with acute progressive glomerulonephritis at the beginning of the disorder (**a**) and 68 days later showing severe neuropathy with rather complete loss of myelinated nerve fibers in the contralateral sural nerve (**b**). **a** × 400; **b** × 420 (see Fig. 199)

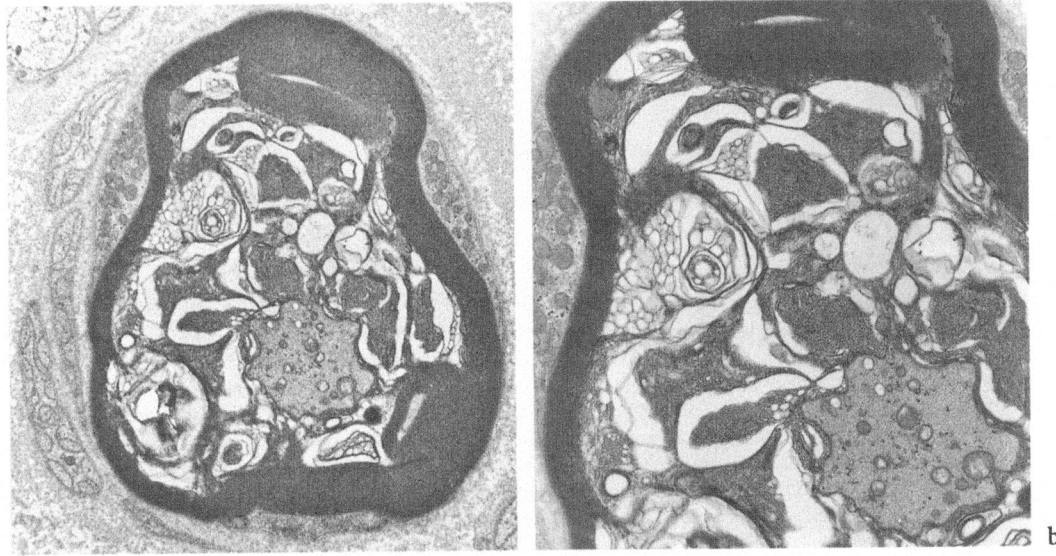

Fig. 88a, b. Uremic neuropathy in a 51-year-old man. The myelin lamellae of a regenerated nerve fiber at the level of a Schmidt-Lanterman incisure show combined microvesicular and vacuolar disintegration. In between are membranous cytoplasmic bodies and electron microscopically empty spaces. **a** × 7,600; **b** × 14,000

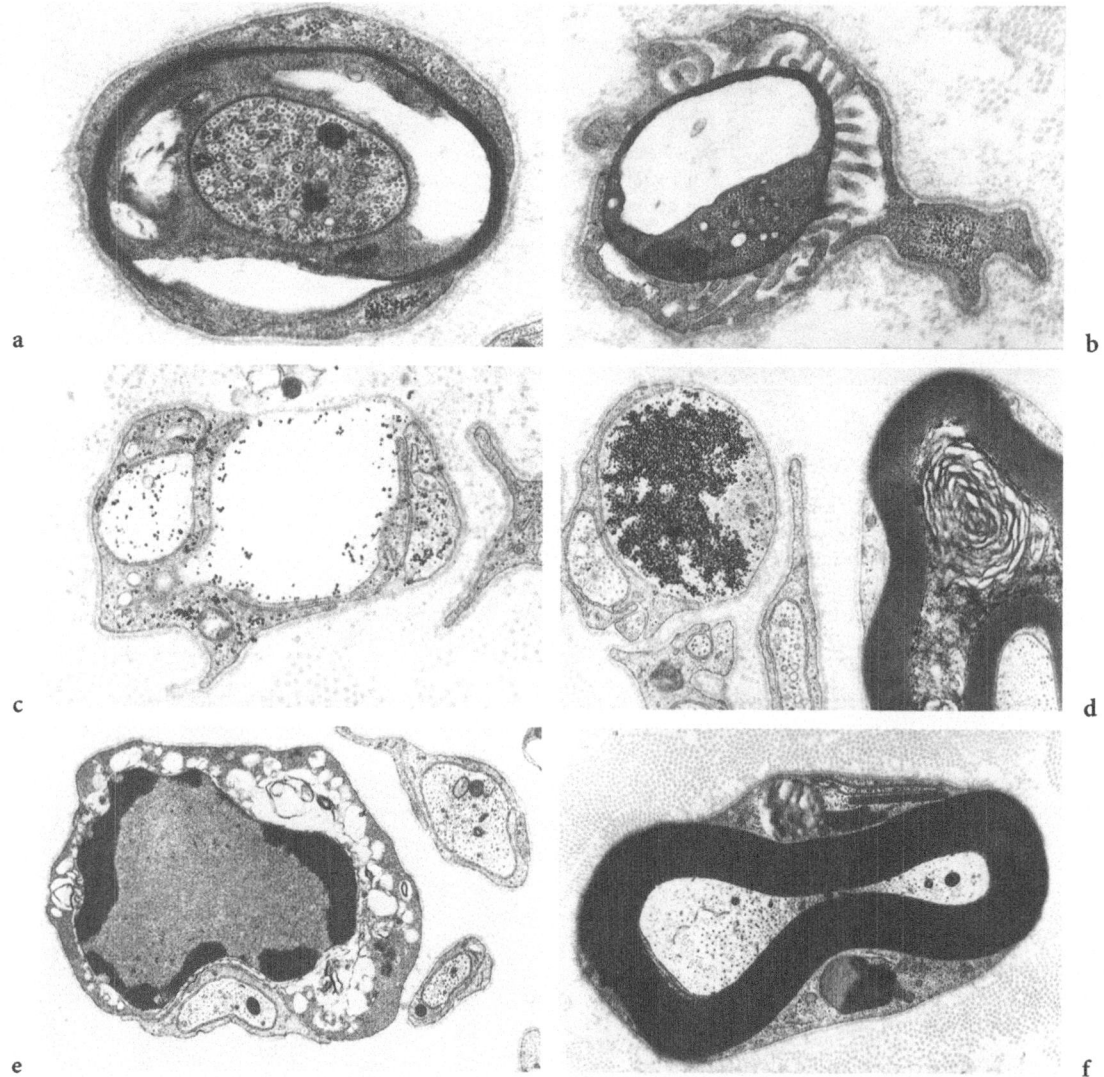

Fig. 89 a – f. Neuropathy in a 35-year-old female with pituitary insufficiency. Vacuoles are apparent in a Schmidt-Lanterman incisure (**a**), in a paranodal axon segment (**b**), in the cytoplasm of presumptive Schwann cell processes (**c**), and in a degenerating cell which is associated with an unmyelinated axon (**e**). The nucleus of the latter shows severe condensation of the heterochromatin beneath the nuclear membrane associated with a homogeneous granular structure of the remaining caryoplasm (apoptosis). Whether this is a degenerating Schwann cell or a macrophage within a common basal lamina is difficult to decide. The axon in **d** is enlarged by glycogen granules. A membranous cytoplasmic body is seen in the Schmidt-Lanterman incisure of a neighboring myelinated nerve fiber. In **f**, the axon appears to be atrophic or shrunken; π-granules and nonspecific lysosomal structures are seen in the cytoplasm of the Schwann cell. **a** × 28,000; **b** × 23,000; **c** × 21,000; **d** × 17,400; **e** × 12,700; **f** × 11,000

CHAPTER 7

Hereditary Motor and Sensory Neuropathies

The number of diseases of the peripheral nervous system in which the underlying molecular genetic defect has been established is rapidly (weekly) increasing.

Diseases already manifesting themselves at birth and showing only minimal progression should be regarded as *developmental disturbances*. The latter include diseases affecting:

- Certain *peripheral neuronal systems*, e.g., (1) large and small myelinated fibers without involving the unmyelinated ones (Figs. 90 a – d, 91) [979], (2) large myelinated fibers only (Figs. 92, 93, 97 a, 106 a – c, 108) [954, 955]), (3) small myelinated fibers of the sensory system (see below), and (4) the unmyelinated fibers of the sensory system (e.g., HSAN III and IV, Fig. 178).
- The *myelin sheath* causing (1) in the most severe form of developmental disturbance *total amyelination in the central and peripheral nervous system* (Figs. 94 – 95) [974], (2) *amyelination in the peripheral nervous system only* [159, 798], (3) *congenital hypomyelination* without apparent progression, or (4) *hypomyelination of some fibers* only (Fig. 96 b, c, Fig. 97 c).

Progressive hereditary neuropathies were classified according to Dyck (1993) [251] as *hereditary motor and sensory neuropathy type I – VI (HMSN I – VI)*, and *as hereditary sensory and autonomous neuropathies (HSAN) type I – V.*

- HMSN I, the most frequent form of inherited neuropathies, is dominantly inherited and demyelinating in type (Fig. 17 f, 20 d, f, 97 b, 98 a, d, 99 a – d, 100).
- HMSN II is also dominantly inherited, but neuronal (axonal) in type (Fig. 107, 111 a, b).
- HMSN III (type Dejerine Sottas) (Fig. 114 a – c) is believed to be recessively inherited and demyelinating in type.
- HMSN IV was originally synonymous with Refsum's syndrome (see below); it is now attributed to severe autosomal recessive (neuronal?) types (HMSN IVa – c) [35].

- HMSN V is characterized by additional spastic components.
- HMSN VI is characterized by additional optic atrophy (type Vizioli) (Figs. 15 f, 20 b, 165 – 166).
- HNPP is the autosomal dominant hereditary neuropathy with liability to pressure palsies.
- HNA is the autosomal dominant hereditary neuralgic amyotrophy [1172].

HMSN I was then further subdivided into type Ia because of its association with the Duffy locus, leaving type Ib without this association. Molecular genetic studies have revealed that:

- *HMSN Ia* [155 – 158, 251, 259, 497, 635, 741, 930, 1001, 1131, 1156, 1157] is caused by mutations in the gene for the peripheral myelin protein with the molecular weight of 22 kDa (PMP22)
- Type Ib, however, is due to mutations in the myelin protein zero (MPZ, Po) (see below).

Geneticists tend to denominate the inherited neuropathies according to the first authors describing a dominantly inherited distal (peroneal) type of neuropathy (Charcot-Marie-Tooth), e.g., CMT 1A, CMT 1B, etc.

The system of classification is confusing because of the phenotypic variability of genotypes. For example, *PMP22 point mutations* may cause HMSN Ia (CMT 1A) or HMSN III (CMT 3, Dejerine Sottas disease), *PMP22 duplication* causes HMSN Ia, *PMP22 deletion* causes *hereditary neuropathy with liability to pressure palsies (HNPP; tomaculous neuropathy* [624]) (Figs. 101 – 105) [2, 37, 48, 101, 102, 313, 446, 447, 449, 545, 592, 593, 626, 636, 728, 731, 743, 809, 873 – 875, 910, 912, 1163, 1169, 1268].

MPZ (Po) mutations may cause HMSN Ib, HMSN II, Dejerine Sottas syndrome (DSS), or congenital hypomyelination neuropathy (CH) [101, 315, 332, 402, 403, 546, 640, 661, 722, 732, 999, 1018, 1023, 1100, 1101, 1209, 1291].

Further confusion in this system of using Roman numerals is caused by designating the dominantly or recessively inherited neuropathies caused by mutations on the *X chromosome* as *HMSN X (or CMT X* which is not: CMT 10!) (Figs. 119–123). Dominant HMSN X is attributed to more than 216 different mutations in the connexin32 gene (*Cx32*) [1, 68, 70, 83, 96, 129, 191, 293, 294, 316, 379, 445, 448, 450, 451, 577, 582, 703, 737, 869, 912, 1015, 1016, 1098, 1232].

Other genes have been detected such as the *early growth response 2 (EGR2)-gene* (krox20) which may cause HMSN Ia or CH [730, 806, 807, 1142, 1210].

Dominantly inherited neuropathies of the demyelinating type that could not be attributed to one of the known mutations are designated as *HMSN Ic (non-a non-b)*.

Recessively inherited neuropathies of the demyelinating type are classified as CMT 4 A-C. These are rare and even more difficult to be identified by molecular genetic techniques [188, 235, 314, 451, 470, 616, 731, 1132]. A severe demyelinating neuropathy is caused by a stop codon in the N-myc downstream regulated gene 1 (*NDRG1*) on chromosome 8q24.3 [481] causing *HMSN L*, taking its name from the town called Lom in Bulgaria where it has been detected in gypsy families (Figs. 111c, d, 112a–g, 113a–c) [38, 482, 511, 665]. A congenital, demyelinating type (*congenital hypomyelination neuropathy, CH*) shows basal laminae surrounding centrally located myelinated or demyelinated nerve fibers (Figs. 115a, b, 116a–f) instead of regular onion bulbs as seen in DSS (Fig. 98c). Unusual changes are illustrated in Fig. 106a–c. *Neuropathy with excessive myelin outfolding* (Figs. 117, 118, 173b) (*hyper-/hypomyelination neuropathy*) [776, 859, 897, 908, 1164] is caused by mutations in the gene encoding *myotubularin-related protein-2* on chromosome 11q22 (CMT4B) [91]. Another form of CMT4 could not be linked to 5q23–33, where mutations in the human neuregulin-2 (*NRG2*) gene have been suggested causing the neuropathy [1303]. CMT4A has been localized to chromosome 8q13–21; CMT4C to chromosome 5q23–33; CMT4E to chromosome 10q21 (early growth response 2, EGR2 gene) [1210], and others will follow.

Another, severe, demyelinating type of *neuropathy with mental retardation and congenital cataract* is characterized by loss of nerve fibers and *dysplastic perineurial cells* (Figs. 109–110) [992]. More severe perineurial changes were noted in another case [1130]. Unusual *Schwann cell inclusions* were noted in another type of neuropathy of unknown cause (Figs. 172a–d, 173a) [1002]. A later muscle biopsy did not offer any elucidating changes.

Inherited neuropathies of the *neuronal type* (HMSN II or CMT2) are attributed to chromosomes 1p35–36 (CMT2A), 3q13–22 (CMT2B), and 7p14 (CMT2D), although no corresponding genes have yet been identified and cloned from these loci. HMSN IIC characterized by additional diaphragm

and vocal cord paralysis has not yet been attributed to any locus. Recently, a CMT2 phenotype was described that is believed to be caused by a mutation in the neurofilament-light gene (*NF-L*) [1302].

Dominantly inherited neuropathies of a severe, progressive, neuronal type are also seen in *familial amyloidoses* (FA type) (Fig. 127a, b) which can be differentiated immunohistochemically from amyloid neuropathies caused by light chain deposits due to paraproteinemias (AL type, primary amyloidosis) (see below) (Figs. 124–126, 128a–c; 238f) [15, 116, 598, 676, 1068, 1139, 1181].

In a large number of diseases, protein components, mainly of other organs, are primarily involved where the peripheral nervous system is only one of several organ systems affected. These include several myopathies such as the following:

- *Myotonic dystrophy* (Figs. 129–132) [196, 228, 1066, 1162, 1197].
- *Oculopharyngeal muscular dystrophy* [389].
- *Dominantly inherited distal myopathies* (Fig. 133b, d) [98–100, 595].
- *Merosin deficiency* [650].
- *Emerin deficiency* [1092].
- *Marinesco-Sjögren syndrome* (Fig. 134a–e) [8, 1294].

Other diseases or syndromes include:

- *Rett syndrome* [229, 468].
- *Chédiak-Higashi disease* [675].
- *Ehlers-Danlos disease* [923].
- *Marfan syndrome* (Fig. 135a–c).
- *Hyperglycinemia* (Fig. 136a–d).

and certain experimental animal models such as:

- *trkB(-/-) mice* which are deficient in motor neurons [1055].
- NT-3(-/-) mouse mutants [275] which are deficient in large spinal ganglia neurons, tendon organs, and muscle spindles.
- Japanese quails which are deficient in neurofilaments [679, 1105, 1258, 1286–1288], and others.

A neuropathy of the dying back type is seen in the various forms of *porphyria* [655, 664]. Yet the histopathological findings are nonspecific.

Several disturbances of *lipid metabolism* may cause more or less severe neuropathies such as:

- *Metachromatic leukodystrophy* (Figs. 137a–d, 138e, 139a–d) [46, 247, 306, 383, 1022, 1027, 1215, 1252], *globoid cell leukodystrophy* (Fig. 138b).
- *Niemann Pick's disease type II* (type C) (Fig. 140a–c) [148, 382, 412, 568, 633, 638, 1179].
- *Cockayne syndrome* (Fig. 141a) [697, 775], *cerebrotendinous xanthomatosis* [24, 236, 494, 548, 674, 777, 841, 1063, 1195].

- *Familial multiple symmetric lipomatosis (Madelung's disease)* [837].
- *Multiple lipomatosis (Krabbe-Bartels syndrome)* (Fig. 142 a – c).
- *Membranous lipodystrophy (Nasu-Hakola disease* [437, 516]).
- *N-acetylgalactosidase deficiency* [1247].
- *Neuraminidase deficiency (Sandhoff's disease)* (Fig. 143 a – e) [890], and *other gangliosidoses*.

The *lipofuscinoses* are characterized by various curvilinear or granular lysosomal inclusions in different cell types including Schwann cells (Figs. 138 c, 144 – 145) [120, 1004, 1181].

A lysosomal, X-chromosomal, recessively inherited disorders is *Fabry's disease* (glycosphingolipid lipidosis; *angiokeratoma corporis diffusum*) (Fig. 146 a – d) [84, 111, 431, 525, 716, 773].

Autosomal recessive proteolipid abnormalities include: *analphalipoproteinemia (Tangier disease)* (Figs. 147 – 148) [90, 123, 331, 524, 794, 838, 892, 893, 932], and *abetalipoproteinemia (Bassen Kornzweig's disease; neuroakanthocytosis)* [388].

Peroxisomal diseases include:

- *Adrenoleukodystrophy* (ADL; called *adrenomyeloneuropathy* in less severely affected cases) (Figs. 25 b, 149 – 153, possibly also Fig. 154 a, b) [59, 282, 362, 377, 677, 700 – 702, 872, 1235, 1236].
- *Infantile Refsum's disease*. In adult *Refsum's disease* (phytanic acid storage disease, heredopathia atactica polyneuritiformis) (Fig. 98 b) no peroxisomal defect has thus far been detected [47, 322, 767, 839, 1140, 1205]. Massive deposits of oxalat crystals may be seen in
- *Oxalosis*: Type I is associated with a defect of the peroxisomal enzyme alanin-glyoxalat-aminotransferase [318].
- *Optico-cochleo-dentate degeneration* (J.M Schröder, personal observation; Hackel, Doctoral thesis, Aachen, 1999; Voit et al., in preparation) appears to be another peroxisomal disease characterized by deficient peroxisomal enzyme activity (J. Wanders, personal communication). The associated peripheral neuropathy is characteriz-

ed by a severe loss of myelinated nerve fibers (unpublished observations). In another case with periodic weakness due to an unidentified peripheral neuropathy, somewhat similar bilaminar inclusions in Schwann cells, as seen in ALD, were detected (Fig. 155 a – d).

Mucopolysaccharidoses are characterized by both deposits of vacuolar material representing mucopolysaccharides (Figs. 138 a, 157 a – d) and membranous cytoplasmic bodies presumably representing gangliosides or other lipids or proteolipids (Fig. 156 a – f) [302, 469, 959]. Similar vacuoles with additional features may be seen in *α-mannosidase deficiency* [589, 1096] (Fig. 158 a – d).

Among the *glycogen storage diseases*, *Anderson's disease* or *polyglucosan body disease* may affect the central and peripheral nervous system (Figs. 23 a, b, 159 – 161) [130, 142, 604, 988, 1046, 1292], and smooth and sketal muscle fibers.

Diseases with defective DNA repair include *ataxia teleangiectatica* [628] and *xeroderma pigmentosum* (Fig. 173 a, b) [628].

In *mitochondrial disorders* caused by mitochondrial or nuclear DNA mutations, peripheral nerves tend to be involved (Figs. 22 b, 28 a – d, 162 – 164) [45, 173, 281, 298, 415, 522, 686, 690, 691, 820, 870, 961, 962, 1000, 1030, 1047, 1069, 1160, 1176, 1202, 1278 – 1280]. However, "abnormal" mitochondria with paracrystalline inclusions may already occur in Schwann cells of normal unmyelinated fibers (Figs. 167 – 168). Significant mitochondrial alterations are apparent in Schwann cells of myelinated fibers in *HMSN VI (type Vizioli)* (Figs. 165 – 166), and *MELAS* (Figs. 169 – 170). Unusual lipids and other inclusions were seen *in myo-, neuro-, and gastrointestinal encephalopathy (MNGIE syndrome)* (Fig. 171 a – f) [45, 805]. Mitochondrial alterations may also occur following application of *2',3'-dideoxycytidine* [286], a drug analogous to *zidovudine* (see above) used for the treatment of AIDS. We have also seen mitochondrial abnormalities in Schwann cells in *adrenoleukodystrophy* where they may be significant [990], in *phosphoglycerate deficiency* [977], and *oculopharyngeal muscle dystrophy*.

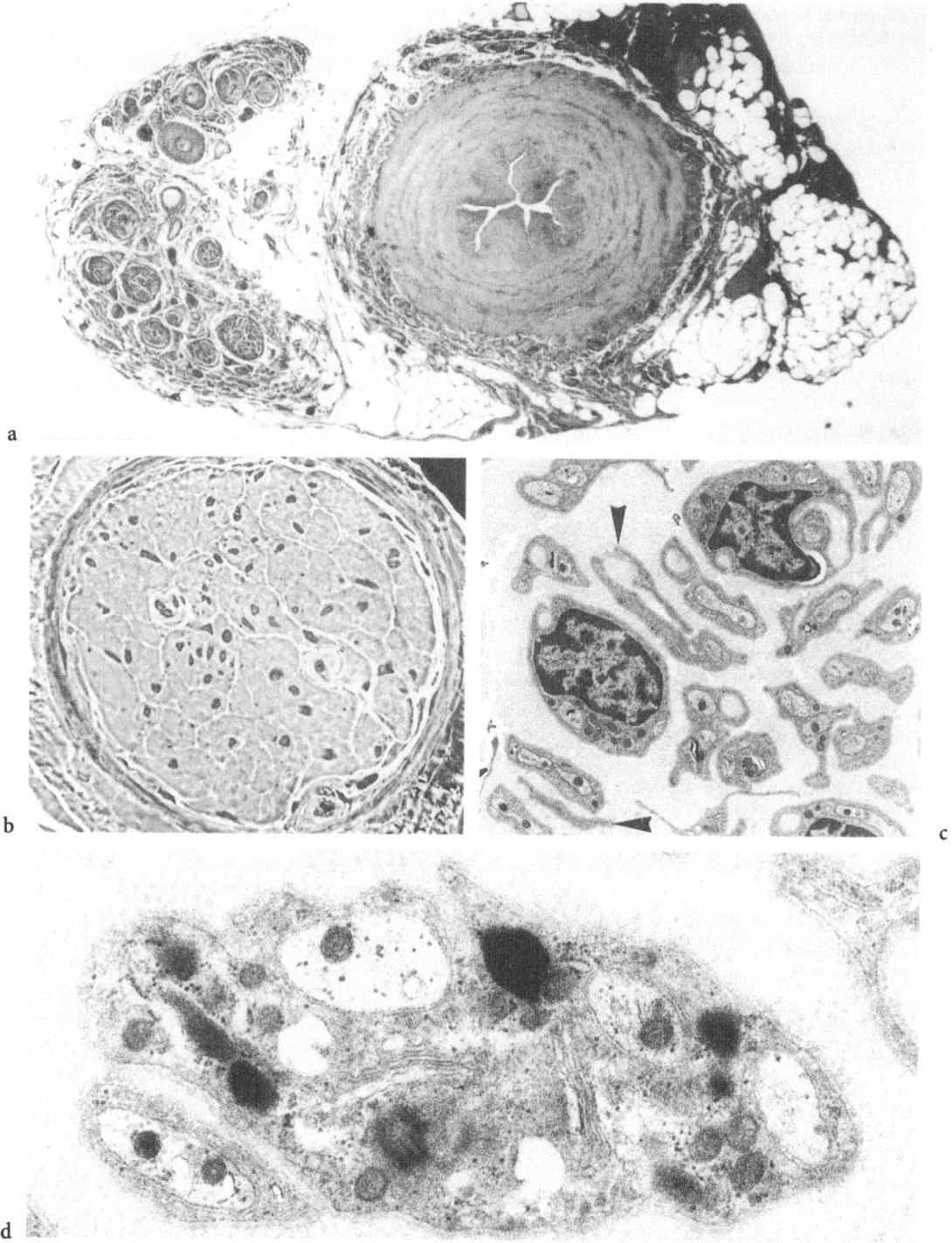

Fig. 90 a–d. Aplasia of myelinated nerve fibers in a 14-year-old girl. (From [979]). **a** Thirteen unusually small nerve fascicles can be seen adjacent to a normal large artery; they are surrounded by a regular epineurium and perineurium. × 33. **b** Most fascicles do not contain any myelinated nerve fibers. The endoneurial connective tissue is not increased. × 500. **c** At electron microscopic magnification there are normal numbers of unmyelinated fibers surrounded by Schwann cells and their processes. Occasional collagen pockets can also be seen. Schwann cells without axons are rare (*arrowheads*). × 6,700. **d** A Schwann cell with three unmyelinated axons contains several electron-dense cytosomes, presumably lysosomes, and some mitochondria. × 31,000

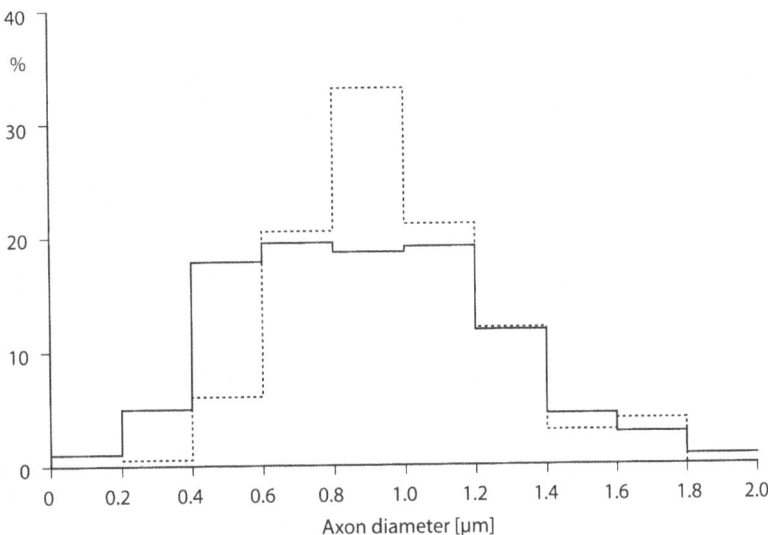

Fig. 91. Histogram of the unmyelinated axons illustrated in Fig. 90. The data are based on measurements on electron microscopic images (*interrupted line*, case with aplasia of myelinated nerve fibers; *solid line*, autopsy case, normal 10-year-old boy). (From [979])

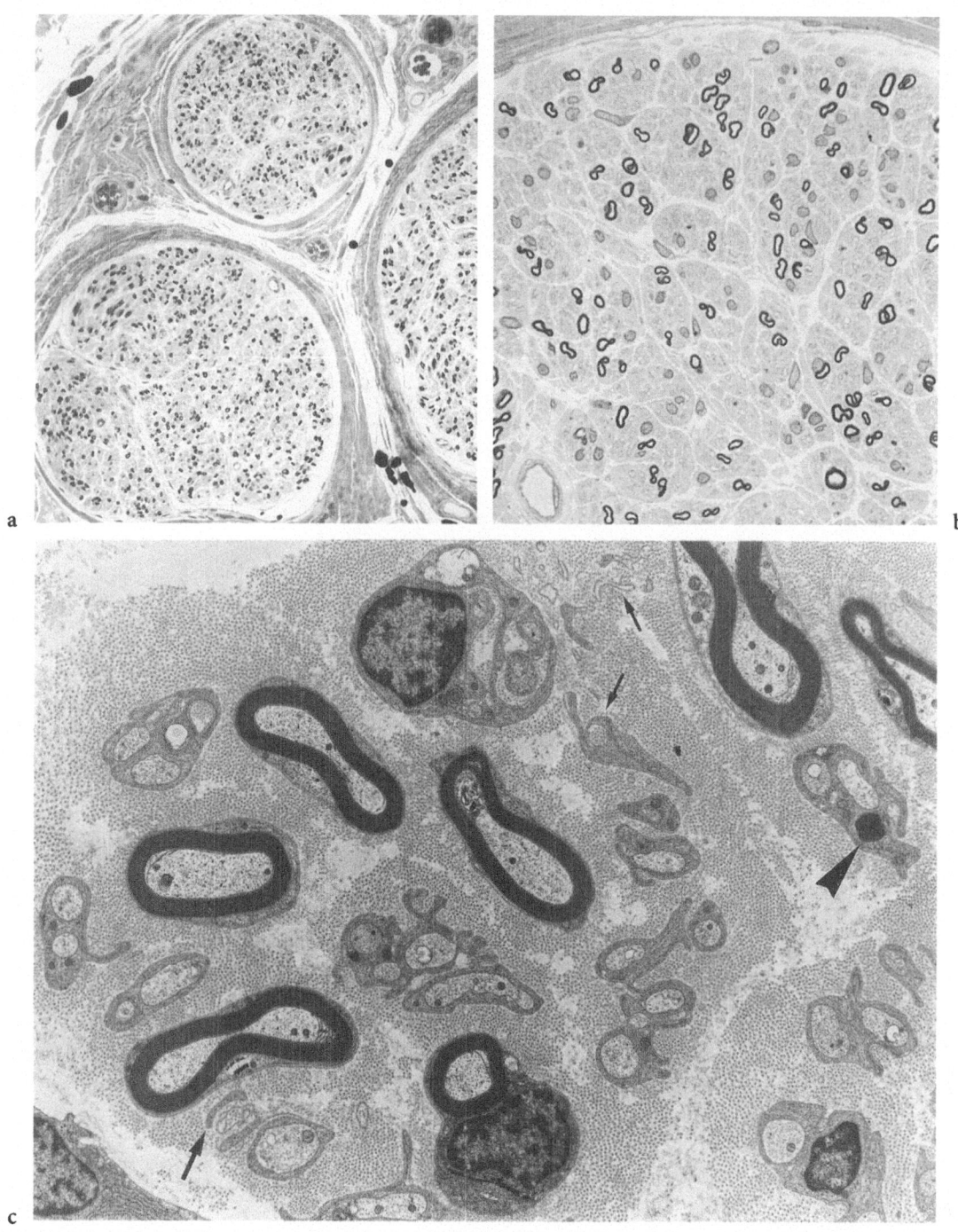

Fig. 92a–c. Sural nerve of a 10-year-old boy with sensorimotor, minimally progressive neuropathy (motor NCV: 19.6 m/s). Aplasia of large myelinated nerve fibers. There are no apparent myelin degradation products or any other signs of progressive degeneration of myelinated nerve fibers although there is some evidence of degeneration of unmyelinated axons (c). The number of unmyelinated axons appears to be reduced and the bands of Büngner are of the unmyelinated type. **a** × 160; **b** × 640; **c** × 7,100. (From [954])

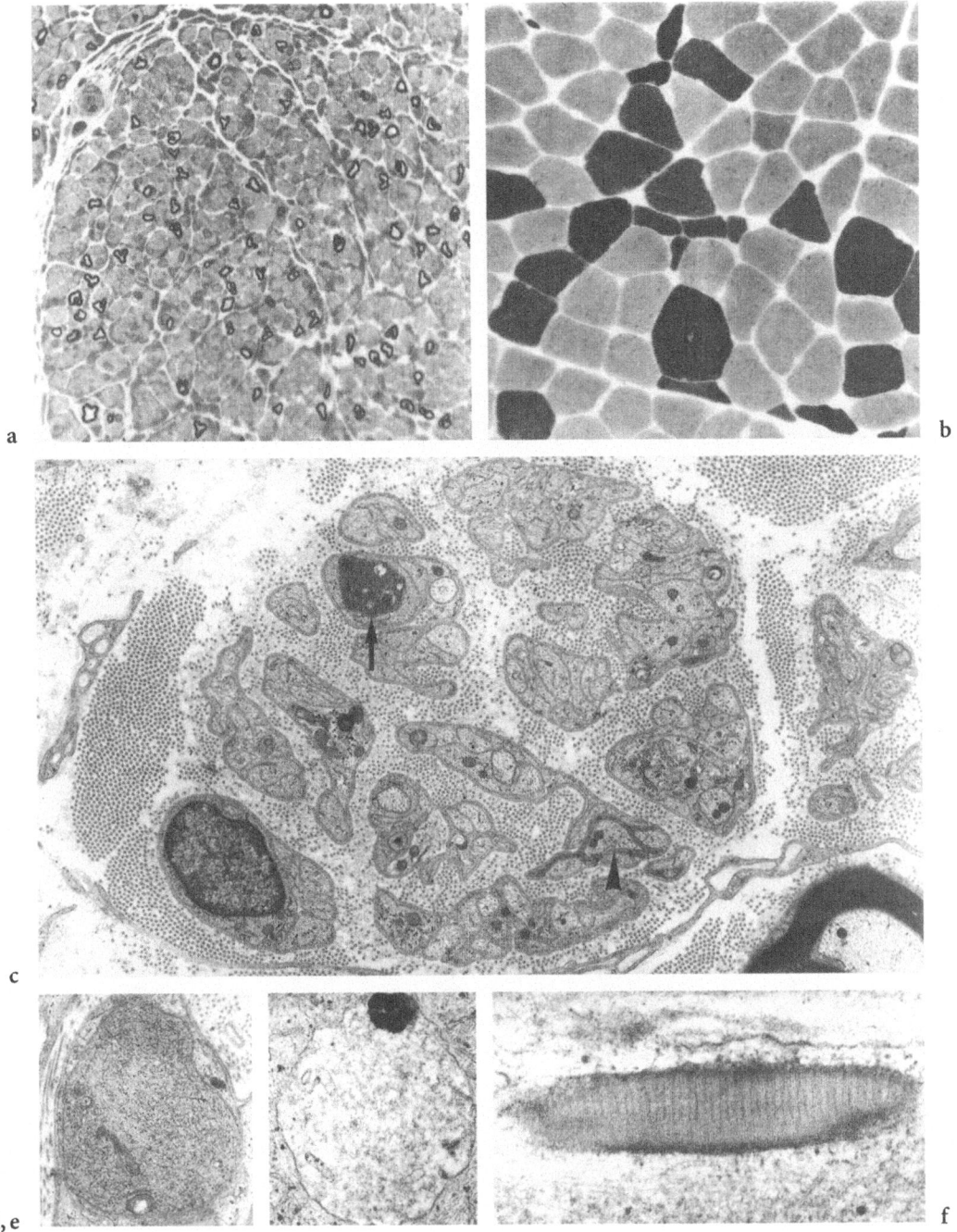

Fig. 93 a – f. Aplasia of large myelinated nerve fibers in a 15-year-old boy with Friedreich's ataxia. **a** Only small myelinated and unmyelinated nerve fibers are preserved in this sural nerve. × 475. **b** In the muscle biopsy there are only a few atrophic muscle fibers which are mainly of type 2. Myofibrillar ATPase after preincubation at pH 9.4. × 176. **c** Electron micrograph of a group of unmyelinated nerve fibers and Schwann cell processes which have partially lost their unmyelinated axons. One axon is enlarged and condensed; it contains an increased number of filaments (*arrow*). Two further axons are surrounded by pycnotic Schwann cell processes (*arrowheads*). × 8,600. **d** Dystrophic axon with increased axoplasmic components. × 10,600. **e** Vacuole within a Schwann cell containing an electron-dense body. × 24,000. **f** Unusual cross-striated mitochondrion in a Schwann cell. × 59,000

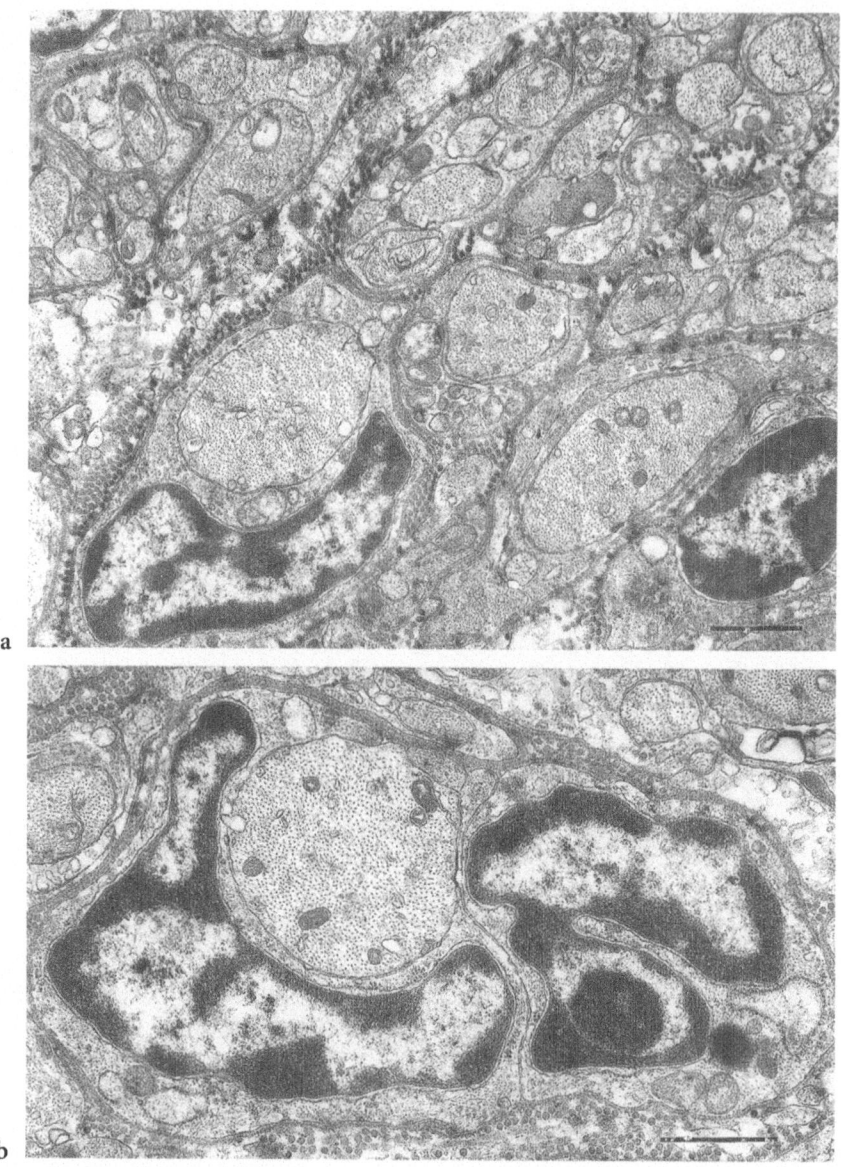

Fig. 94 a, b. Total absence of myelin sheaths (amyelinization) in the peripheral and central nervous system in an 8-day-old, otherwise mature newborn with hydrocephalus internus (autopsy, case 5 in [939]). The maximal thickness of promyelin fibers (numerical relation of axon: Schwann cell = 1:1) is 3 µm. These fibers contain an increased number of neurofilaments (see Fig. 95). The Schwann cells also contain an increased number of filaments. **a** 12,300; **b** × 16,700. (From [974])

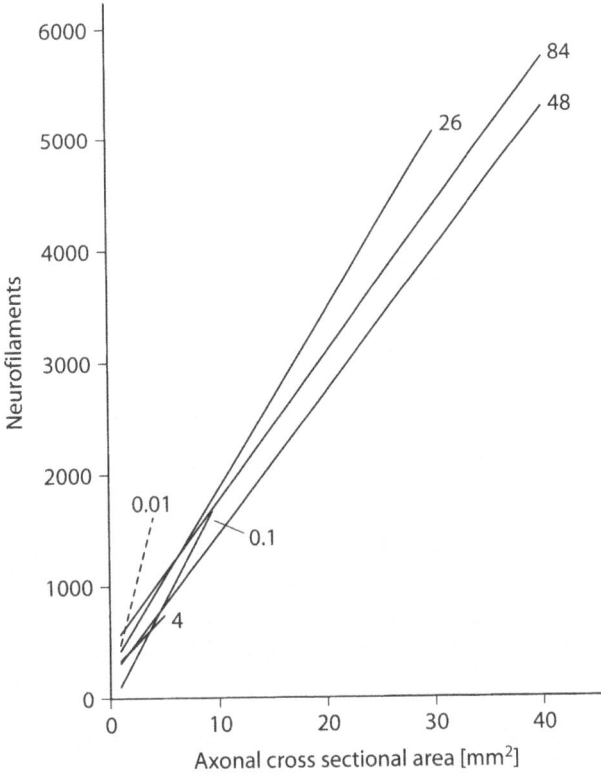

Fig. 95. Same case as in Fig. 94. The number of neurofilaments per axon (*ordinate*) are related to the axonal cross-sectional area in μm² (*abscissa*) of four control cases at the age between 4 months before term and 84 months thereafter (*solid line*) in comparison to the 8-day-old newborn with complete absence of myelin sheaths (*dotted line*). The age of the individuals is indicated in months at the *upper right end* of the lines. The slope of the *dotted line* is considerably steeper than that of the *solid lines* for the normal cases thus indicating the increased neurofilament density in the axons without myelin sheaths. (From [958])

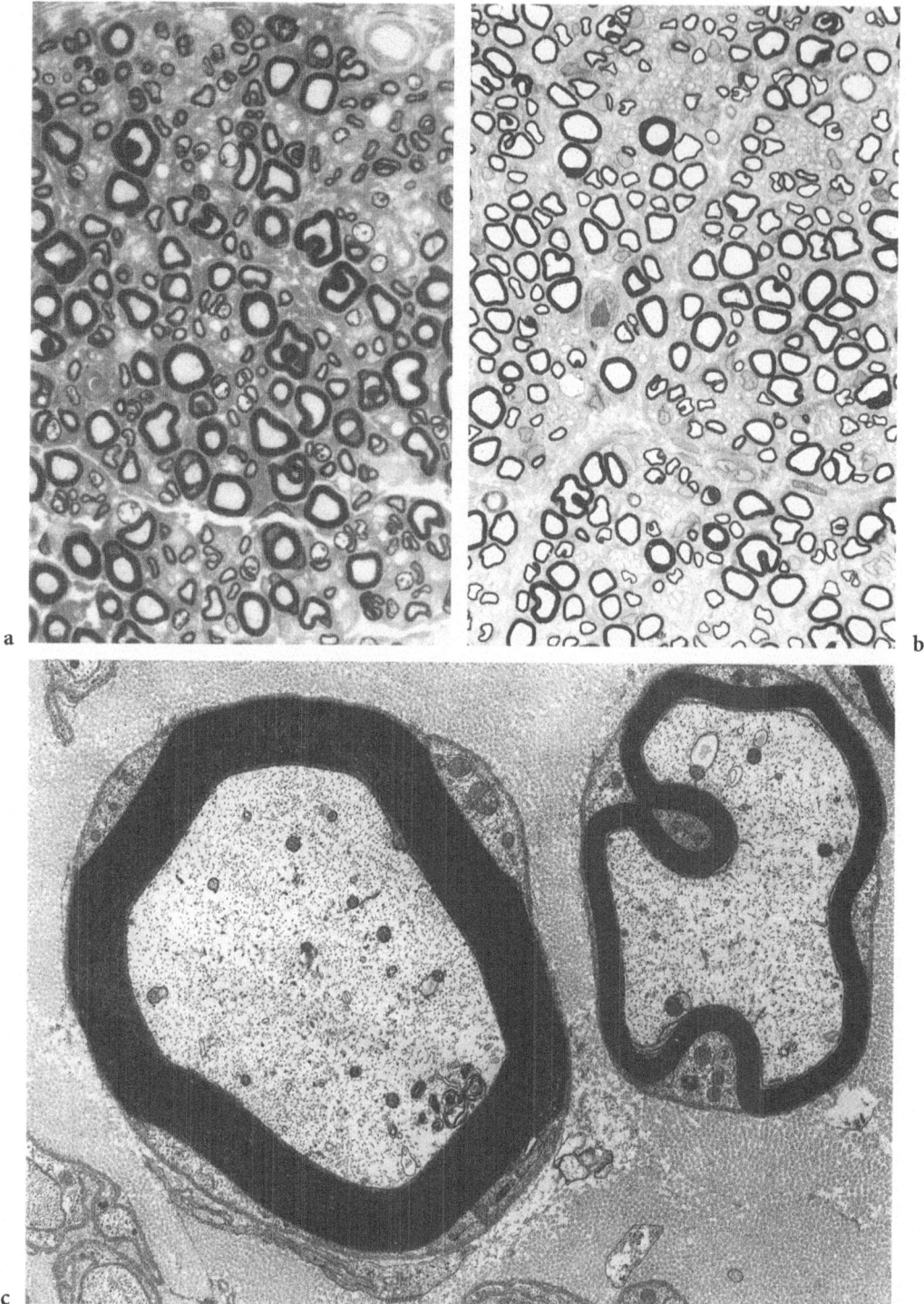

Fig. 96 a, b. Primary hypomyelination (**b**) without signs of demyelination or remyelination in a 39-month-old child in comparison to a 32-month-old control case studied at autopsy (**a**). Most of the myelin sheaths in **b** are too thin in relation to the age as well as to the axonal caliber. **a** × 928; **b** × 912. **c** On the *left*, there is one of the rare nerve fibers with a nearly normally thick myelin sheath, whereas on the *right* a hypomyelinated axon without any signs of prior demyelination or remyelination is shown. (This case was clinically suggestive of Leigh's disease.) × 25,560. (From [953])

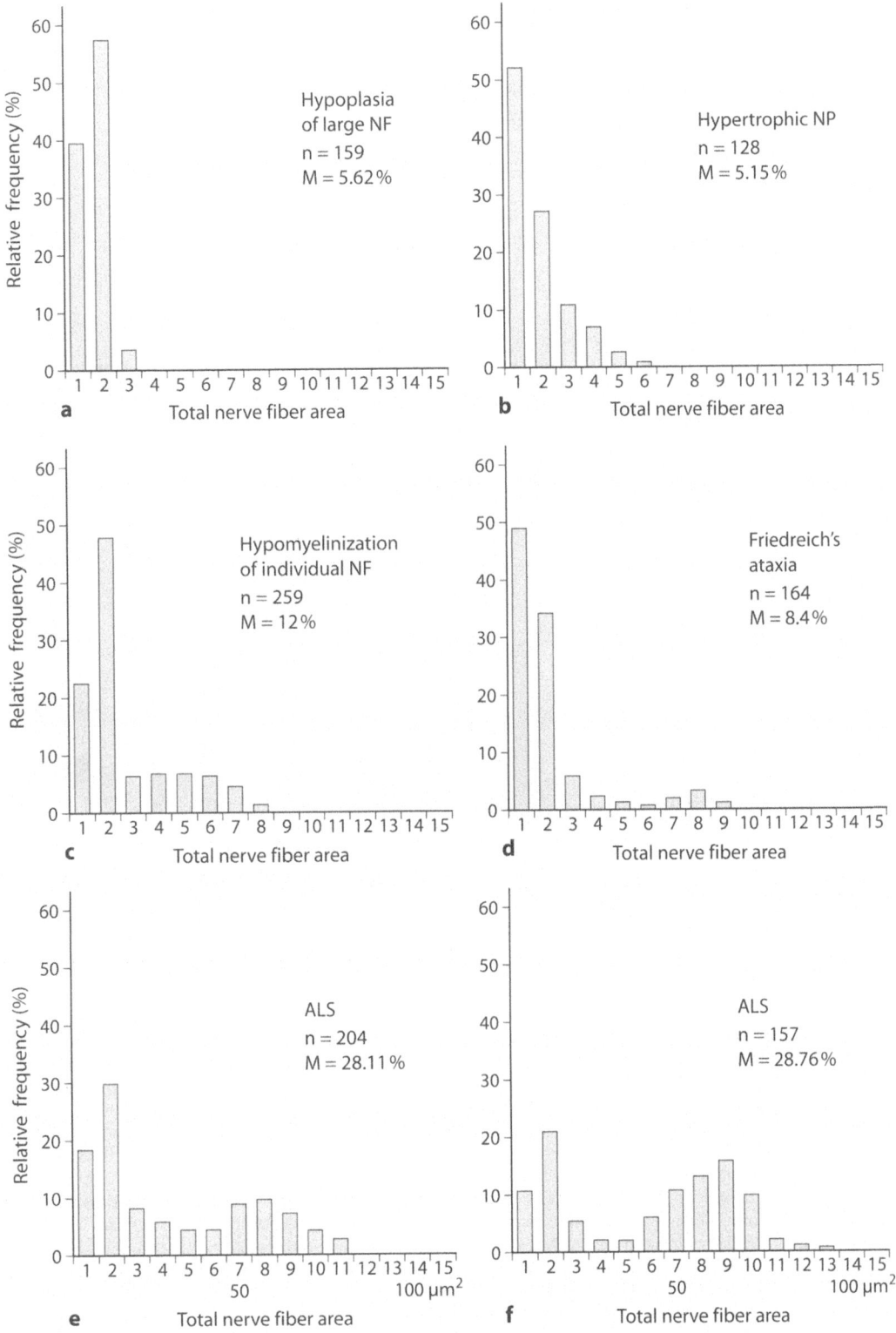

Fig. 97a–f. Characteristic histograms of the total nerve fiber areas in a variety of different neuropathies (**a–d**) in comparison to ALS cases with a nearly normal caliber spectrum (**e, f**) (*n* = number of nerve fibers measured optic-electronically; *M* = area of myelin sheaths per endoneurial area in percent)

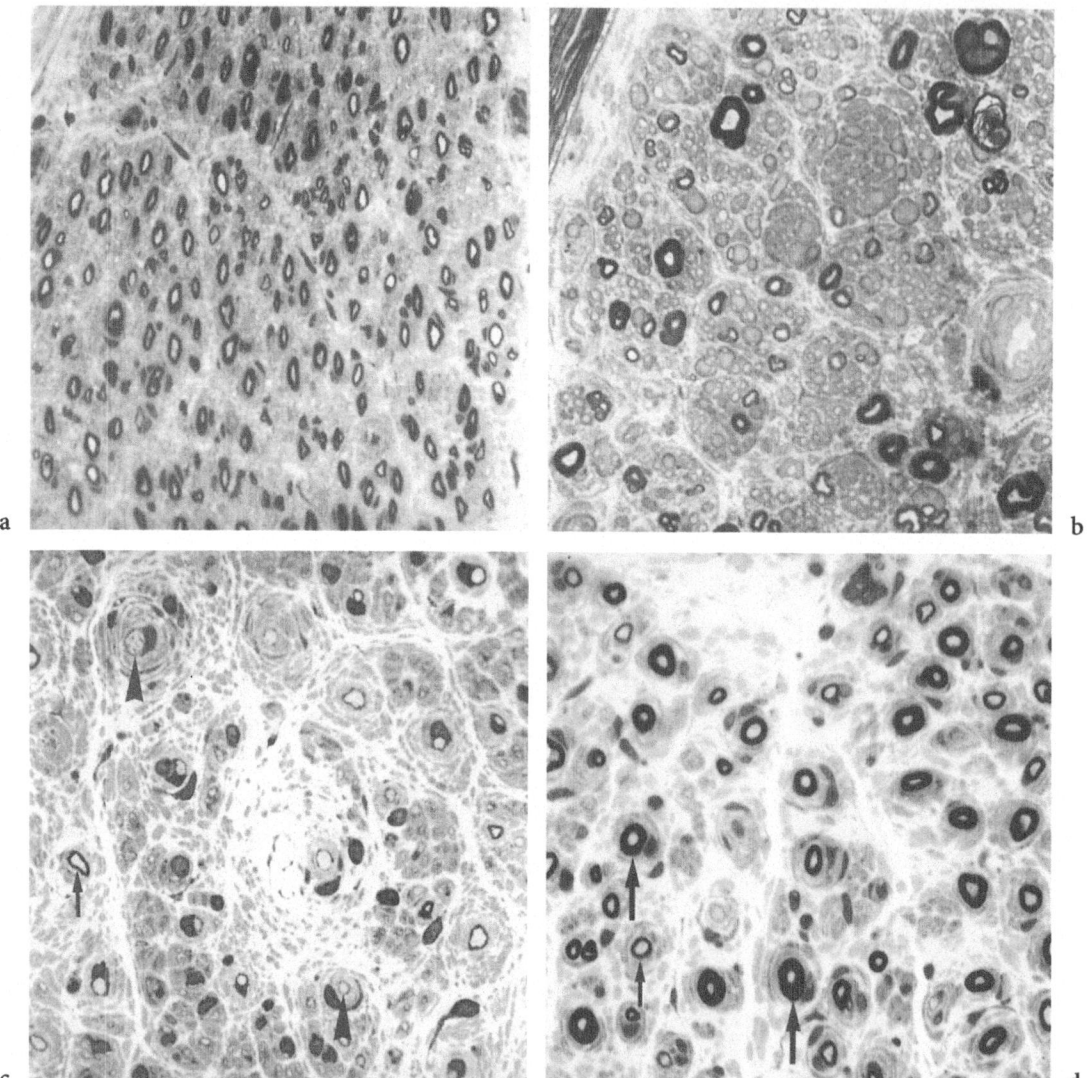

Fig. 98 a – d. Hypertrophic neuropathies in different developmental stages of onion bulb formation, i.e., concentrically arranged Schwann cell processes around demyelinated (*arrowheads*), thinly remyelinated (*small arrows*), and hypermyelinated (*large arrows*) nerve fibers. The endoneurial collagen is unevenly increased (pseudohypertrophy), the endoneurial edema in **c**, **d**, and **f** is prominent. **a** Seven-year-old boy with HMSN I. There are some hypomyelinated nerve fibers, rare onion bulb formations at an early stage, and moderately increased endoneurial connective tissue. **b** Fifty-one-year-old male with Refsum's disease. The number of large and small myelinated nerve fibers is considerably reduced, the number of Schwann cell nuclei is clearly increased. Focal proliferations of Schwann cells are more prominent than typical onion bulb formations. The endoneurial connective tissue is clearly increased. **c** Sixteen-year-old girl with an early stage of hypertrophic neuropathy (probably Dejerine-Sottas disease). Sensory NCV was 2 m/s. Prominent onion bulb formations are apparent around demyelinated nerve fibers (*arrowheads*). The endoneurial connective tissue is increased; there is considerable endoneurial edema. A vacuolated macrophage can also be seen. **d** Ten-year-old girl with advanced, probably autosomal dominant hypertrophic neuropathy (HMSN Ia). Onion bulb formations around demyelinated, thinly remyelinated (hypomyelinated) fibers, and nerve fibers with disproportionately thick myelin sheaths (hypermyelinated fibers) are apparent. The endoneurial connective tissue is increased and edematous. **e, f** s. p. 113

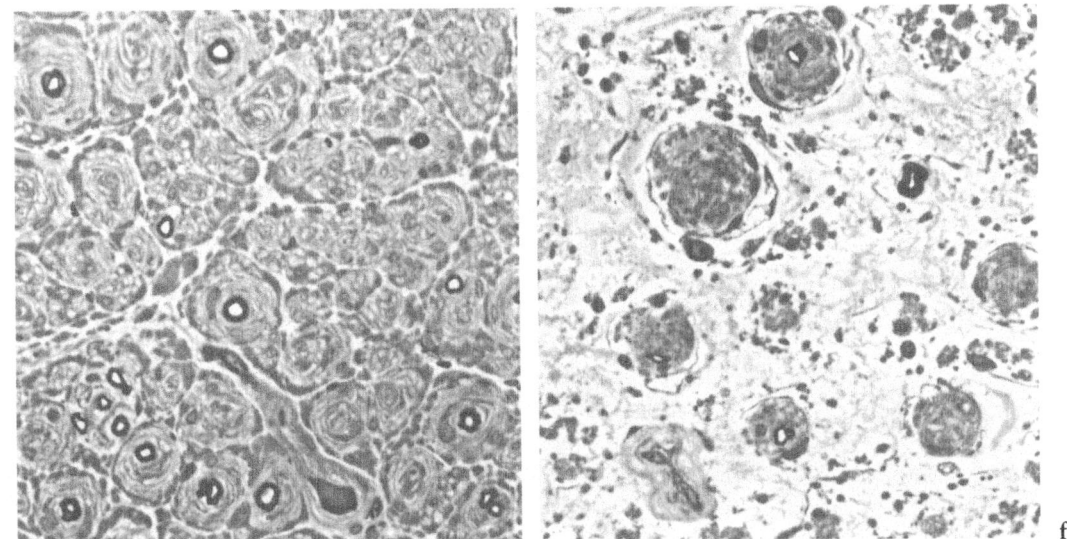

Fig. 98 e, f. e Twenty-two-year-old male with chronic recurrent Guillain-Barré syndrome and involvement of cranial nerves (Miller-Fisher syndrome). Prominent, multilayered onion bulb formations can be seen with a clear increase of the endoneurial connective tissue and a reduction in the number of large and small myelinated fibers. **f** Same nerve as in **e**, but another fascicle with more severe endoneurial edema

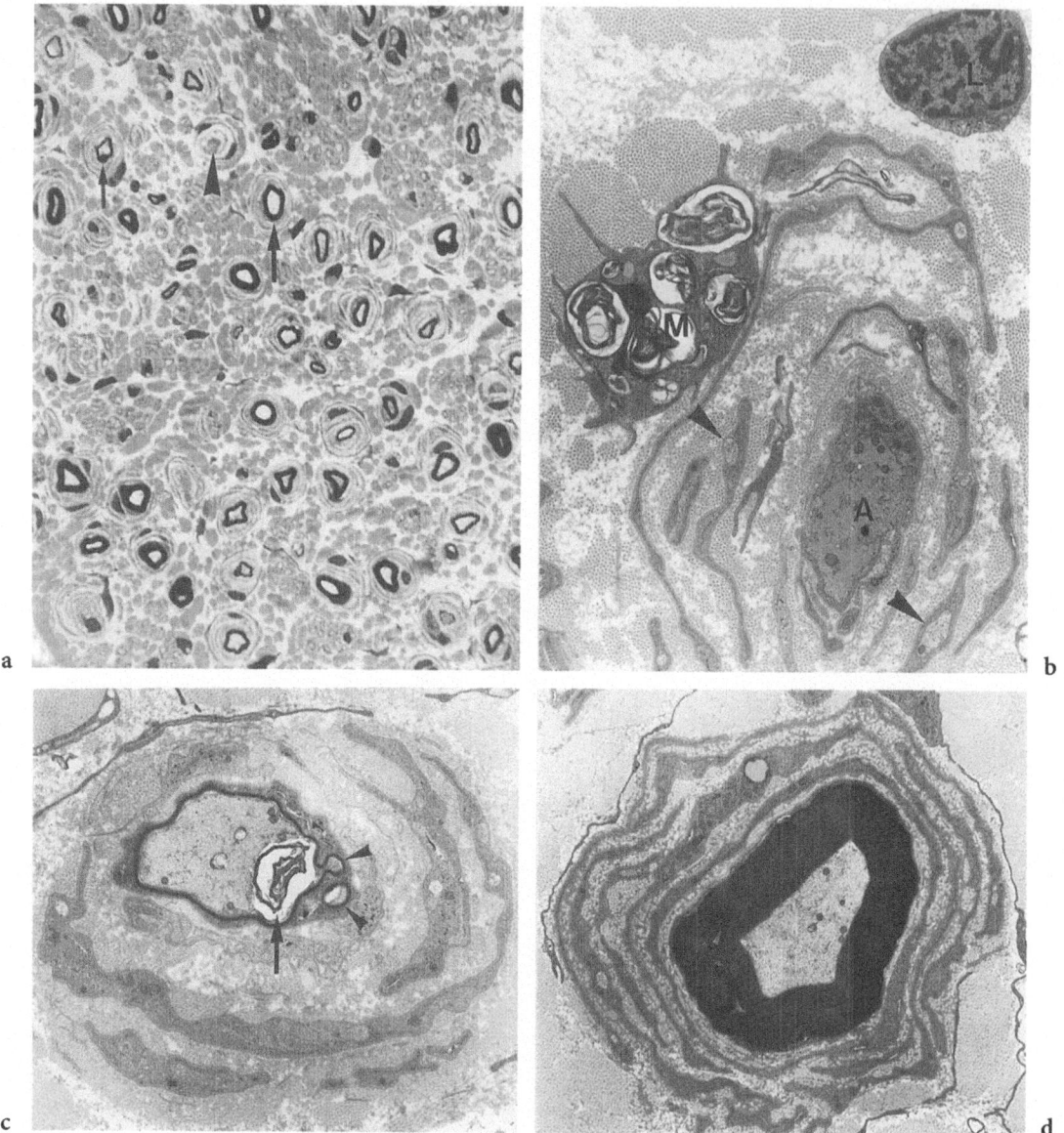

Fig. 99 a–d. Hypertrophic neuropathy in a 10-year-old girl (presumably type HMSN Ia). **a** Prominent onion bulb formations around thickly remyelinated (*thick arrow*), thinly remyelinated (*thin arrow*), or demyelinated (*arrowhead*) nerve fibers. The endoneurial connective tissue is increased. × 648. **b** Onion bulb formation around a demyelinated axon (*A*). Unmyelinated axons can be repeatedly seen in the Schwann cell processes of the onion bulb (*arrowheads*). Between these processes are flattened processes presumably of a macrophage, which are not surrounded by a basal lamina. Adjacent lies a large macrophage with myelin degradation products (*M*) and a lymphocyte (*L*). Between the various cell processes there are numerous collagen filaments. × 5,800. **c** Thinly remyelinated nerve fiber with myelin loops (*arrowheads*) and an adaxonal membranous cytoplasmic body (*arrow*) surrounded by Schwann cells and a fibroblastic cell process. × 5,900. **d** Thickly myelinated nerve fiber with 3–5 circumferentially arranged Schwann cell processes. These are remarkably flat and electron dense separated by basal lamina-like material as well as collagen fibrils. × 4,800

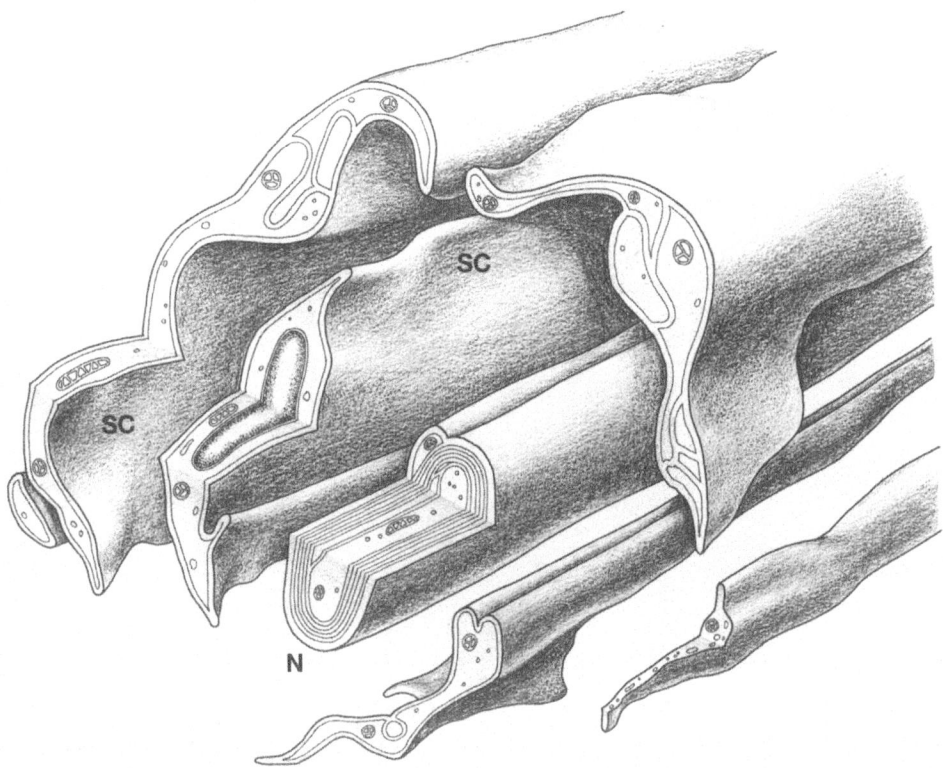

Fig. 100. Three-dimensional reconstruction of a typical "onion bulb formation" with concentrically arranged, multiple inter-digitating Schwann cell processes (*SC*) around a centrally located small myelinated nerve fiber (*N*) in hypertrophic neuropathy. (From [940, 1217]: unpublished drawing)

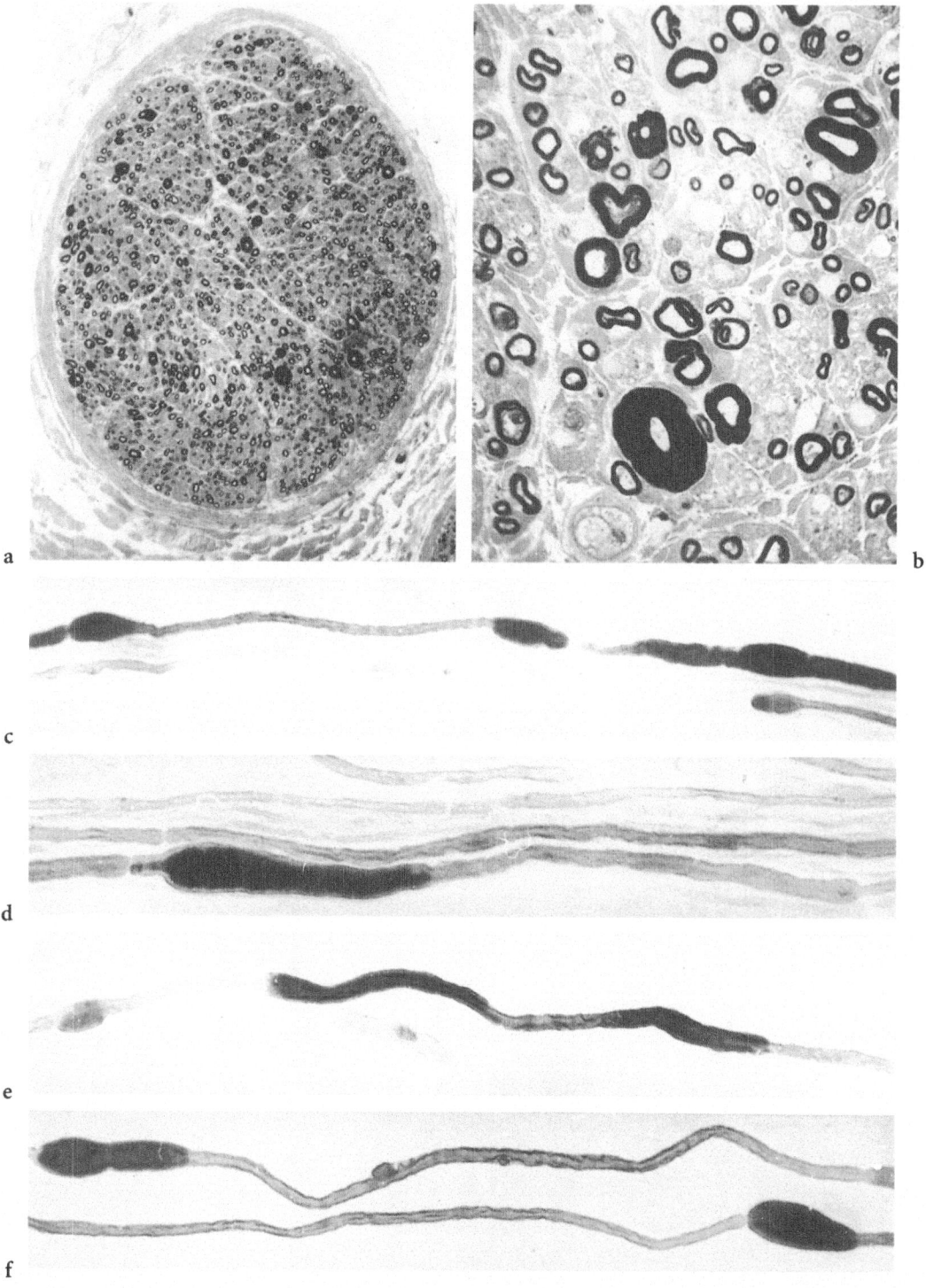

Fig. 101 a–f. Tomaculous neuropathy (hereditary neuropathy with liability to pressure palsies; HNPP) in a 37-year-old patient. The sausage-like distensions of the myelin sheaths ("tomacula") are already visible at low magnification (**a**). **b** At higher magnification there is considerable narrowing of the axonal cross-sectional area. In teased fiber preparations of isolated nerve fibers, the distensions are mainly localized at paranodal segments. The internodes shown are shortened to approximately 250–300 μm (see Fig. 102). **a** 021596; **b** × 600; **c–f** × 140. (From [958])

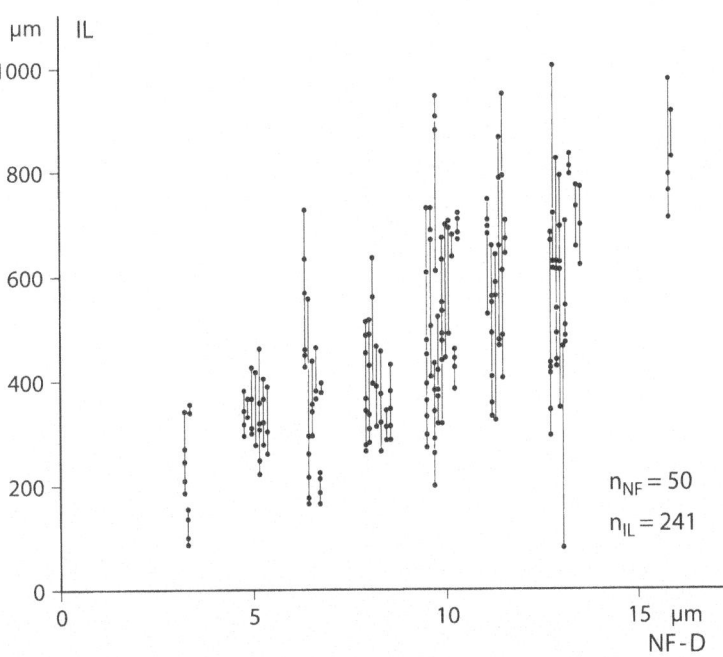

Fig. 102. Internodal lengths (IL) of the internodes of isolated ("teased") nerve fibers in a patient with tomaculous neuropathy with unusual colicy pain (case of [1145]). Some nerve fibers show subsequent short and long internodes as a sign of prior demyelination and remyelination, or paranodal demyelination when only one internode is shortened (intercalated segment, "Schaltstück"). n_{NF}, number of evaluated nerve fibers; n_{IL}, number of internodes measured; *NF-D*, nerve fiber-diameter

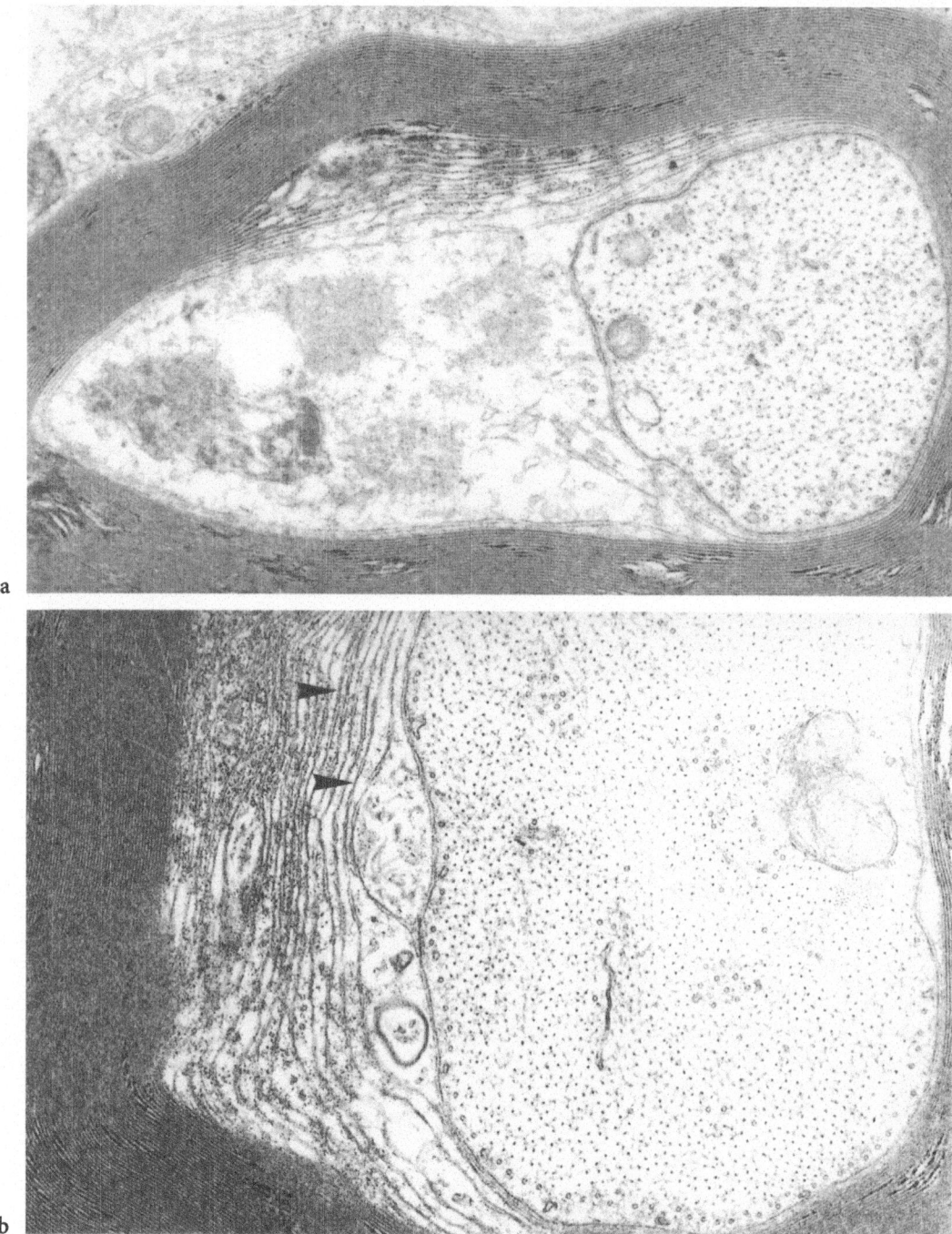

Fig. 103 a, b. Same case as in Fig. 102. **a** Severely distended adaxonal myelin loop at the inner mesaxon with several adjacent uncompacted myelin lamellae at the site of a Schmidt-Lanterman incisure. Amorphous substances which are not surrounded by a membrane and some vesicular components can be seen in the cytoplasm of the adaxonal myelin loop. **b** The innermost myelin lamellae of this presumably regenerated small nerve fiber are not compacted. At several sites, the extracellular spaces between adjacent noncompacted myelin lamellae appear to be obliterated (*arrowheads*). In the axoplasm the microtubules are unevenly distributed. **a, b** × 34,000. (Modified from [1145])

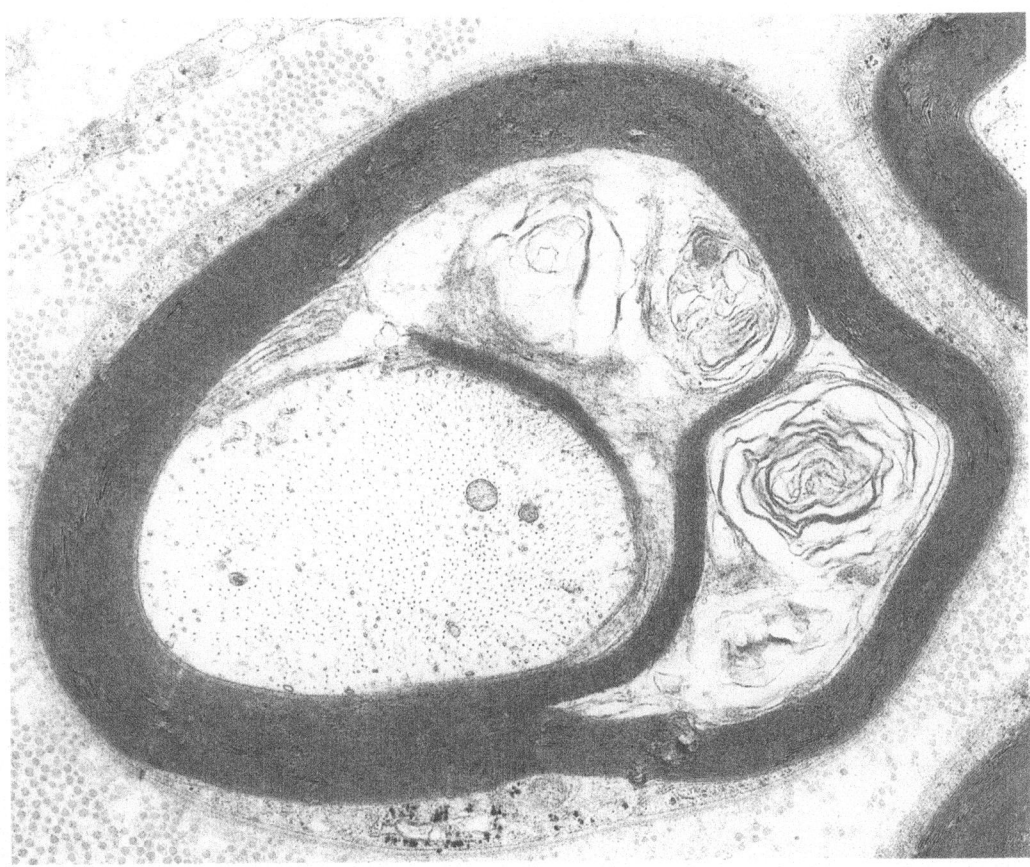

Fig. 104. Same case as in Figs. 102 and 103. Several compact myelin lamellae are interrupted at the border zone to the noncompacted part of the myelin sheath. In the Schmidt-Lanterman incisures are several membranous, concentrically lamellated figures with loose arrangement of the lamellae. × 21,000

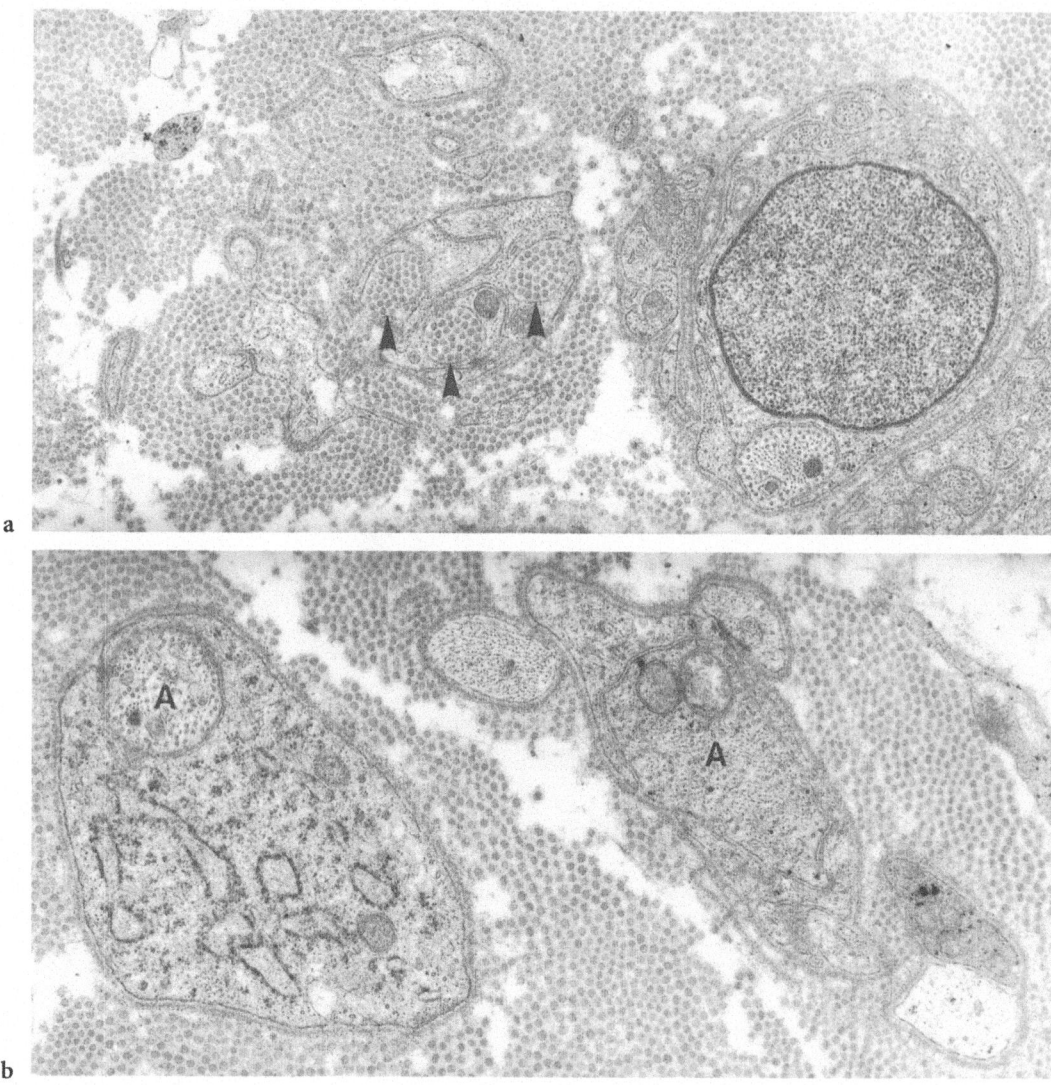

Fig. 105. Same case as in Figs. 102–104. **a** The unmyelinated axons are focally replaced by collagen fibrils (so-called collagen pockets; *arrowheads*). In addition there are several empty Schwann cell processes with no contact to axons, indicating prior degeneration of unmyelinated axons. × 17,000. **b** In this group of Remak fibers only two unmyelinated axons (*A*) are left. The number of the Schwann cell processes is considerably increased on the *right side*. On the *left side* there are granular substances in the endoplasmic reticulum and numerous polyribosomes indicating active protein synthesis in the Schwann cell. × 21,000

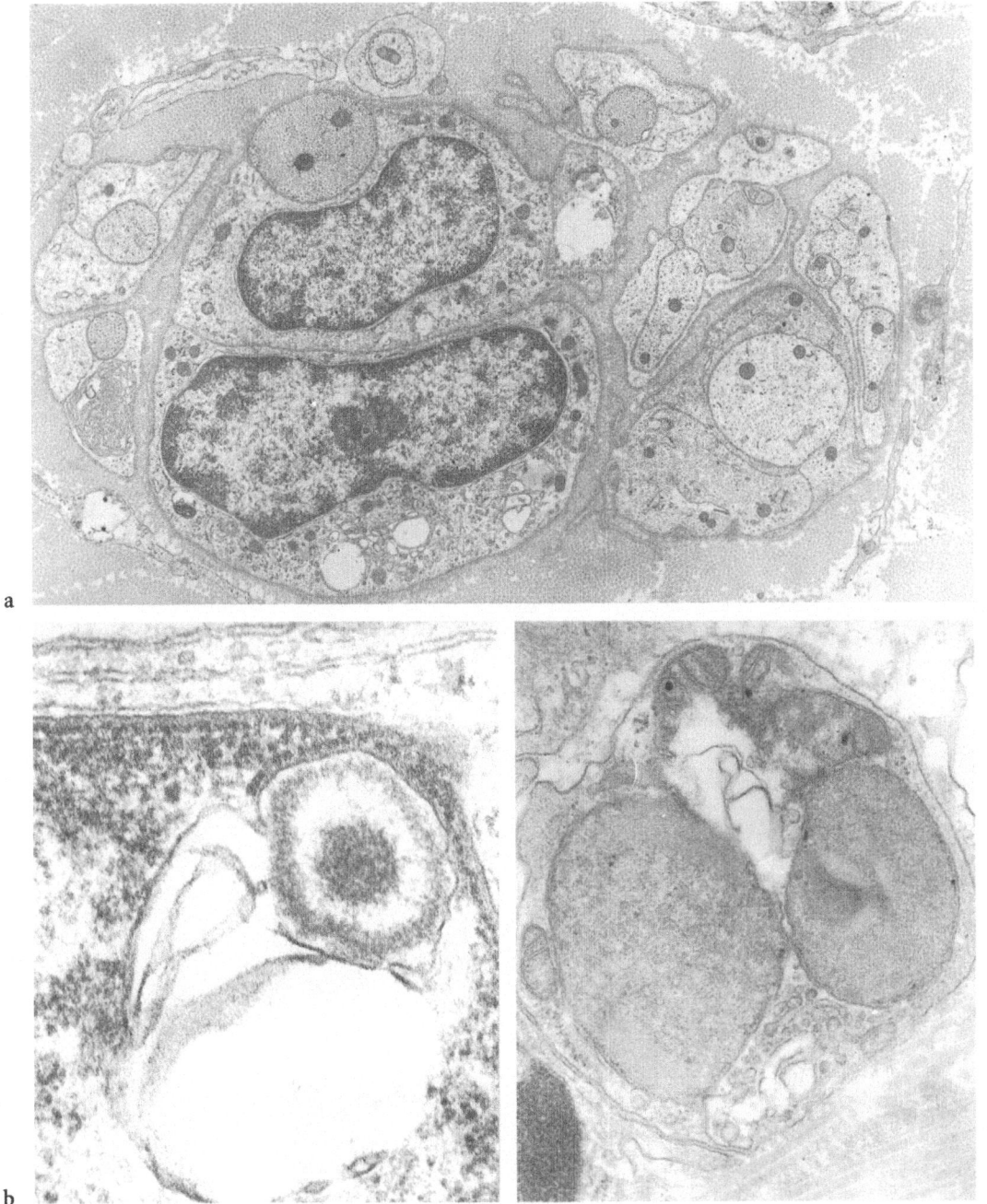

Fig. 106a–c. Severe form of a congenital neuropathy in a 15-year-old girl. **a** Aplasia of large myelinated nerve fibers in clinically suggested Friedreich's ataxia with Roussy-Levy syndrome showing an axon Schwann-cell complex with some very large, presumably regenerated (or demyelinated) axons. × 11,100. **b** Unusual nuclear inclusion in a Schwann cell with vacuoles and concentric rings (presumably incipient calcospherite) which are surrounded by a membrane. × 73,000. **c** Unusual, abnormally large cytosomes, presumably of mitochondrial origin because of the surrounding double membranes, with filaments or lamellae focally arranged in parallel, and granular, homogeneous or finely vesicular inclusions in the matrix, adjacent to largely inconspicuous mitochondria in an endoneurial fibroblast. Two mitochondria show artificial vacuoles. × 36,000

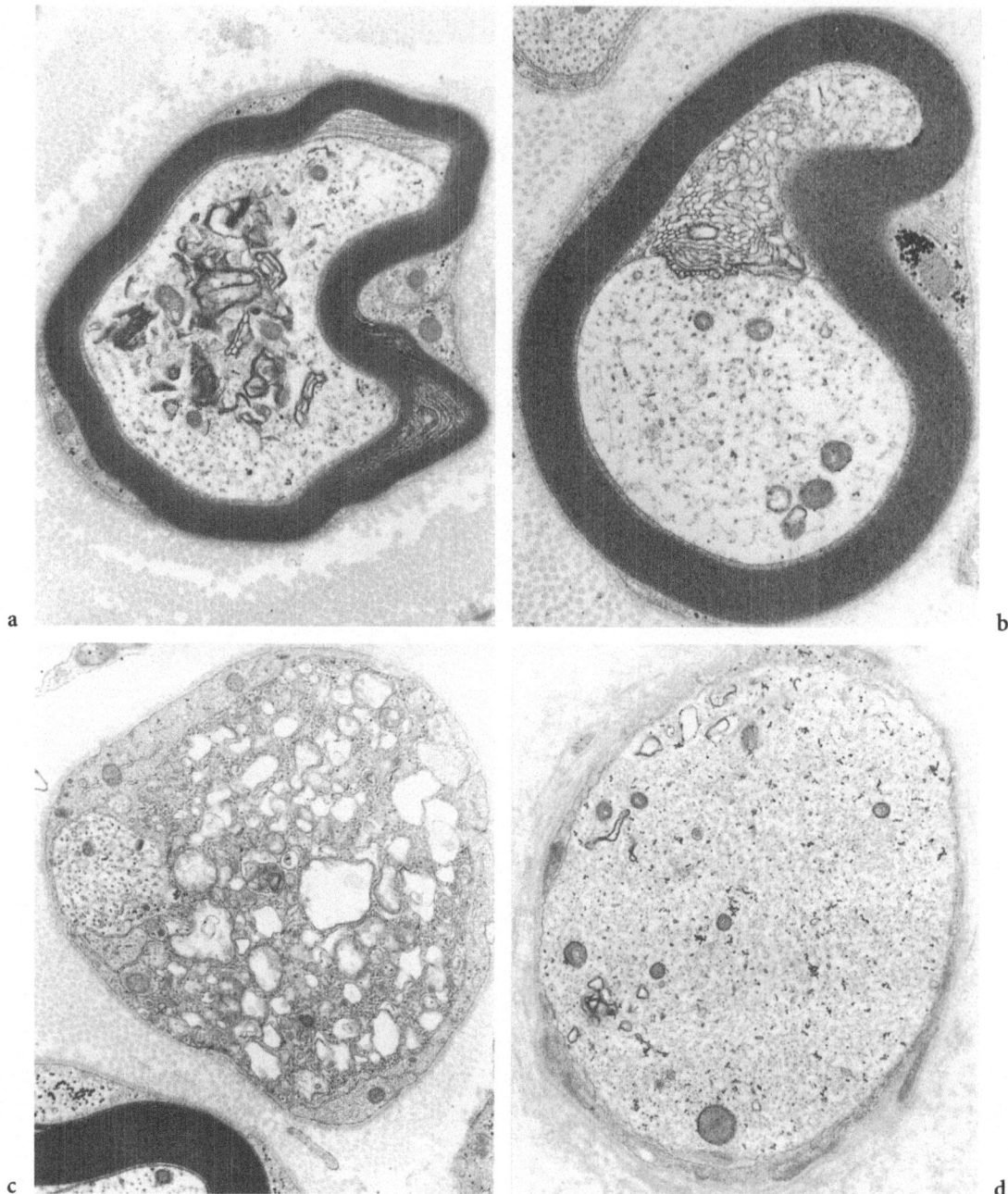

Fig. 107 a – d. Chronic neuropathy of the axonal type, presumably HMSN II, in a 55-year-old man. **a** Multiple membranous axoplasmic phospholipid precipitates in the center of the axons, as they may also occur as an artifact after prolonged fixation in phosphate buffered glutaraldehyde (From [960]). × 19,000. **b** Multivesicular disintegration of adaxonal myelin lamellae in an otherwise inconspicuous nerve fiber. × 22,000. **c** Unusual axon-Schwann cell complex with multivesicular components in a degenerating Schwann cell. × 17,000. **d** Severely enlarged axon partially surrounded by Schwann cell processes. In addition to glycogen granules, it contains several vesicles, mitochondria, an increased number of neurofilaments, microtubules, and finely granulated substances. × 16,000

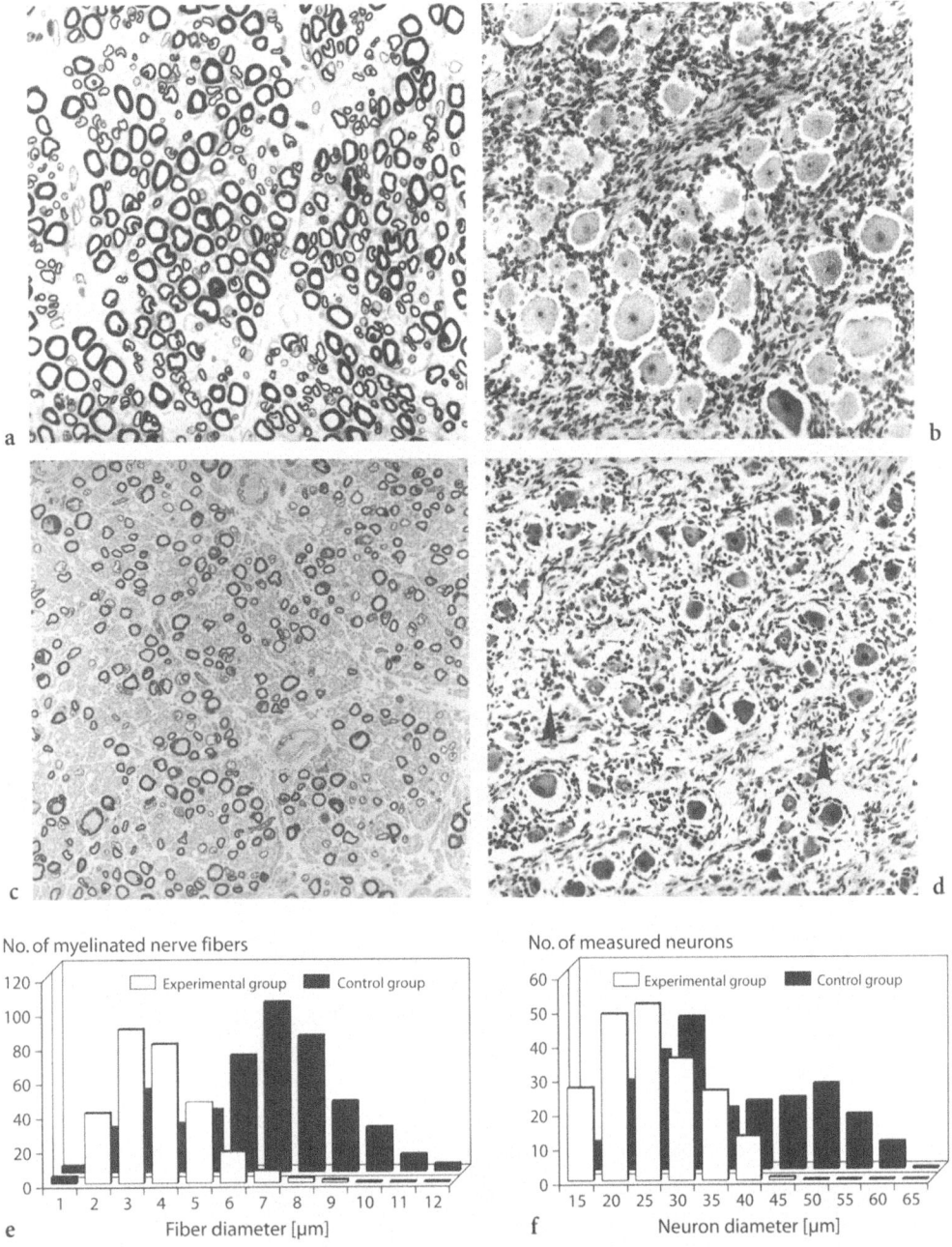

Fig. 108 a–f. HMSN with deafness, mental retardation, and absence of large myelinated nerve fibers in a 2 1/2-year-old girl [707]. **a, b** Sural nerve (**a**), and spinal ganglion (**b**) of an age-matched control (26 months of age). **a, b** × 417. **c** Sural nerve of the patient. It is apparent when compared to **a** that there is a complete absence of large myelinated nerve fibers. The number of small myelinated nerve fibers is not reduced and there are many unmyelinated axons. Some of these are artificially swollen as a result of advanced autolysis of this autopsy specimen. × 239. **d** There is a deficiency of large neurons in the spinal ganglion. At the possible site of degenerated neurons there are presumably some nodules of Nageotte (*arrowheads*) although the number of nuclei is not significantly increased when compared to the control ganglion (**b**). × 239. **e** Comparison of the histograms for the myelinated nerve fibers of the control case and the patient reveals a shift to the left resulting from the absence of large myelinated nerve fibers in the patient. **f** The histograms for the neurons in the spinal ganglia show a corresponding lack of large neurons with a shift to the left in the patient

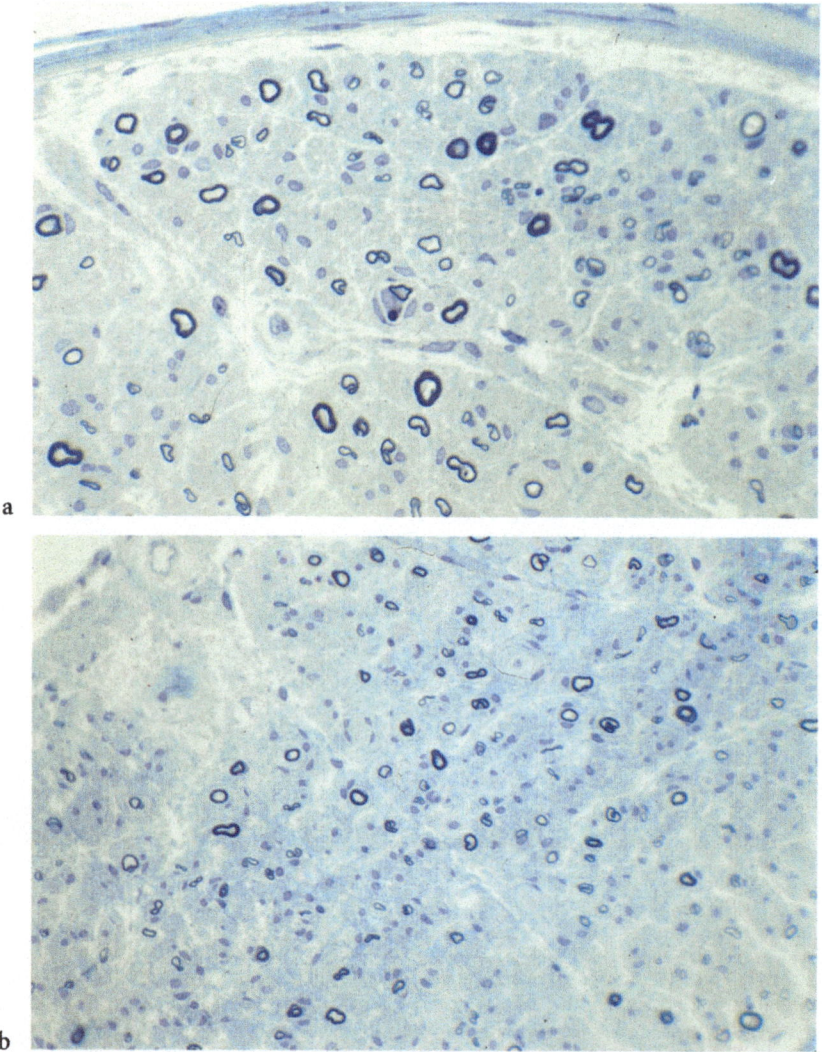

Fig. 109a–d. Unusual sensorimotor neuropathy in a 20-year-old female with mental retardation and a congenital cataract (From [992]). **a, b** The number of myelinated nerve fibers is severely reduced. Demyelinating alterations and small onion bulb formations dominate. Toluidine blue. **c, d** s. p. 125

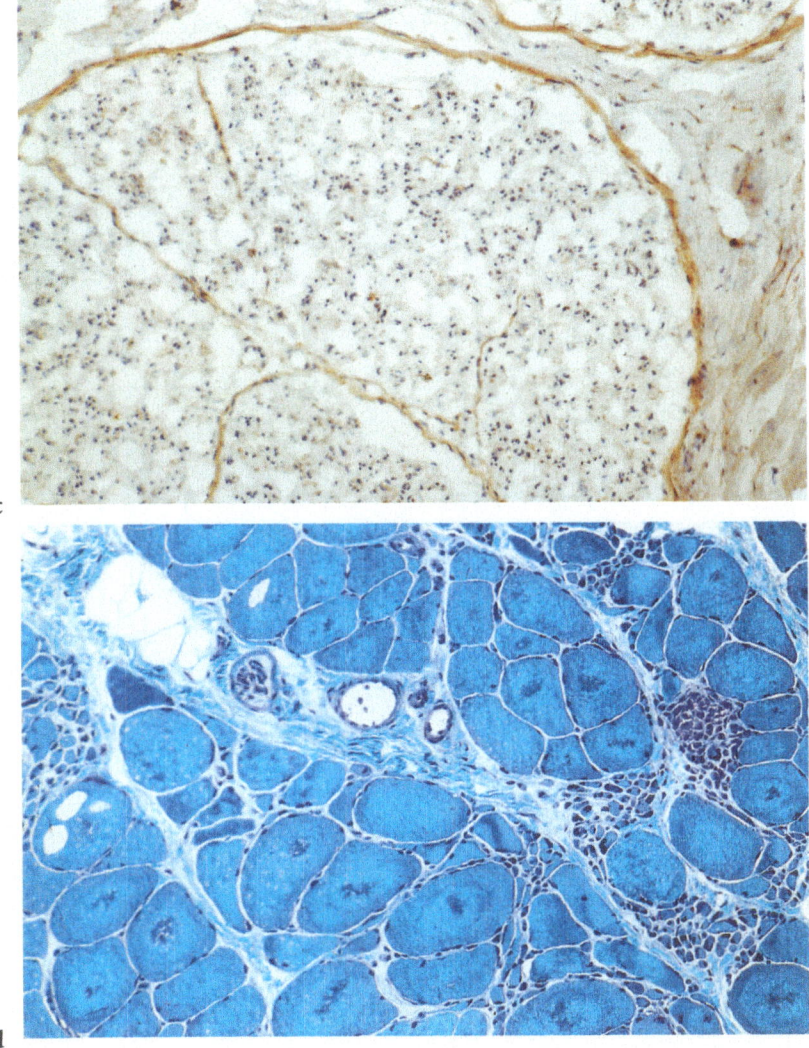

c

d

Fig. 109. **c** In the endoneurium there are epithelial membrane antigen (EMA)-positive cell processes of abnormally branched perineurial cells. **d** The muscle biopsy shows considerable chronic neurogenic atrophy with many target fibers and a focal myophagic reaction subsequent to muscle fiber necrosis

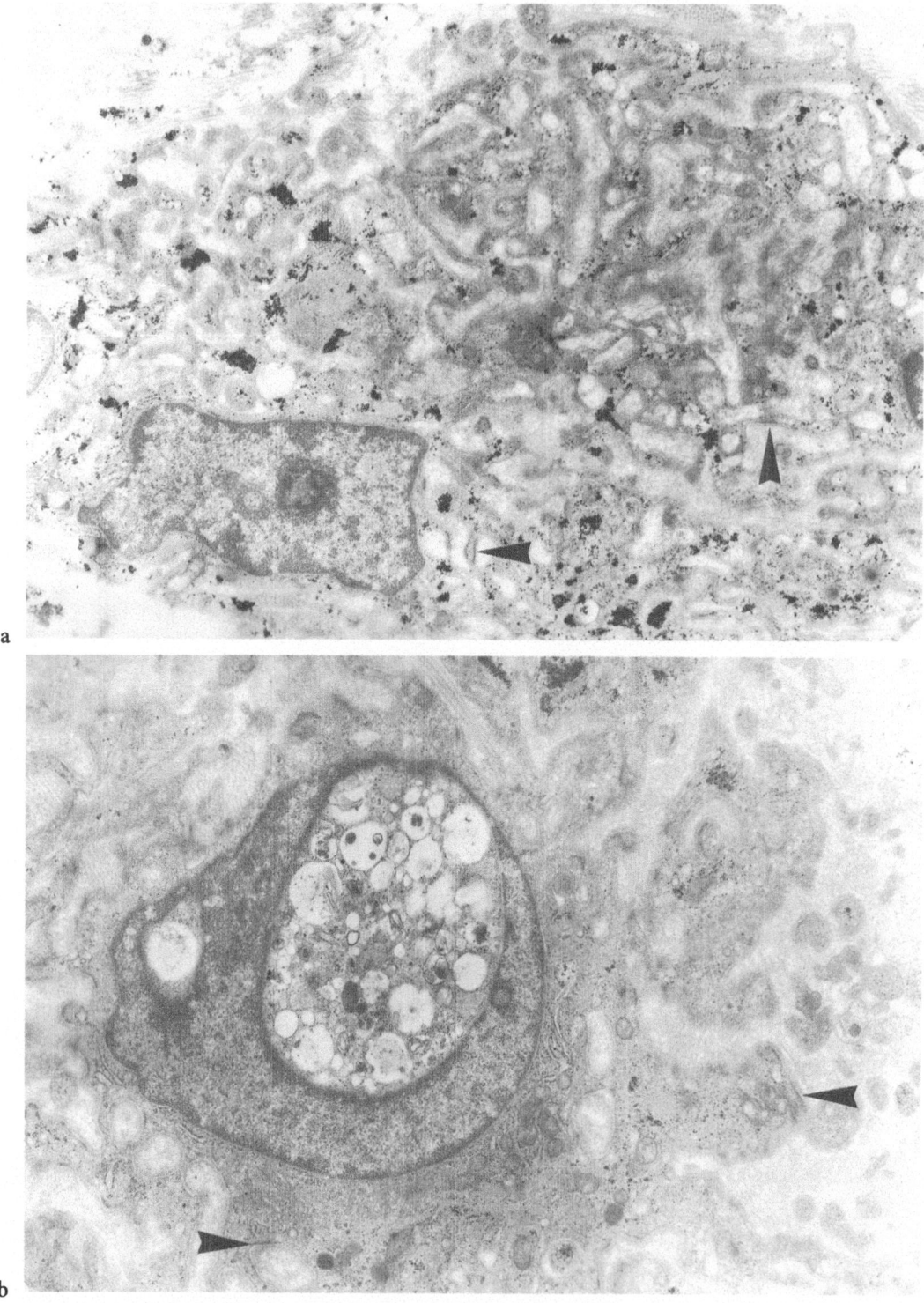

Fig. 110 a, b. Same case as in Fig. 109. Electron microscopic images of atypical perineurial cells within the endoneurium showing abnormally branched cell processes and multiple invaginations filled with reticulin fibers (immature collagen fibrils) and an inconspicuous nucleus in **a**, but with a nucleus indented by cytoplasmic invaginations containing numerous vesicles in **b**. Hemidesmosome-like structures are apparent at several sites (*arrowheads*). Glycogen granules and intermediate filaments are more or less focally accumulated. **a** × 10,000; **b** × 13,000

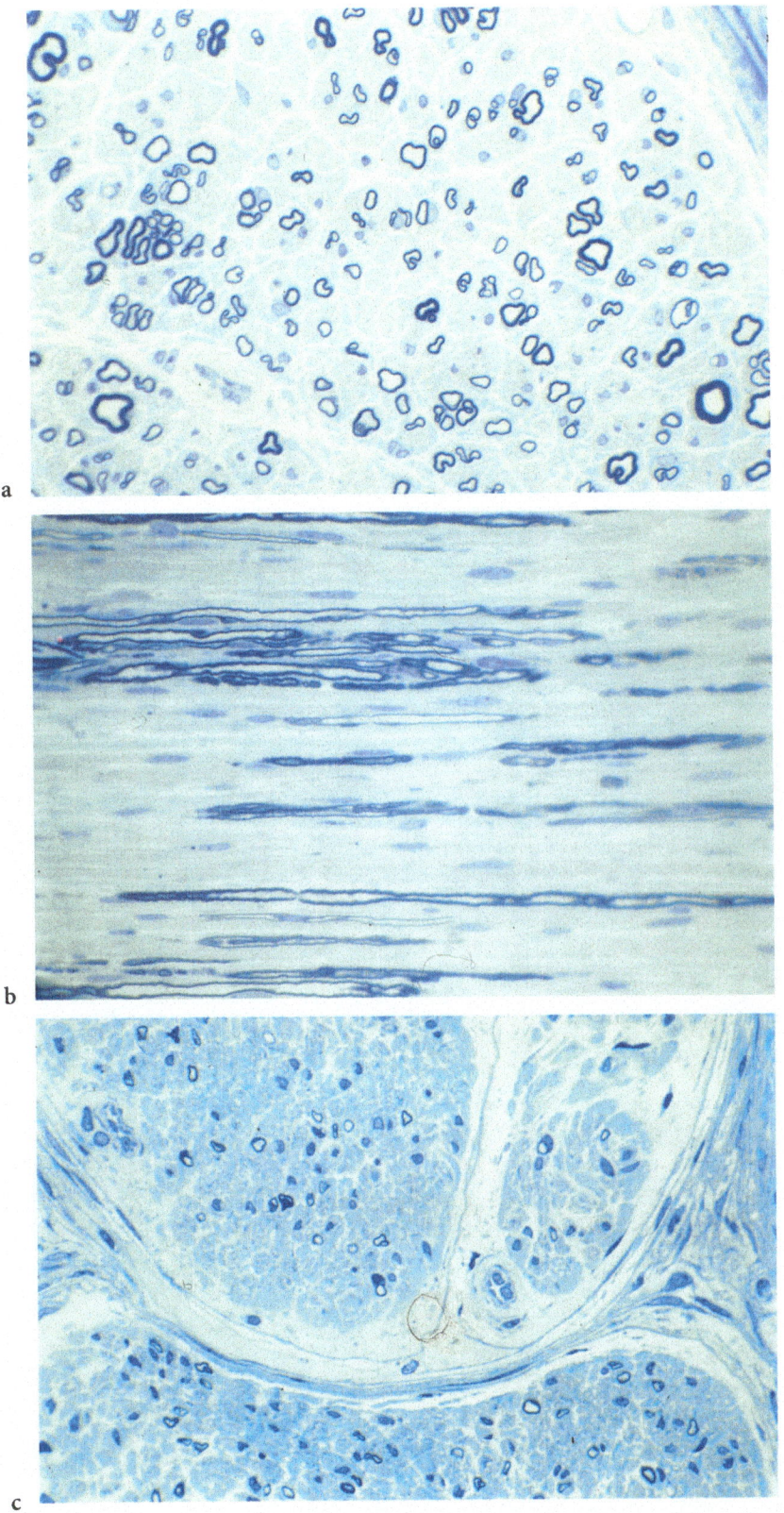

Fig. 111. Legend s. p. 128

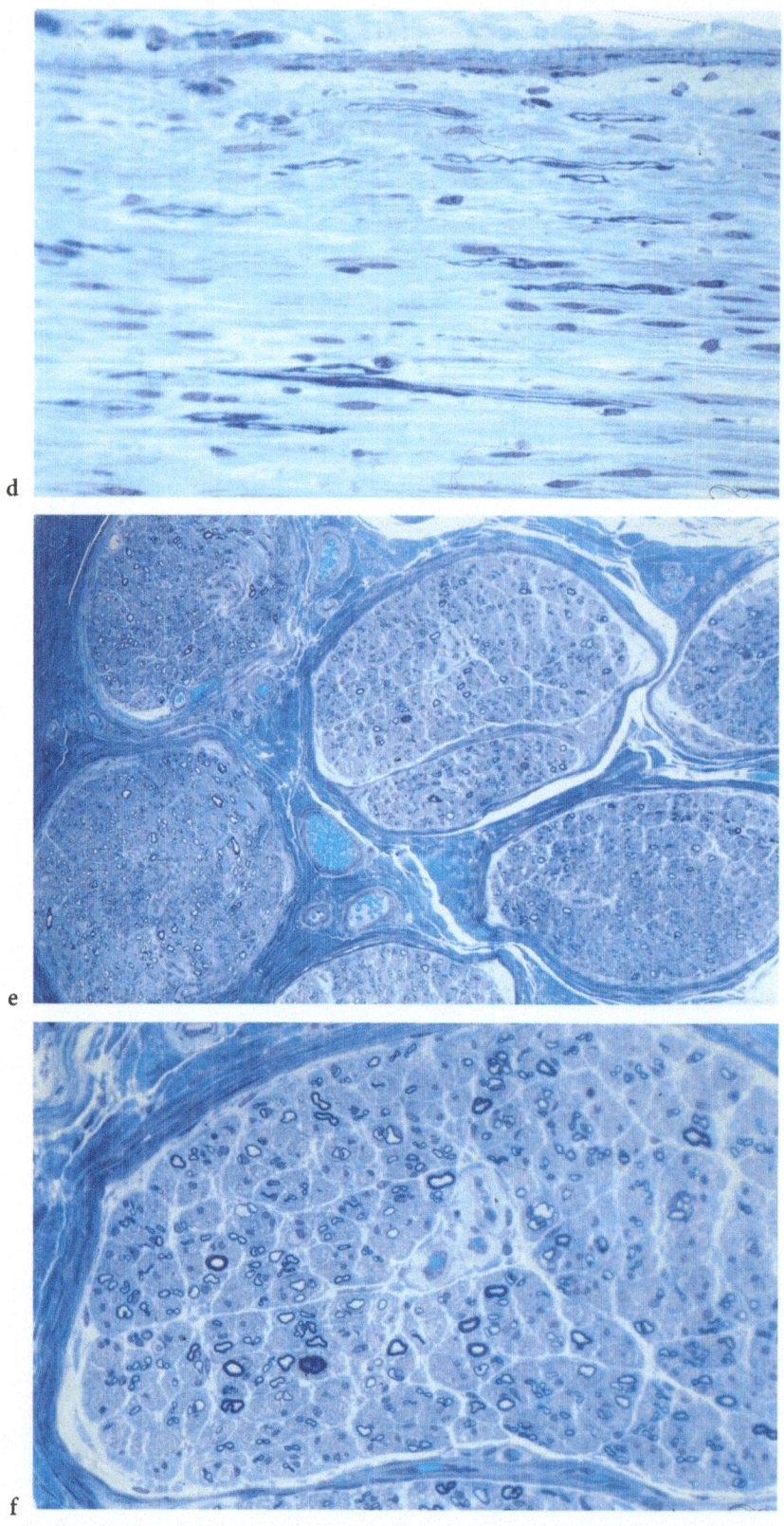

Fig. 111. a, b HMSN II showing loss of large and small myelinated nerve fibers and numerous clusters of regenerated fibers. **c, d** HMSN-Lom in a 13-year-old girl of Bulgarian origin (From [38]). The number of myelinated nerve fibers is severely reduced. **e, f** Dominantly inherited HMSN X in a 29-year-old man with a new point mutation in codon 39 of the connexin32 gene. There is a prominent neuropathy of a combined axonal/neuronal and demyelinating type. (From [1016])

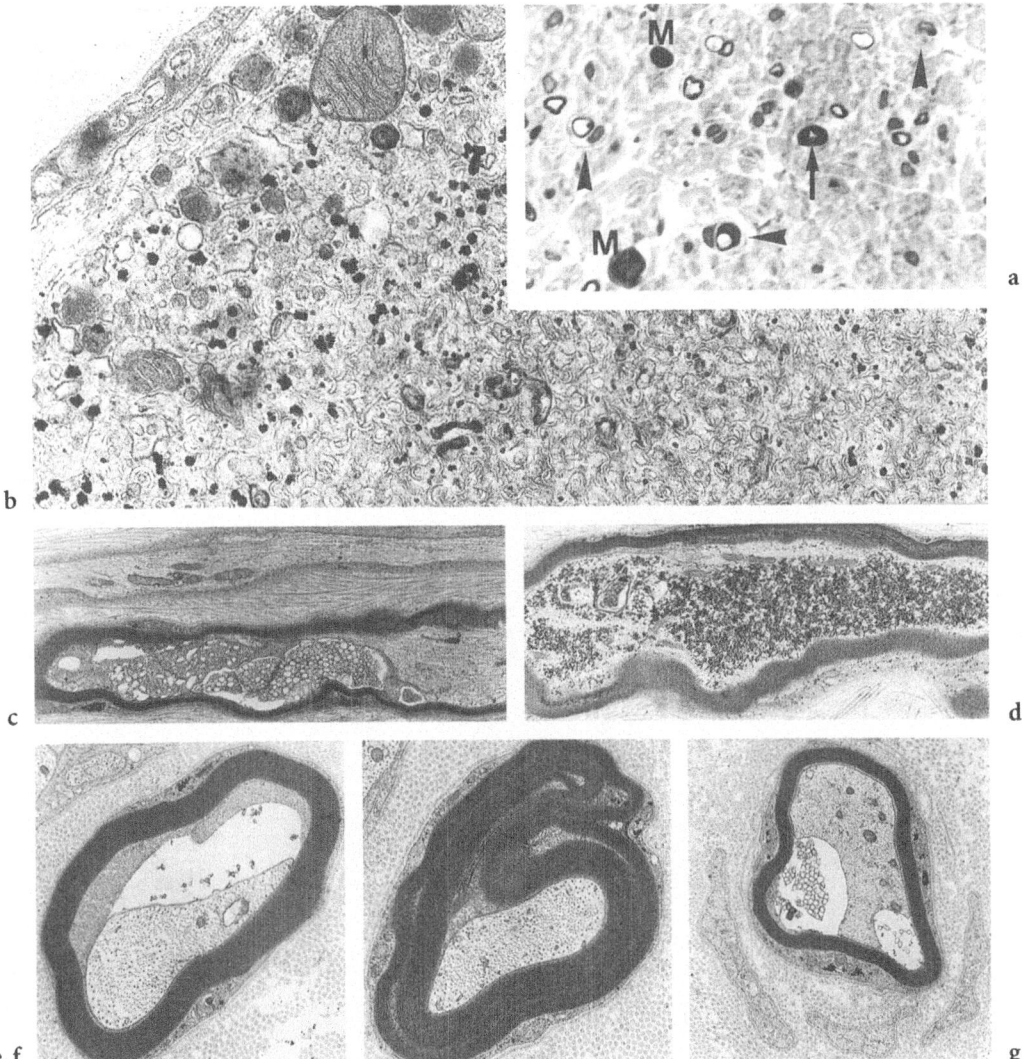

Fig. 112 a – g. Same case as in Fig. 111 c, d (HMSN L). **a** Cross section of the sural nerve with complete absence of large myelinated nerve fibers. The number of small myelinated nerve fibers is considerably reduced. Incipient onion bulb formation can occasionally be seen (*arrowheads*). An atrophic axon is hypermyelinated (*arrow*). A myelin ovoid is indicated by *M*. The unmyelinated nerve fibers appear to be relatively well preserved. × 800. **b** This unusual axon is severely enlarged and filled with numerous curvilinear structures, dense bodies, glycogen-like granules, and small vesicles in addition to mitochondria. Many curvilinear structures with a double contour resemble cup-like indented vesicles. The axon is covered by a thin cellular layer with a basal lamina (Schwann cell processes). × 39,000. **c** Microvesicular disintegration of a thin myelin sheath of a small myelinated nerve fiber adjacent to a well-preserved unmyelinated axon. × 7,000. **d** The axon of this myelinated nerve fiber is filled with glycogen granules. × 7,000. **e** The adaxonal cytoplasm of the Schwann cell (inner loop of the myelin sheath) is filled with filamentous material. An adjacent vacuole contains glycogen-like granules. The axon appears somewhat compressed. × 12,000. **f** The myelin loop of this axon is subdivided by several Schmidt-Lanterman incisures. × 12,600. **g** The innermost myelin lamella of this myelin sheath shows finely vesicular lysis at two sites. This thinly remyelinated nerve fiber is surrounded by several concentrically arranged Schwann cell processes and remnants of a basal lamina (early stage of an onion bulb formation). × 8,700

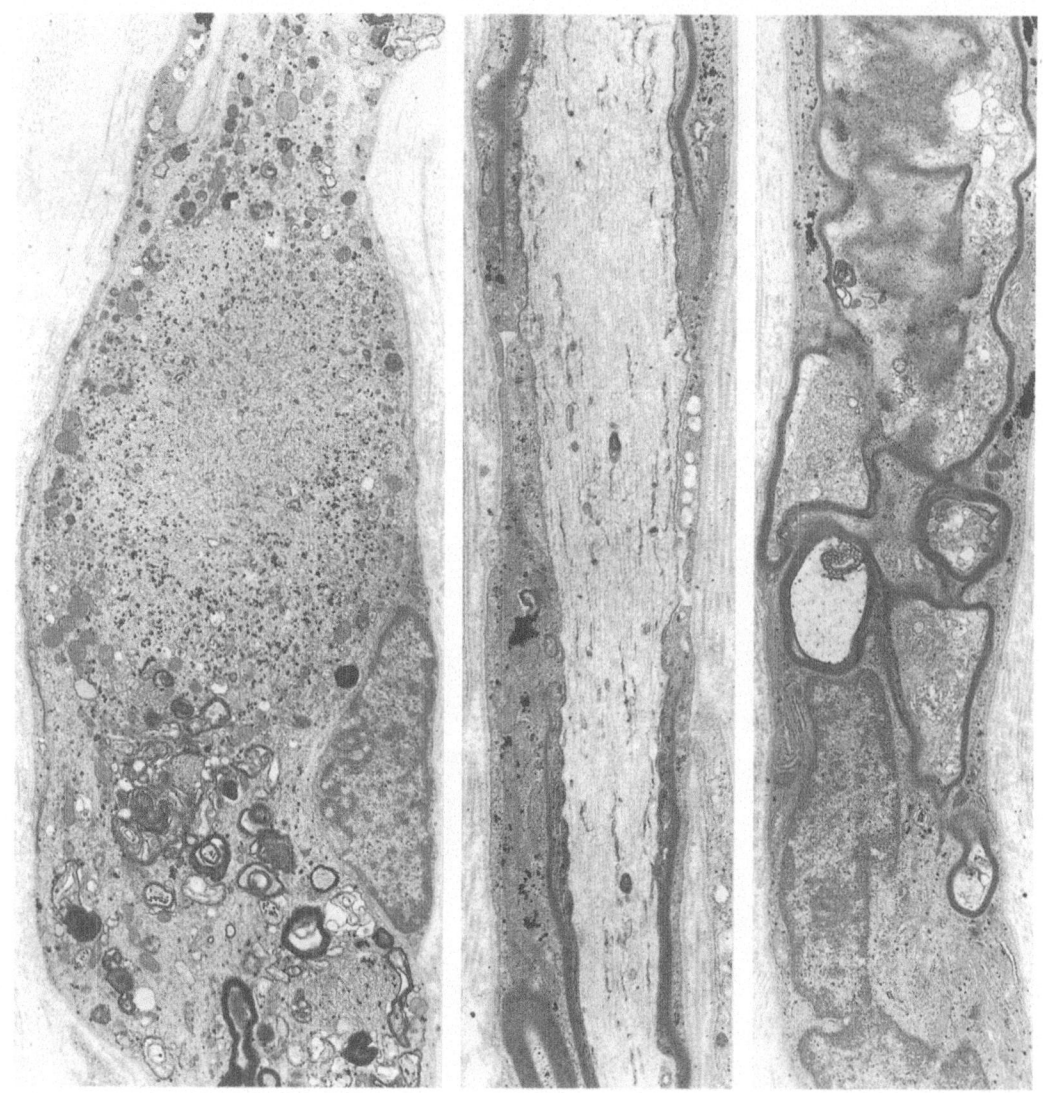

a, b   c

Fig. 113 a – c. Same case as in Fig. 112. **a** This enlarged, dystrophic axon contains pleomorphic organelles in which membranous cytoplasmic bodies focally predominate. It is surrounded by thin Schwann cell processes and a moderately shrunken Schwann cell nucleus. × 7,400. **b** The nodal segment of this node of Ranvier of a thin myelinated nerve fiber appears distended; the axon shows a normal number of organelles. × 16,000. **c** Tangential section through a thinly remyelinated nerve fiber with irregular myelin loops and multiple vesicular cytoplasmic components of different size. × 9,500

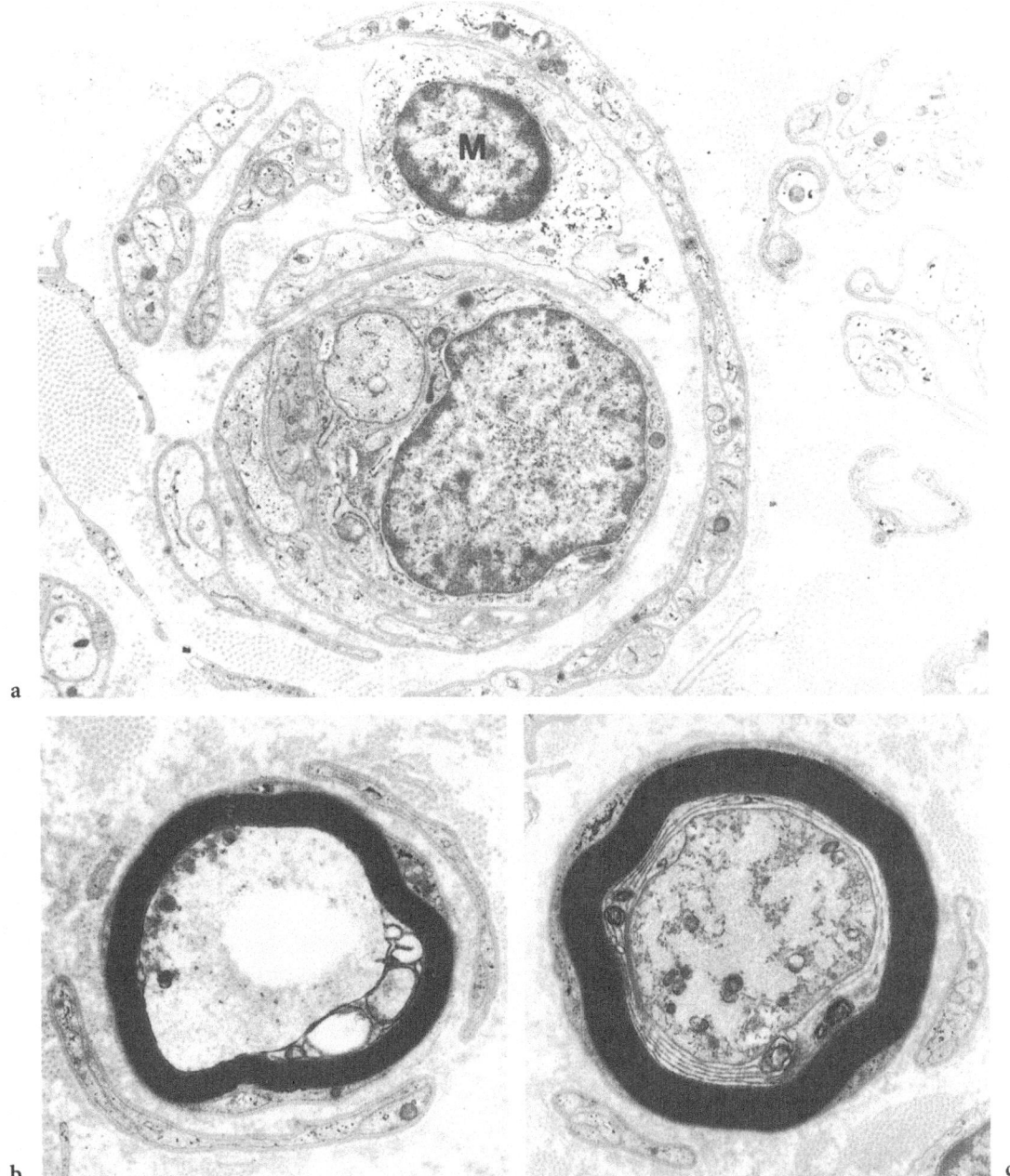

Fig. 114a–c. Hypertrophic neuropathy, presumably HMSN III, in a 3-year-old girl and an 8-month-old girl. **a** A demyelinated axon is surrounded by multiple Schwann cell processes enclosing a macrophage (*M*). × 11,000. **b** Unusual form of an axonal degeneration in an obviously de- and remyelinated nerve fiber with concentrically arranged Schwann cell processes in the periphery. The axoplasm in the center appears partly amorphous and partly dissolved. At its periphery there are some dense bodies. The myelin sheath shows several adaxonal vacuoles as a sign of incipient degeneration. × 12,000. **c** Demyelinated and remyelinated axon with irregularly distributed neurofilaments as well as multiple components of the axoplasmic reticulum and several mitochondria, surrounded by a compact myelin sheath. Its two to five inner lamellae are not compacted and include some membranous cytoplasmic bodies. × 9,000

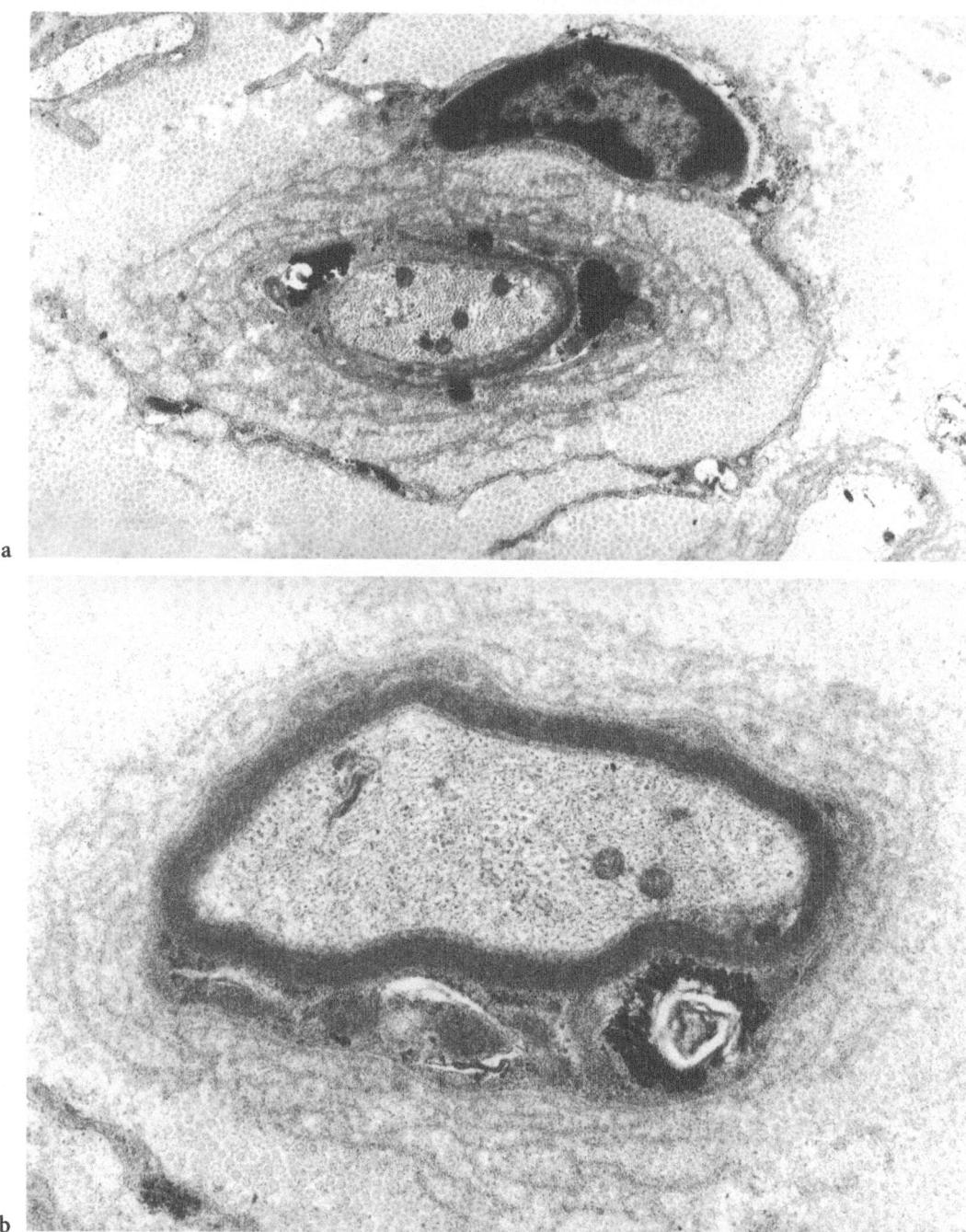

Fig. 115. a, b Basal lamina type of onion bulb formation (Lyon-type of hypomyelination neuropathy). In **a** up to five layers of basal laminae can be seen around a central, small, thinly remyelinated fiber with focal accumulation of glycogen granules in the cytoplasm of its Schwann cell which is cut at the level of the paranode. In the periphery a fibroblast can be seen with very thin processes surrounding the central nerve fiber rather completely. The basal laminae appear to be irregularly interwoven in **a** and **b**. The cell processes between the basal laminae are presumably degenerated. **a** × 18,000; **b** × 31,000

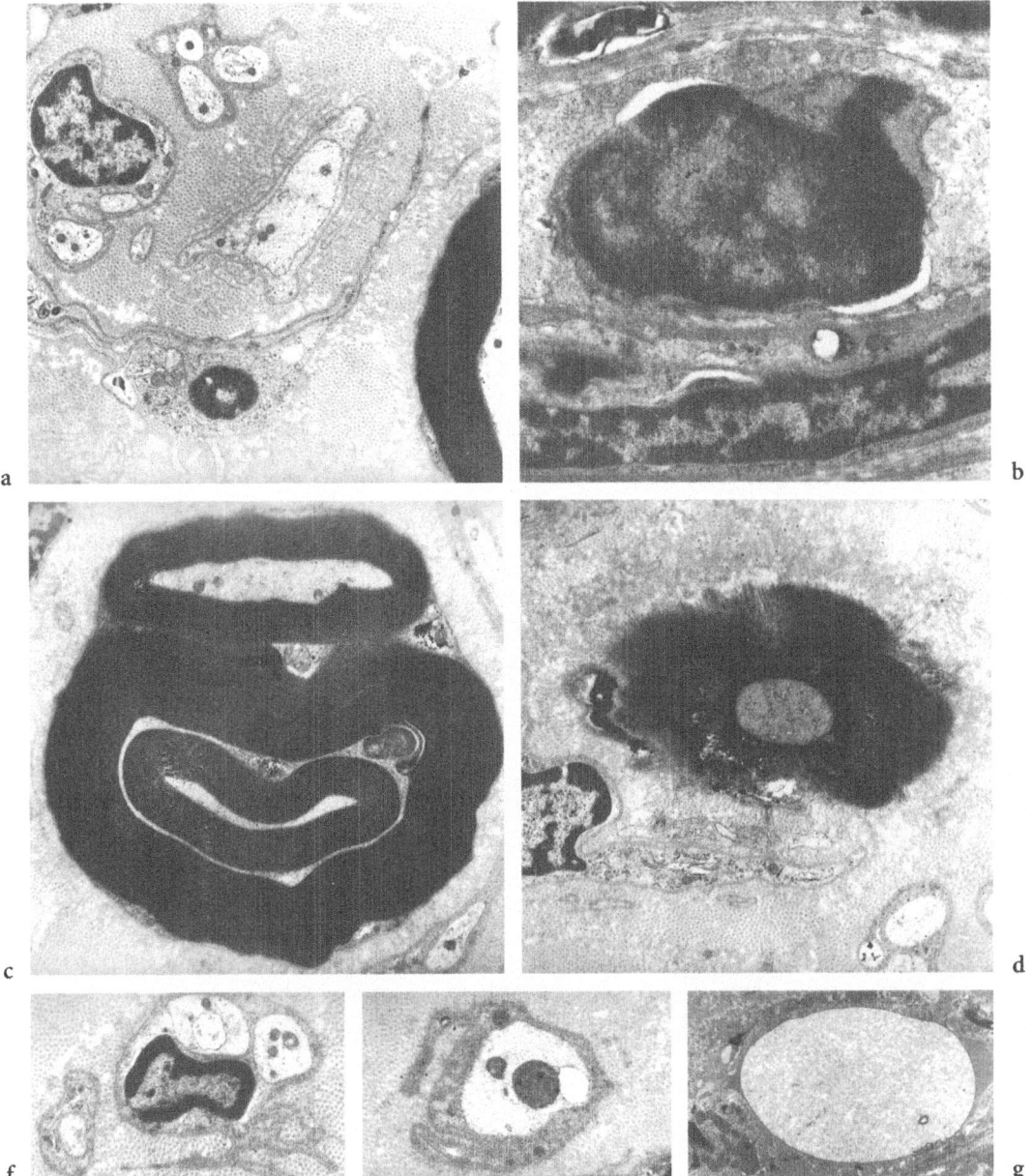

Fig. 116 a–g. Same case as in Fig. 115. **a** An obviously demyelinated large axon is surrounded by several empty basal laminae whereas the neighboring unmyelinated axons do not show this phenomenon. Adjacent lies a semi-circumferentially arranged Schwann cell. A macrophage with finger-like processes is apposed to its surface. × 8,400. **b** In the perineurium a rounded cell is obviously altered: its cytoplasm appears to be shrunken and the outer nuclear membrane is focally distended. × 18,000. **c** Unusually extensive and reduplicated myelin loops within the Schwann cell can be seen adjacent to a clearly compressed, myelinated nerve fiber. × 9,200. **d** Paranodal nerve fiber segment with several empty Schwann cell processes and basal lamina-like substances above the nerve fiber. × 9,000. **e** Abnormal Schwann cell nucleus with marginal condensation of the nuclear chromatin (apoptosis) including one unmyelinated axon with a vacuole and another inconspicuous axon with four mitochondria. At the surface of this Schwann cell, collagen fibrils are incompletely enclosed. × 11,500. **f** Unmyelinated axon which is surrounded by several Schwann cell processes and contains an unusually large mitochondrion with a vacuole. × 11,500. **g** Conspicuous swollen cell process, presumably an axon, with floccular material. × 4,400

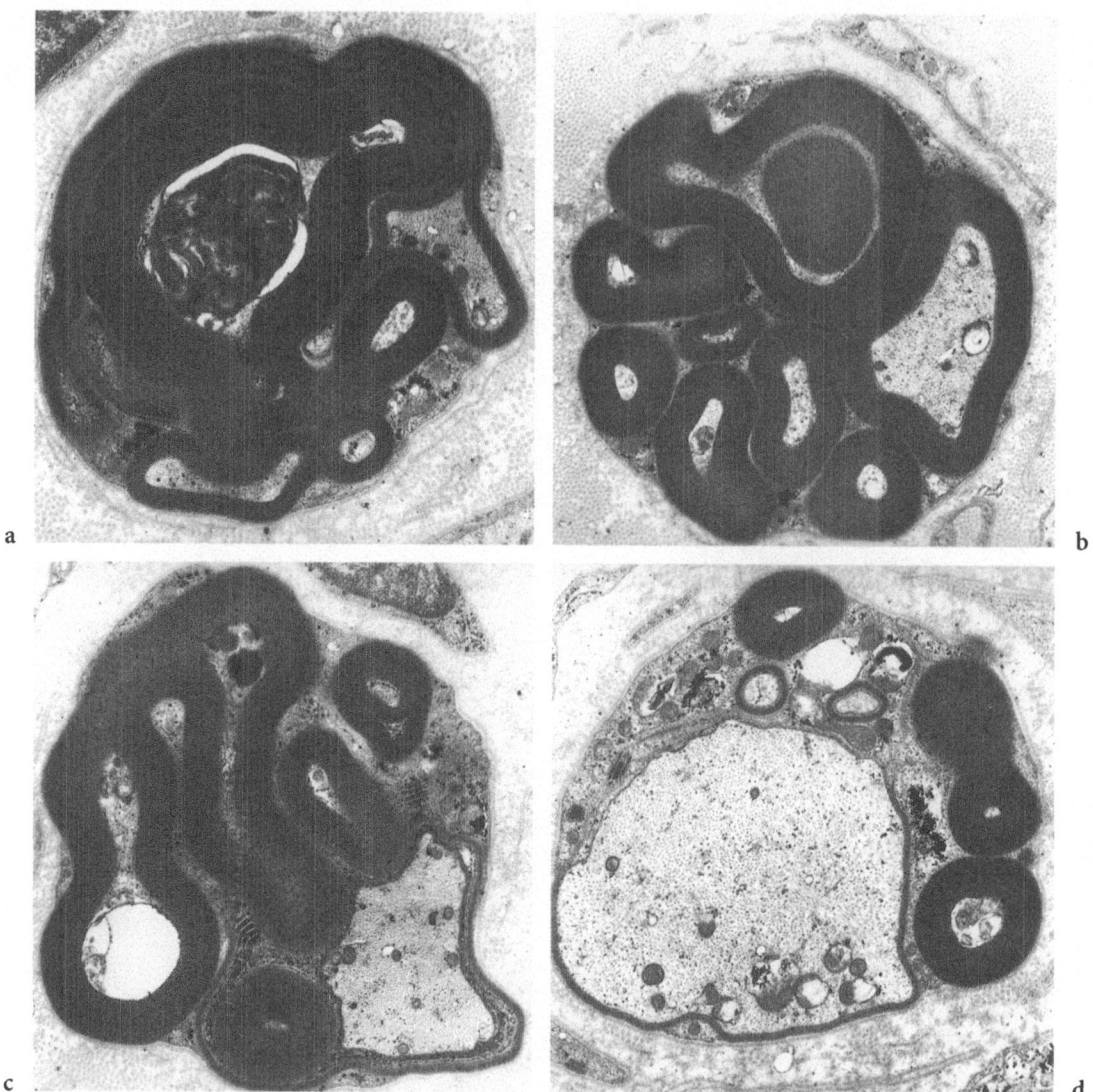

Fig. 117 a – d. Congenital hypo-/hypermyelinisation neuropathy (neuropathy with focally folded myelin) in an 11-year-old boy. Internodal and paranodal myelin loops are formed in excess although the myelin sheath around the axon itself tends to be quite thin (**a, c, d**). **a, c** × 12,600; **b** × 9,700; **d** × 13,600

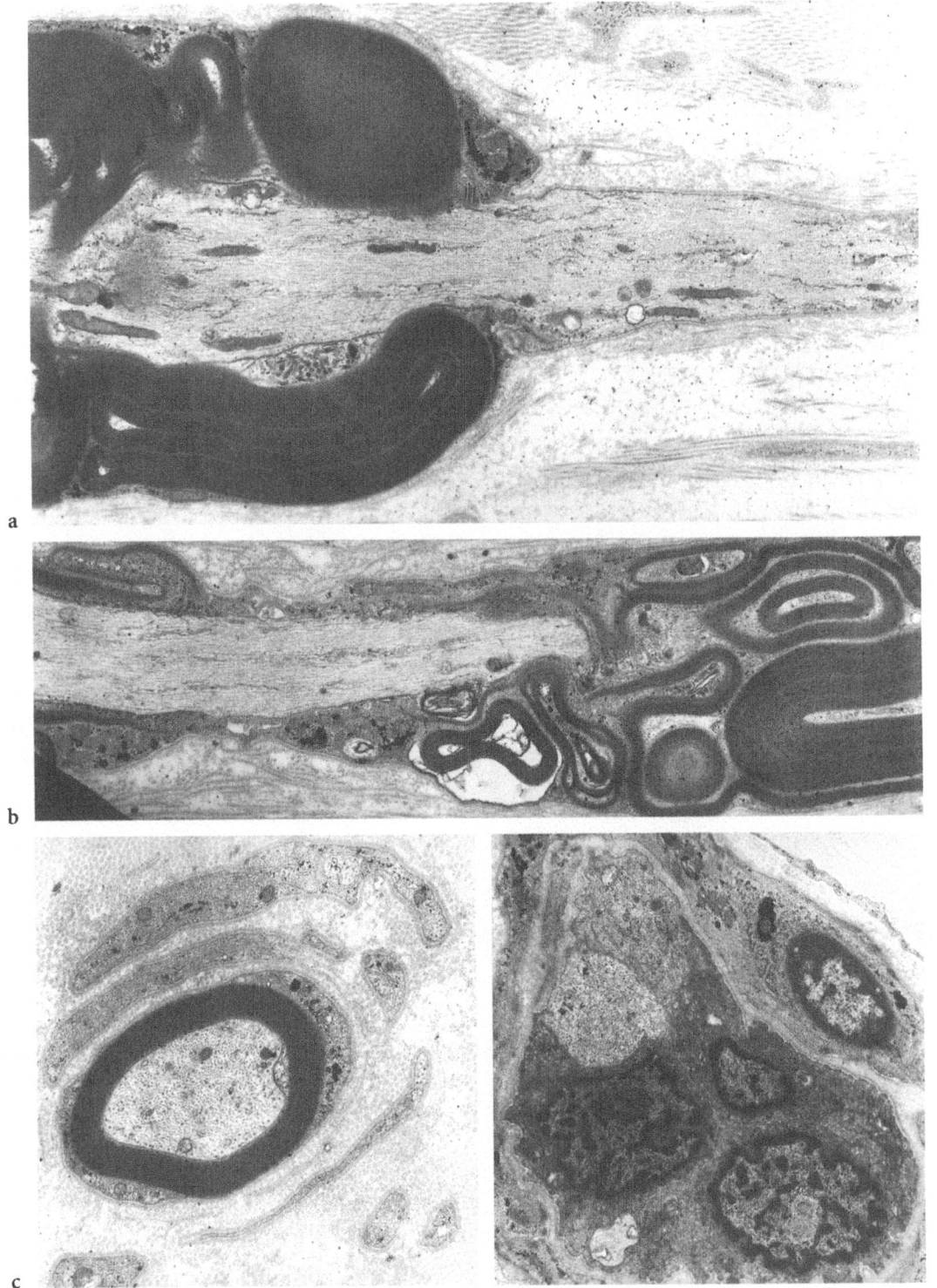

Fig. 118 a–d. Same case as in Fig. 117. Adjacent to a demyelinated segment (**a**) paranodal myelin loops appear to be retracted (**a, b**). Onion bulb formation (**c**) and an increased number of Schwann cells with irregular nuclear shape (**d**) are also apparent.
a × 16,600; **b** × 12,200; **c** × 9,800; **d** × 17,600

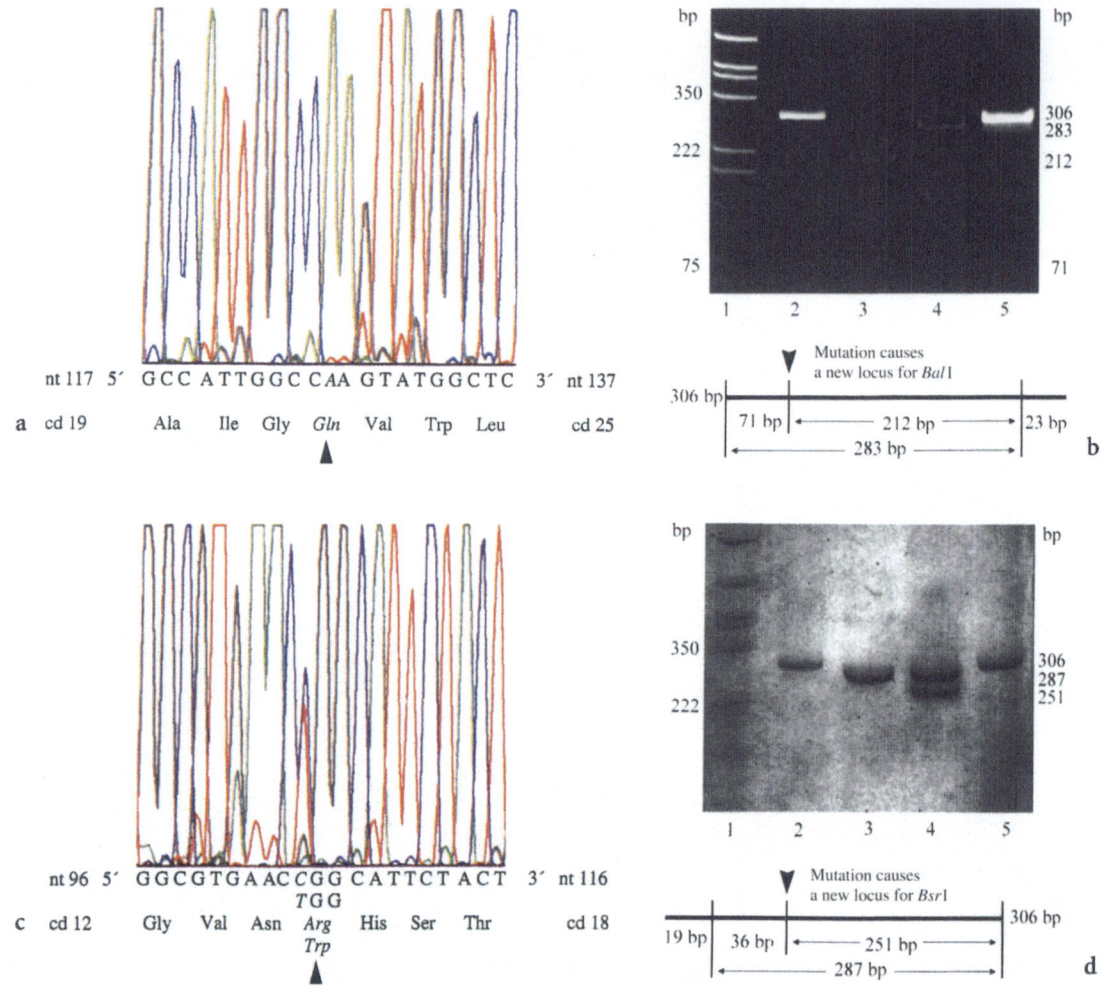

nt 117 5′ GCC ATTGGC CAA GTATGGCTC 3′ nt 137

a   cd 19   Ala   Ile Gly *Gln* Val Trp Leu   cd 25

Mutation causes
a new locus for *Bal*I

306 bp |←71 bp→|←————— 212 bp —————→|23 bp|
       |←—————————— 283 bp ——————————→| b

nt 96 5′ GGCGTGAAC*CGG* CATTCT ACT 3′ nt 116
                     TGG

c   cd 12   Gly Val Asn *Arg* His Ser Thr   cd 18
                             Trp

Mutation causes
a new locus for *Bsr*I

                                                  306 bp
19 bp| 36 bp |←————— 251 bp —————→|
     |←—————————— 287 bp ——————————→| d

Fig. 119 a – d. Mutation analysis in both HMSN X-patients of Figs. 120 – 122. **a, b** Fifteen-year-old boy with HMSN X. **a** Automated sequencing revealed a G → A-transition at position 127 in exon 2 of the Cx32 gene (*arrowhead*). **b** The mutation was confirmed by restriction enzyme analysis with *Bal*I. *Lane 1:* pGEM-DNA-standard, *lane 2:* undigested patient-DNA. *Lane 3:* patient-DNA after digestion; the 283-bp-fragment is digested into a 212- and a 71-bp-fragment. *Lane 4:* digestion of the normal control-DNA. *Lane 5:* undigested control-DNA. **c, d** Forty-four-year-old female with HMSN X. **c** The DNA-sequencing reveals a C → T-transition at position 105 (*arrowhead*). **d** The restriction enzyme analysis with *Bsr*I confirms the mutation. *Lane 1:* pGEM-DNA-standard. *Lane 2:* undigested normal control-DNA. *Lane 3:* digested control-DNA. *Lane 4:* patient's specimen after *Bsr*I-digestion reveals an additional 251-bp-fragment. *Lane 5:* undigested patient's specimen. The short 23- and 71-bp-fragments (1st case) and the 19- and 36-bp-fragments (2nd case) cannot be seen in the figures (*nt*, nucleotide; *cd*, codon; *bp*, base pairs). (From [1015])

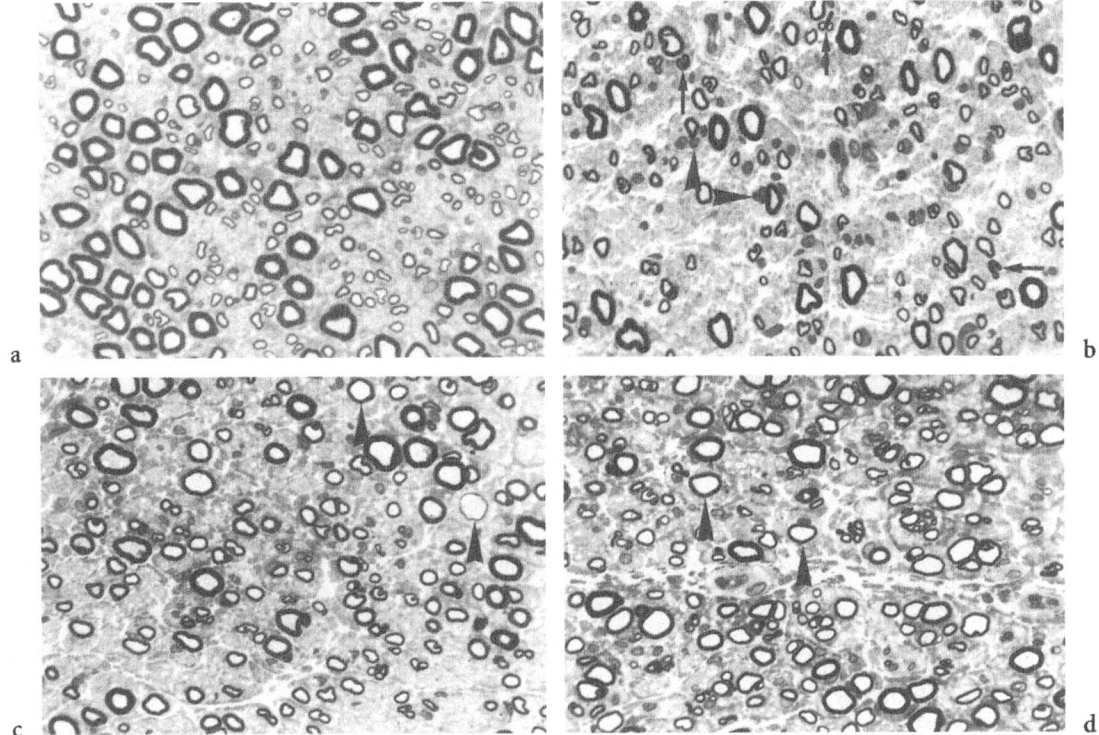

Fig. 120 a – d. Cross sections of sural nerve biopsies. **a** Regular distribution of large and small myelinated and unmyelinated nerve fibers in a 12-year-old boy (control). **b** Fifteen-year-old boy with HMSN X. The number of the large myelinated nerve fibers is considerably reduced. Fibers lying closely adjacent to each other indicate prior degeneration and regeneration. Occasionally there are supernumerary Schwann cells, indicated by *arrowheads*, which correspond to incipient onion bulb formation. Some small fibers are obviously atrophic, their myelin sheaths collapsed (*arrows*). **c, d** Forty-four-year-old female with HMSN X. Two different fascicles show considerable reduction in the number of large myelinated nerve fibers and a variable number of groups of regenerated nerve fibers. Some isolated, thinly myelinated fibers indicate preceding demyelination and remyelination (*arrowheads*). These and the regenerated fibers show conspicuously thin myelin sheaths in relation to axonal diameter, but atrophic axons with collapsed or relatively thick myelin sheaths can also be seen. Myelin degradation products are rare. **a – d** Toluidine blue, × 530. (From [1015])

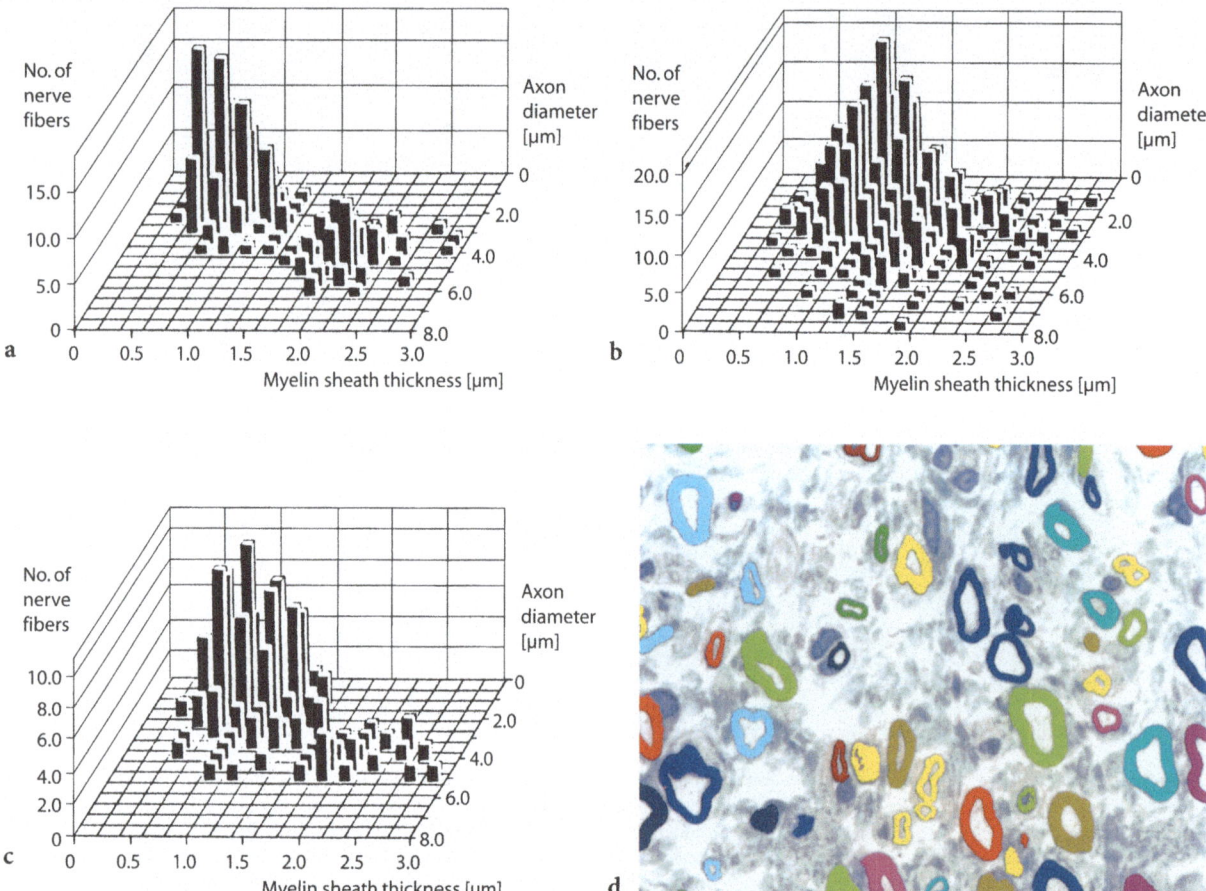

Fig. 121a–c. Three-dimensional diagrams of the myelinated fibers of the cases in Fig. 120. **a** Twelve-year-old boy as a control. **b** Fifteen-year-old boy with HMSN X. **c,d** Forty-four-year-old female with HMSN X. The number of nerve fibers is indicated at the ordinate (*y-axis*), the thickness of the myelin sheaths at the abscissa (*x-axis*), and the thickness of the axons at the *z-axis*, the last two in micrometers. The number of large myelinated nerve fibers in **b** and **c** is clearly reduced, the number of small myelinated nerve fibers relatively increased. The evaluation of the nerve fiber density revealed a 15% reduction of myelinated nerve fibers in **b** and a 45% reduction in **c**. **d** Documentation of an optic-electronic, digital evaluation image of the number and size of myelinated nerve fibers in the case of **b** using pseudocolors. The myelinated nerve fibers with the usual irregularities of the myelin sheaths are quite accurately represented

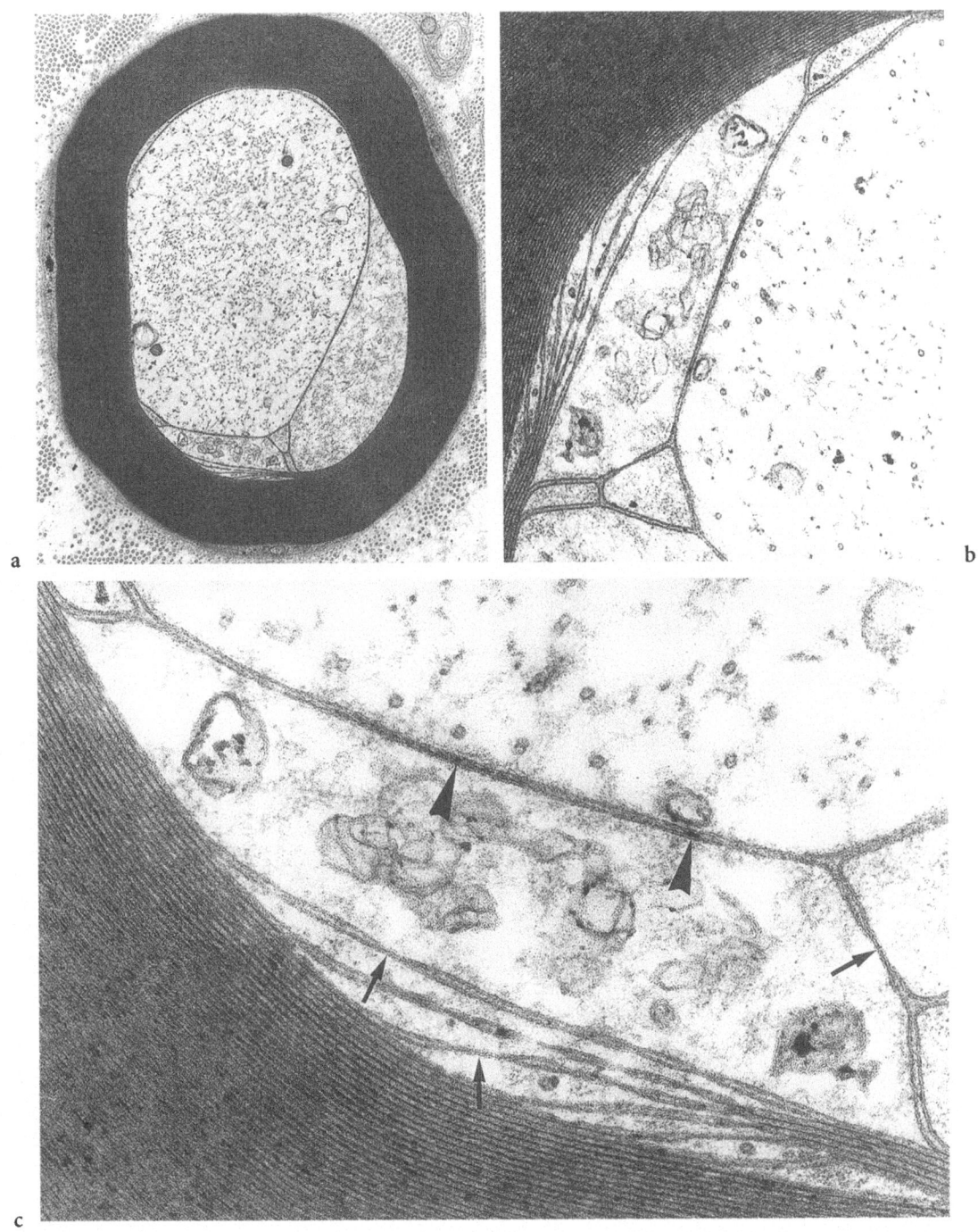

Fig. 122. Same case as in the Figs. 119a, 120b, and 121b. The adaxonal myelin loops are considerably distended. There are unusual contacts between adjacent membranes which focally form transverse bands similar to those seen in normal paranodes though at an abnormal site (*arrowheads*). The *arrows* indicate fusion of adjacent processes of Schwann cells. **a** × 12,600; **b** × 49,000; **c** × 95,000

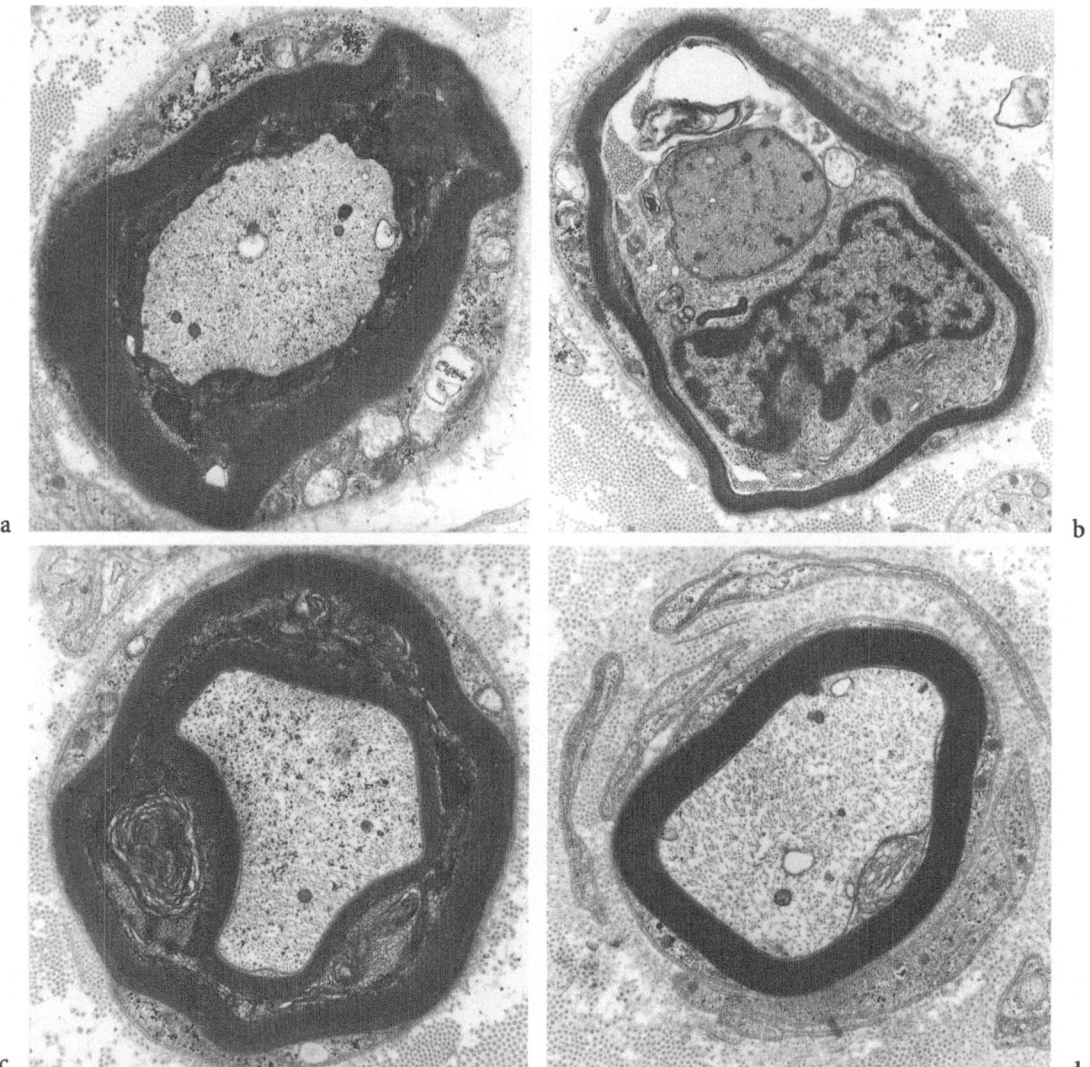

Fig. 123 a – d. Same case as in Fig. 122. **a** Shrivelling, microvesicular lysis, and condensation of inner myelin lamellae adjacent to a Schmidt-Lanterman incisure with membranous cytoplasmic bodies and a myelin loop in a myelinated nerve fiber, the outer myelin lamellae of which appear to be regularly structured. × 9,900. **b** Adaxonal macrophage situated between the axon and a thin, newly formed myelin sheath. There is microvesicular disintegration of inner myelin lamellae at several sites. × 9,300. **c** Abnormalities in the Schmidt-Lanterman incisure of a myelinated nerve fiber with membranous cytoplasmic bodies, microvesicular disintegration of myelin lamellae, and somewhat loosely arranged, less densely structured outer myelin lamellae. × 13,000. **d** Early stage of an onion bulb formation with several concentrically arranged interdigitating Schwann cell processes of uneven thickness around a centrally located myelinated nerve fiber. × 11,000

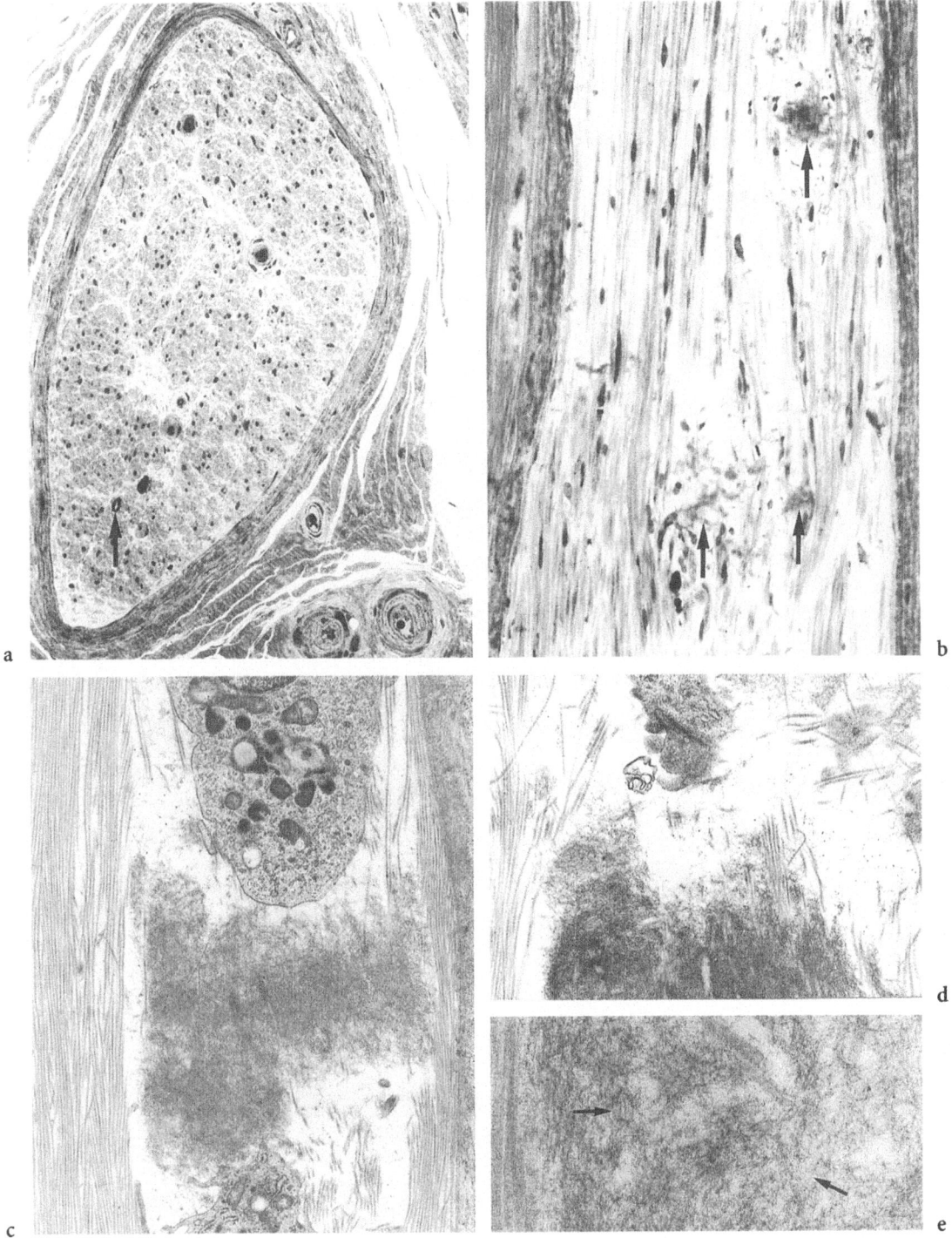

Fig. 124a–e. Amyloid neuropathy in a 64-year-old man. The amyloidosis could not be diagnosed by a previous rectum biopsy. **a** The number of myelinated (and unmyelinated) nerve fibers is severely reduced. In the area shown there is only one large fiber left (*arrow*). × 155. **b** The amyloid deposits are indicated in this nerve fascicle by *arrows*. × 170. **c–e** Electron microscopic evidence of endoneurial amyloid, **c** between endoneurial collagen fibrils and 2 fibroblasts. × 5,800. **d** Interlacing of endoneurial collagen fibrils and amyloid. × 6,900. **e** Individual amyloid filaments are detectable at higher magnification (*arrows*). × 32,900

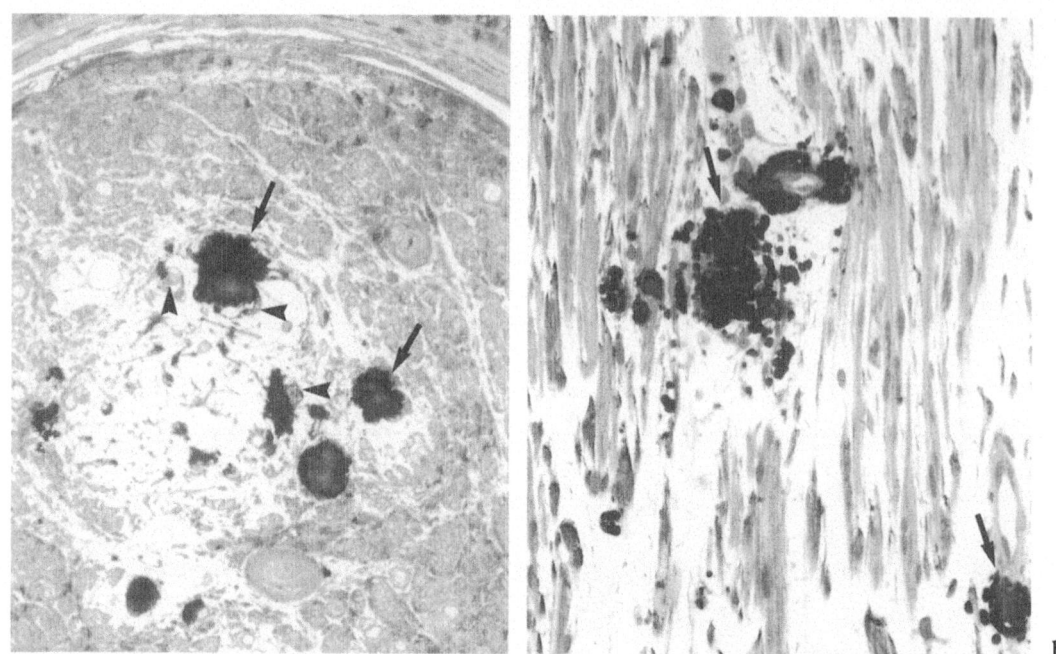

Fig. 125. a Amyloid neuropathy of the lambda-light-chain type in a 65-year-old case with predominantly sensory neuropathy, diarrhoea, hypotension, vagovasal syncopes, and nocturnal apnoeas associated with proven plasmocytoma (case 7 of [1068]). The amyloid deposits are selectively immunoreactive for antibodies against lambda-light chains (AL-amyloid) (*arrows*). Endoneurial macrophages in close contact with amyloid plaques are indicated by *arrowheads*. × 430. **b** Chronic progressive sensorimotor neuropathy in a 67-year-old case with kappa-light chain-gammopathy (case 10 in [1068]). The amyloid has reacted with anti-kappa-antibodies (*arrows*). × 800

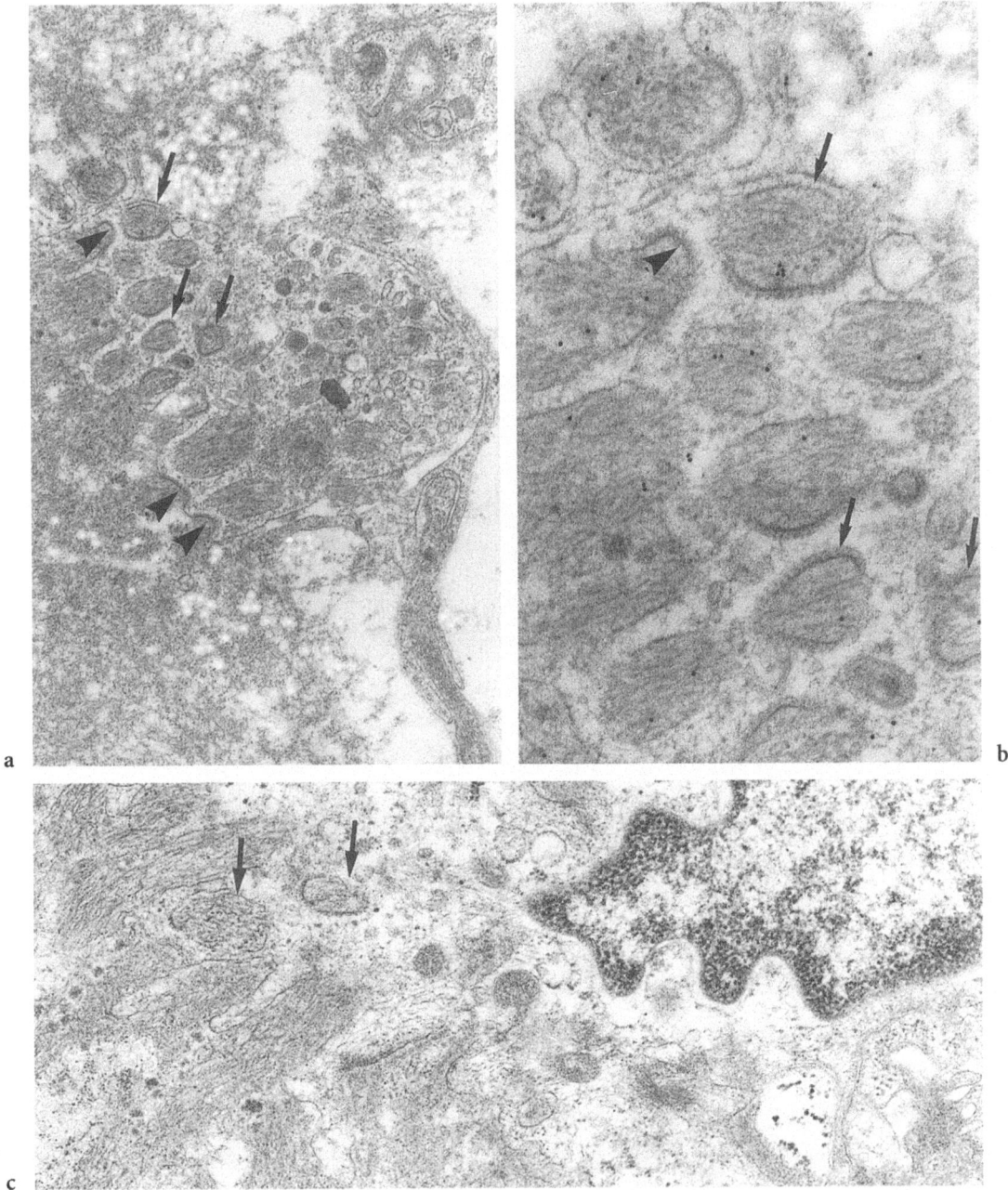

Fig. 126. a, b Macrophage in contact with amyloid shows condensation of some material on the cytoplasmic side of the vacuoles such as can be seen around coated vesicles (*arrows*) or in hemidesmosomes (*arrowheads*); the vacuoles contain bundles of immunogold-labeled amyloid filaments. **a** × 23,000; **b** × 75,000. **c** Perineurial cell with similar vacuoles that are filled with immunogold-labeled amyloid. Some of the vacuoles are coated by electron dense material. × 32,000. (From [1068])

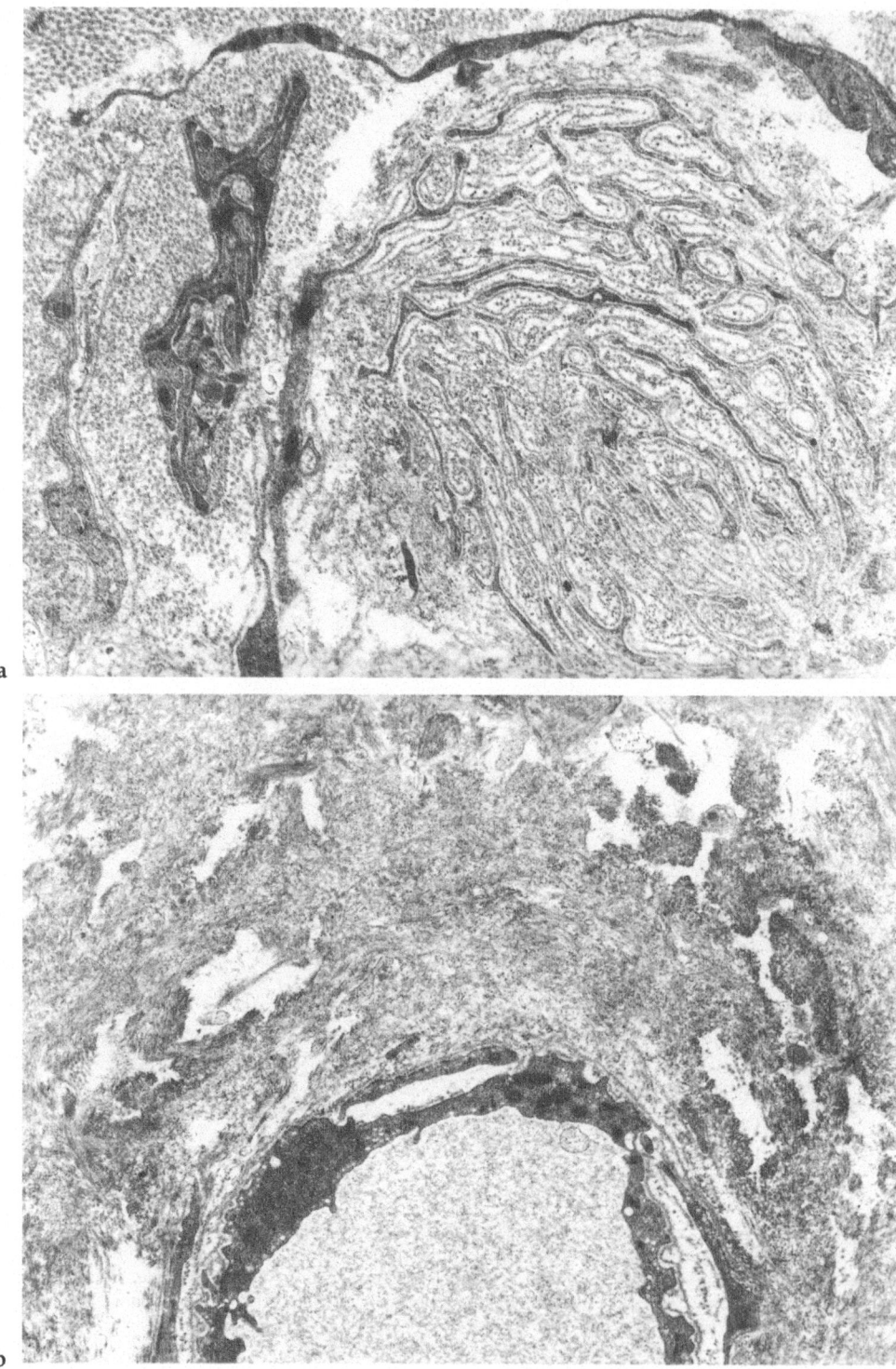

Fig. 127 a, b. Amyloid neuropathy in familial amyloidosis of the Portuguese type in a 32-year-old male. **a** All unmyelinated axons are lost; the remaining empty Schwann cell processes enclose collagen fibrils. × 15,120. **b** Pericapillary endoneurial amyloid deposits the filaments of which show diameters between 3.5 – 8 nm and are thus considerably thinner than those of collagen fibrils. × 11,300. (From [958])

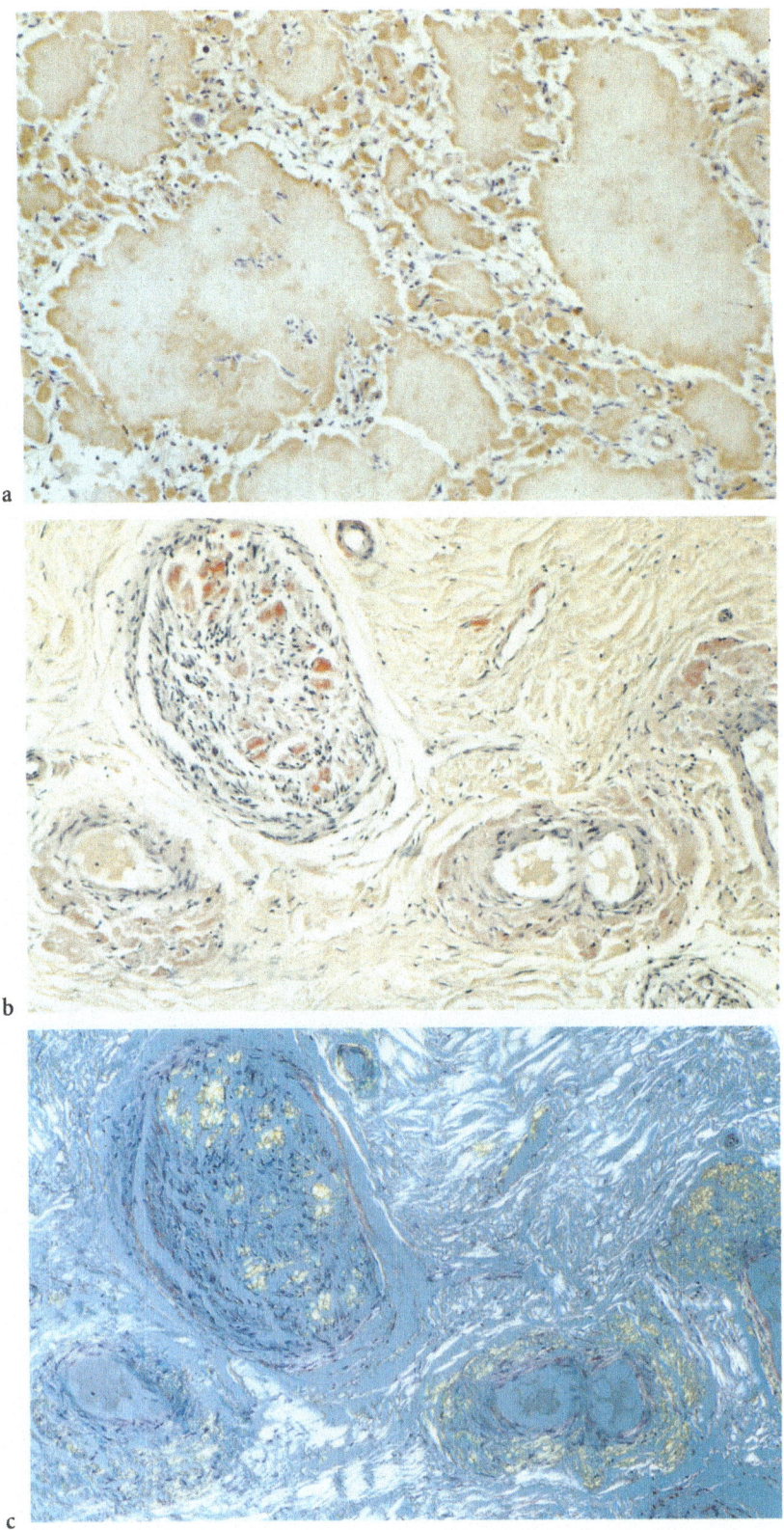

Fig. 128a–c. Amyloidoma of the ganglion Gasseri, which clinically was suggestive of a neurinoma in a 55-year-old female. **a** Extensive homogeneous amyloid deposits which are not immunoreactive for antibodies against kappa-light chains. **b** The congo red stain reveals a large number of endoneurial amyloid deposits in an adjacent nerve fascicle. **c** Polarized light reveals the characteristic green dichroism of the congophilic depositions shown in **b** whereas the epineurial collagen fibrils appear whitish in polarized light

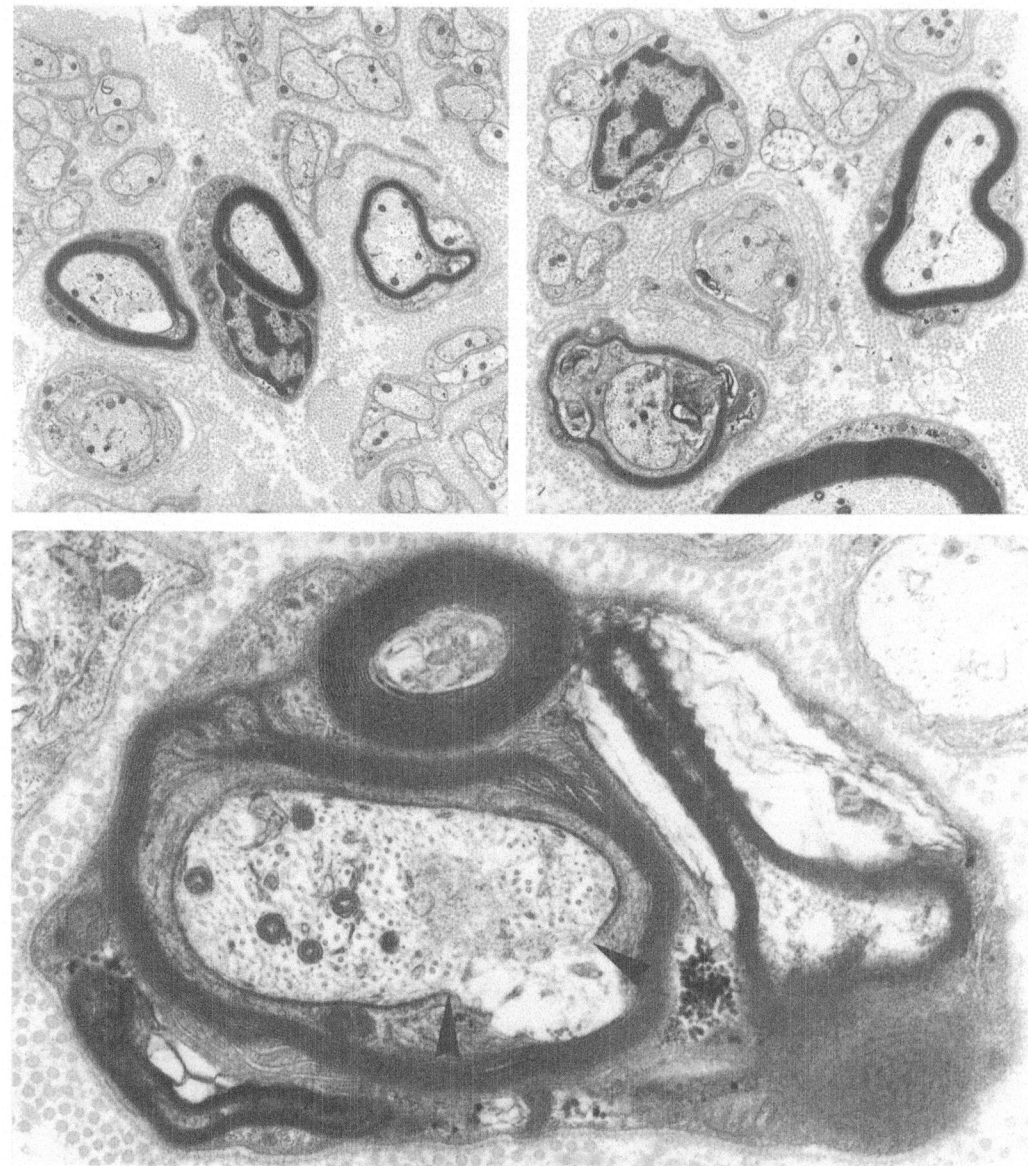

c

Fig. 129 a–c. Neuropathy in a two-month-old newborn with congenital myotonic dystrophy. **a** Concentrically arranged Schwann cell processes and basal laminae around a demyelinated or promyelin fiber in the *lower left* and an adaxonal vacuole in the myelinated nerve fiber above. × 7,800. **b** Demyelinated nerve fiber with surrounding Schwann cell processes and empty basal laminae in the *center*; several myelin-like bodies in the adaxonal cytoplasm, and a Schmidt-Lanterman incisure in the paranodal part of a myelinated fiber with a disproportionately thin myelin sheath in the *lower left*. × 9,700. **c** Complex paranodal myelin sheath associated with myelin loops and focal lysis of myelin lamellae. The axon contains a focal accumulation of amorphic and microvesicular structures. Focal lysis of the axolemma and the neighboring myelin sheath is indicated by *arrowheads*. × 38,000

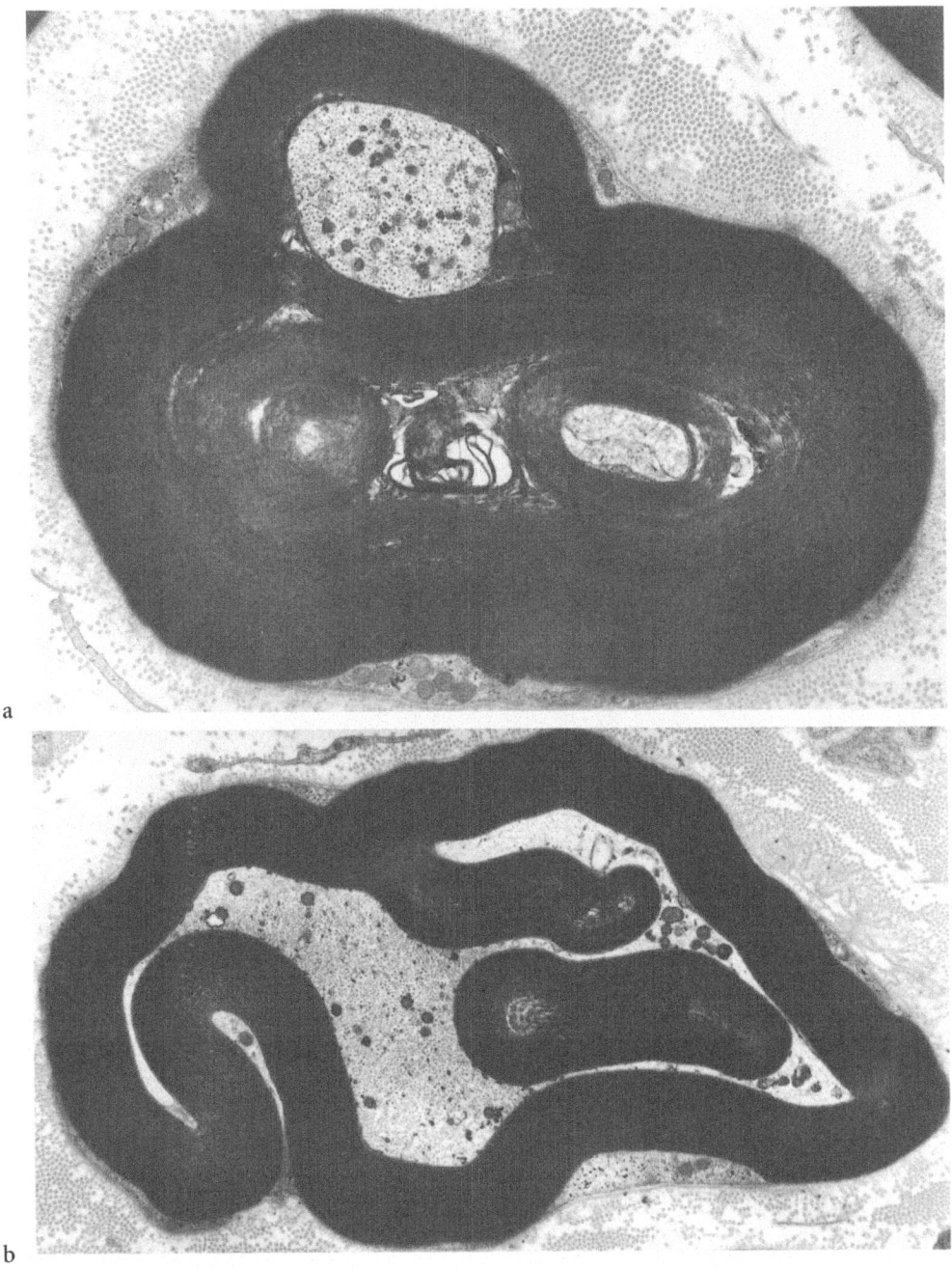

Fig. 130 a, b. Unusually extensive inner and outer myelin loops in the paranode of a 48-year-old female with myotonic dystrophy. **a** × 14,500; **b** × 9,800

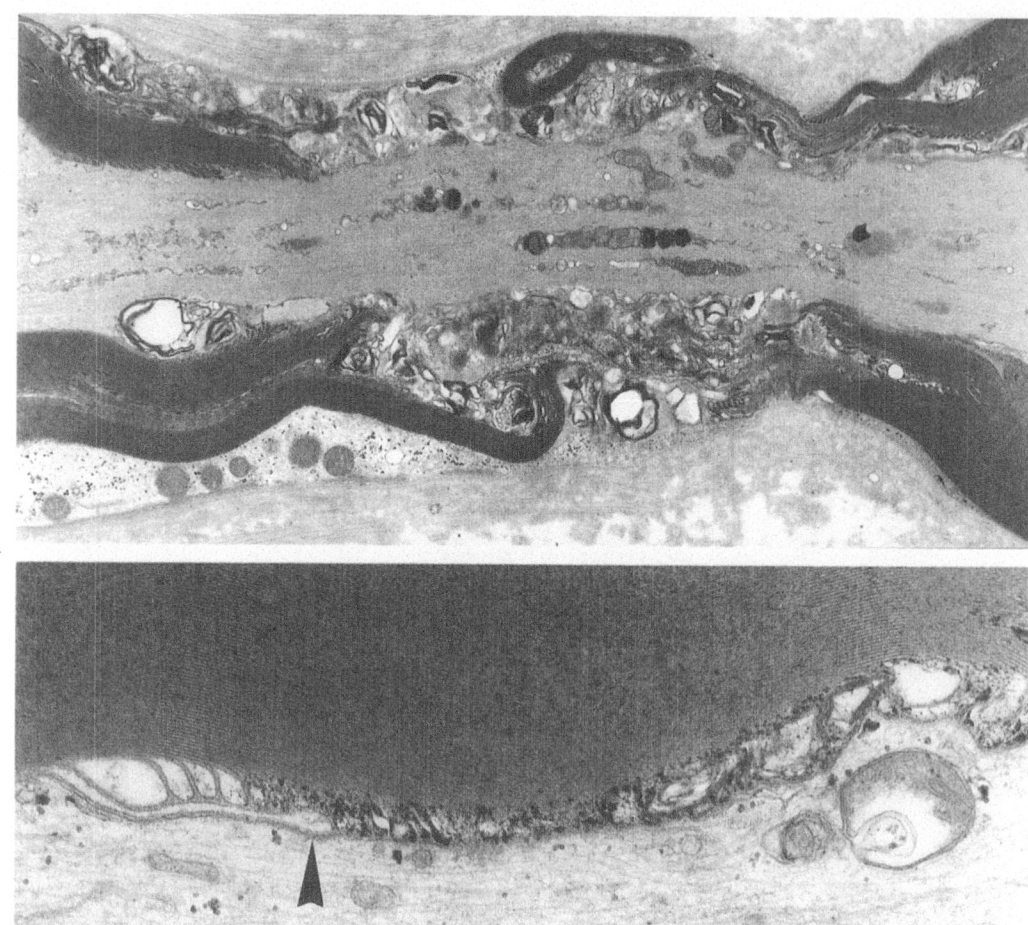

Fig. 131 a, b. Partly demyelinating, partly axonal type of neuropathy in a 61-year-old man with myotonic dystrophy. **a** At the level of the node of Ranvier there are multiple membranous cytoplasmic bodies in the axon and in the cytoplasm of the Schwann cell. The distinction between vesicular disintegrating processes at the myelin sheath and abnormal inclusions is focally difficult. In the center of the axon, mitochondria and dense lamellated bodies are accumulated in a row. **b** Irregularly arranged myelin loops with or without contact to the axon are seen at some distance from the node of Ranvier. A terminal myelin lamella has extended below several other terminal loops (*arrowhead*)

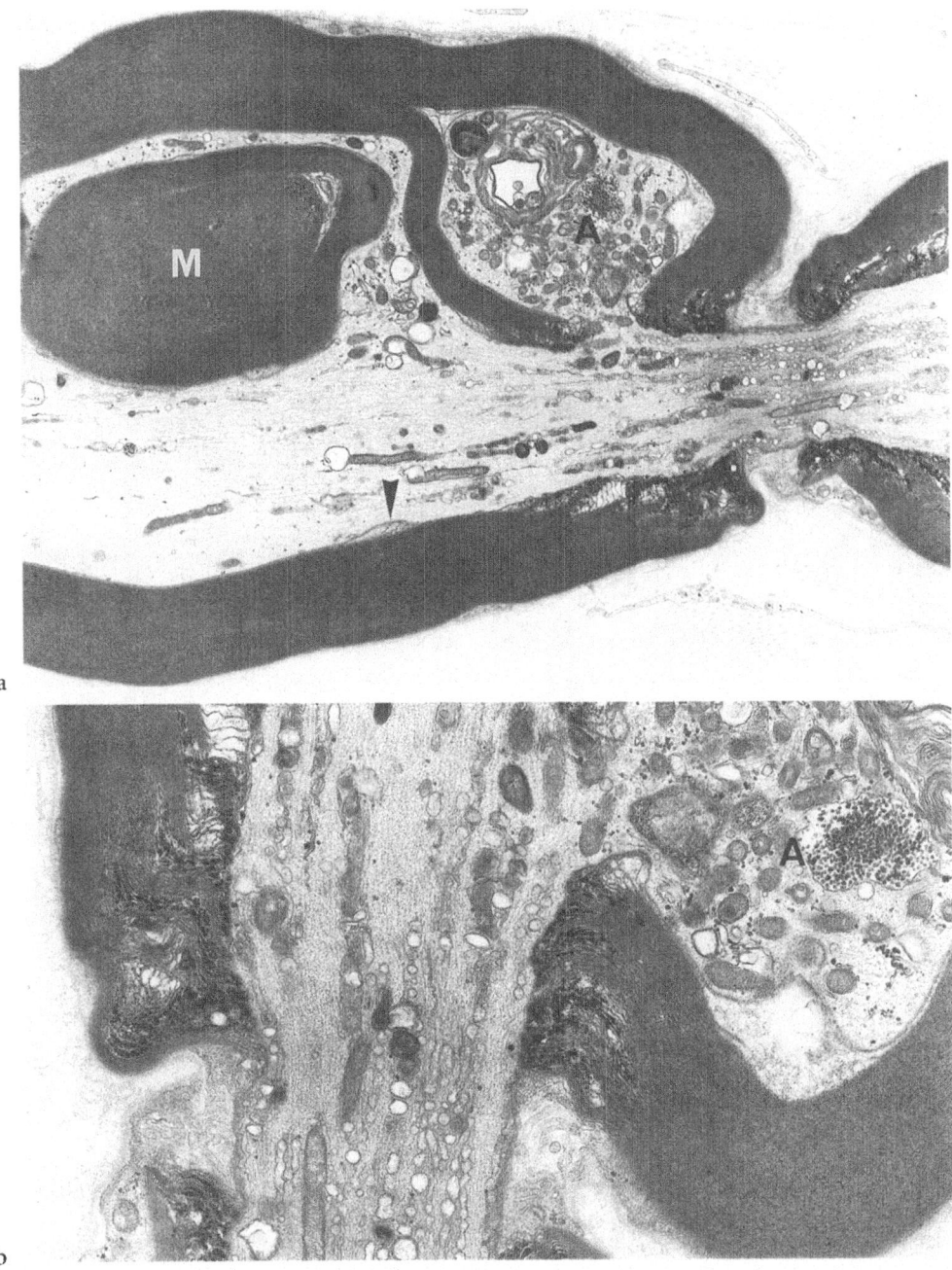

Fig. 132 a, b. Peripheral neuropathy in a 40-year-old female with myotonic dystrophy. **a** Unusually extensive axonal projections can be seen at a paranodal myelin segment (*A*) with accumulation of numerous mitochondria, myelin-like figures, glycogen granules, and vesicular components adjacent to an inner myelin loop (*M*). Some myelin lamellae terminate at some distance from the node of Ranvier (*arrowhead*). Numerous fine vesicles are accumulated in the nodal axoplasm in addition to mitochondria and electron-dense bodies. The nodal area is shown in **b** at higher magnification. There is no axon–Schwann-cell network detectable at this site. Mitochondria are rare in the abaxonal cytoplasm of the corresponding Schwann cell. Many myelin lamellae are not terminating on the axon, but are displaced at some distance from the axolemma into the myelin sheath corresponding to the spines on the doubled bracelet ("double bracelets épineux") of Nageotte. **a** × 9,000; **b** × 21,000. (Modified from [966])

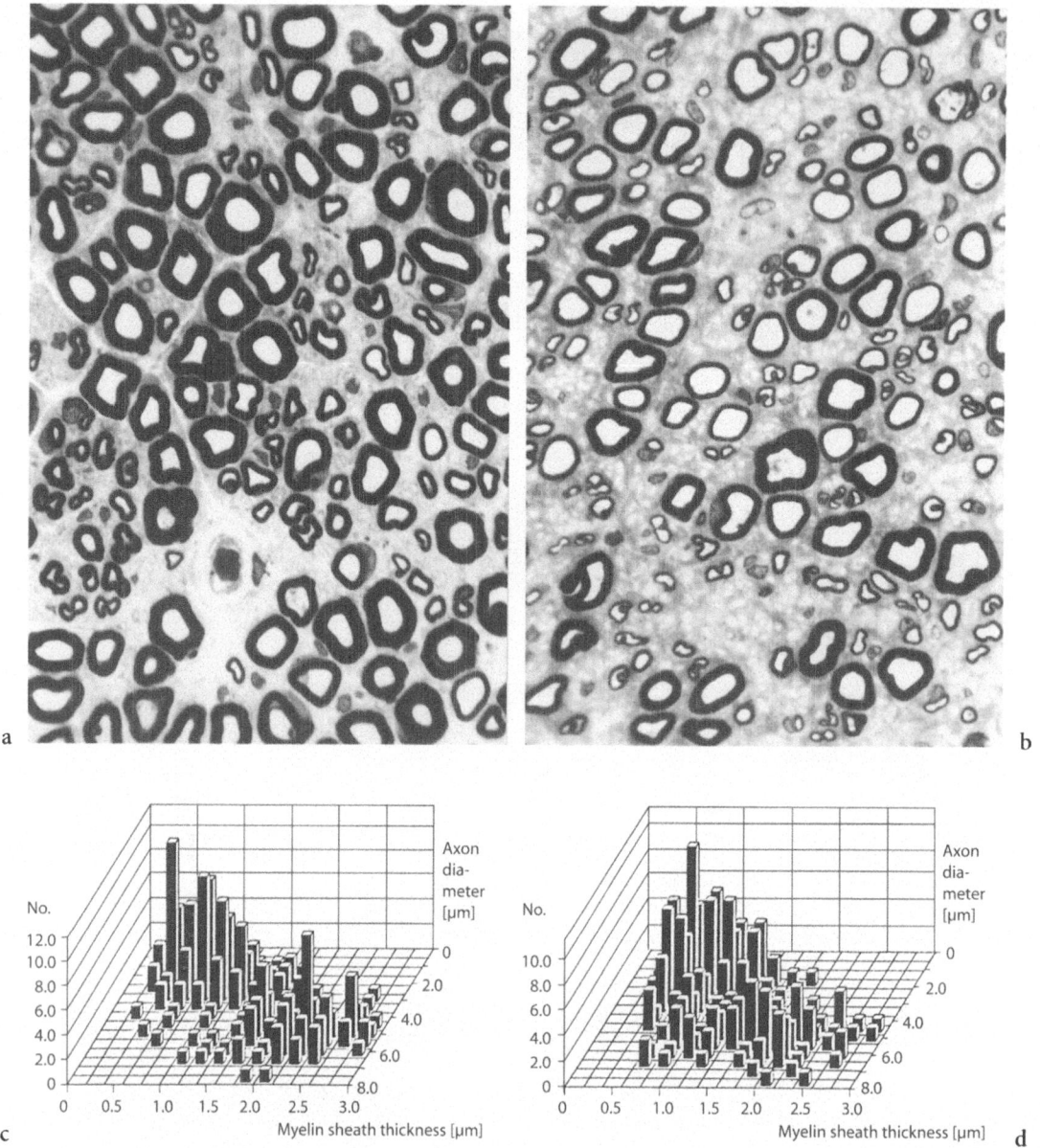

Fig. 133 a–d. Forty-five-year-old male with autosomal dominant distal myopathy, type Laing (Voit et al., in preparation) (**b, d**) in comparison to a control case with myotonic dystrophy (**a, c**). **a, b** In the sural nerve of the case with distal myopathy (**b**) there are numerous large myelinated axons with disproportionately thin myelin sheaths whereas the case with myotonic dystrophy (**a**) shows normally large myelinated nerve fibers with remarkably thick myelin sheaths. **a, b** Toluidine blue × 864. **c, d** The corresponding 3D-diagram of the myelinated nerve fibers reveals an increase in thinly myelinated large axons in **d** combined with a reduction in the number of large, thickly myelinated nerve fibers when compared to the control (**c**) (evaluation by using the KS300-system of Zeiss/ Kontron, Munich, Germany)

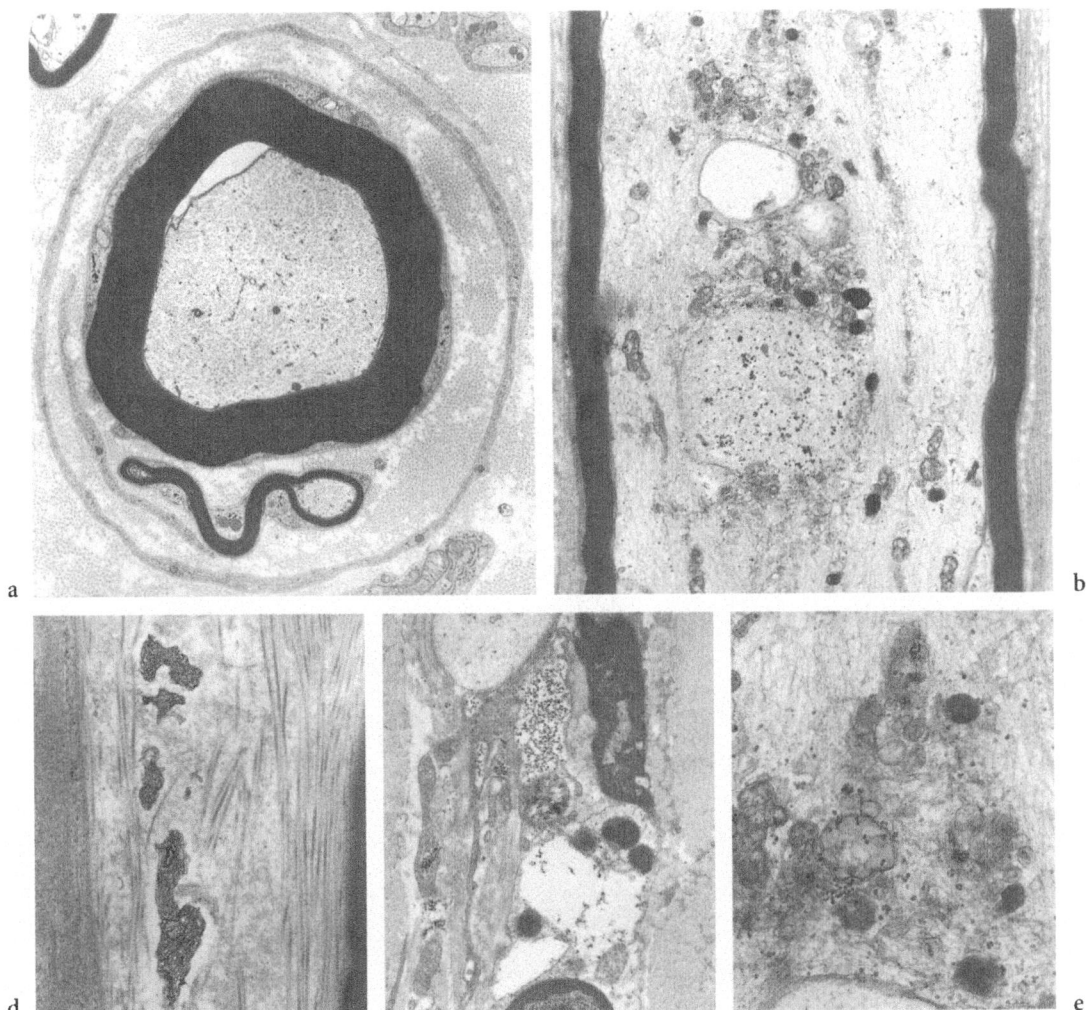

Fig. 134a–e. Demyelinating neuropathy in Marinesco-Sjögren syndrome in a 9-year-old girl. **a** A large and a small, atrophic nerve fiber are surrounded by a complete ring of Schwann cell processes and an incomplete, circumferentially arranged inner layer of Schwann cell processes. In between there are collagen fibrils which are not much thinner than those in the surrounding endoneurium as an indicator of the long time interval since the prior process of degeneration and regeneration. × 7,600. **b** Unusual myelinated axon with disproportionately thin myelin sheath and focal accumulation of mitochondria, electron dense bodies, vesicles, an electron optically empty vacuole, and a vacuole with amorphous material and glycogen granules. The orientation of the neurofilaments is focally disturbed. × 9,400. **c** Extracellular, finely vesicular membranous complexes corresponding to phospholipid precipitates. × 9,400. **d** Group of cells with focal microcystic degeneration, nuclear pycnosis, accumulation of dense bodies, calcium precipitates in a mitochondrion, and focal accumulation of glycogen granules in a fibroblast-like cell. × 12,000. **e** Accumulation of vesicular structures, mitochondria, and dense bodies within an axon. × 27,000

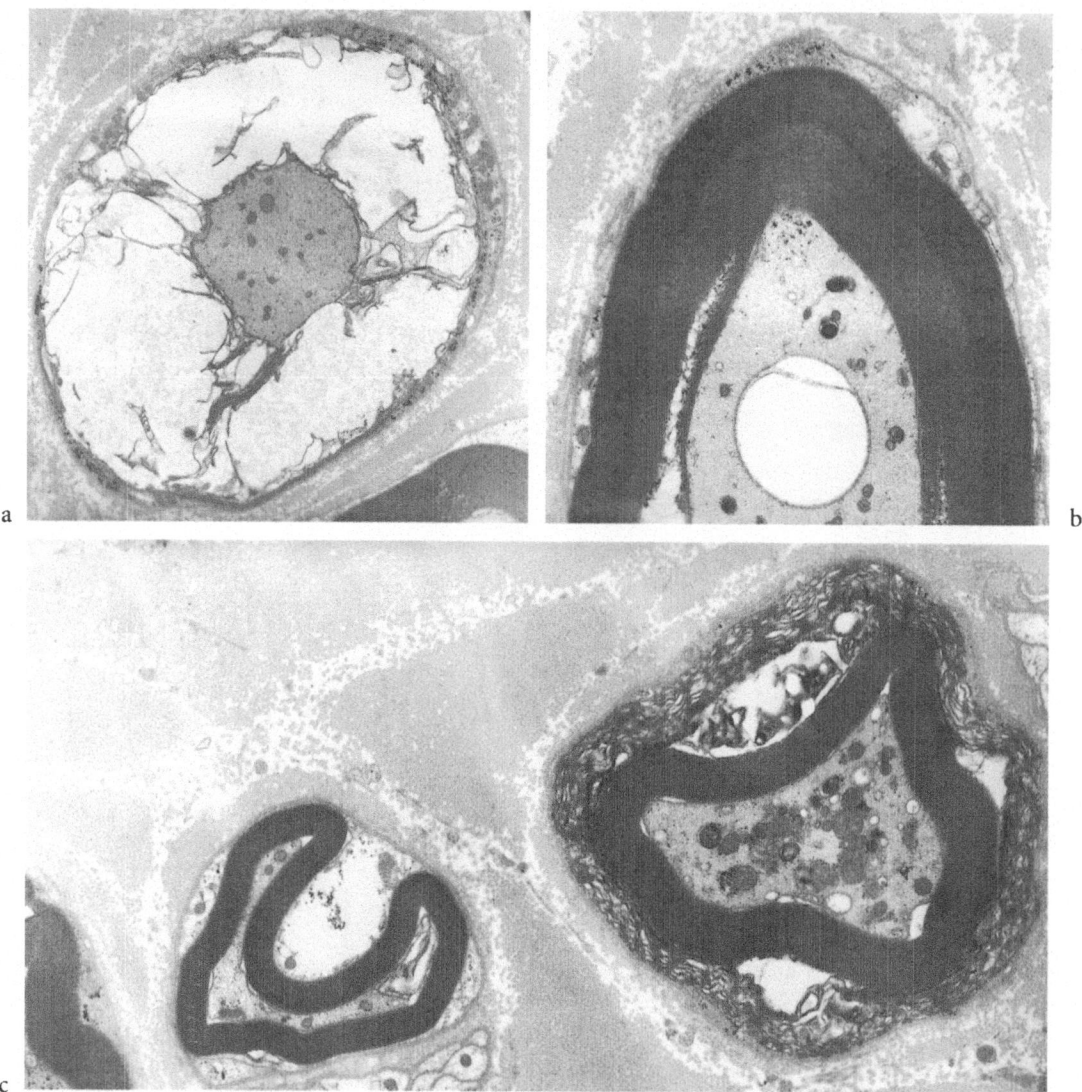

Fig. 135 a–c. Chronic neuropathy in a 40-year-old female with Marfan syndrome. **a** The paranode shows multivacuolar distension and the enclosed axon appears to be shrunken. × 5,800. **b** Myelinated nerve fiber with a central vacuole and small membranous cytoplasmic bodies in the axon. The inner lamellae of its myelin sheath appear to be lighter than the outer ones.
× 9,700. **c** In the center of the nerve fiber on the right, some abnormal organelles appear to be accumulated. Its myelin sheath
is wrinkled and split only in the periphery. On the *left* there is conspicuous vacuolization of the cytoplasm of a Schwann cell;
its axon appears to be shrunken. × 9,700

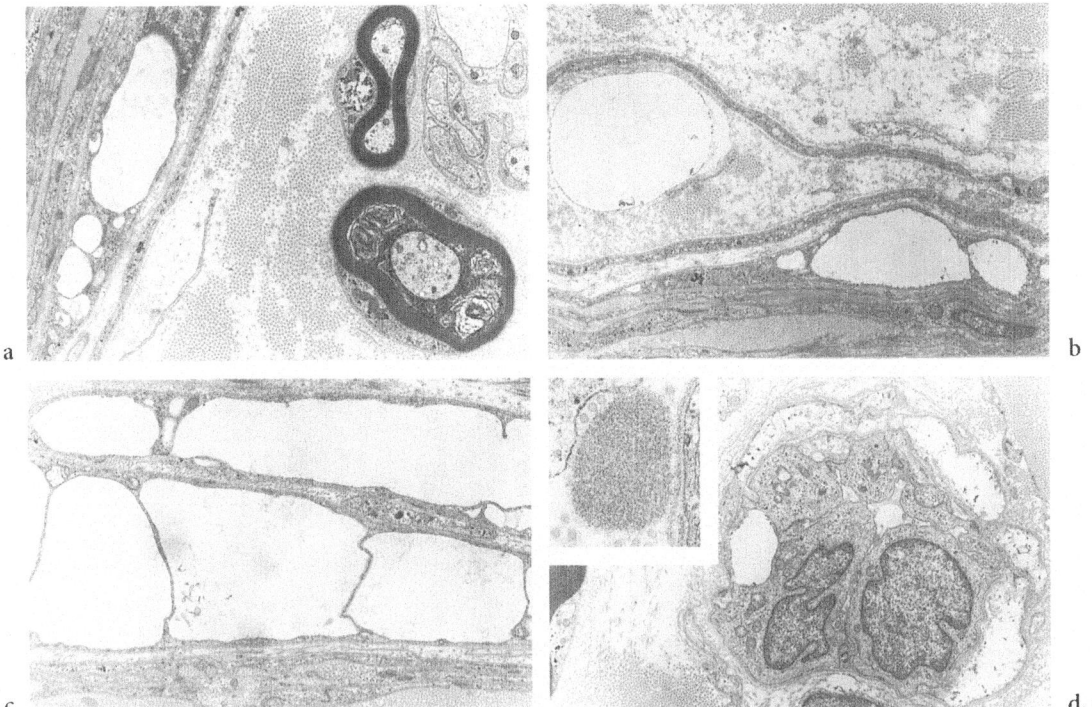

Fig. 136 a – e. Sural nerve biopsy in a 3-year-old girl and a 7-month-old girl with hyperglycinemia. **a** Vacuoles of large uneven size with electron optically lucent content, aside from moderately floccular precipitates, can be seen adjacent to the nucleus and at other sites in the cytoplasm of a perineurial cell. An unmyelinated axon is enlarged. The number of glycogen granules in the cytoplasm of a Schwann cell is increased. The Schmidt-Lanterman incisure in the nerve fiber in the lower right contains several membranous cytoplasmic bodies. × 6,500. **b** Some of the vacuoles are located intracytoplasmatically, another one is surrounded by a membrane but nevertheless is located extracellularly. × 5,800. **c** Some of the vacuoles are separated by very thin cytoplasmic bridges. × 7,500. **d** Several perithelial cells of a small endoneurial arteriole appear to be vacuolated. Another vacuole is located extracellularly adjacent to endothelial cells. × 5,500. **e** A bundle of oxytalan-fibrils is located in the extracellular space between collagen fibrils. × 28,000

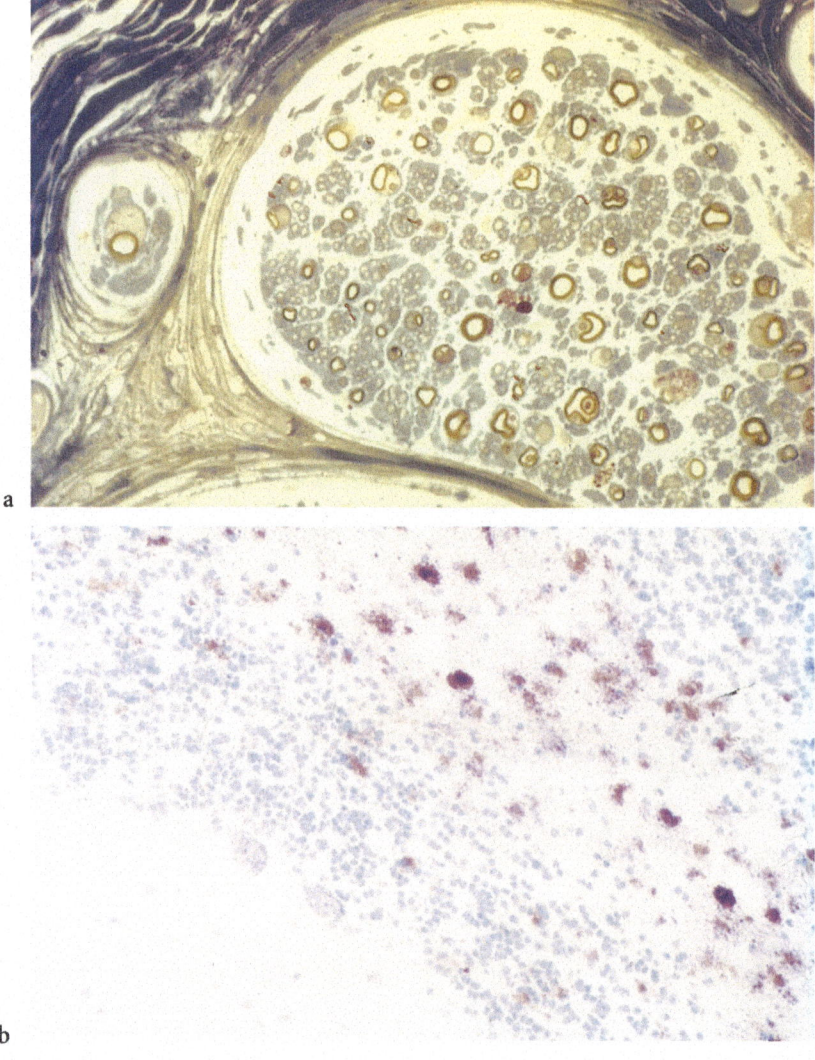

a

b

Fig. 137 a–d. Metachromatic leukodystrophy. **a–c** Infantile type, **d** juvenile type. **a, c, d** Toluidine blue. **b** Cerebellum Hirsch-Peiffer stain with acid cresylviolet. The metachromatic substances are stained reddish-brown; they are considerably more numerous in the infantile type than in the juvenile type. They occur in the cytoplasm of Schwann cells and oligodendroglial cells of myelinated nerve fibers as well as in macrophages, the latter mainly in a perivascular location

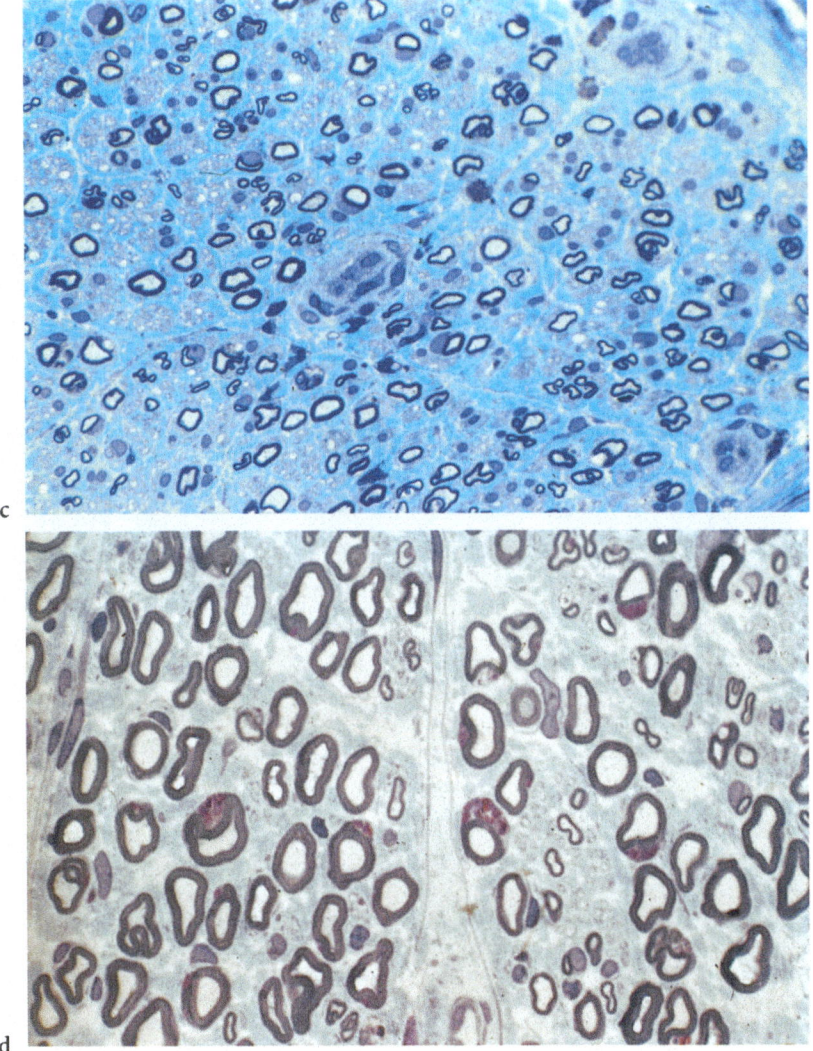

c

d

Fig. 137 c, d. Legend s. p. 154

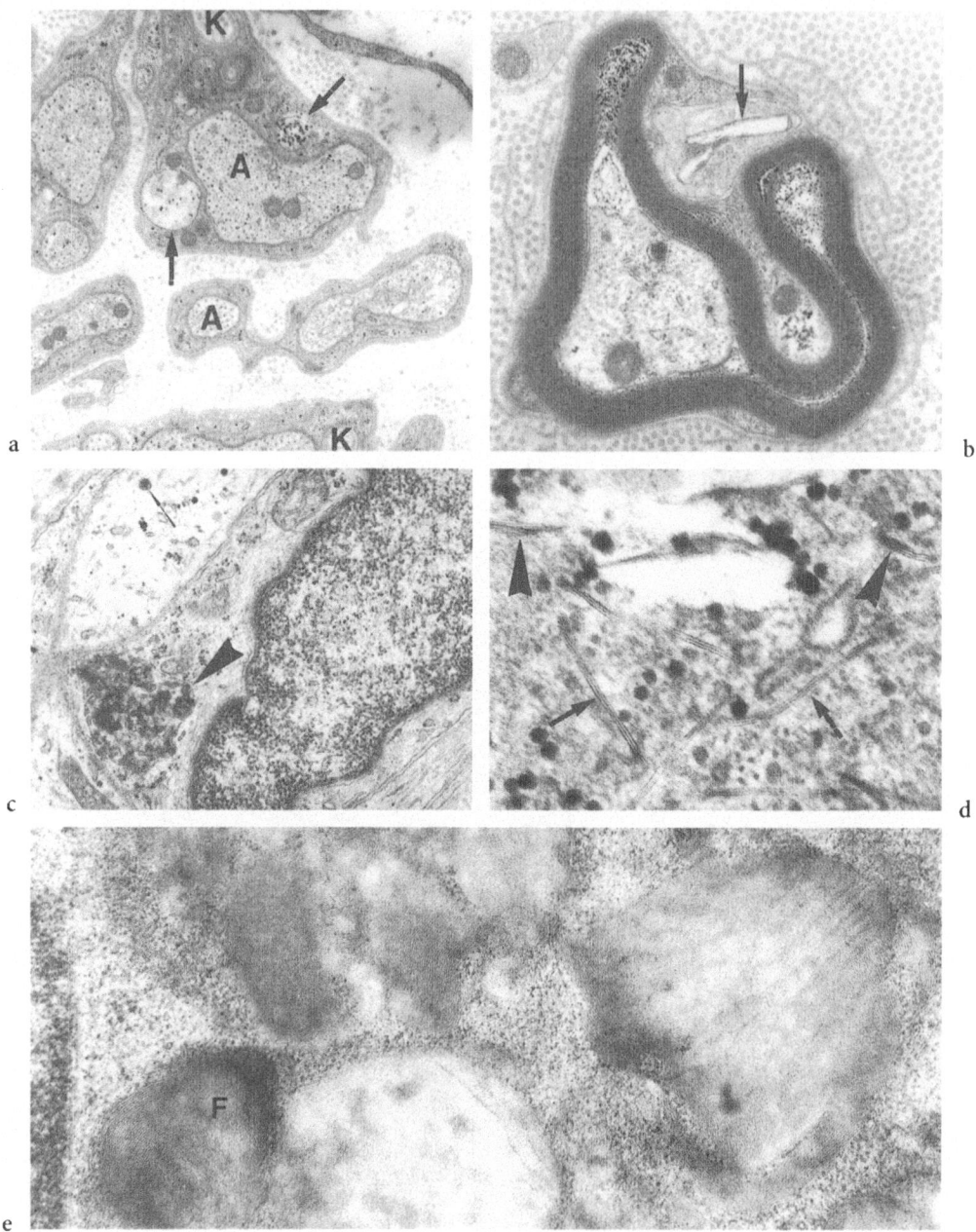

Fig. 138a–e. Pathognostic Schwann cell inclusions. **a** Mucopolysaccharidosis with typical vacuoles (*arrows*) which may contain mucopolysaccharides together with some glycogen granules, in an 8-year-old girl with Sanfilippo's disease, type A. The vacuoles are clearly distinguishable from unmyelinated axons (*A*) and collagen pockets (*K*). × 12,500. **b** Prismatic Schwann cell inclusions (*arrow*) in Krabbe's leukodystrophy. × 21,000. **c** Curvilinear cytosome (*arrowhead*) typical for ceroidlipofuscinosis in a Schwann cell within an autonomous nerve fiber of the plexus submucosus (Meissner) from a rectum biopsy. A catecholamine granulum is indicated by a *thin arrow*. × 23,400. **d** Adrenomyeloneuropathy in a 41-year-old female whose son is more severely affected. The trilaminar, i.e., threefold (*arrows*) or manifold (*arrowheads*) lamellated structures occur in large numbers in this Schwann cell and are unevenly oriented. × 92,400. **e** Fingerprint-like (*F*) and irregularly lamellated body in a Schwann cell of a 32-year-old female with adult metachromatic leukodystrophy. × 81,500. (From [958])

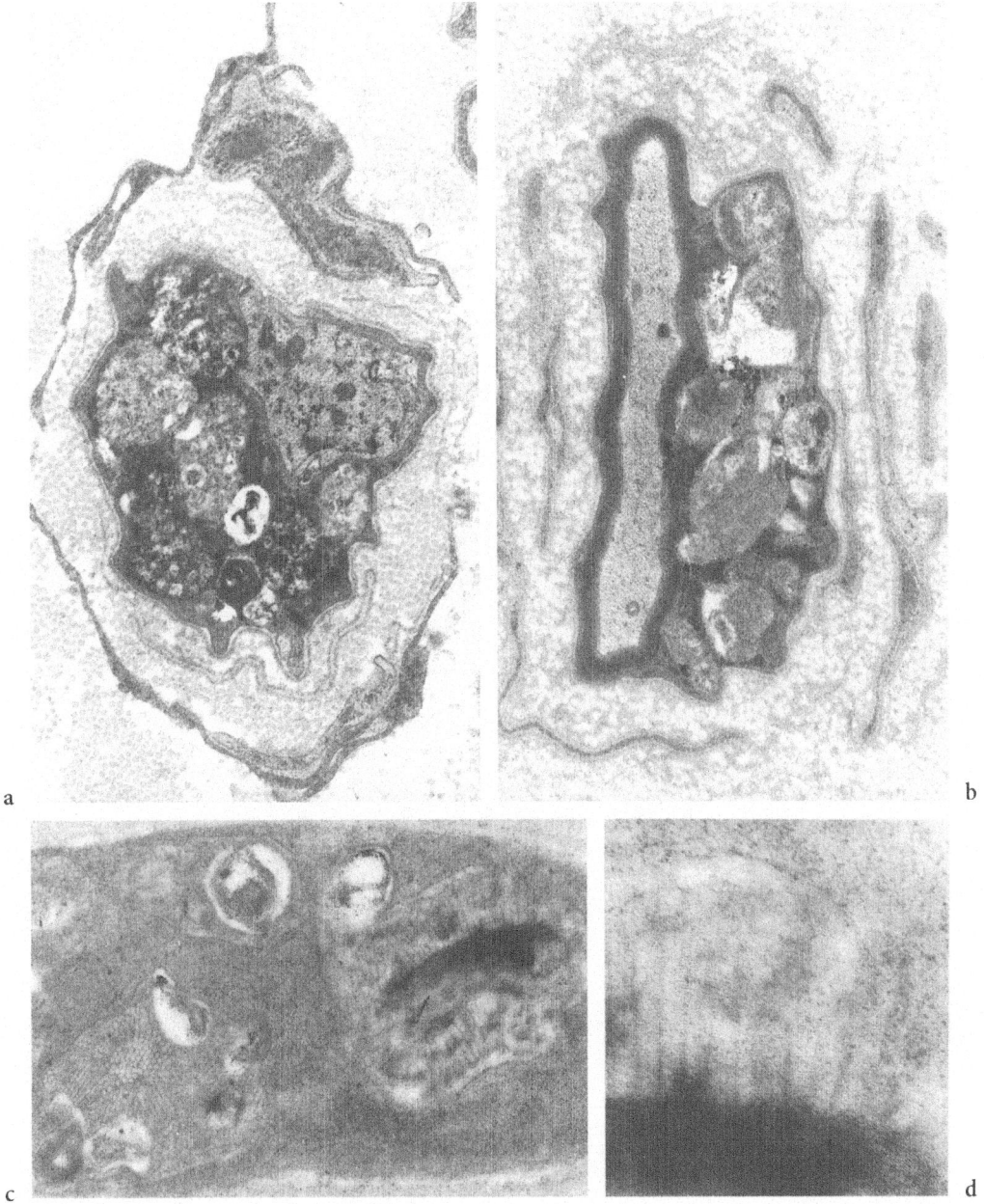

Fig. 139 a – d. Different Schwann cell inclusions in a 2-year-old boy with infantile metachromatic leukodystrophy. **a** Aside from a demyelinated axon there are pleomorphic Schwann cell inclusions of variable shape. This demyelinated nerve fiber is surrounded on one side by an empty collapsed basal lamina, and on the other side by a fibroblast and thin fibroblastic processes, but not by Schwann cell processes. **b** This presumably artificially shrunken axon with a disproportionately thin myelin sheath is surrounded by a Schwann cell with multiple inclusions. In the periphery are several flattened Schwann cell processes which are also covered by basal laminae. **a, b** × 18,100. **c** Higher magnification of Schwann cell inclusions with typical stacks of lamellar structures. Membranous cytoplasmic inclusions are also apparent. × 26,000. **d** Higher magnification of the parallel lamellae showing a periodicity of approximately 5 – 6 nm. × 90,000

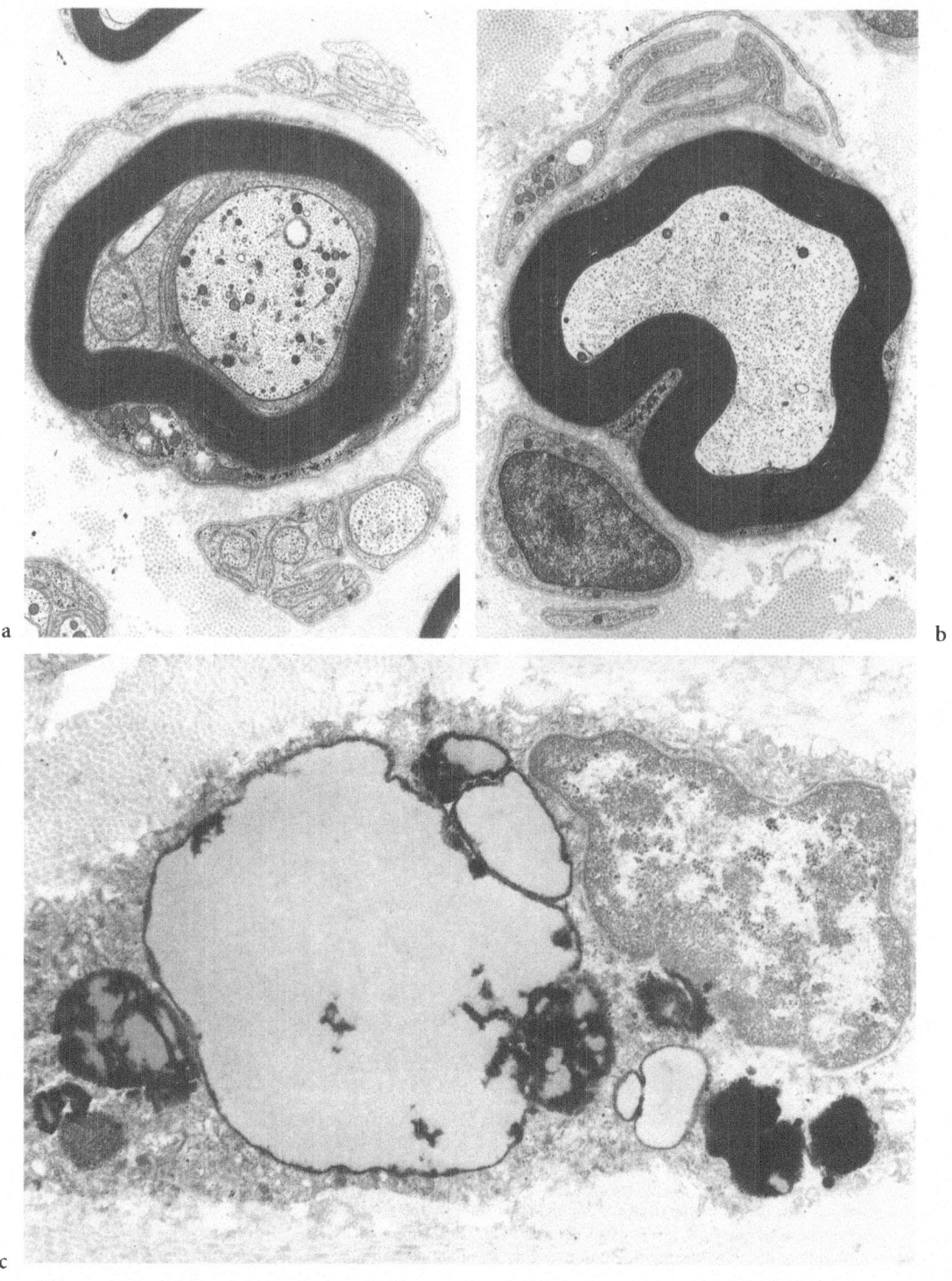

Fig. 140 a, b. Niemann-Pick disease type II in a 42-year-old female. **a, b** Nerve biopsy, 4 years before death. Incipient onion bulb formations with a myelinated nerve fiber in the center and a single unmyelinated axon in the periphery. **a** × 11,500; **b** × 9,000. **c** Autopsy revealed perivascular macrophages in skeletal muscles with lipofuscin showing an extensive lipid component. × 16,600

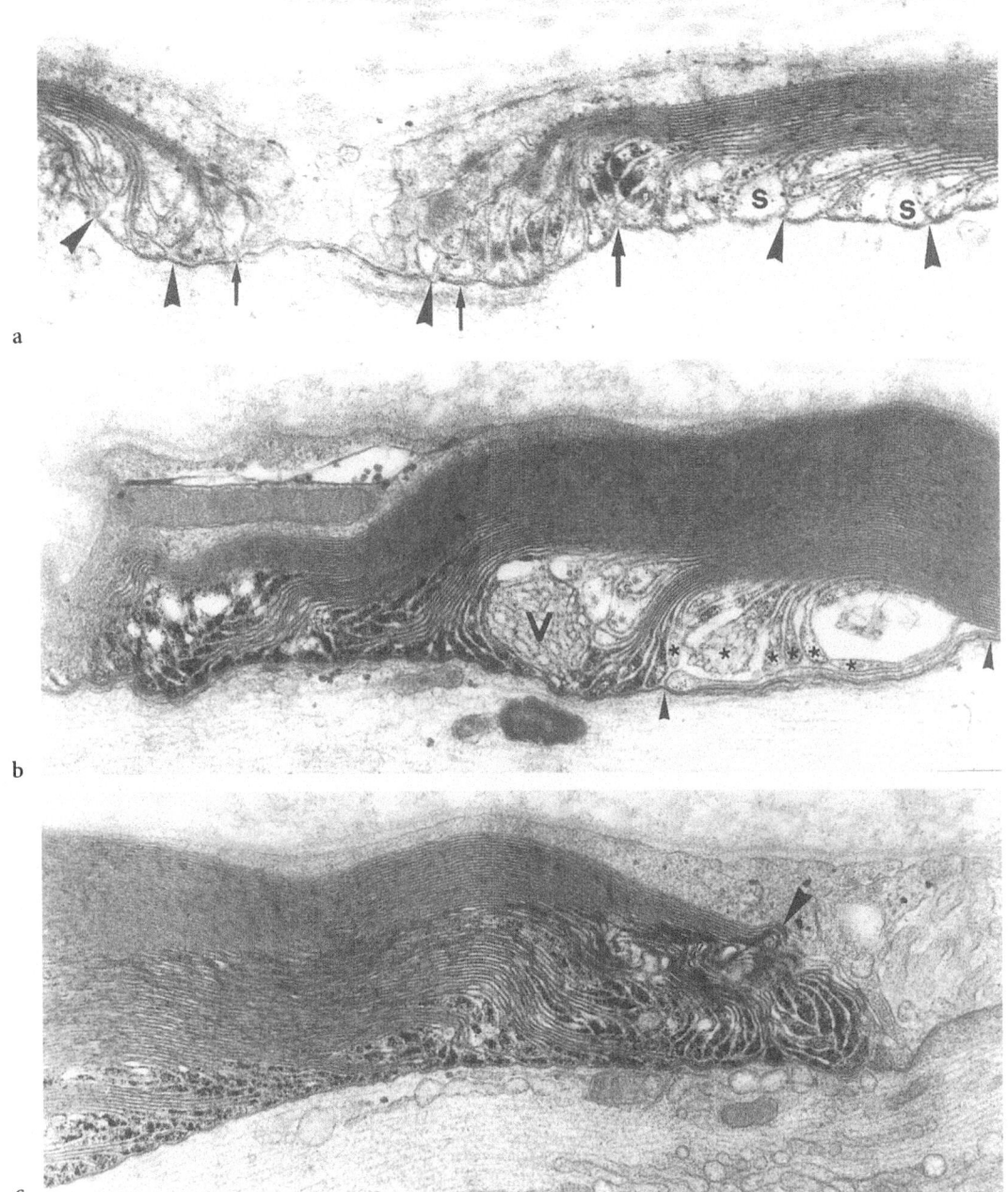

Fig. 141 a – c. Various alterations in the paranodal myelin loops in (**a**) a patient with Cockayne syndrome (5-year-old girl) in comparison to (**b**) a 5-month-old newborn with glomerulonephritis, and (**c**) a normal sural nerve of a 17-year-old boy who succumbed to a necrotizing myopathy of unknown cause. **a** Several terminal myelin loops are separated from the axolemma (*arrowheads*). At some sites there are desmosome-like structures (*large arrow*). Some loops are artificially swollen (*s*). *Small arrows* indicate terminal myelin loops in the paranode where there are no transverse bands. **b** The innermost myelin lamella between the *arrowheads* separates 6 other terminal myelin loops from the axon which are indicated by *asterisks*. Another group of lamellae is displaced from the axon adjacent to an area with focal, finely vesicular myelin degeneration (*V*). Other terminal myelin loops are regularly displaced into the myelin sheath. The abaxonal cytoplasm of the Schwann cell shows a split-like gap with some glycogen granules above a single mitochondrion. A small membranous cytoplasmic body can be seen in the axoplasm. **c** A double row of terminal myelin loops is separated from the axolemma at several sites (ultrastructural correlate of the thorns in the "double bracelets épineux" of Nageotte). An artificial deformation of the myelin lamellae, presumably caused by a moderate mechanical trauma, is indicated by an *arrowhead*. **a – c** × 40,000. (Modified from [966])

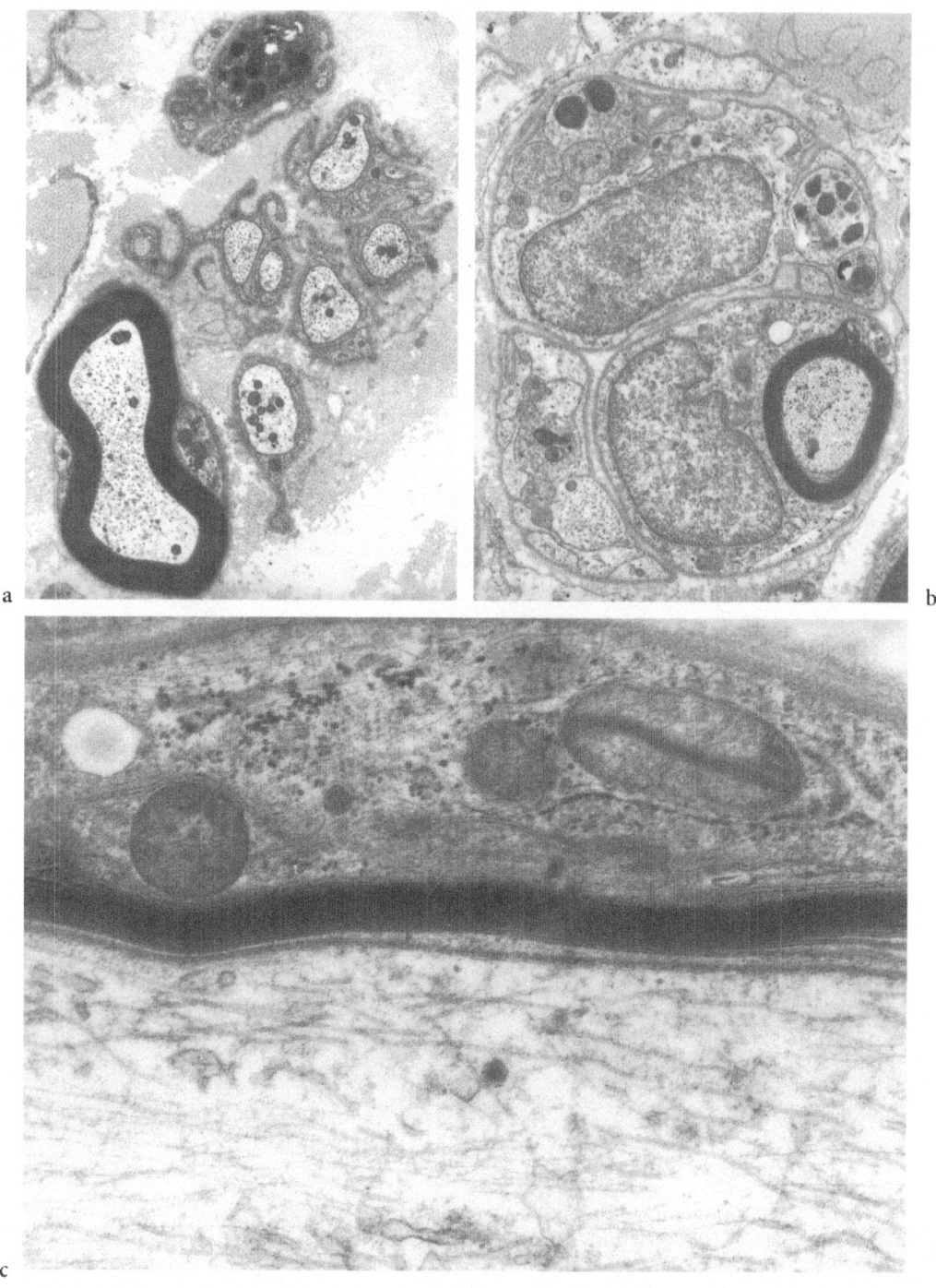

Fig. 142 a–c. Moderate neuropathy in multiple lipomatosis (Krabbe-Bartels syndrome) in a 59-year-old female. **a** Along with a group of partly preserved, partly deleted unmyelinated axons an abnormal axon can be seen with numerous dense bodies and some vacuoles. × 9,800. **b** Group of regenerated unmyelinated axons and a myelinated nerve fiber. Two axons contain large numbers of unusually homogeneous osmiophilic bodies. Some axons border immediately on each other. × 11,400. **c** Abnormal mitochondrion with parallel arranged mitochondrial cristae in the abaxonal cytoplasm of the Schwann cell of a myelinated nerve fiber. The microtubules and neurofilaments in the axon are partly irregularly oriented. × 45,000

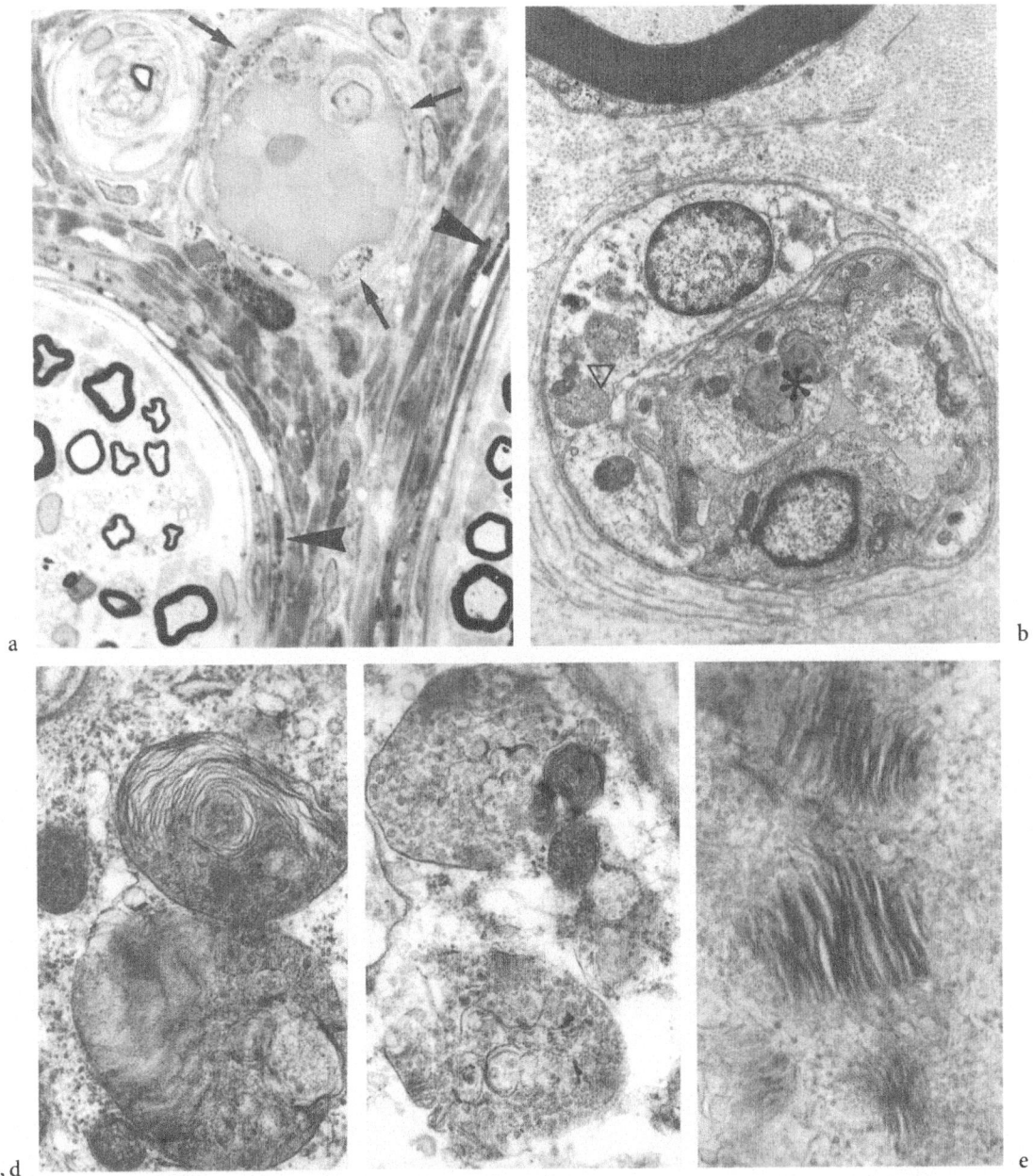

Fig. 143 a–d. Sandhoff's disease in a 16-month-old boy with cardiomyopathy. **a** Sural nerve with numerous osmiophilic endo-thelial cell inclusions in epineurial and endoneurial blood vessels (*arrows*) as well as in perineurial cells (*arrowheads*). × 1,175. **b** Endoneurial capillary with pleomorphic endothelial cell inclusions which are indicated by an *asterisk* in **b** and enlarged in **c**. The lamellated and multivesicular structures located in the adjacent pericytes are shown at higher magnification in **d**. The parallel lamellated membranous bodies in **e** are located in another endothelial cell. **b** × 9,300; **c, d** × 37,600; **e** × 45,100. (From [958])

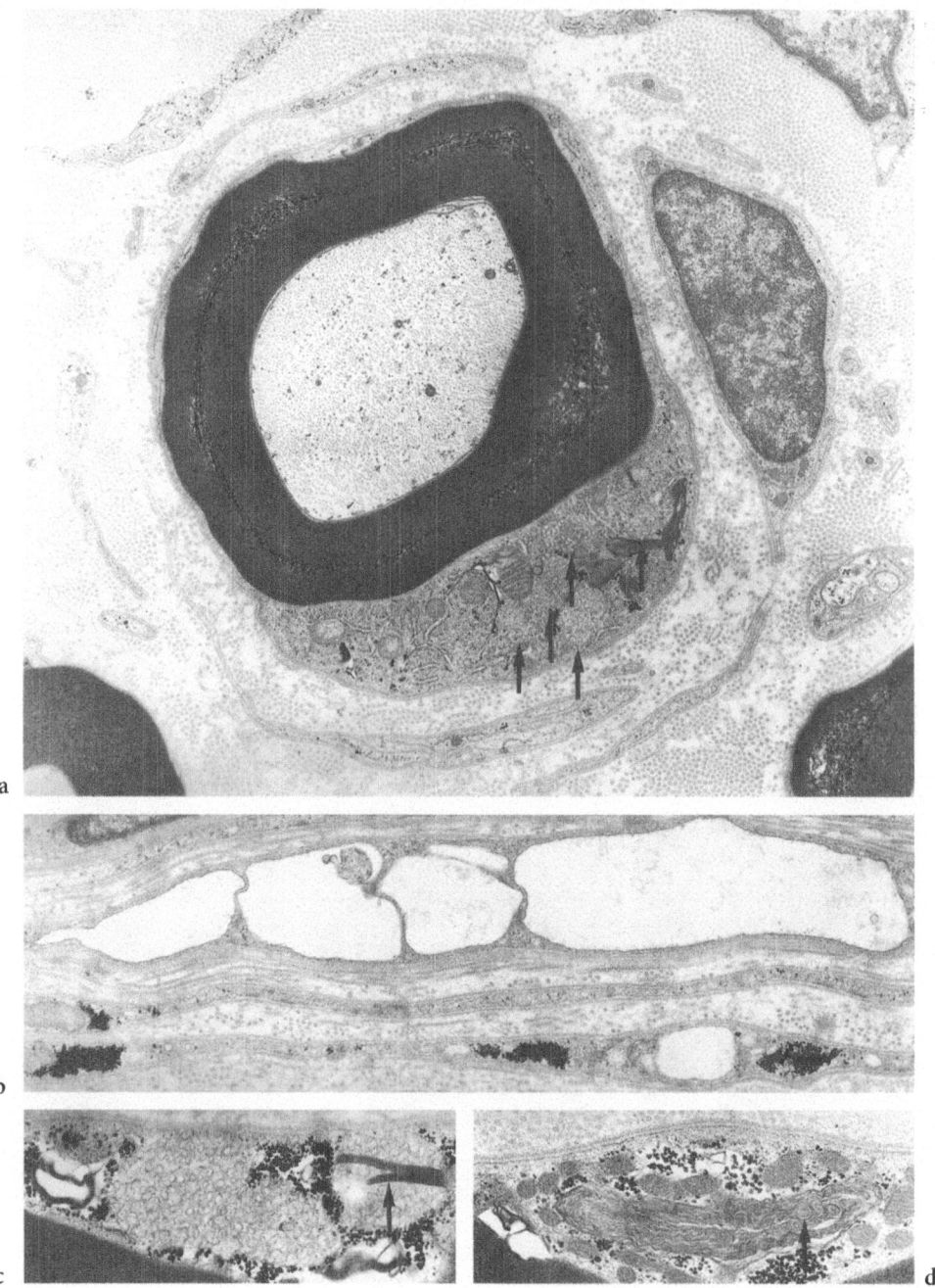

a

b

c   d

Fig. 144a–d. Severe ceroidlipofuscinosis in a 4-year-old girl with unusually numerous curvilinear cytosomes in the cytoplasm of Schwann cells. **a** Regularly remyelinated nerve fiber of intermediate size with a Schmidt-Lanterman incisure and numerous curvilinear cytosomes in the cytoplasm (*arrows*). This nerve fiber is circumferentially surrounded by multiple flattened Schwann cell processes (early stage of an onion bulb formation). × 11,000. **b** Multiple vacuoles in a perineurial cell. The vacuoles are surrounded by thin cytoplasmic bridges and appear electron optically empty. × 17,800. **c** There are two curvilinear cytosomes adjacent to a myelin sheath. One of the cytosomes contains lamellated membranes corresponding to π-granules. In addition, there are two small concentric membranous cytoplasmic bodies and numerous glycogen granules. × 21,000. **d** Loosely lamellated membranous cytoplasmic bodies (*arrow*) can also be seen in the cytoplasm of another myelinated nerve fiber. × 21,600

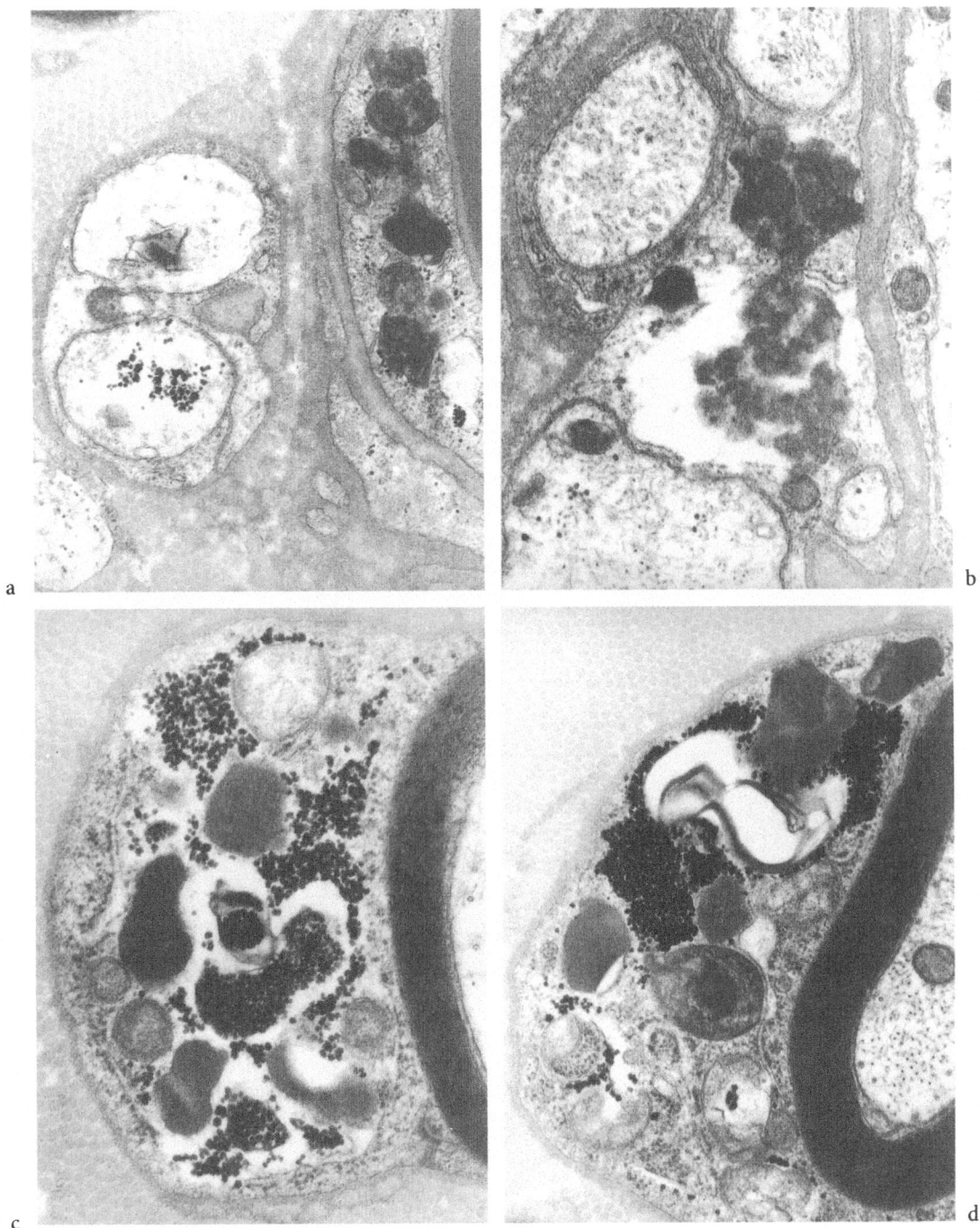

Fig. 145 a–d. Ceroidlipofuscinosis in a 2½-year-old boy. **a** Curvilinear cytosomes in an endothelial cell. The neighboring unmyelinated axons are clearly altered, the upper axon contains needle-like membranous inclusions, the lower one glycogen-like granules. × 28,600. **b** Finely granulated or amorphous Schwann cell inclusions in a Remak fiber with a tendency towards vacuolization. × 32,500. **c** Several irregular lysosomal Schwann cell inclusions without a characteristic structure between glycogen granules and mitochondria in the cytoplasm of a Schwann cell of a myelinated nerve fiber. × 40,300. **d** Further uncharacteristic lysosomal Schwann cell inclusions together with a vacuolated membranous body and a microperoxisome (or "microbody") with central dense inclusion. × 33,200

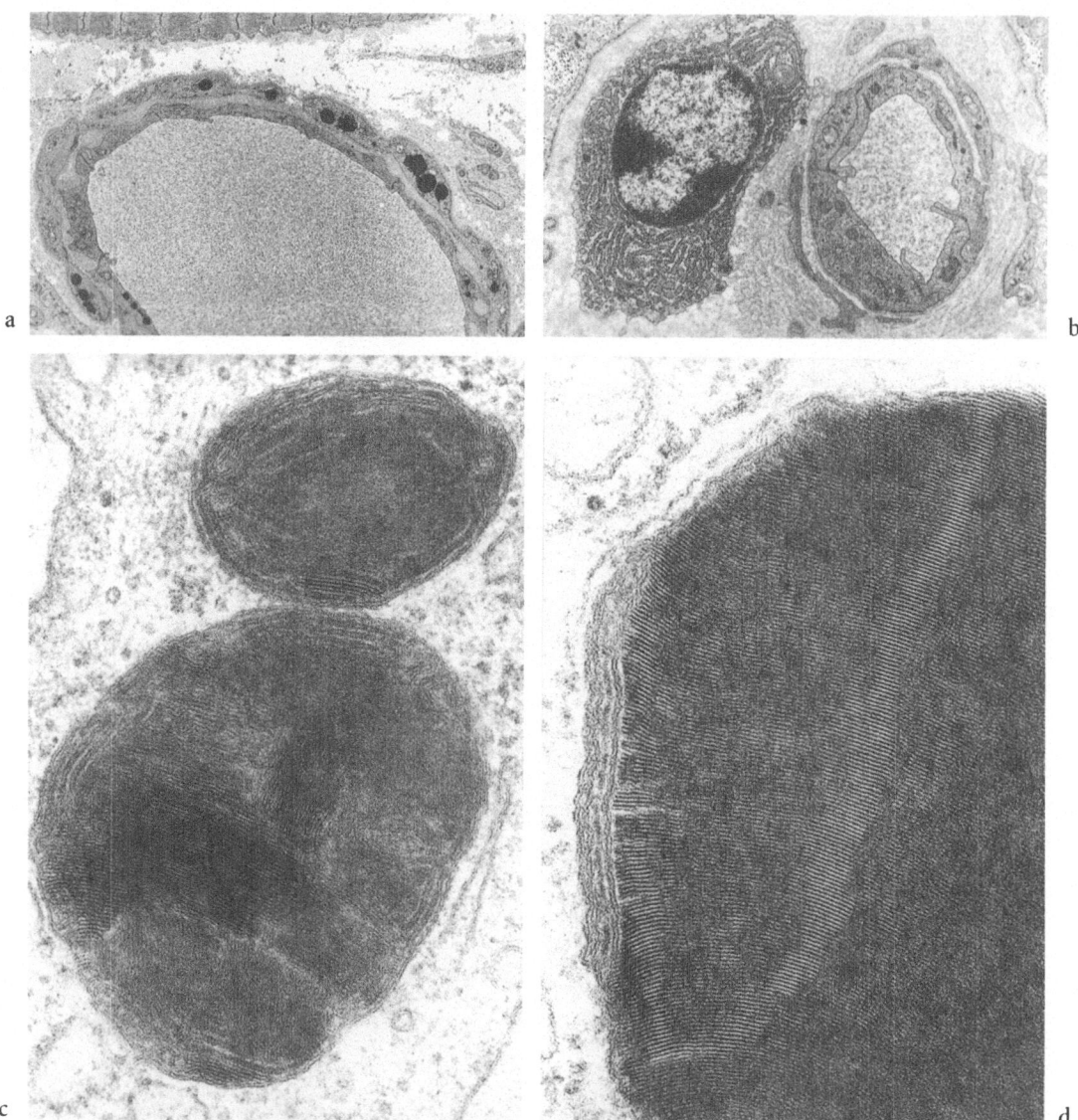

Fig. 146 a – d. Fabry's disease with characteristic membranous endothelial cell inclusions in a muscle biopsy (analogous to those seen in the nerve) in a 20-year-old female. **a, c, d** Partly parallel lamellated, partly concentric cellular inclusions with a lamellae periodicity of roughly 5 nm. **a** × 3,000; **c** × 100,000; **d** × 128,000. **b** A plasma cell with highly differentiated ergastoplasm can be seen close to the capillary. × 12,000

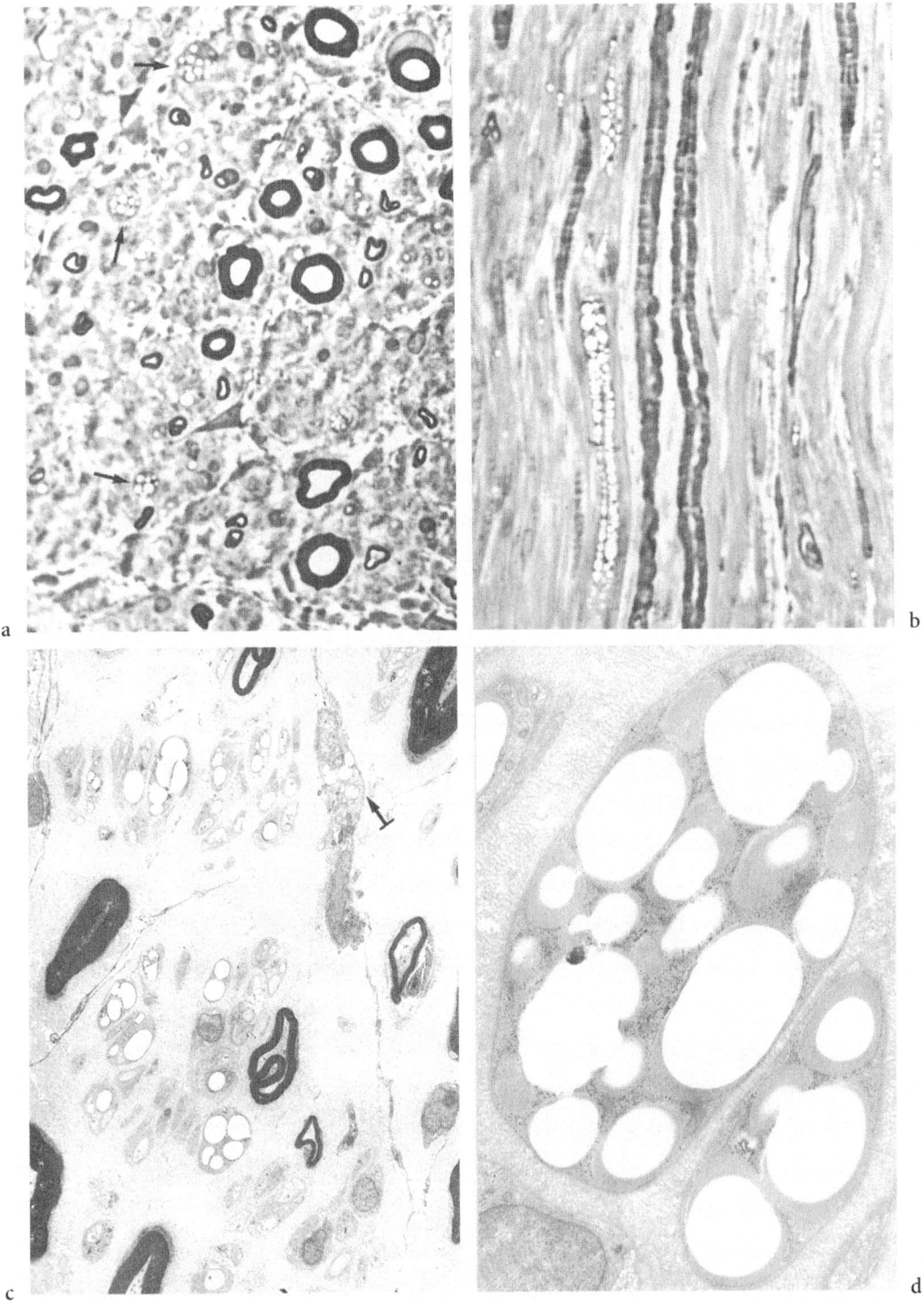

Fig. 147 a–d. Analphalipoproteinemia (Tangier disease) in a 32-year-old patient. **a, b** The number of myelinated nerve fibers is clearly reduced. At several sites there are multiple intracellular vacuoles (*arrows*). × 765. **c, d** Electron micrographs with numerous lipid droplets which are largely extracted (vacuoles) in Schwann cells and in a fibroblast-like cell which is indicated in **c** by an *arrow* and shown in **d** at higher magnification. **c** × 2,160; **d** × 8,640

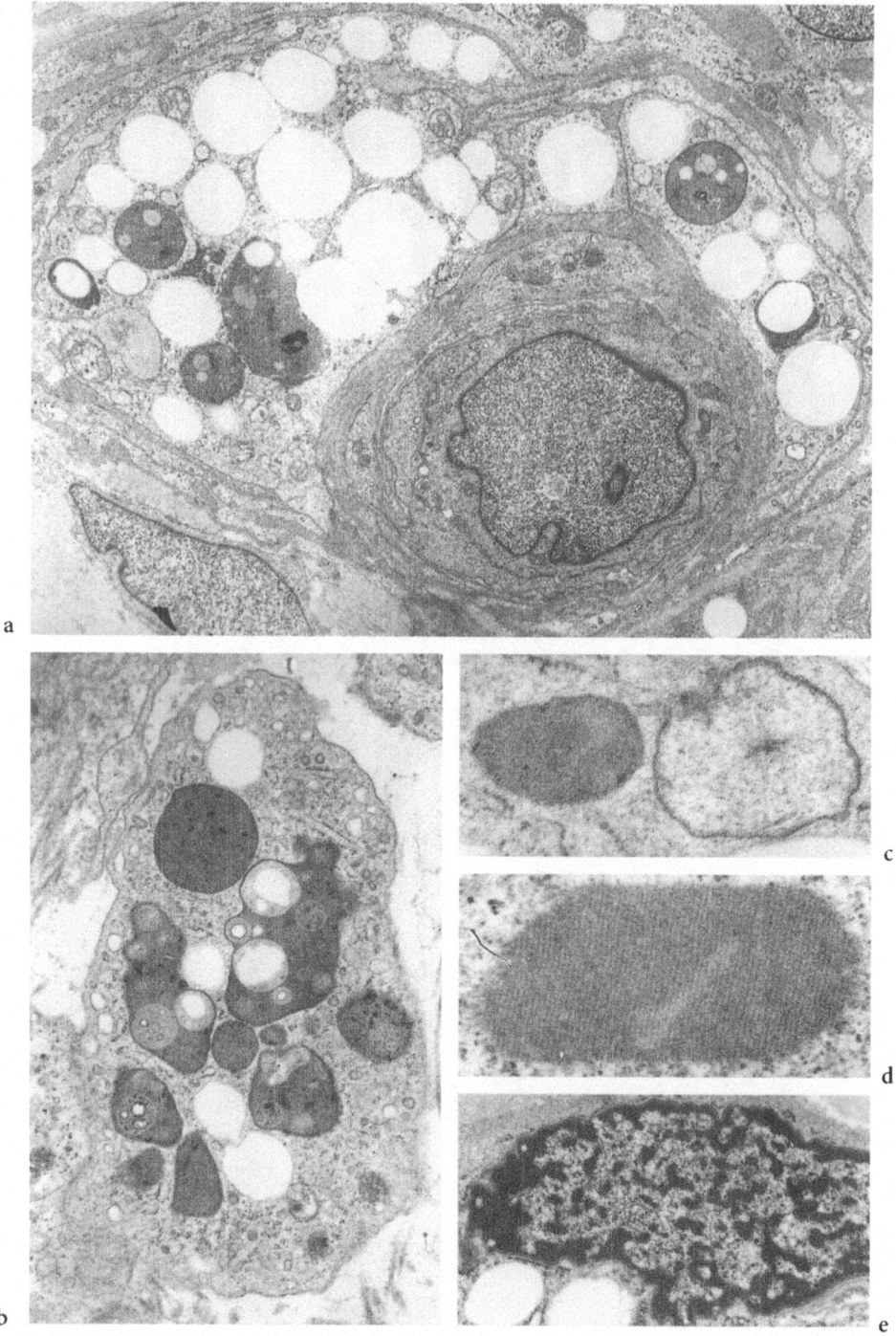

Fig. 148 a – e. Skin biopsy from the same patient as in Fig. 147. **a** Pericapillary histiocyte with numerous vacuoles and various phagolysosomes. × 9,810. **b** Histiocyte in the corium with pleomorphic phagolysosomes and some vacuoles. × 10,700. **c** Adjacent to a lysosomal body is an abnormally dilated mitochondrion which can be identified by the surrounding double membrane. It contains only rudimentary mitochondrial cristae. × 25,800. **d** Unusual periodically structured filamentous body with a dimension of 2.4 × 1.1 μm in a histiocyte. The structure corresponds to intracellular fibrin. The filaments measure about 6 – 8 nm in diameter, the striation shows a periodicity of about 35 nm. × 27,700. **e** Incipient karyorrhexis with aggregated heterochromatin and two vacuoles in the cytoplasm of a histiocyte. × 13,200. (From [331]

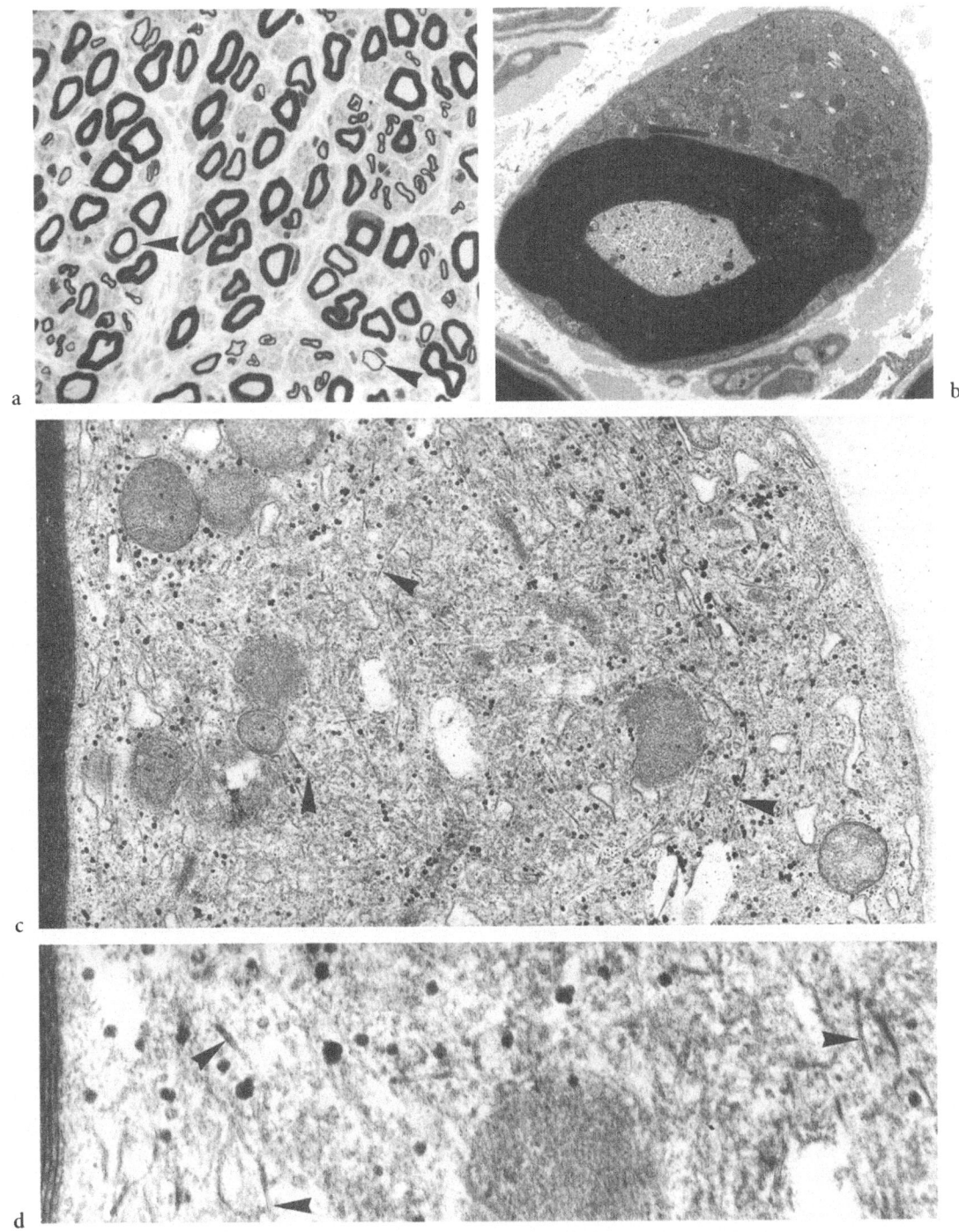

Fig. 149a–d. Adrenoleukodystrophy in a 44-year-old female. **a** Some nerve fibers are hypomyelinated and surrounded by circumferentially arranged Schwann cell processes (*arrowheads*) (case of [990]). Toluidine blue, × 340. **b** Regularly myelinated nerve fiber with conspicuously broad cytoplasm which is shown at higher magnification in **c** and **d**. There are masses of two-, three-, or multilayered, usually trilaminar structures in the cytoplasm (*arrowheads*) representing rather pathognomonic storage products of adrenoleukodystrophy. **b** × 5,600; **c** × 31,000; **d** × 76,000

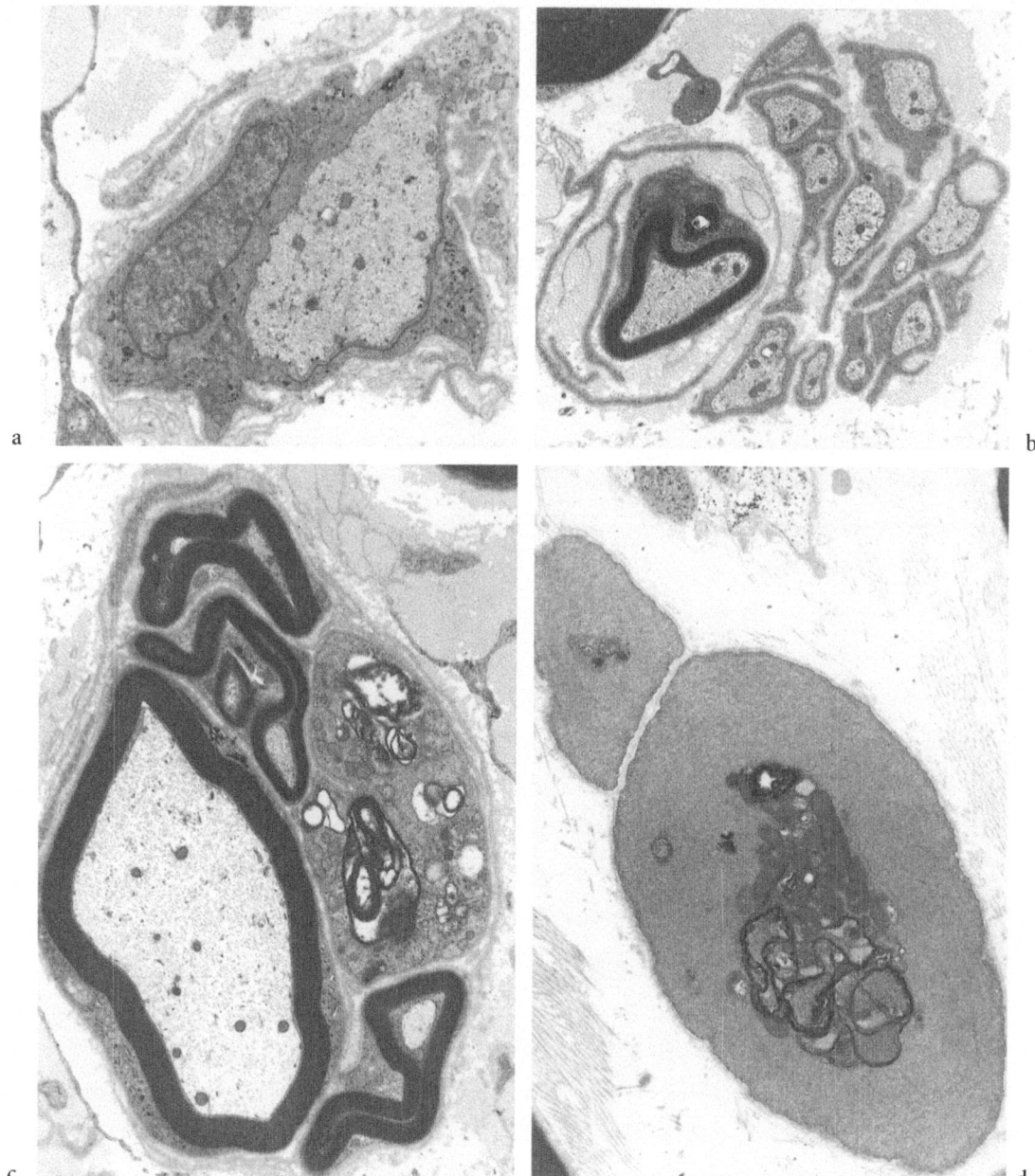

Fig. 150 a–d. Same case as in Fig. 149. **a** Demyelinated axon in a stage of incipient remyelination surrounded by several Schwann cell processes and basal laminae. × 9,300. **b** Myelinated nerve fiber which is completely encircled by thin Schwann cell processes and basal laminae adjacent to a group of unmyelinated axons. × 8,000. **c** Group of regenerated nerve fibers with adjacent Schwann cell processes and myelin degradation products within one of the cells. Only one myelinated fiber has become large, the others are atrophic presumably because they have not found contact to an adequate end organ. × 9,300. **d** Unidentified endoneurial cells with fine actin-like filamentous content and central accumulation of mitochondria and membranous cytoplasmic bodies. × 9,500

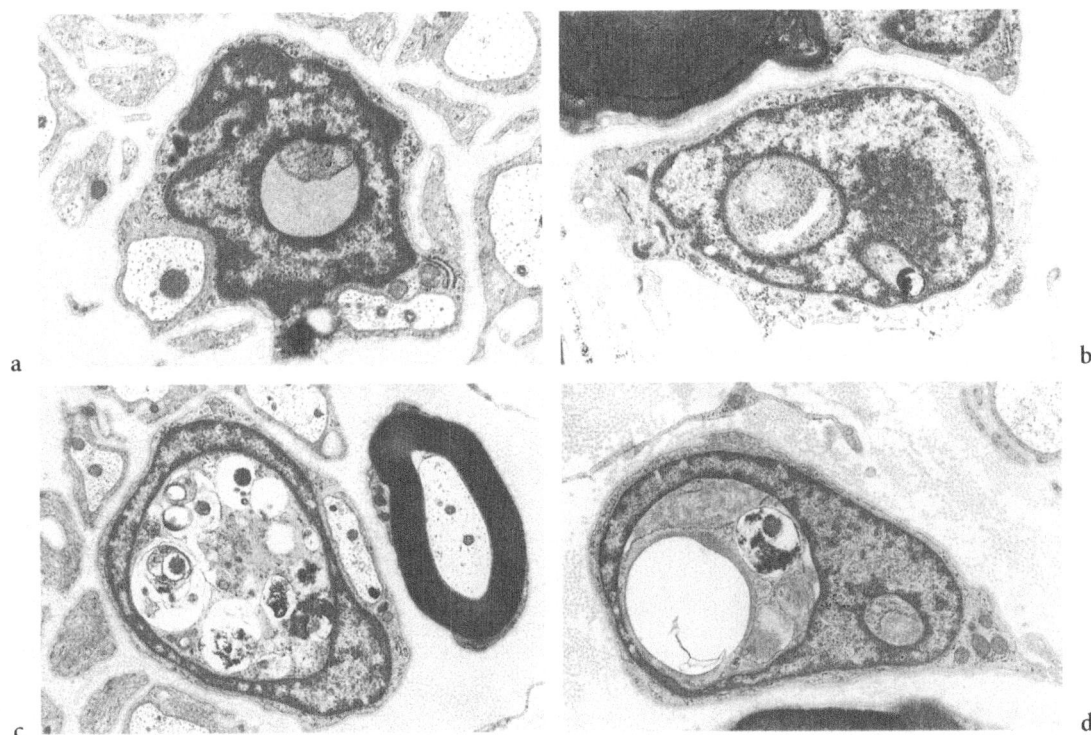

Fig. 151a–d. Same case as in Figs. 149 and 150. Unusual nuclear inclusions in Schwann cells with partly granular, partly amorphous, partly vacuolar or membranous content in combination with unmyelinated axons (**a, c**) or after loss of axons (**b, d**). The inclusions in **b–d** are associated with cytoplasmic invaginations. **a** × 13,300; **b** × 11,100; **c** × 8,700; **d** × 9,200

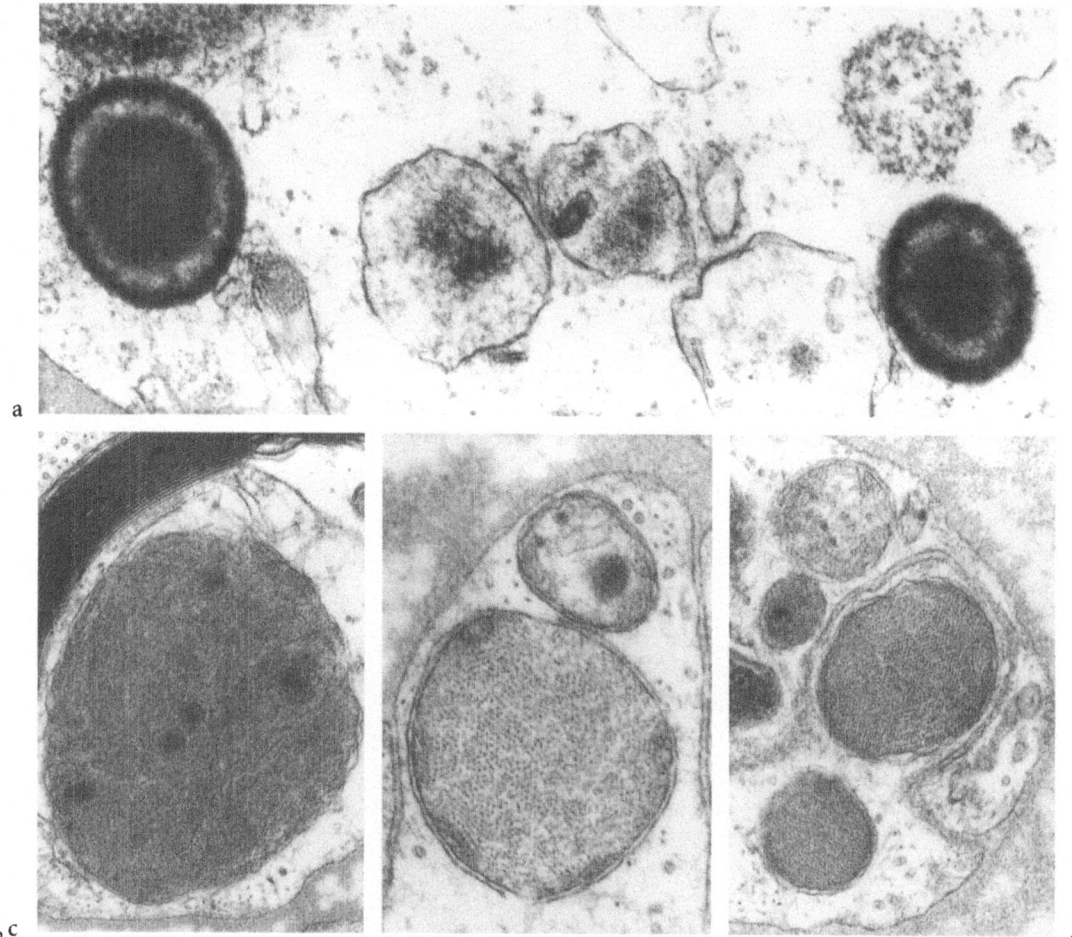

Fig. 152a–d. Twenty-four-year-old son of the 48-year-old female represented in Figs. 149–151. **a** Calcospherites and membrane-limited peroxisome-like swollen cellular inclusions in watery cytoplasm adjacent to a nucleus. × 54,400. **b–d** Abnormal mitochondria in the cytoplasm of Schwann cells; the mitochondrion in **b** is exceptionally large, showing several enlarged matrix granules, irregularly distributed mitochondrial cristae, and a condensed granular or amorphous matrix. By contrast, the granular or amorphous inclusions in the mitochondria of **c** and **d** are uncharacteristic and may occur in many different neuropathies. **b** × 46,000; **c** × 71,000; **d** × 59,000

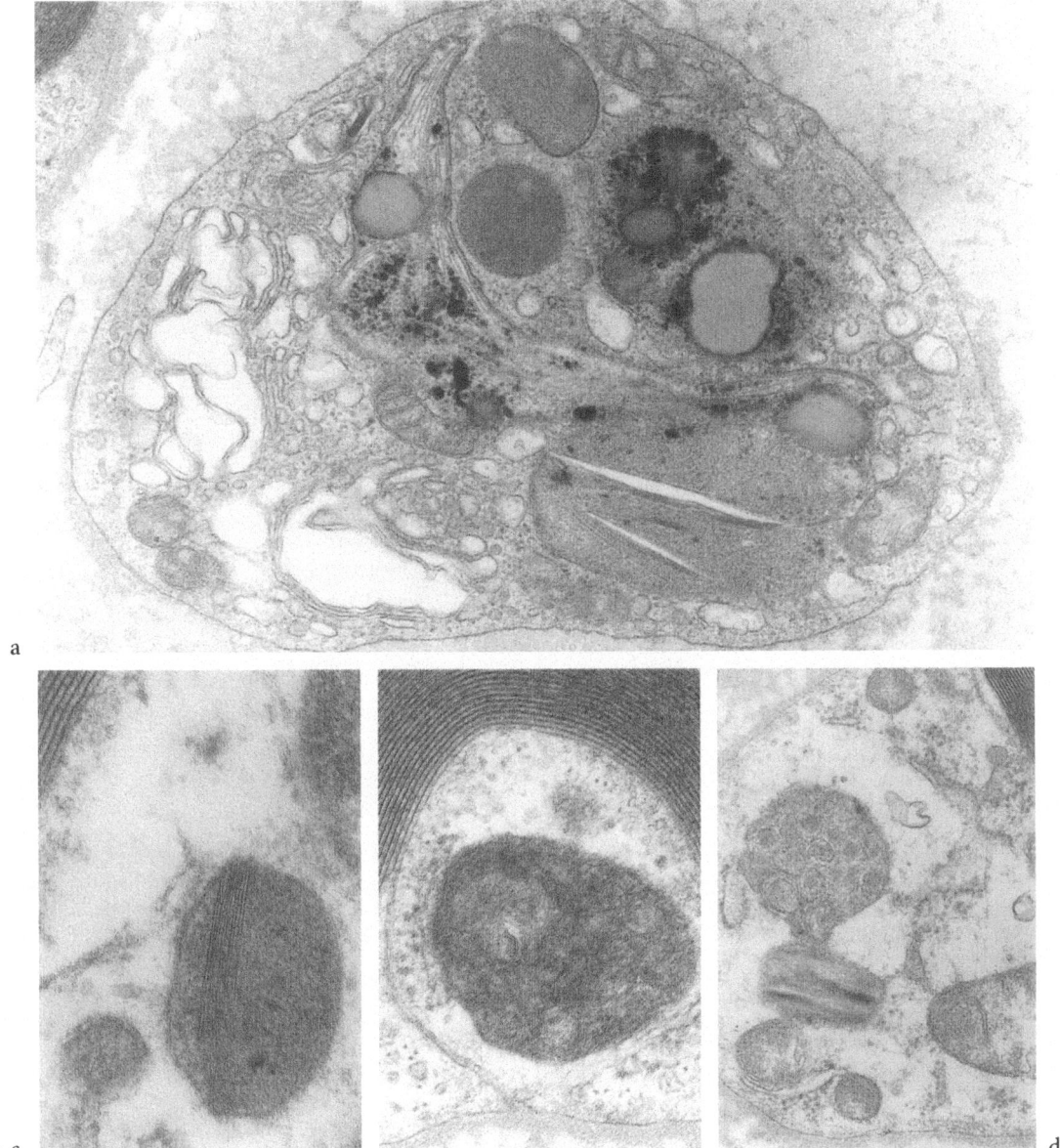

Fig. 153 a–d. Same case as in Fig. 152. **a** Endoneurial macrophage with increased, enlarged, and swollen Golgi complexes, needle-like or slit-like inclusions as well as nonspecific lipofuscin bodies and lysosomes. × 34,400. **b** Abnormal mitochondrion with a few centrally located parallel mitochondrial cristae and an otherwise amorphous matrix structure. × 95,000. **c** Lysosome-like bodies with only indistinct membranous structures. × 70,000. **d** Complex cytosome with partly parallel lamellated, partly concentrically arranged membranes within two seemingly connected components in the cytoplasm of a Schwann cell of a myelinated nerve fiber. × 38,500

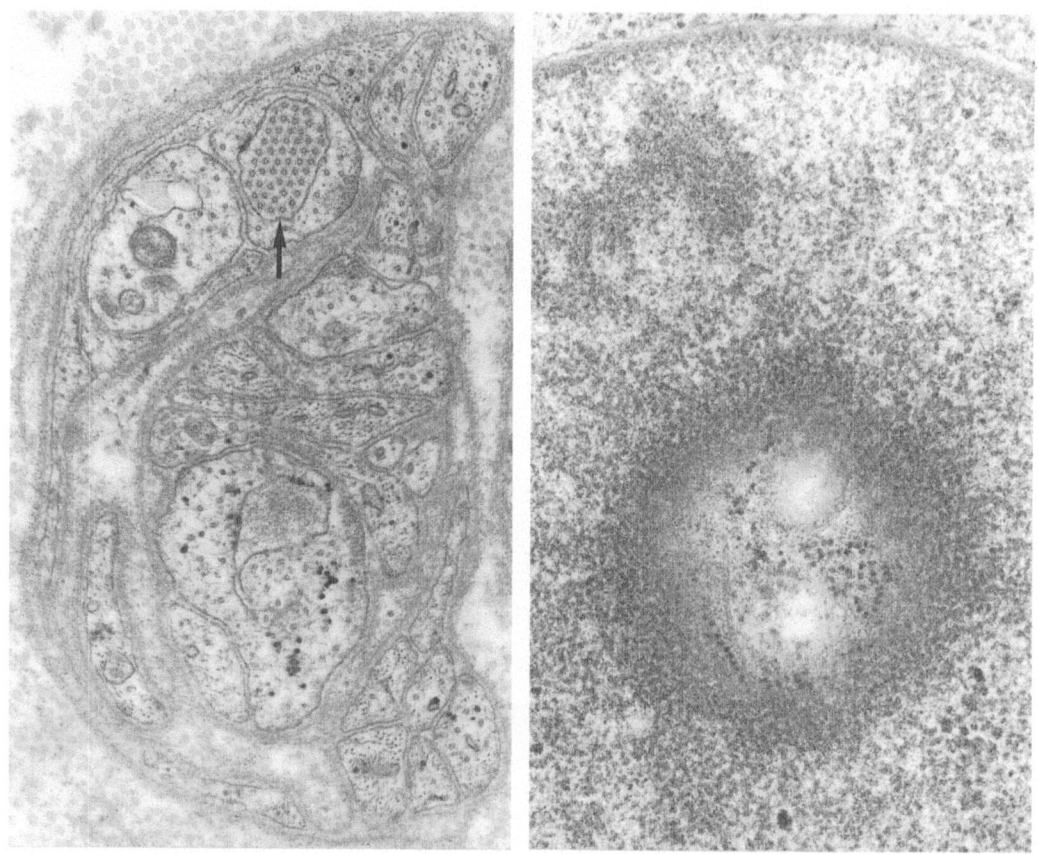

a   b

Fig. 154 a, b. Unusual cytoplasmic and nuclear inclusions in a 59-year-old man with adrenomyeloneuropathy according to clinical data. **a** In a presumptive Schwann cell process adjacent to a similarly structured axon (which, however, shows a somewhat more electron dense surface membrane) is a membrane-bound hexagonally arranged aggregate of microtubules. The tubules are slighly larger than the microtubules in the surrounding cytoplasm and adjacent axoplasm. × 36,000. **b** Central alteration of a nucleus with a microtubule and several granules. This area is surrounded by other less electron dense chromatin granules. × 47,000

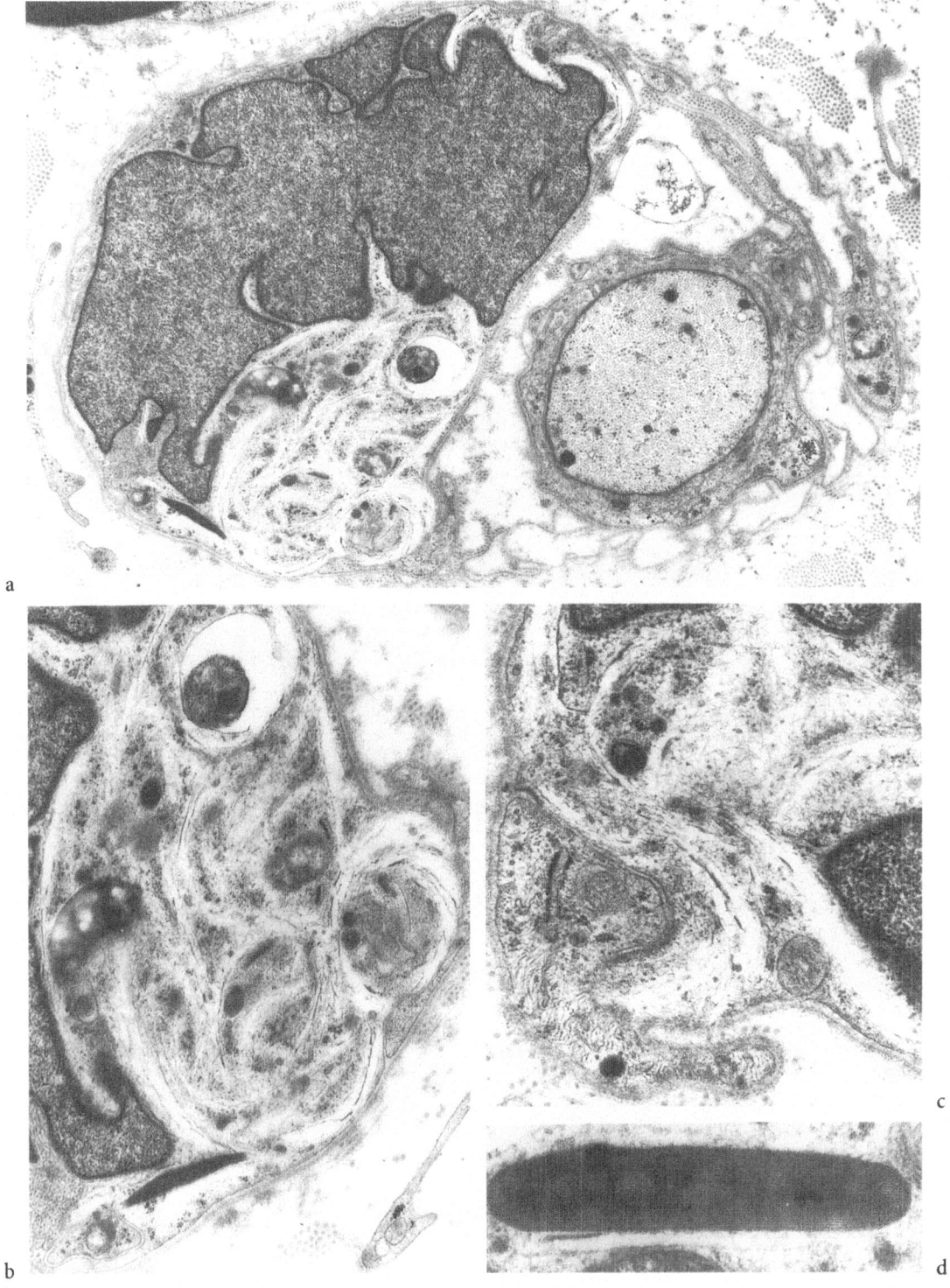

Fig. 155a–d. Unidentified, predominantly demyelinating type of neuropathy in a 38-year-old female with episodic weakness (years after a tick bite with focal inflammatory reaction: Lyme borreliosis?). The Schwann cell inclusions are partly lamellar, partly vacuolar, or electron dense and amorphous. They differ from typical trilaminar or prismatic inclusions such as seen in adrenomyeloneuropathy or Krabbe's disease and from π-granules such as those seen in **d. a** × 11,300; **b** × 22,500; **c** × 38,000; **d** × 70,000

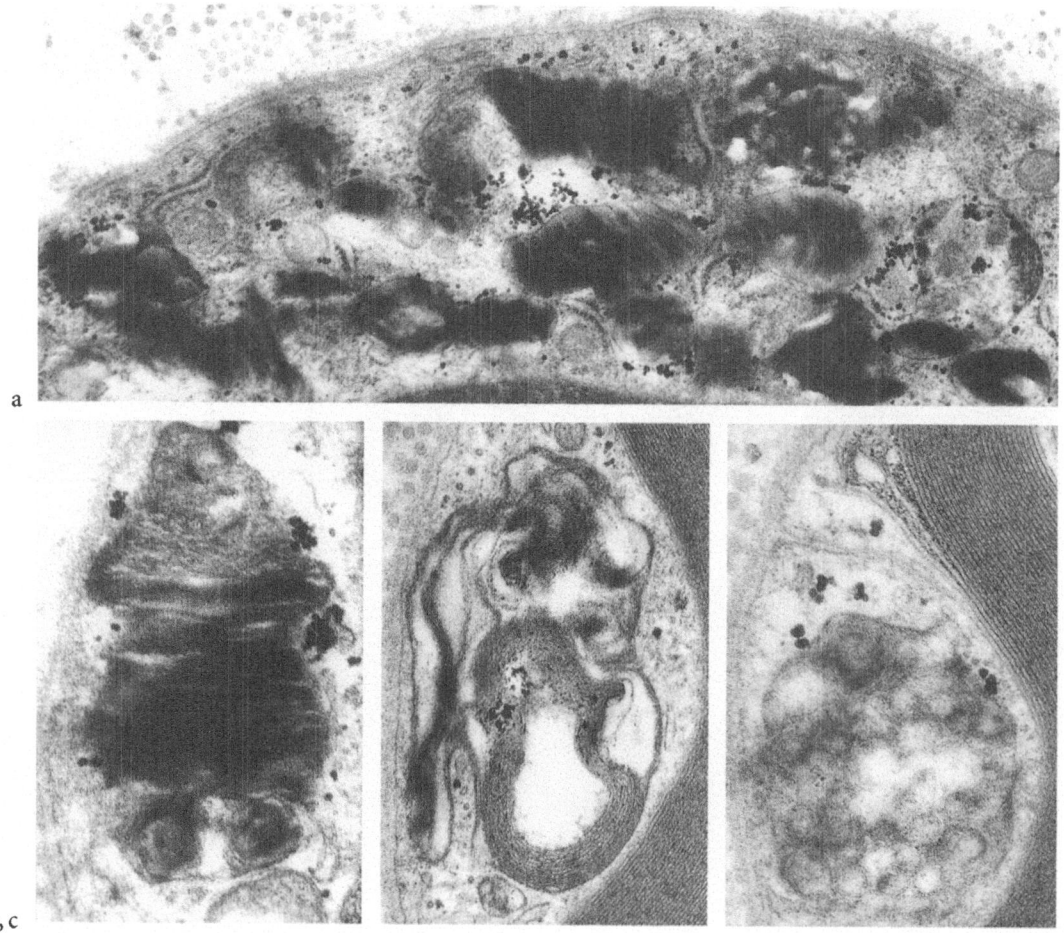

Fig. 156a–f. Same case as in Fig. 138a, Sanfilippo's disease, type A. **a, b** The pleomorphic bodies with amorphous or membranous inclusions presumably correspond to the ganglioside storage material in this disease. They need to be distinguished from π-granules (Reich). **a** × 30,000; **b** × 55,000. **c** This μ-granule (Elzholz) shows incomplete lysis and needs to be distinguished from usual myelin ovoids. × 100,000. **d** This nonspecific cytosome is composed of multiple concentrically arranged membranous structures and surrounded by a unit membrane. × 35,000. **e, f** s. p. 175

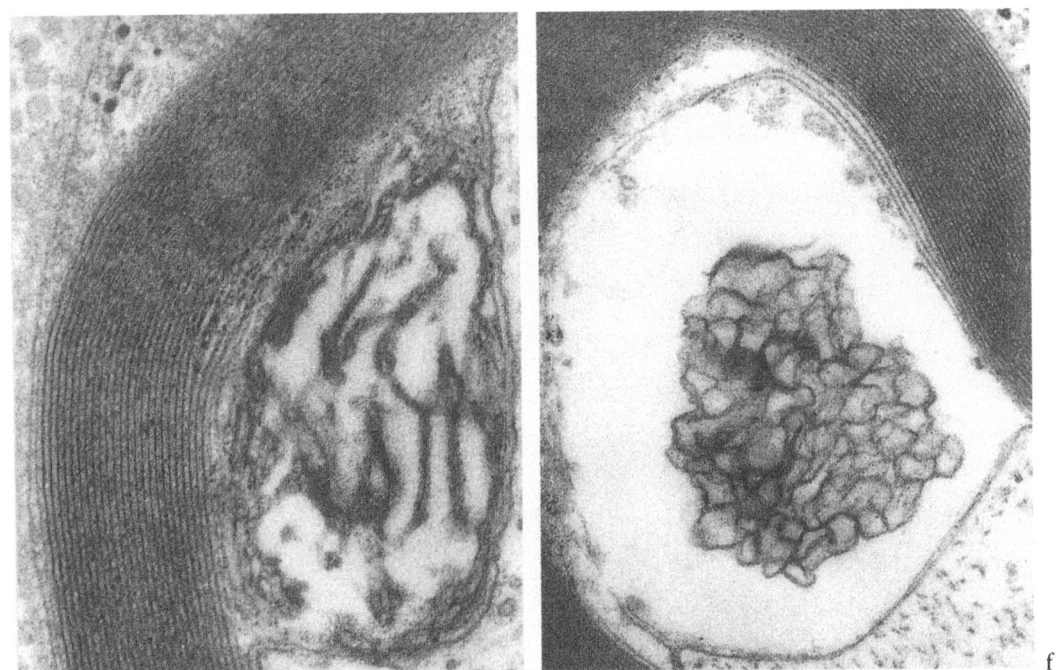

Fig. 156 e, f. Divergent lytic changes of inner myelin lamellae. **e** × 48,000, **f** × 33,000. (From [958])

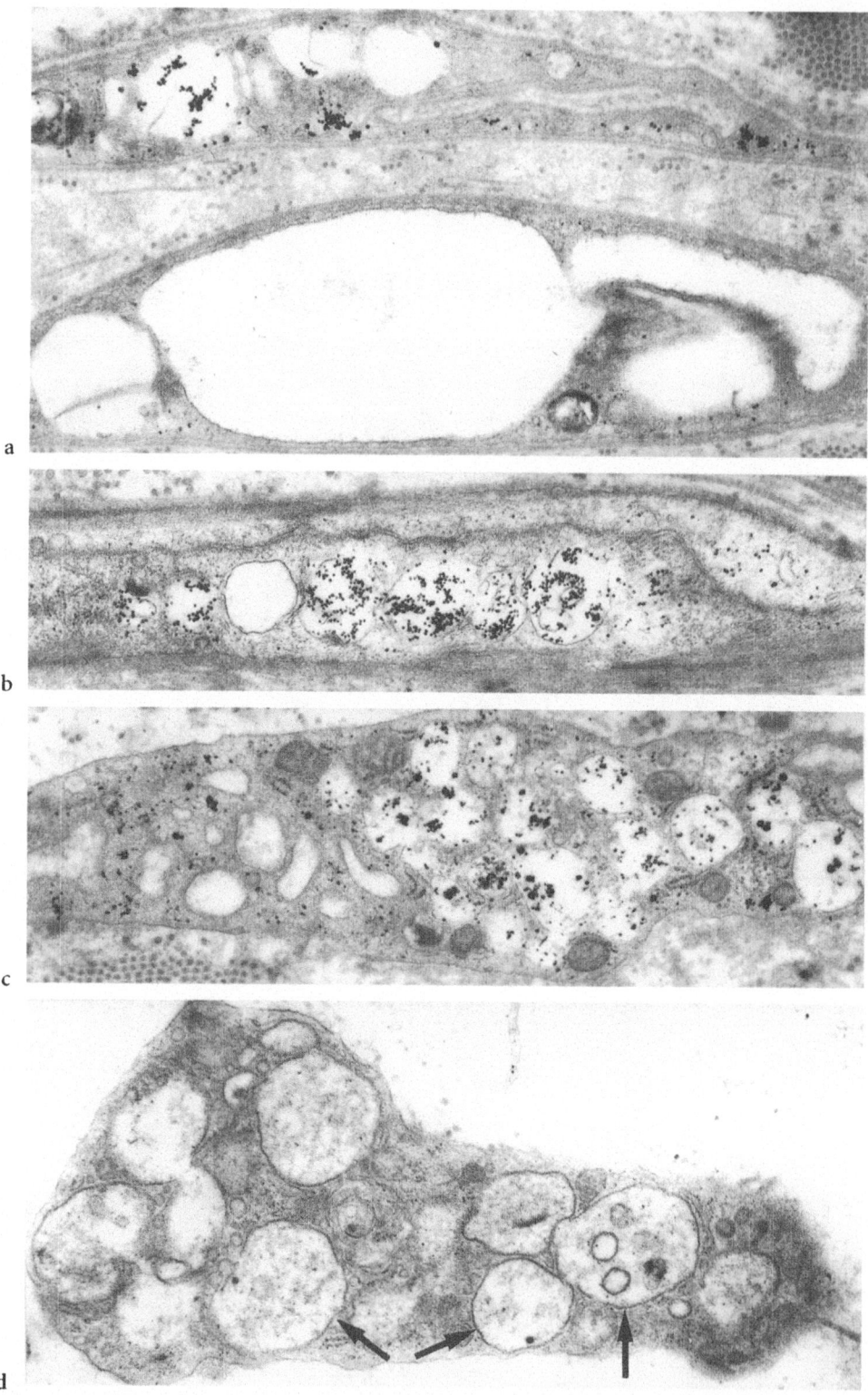

Fig. 157 a – d. Same case as in Fig. 156. Vacuoles (**a**, **b**) and vesicles containing glycogen are nonspecific inclusions in perineurial (**a**, **b**) and subperineurial cells (**c**). The vacuoles with mucopolysaccharide-like amorphic or fine floccular substances with single osmiophilic granules, surrounded by an electron dense unit membrane, in an endoneurial perivascular fibroblast (*arrows* in **d**) are pathognomonic. **a** × 14,000; **b** × 15,000; **c** × 13,000; **d** × 14,500

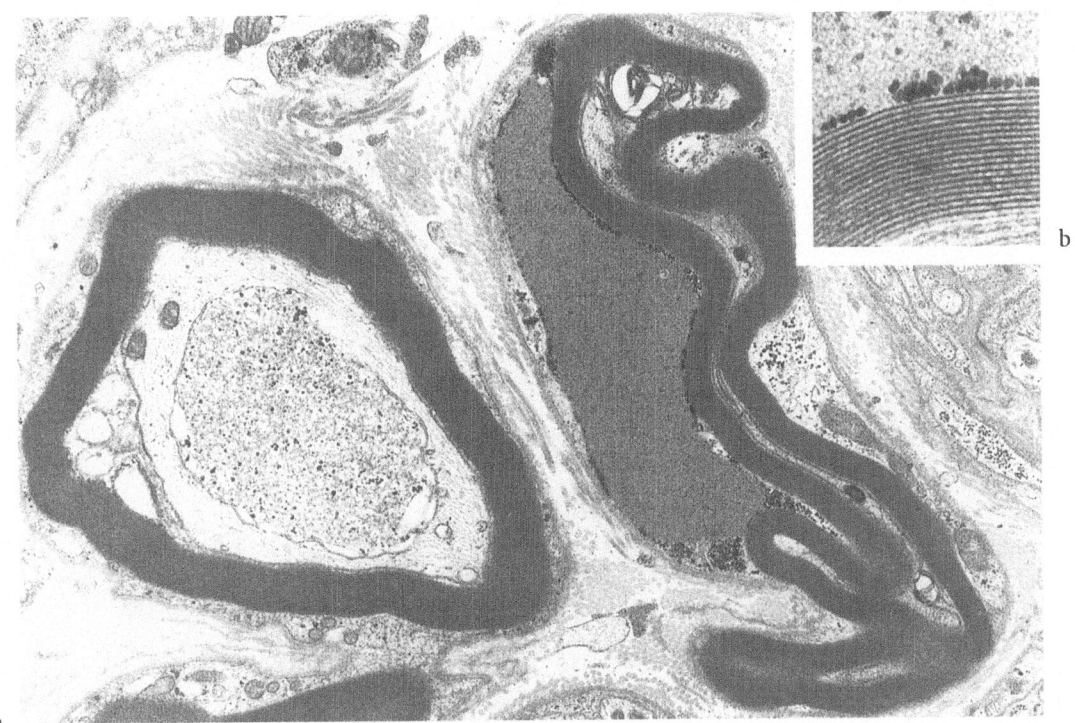

a

b

Fig. 158 a–d. α-Mannosidosis in a 4-year-old boy. **a** Unusual large intra-axoplasmatic inclusion with a double membrane at the surface and partly finely granulated, partly glycogen-like granules. There are several vacuoles in the adjacent axon–Schwann cell network from which it may be derived. The axon on the right is atrophic and is surrounded by a myelin sheath with prominent myelin loops. In the corresponding cytoplasm of the Schwann cell is an unusual, electron dense, homogenous inclusion which is not surrounded by a nuclear membrane; glycogen granules are closely attached. × 15,000. **b** The fine structure of the large homogeneously granular cytoplasmic inclusion in **a** is here shown with the myelin sheath and the glycogen granules in between at higher magnification. × 40,000 **c, d** s. p. 178

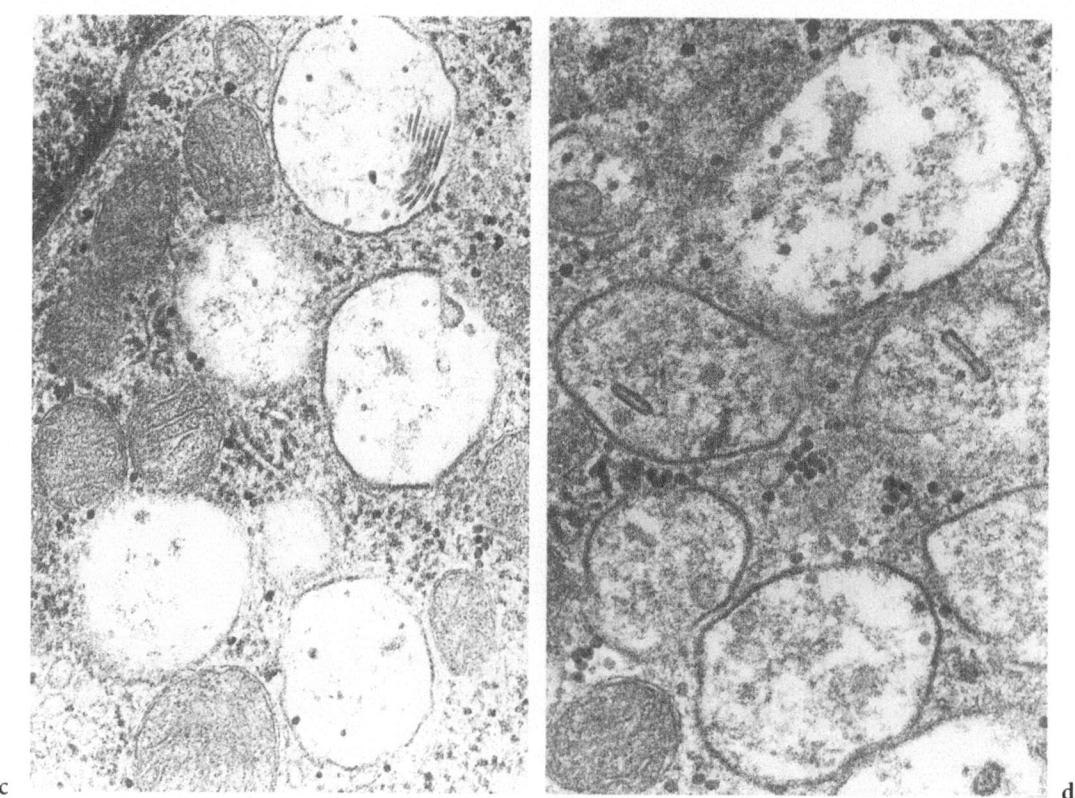

c

d

Fig. 158 c, d. **c** Several membrane-bound vacuoles contain partly osmiophilic granules, partly tubular or membranous components; otherwise they appear electron optically empty. They are easily distinguishable from adjacent mitochondria which are surrounded by a double membrane, here in an endoneurial fibroblast. × 58,000. **d** Higher magnification of the membrane-bound vacuoles. These contain flat, seemingly collapsed vesicles among amorphic and granular components. × 73,000

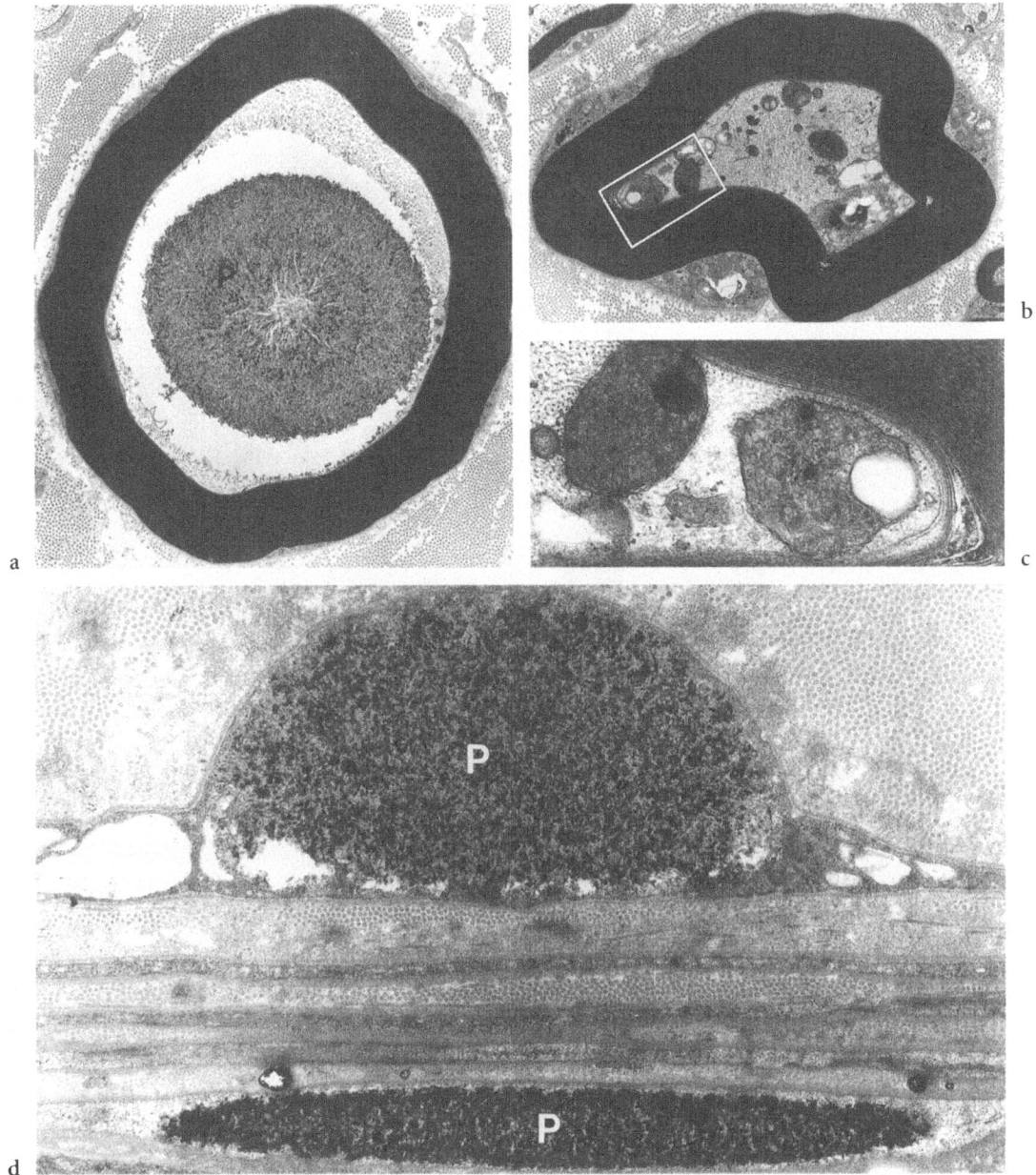

Fig. 159 a–d. Branching enzyme deficiency in a 19-year-old patient. (From [988]). **a** Non-membrane-bound polyglucosan body in an axon of a myelinated fiber. × 6,100. **b, c** Pleomorphic membrane-bound lysosomal structures which in **c** are illustrated at higher magnification. **b** × 6,300; **c** × 33,200. **d** Polyglucosan bodies in perineurial cells one of which is severely enlarged. × 13,700

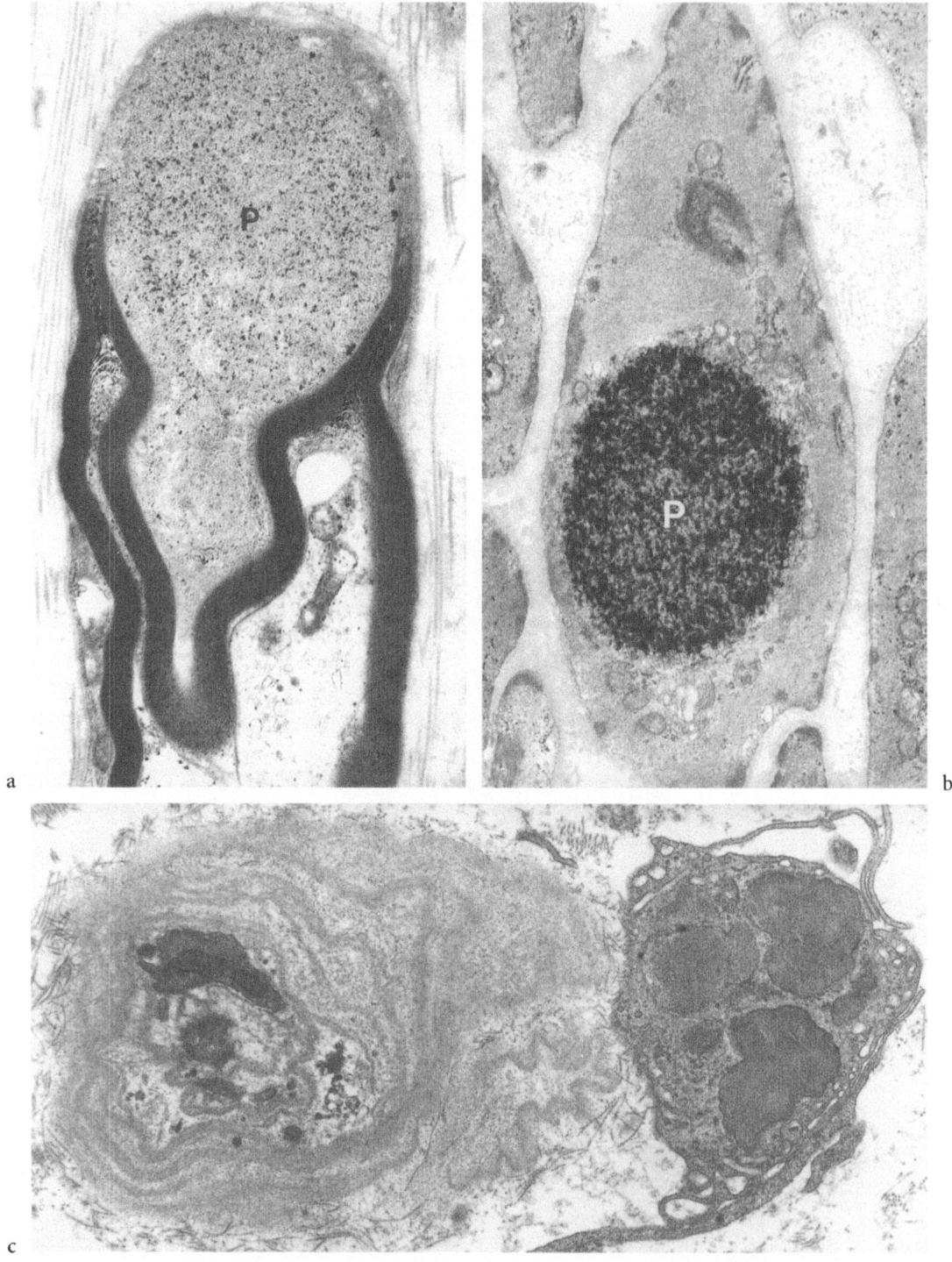

Fig. 160 a–c. Same case as in Fig. 159. **a** Polyglucosan body in a Schwann cell of a myelinated fiber. × 14,400. **b** Polyglucosan body (*P*) in a smooth muscle cell of an epineurial artery. The polyglucosan bodies in **a** and **b** are not membrane-bound. × 17,700. **c** Degenerated endomysial capillary with alternating layers of cell processes and basal laminae adjacent to a fibroblast which contains three membrane-bound polyglucosan bodies. × 11,400

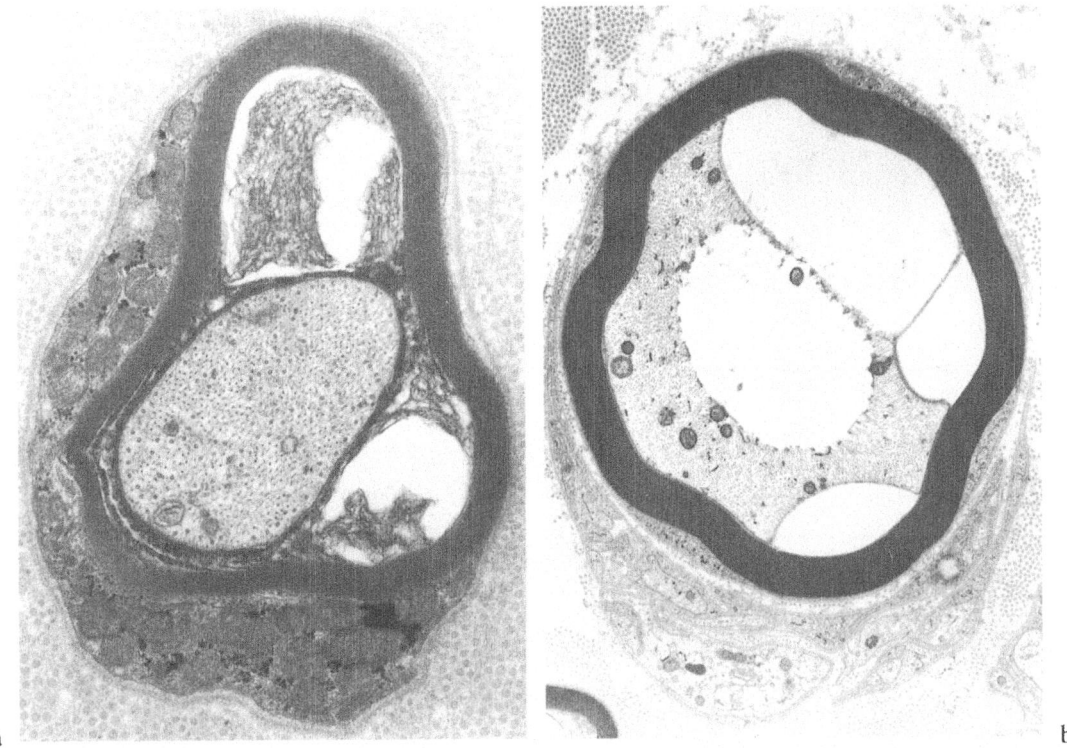

a

b

Fig. 161a,b. Same case as in Figs. 159 and 160. **a** Vesicular myelin sheath degradation in a paranodal myelin segment. × 26,400. **b** Intraaxonal non-membrane-bound vacuole in a myelinated fiber showing additional adaxonal vacuoles. The fiber is surrounded by several Schwann cell processes with a single unmyelinated axon. × 8,600

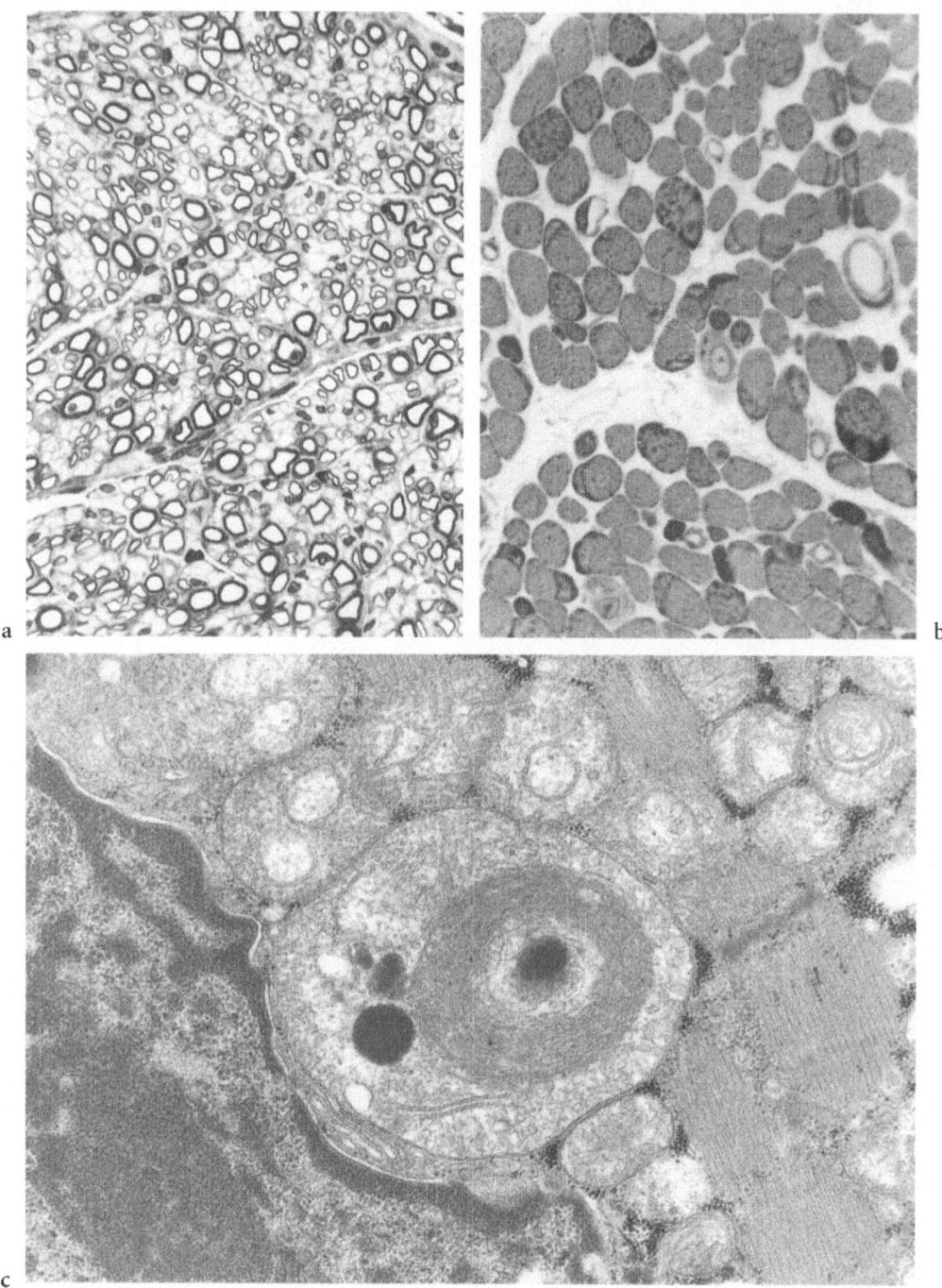

Fig. 162a–c. Myelinated nerve fibers with disproportionately thin myelin sheaths in a 9-month-old girl with mitochondrial myopathy characterized by a cluster of multiple, focally accumulated point mutations in the mitochondrial genome at nt 3259, 3261, 3266, and 3268. (From [1278, 1280]). **a** Aside from normally myelinated nerve fibers there are numerous fibers with the myelin sheath too thin for the axonal caliber, indicating a developmental disturbance of myelination. × 6,900. **b** Numerous muscle fibers show an intermyofibrillar or subsarcolemmal accumulation of osmiophilic substances (mitochondria). × 1,000. **c** Electron microscopic illustration of abnormal mitochondria between a nucleus and myofibrils. Several mitochondria are considerably enlarged (megaconial forms) and contain concentrically or irregularly arranged mitochondrial cristae and amorphous, globoid inclusions. × 3,900

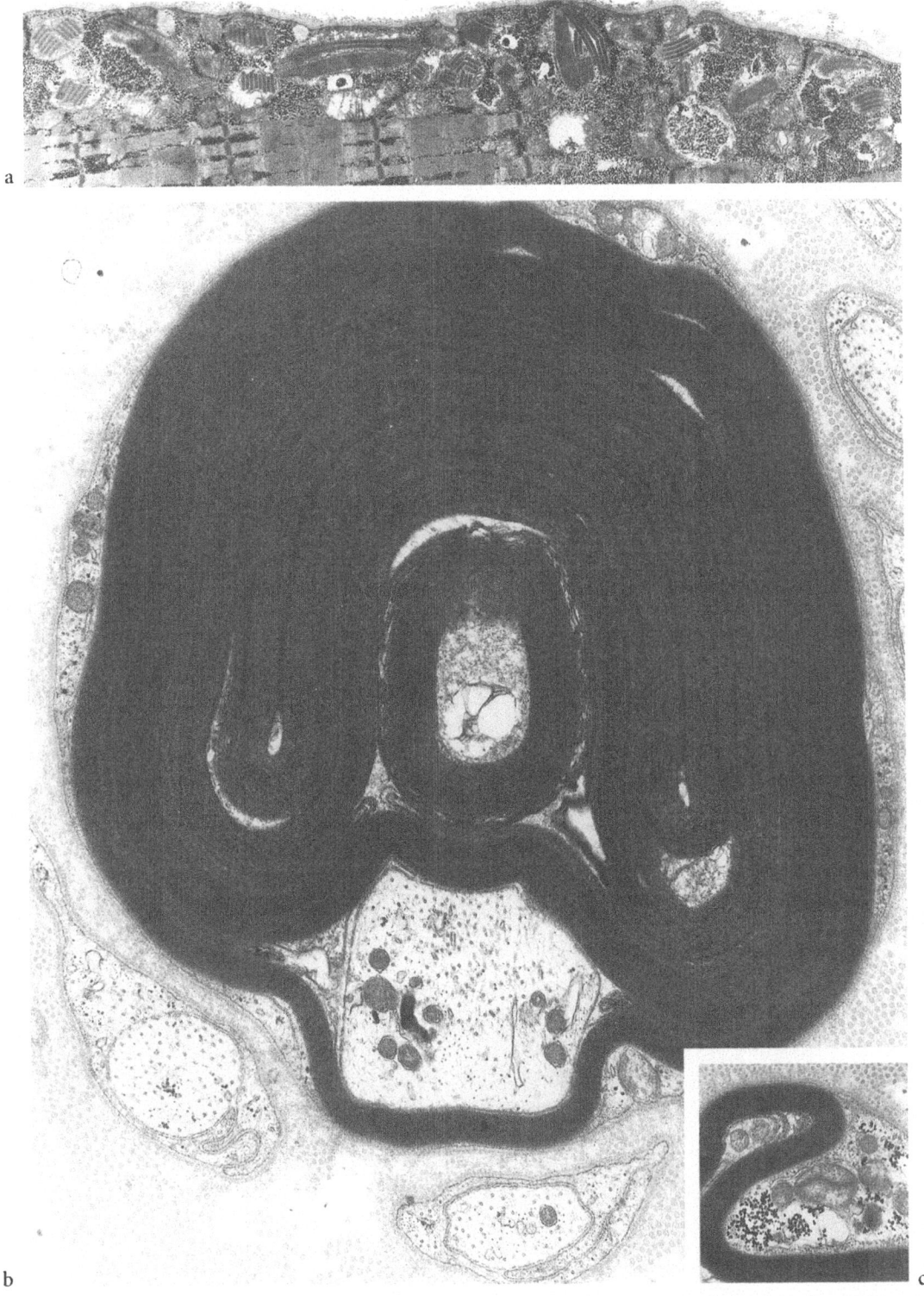

Fig. 163 a – c. Mitochondrial myopathy in a 57-year-old man (**a**) with chronic-progressive neuropathy indicated by nerve fiber loss and extensive myelin loops (**b**). There are only rare abnormal mitochondria in the cytoplasm of Schwann cells (**c**). **a** × 10,400; **b** × 24,000; **c** × 16,000

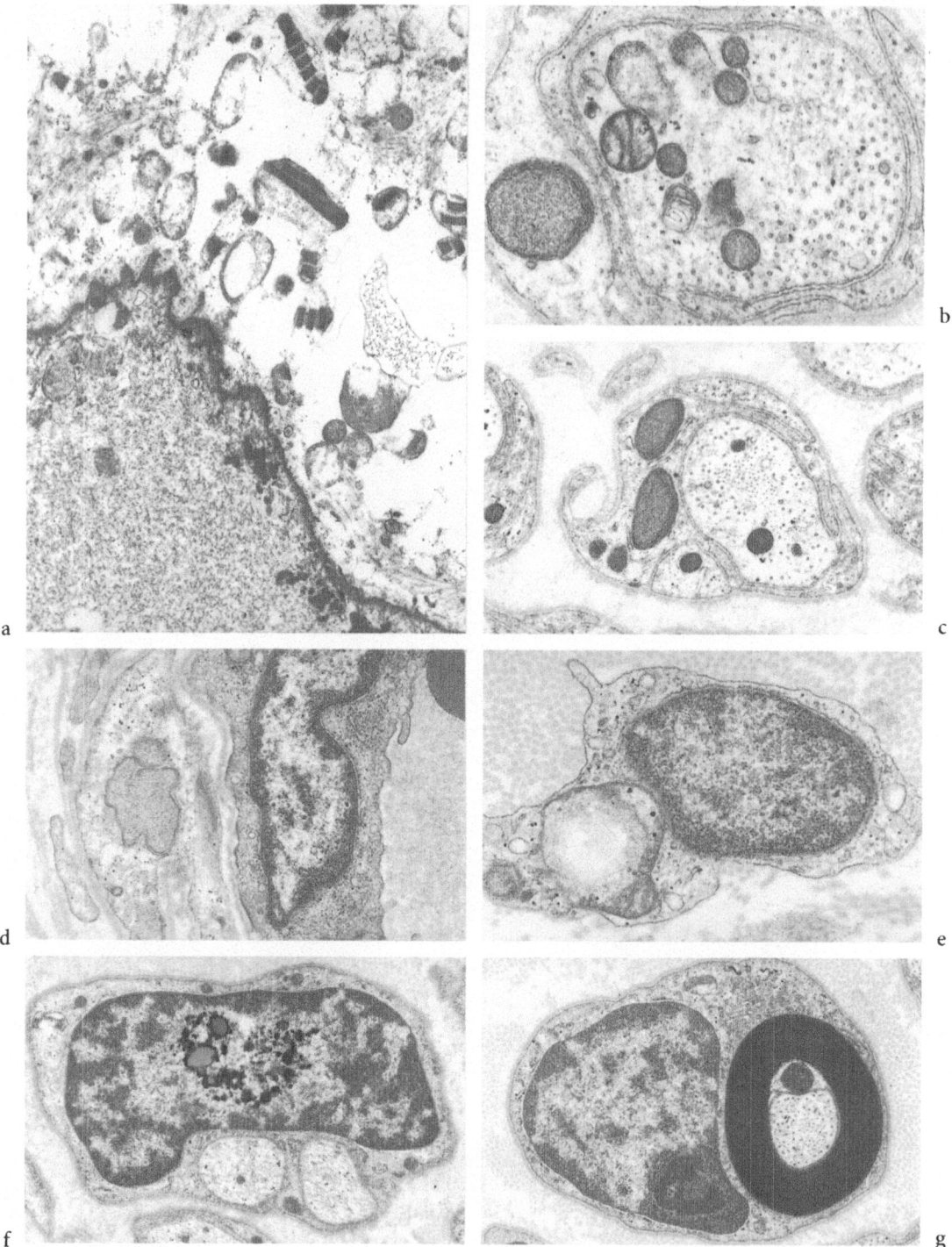

Fig. 164a–g. Mitochondrial myopathy in a 56-year-old man with abnormal mitochondria in muscle fibers (**a**), in Schwann cells of unmyelinated nerve fibers (**b, c**), in a pericyte (**d**), and in an endoneurial fibroblast (**e**). An abnormal Schwann cell nucleus with lipid-like uneven osmiophilic inclusions is illustrated in **f**, an abnormally arranged nucleolus in **g**. **a** × 9,400; **b** × 32,000; **c** × 19,400; **d** 16,400; **e** × 18,000; **f** × 11,300; **g** × 13,000

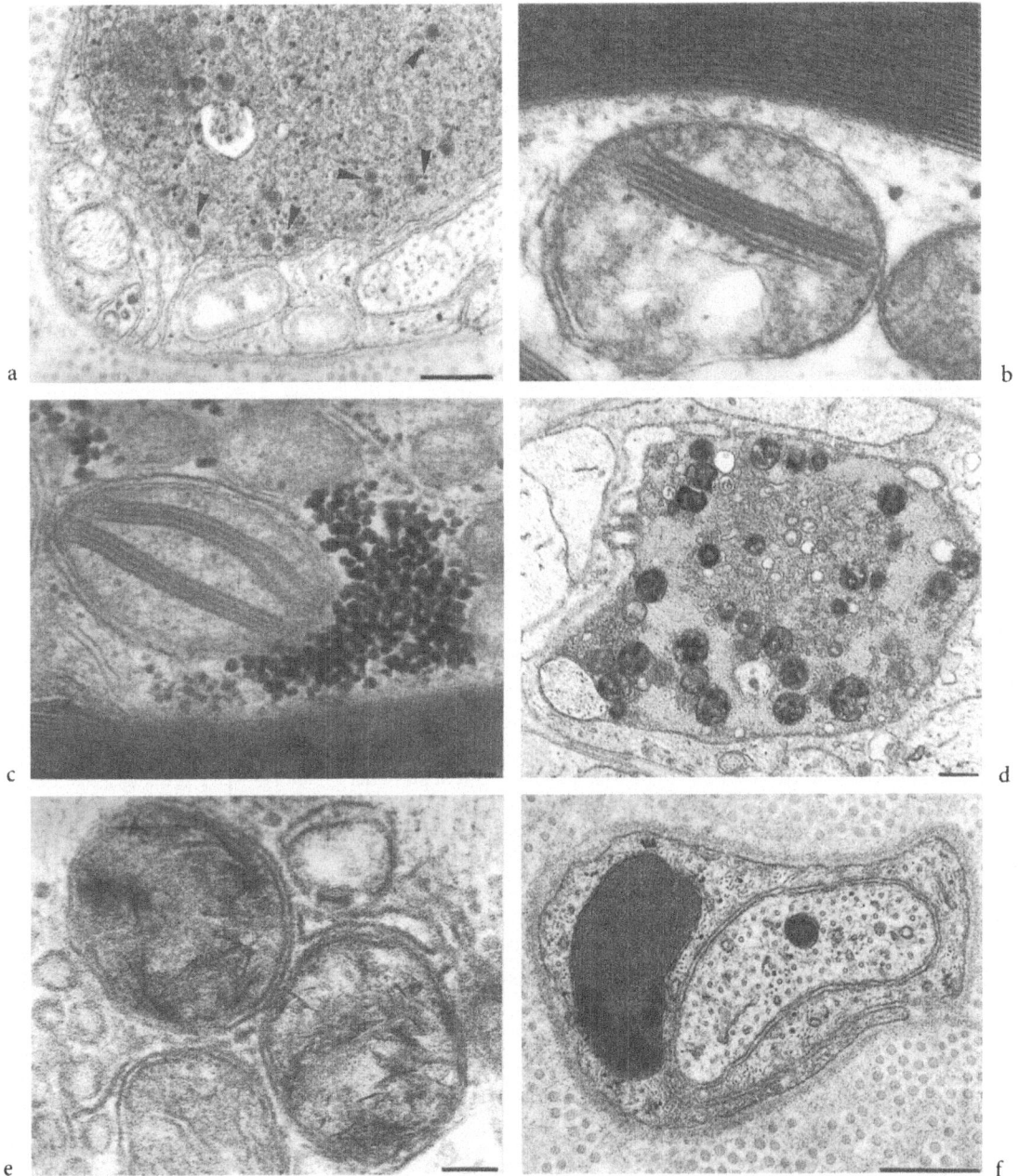

Fig. 165a–f. Neuropathy in Leber's optic atrophy (HMSN VI, type Vizioli; Figs. 165–168; modified from [1069]). **a** One axon with numerous neurosecretory granules (*arrowheads*) is severely distended. × 26,400. **b, c** In the cytoplasm of Schwann cells of myelinated fibers there are conspicuous electron dense mitochondrial cristae adjacent to each other containing paracrystalline material. **b** Fifteen-year-old boy with autosomal dominant HMSN VI. × 83,000. **c** Nineteen-year-old male, sporadic case. × 71,400. **d** Needle-like calcium precipitates in mitochondria of a severely distended dystrophic axon. × 14,300. **e** Higher magnification of the mitochondria in **d**. × 10,500. **f** Enlarged mitochondrion in the cytoplasm of the Schwann cell of an unmyelinated nerve fiber. The mitochondrion contains partly granular, partly amorphous globoid osmiophilic inclusions (which is a nonspecific change in unmyelinated nerve fibers). × 35,000

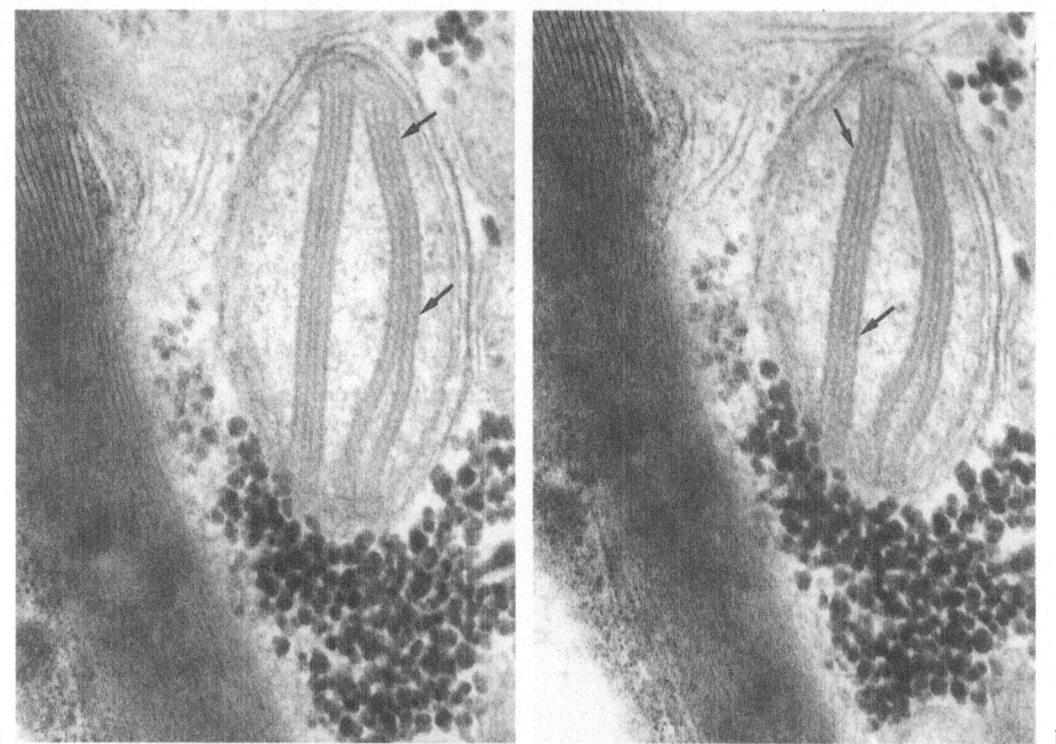

Fig. 166 a, b. Same case as in Fig. 165 c. The paracrystalline inclusions between the mitochondrial cristae are illustrated at different goniometer positions in the electron microscope (**a, b** with an angle difference of 36°). The *arrows* indicate regularly arranged inclusions which can be clearly determined after changing the angle of the goniometer stage. **a, b** × 99,400

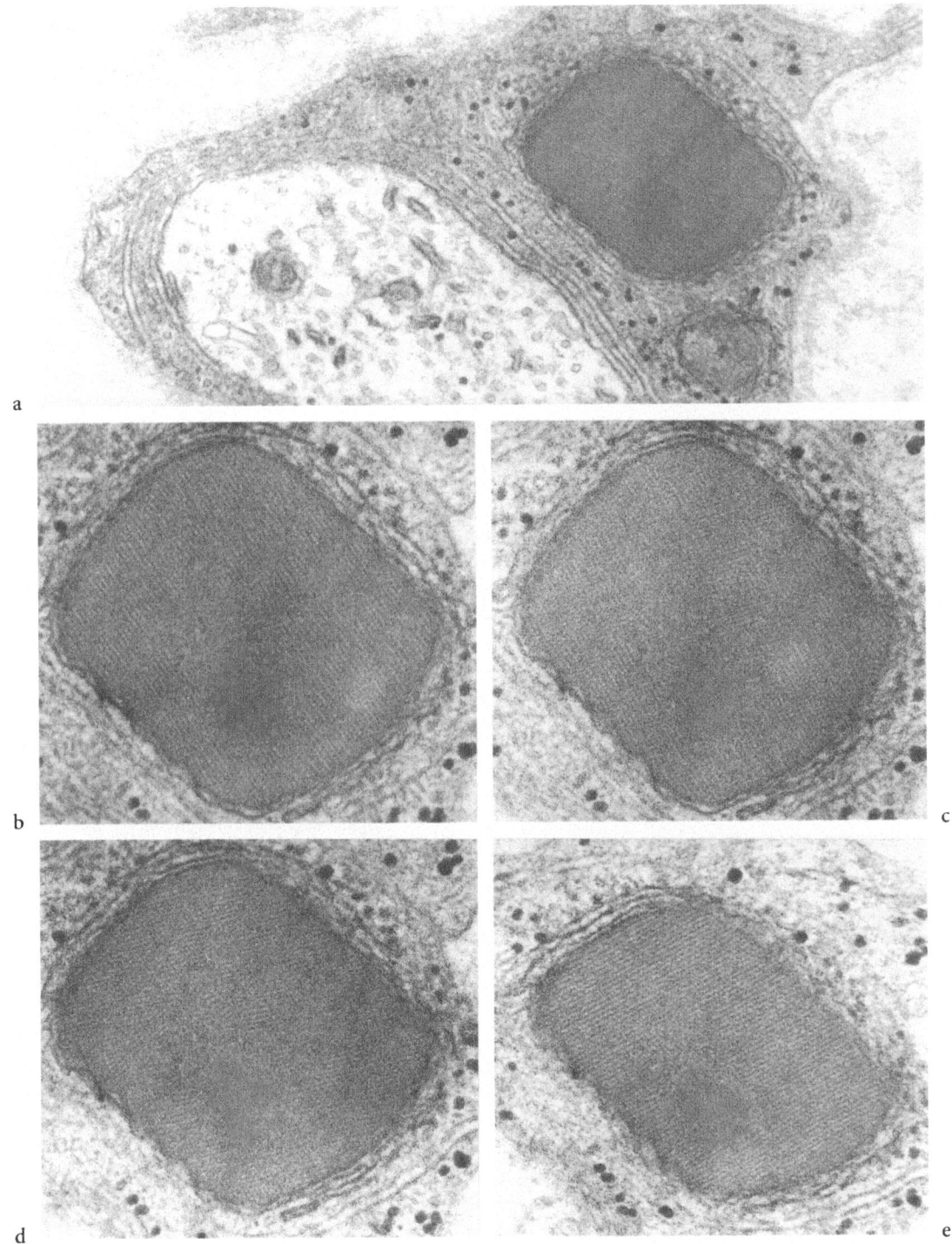

Fig. 167a–e. The paracrystalline granules of the mitochondria seen in the cytoplasm of a Schwann cell with an unmyelinated axon shows a typical pattern of striation. The lines are oriented in different directions depending on the angle position of the goniometer stage in the electron microscope despite identical orientation of the specimen indicating a granular fine structure (a–e). **a** × 66,400; **b–e** × 95,200

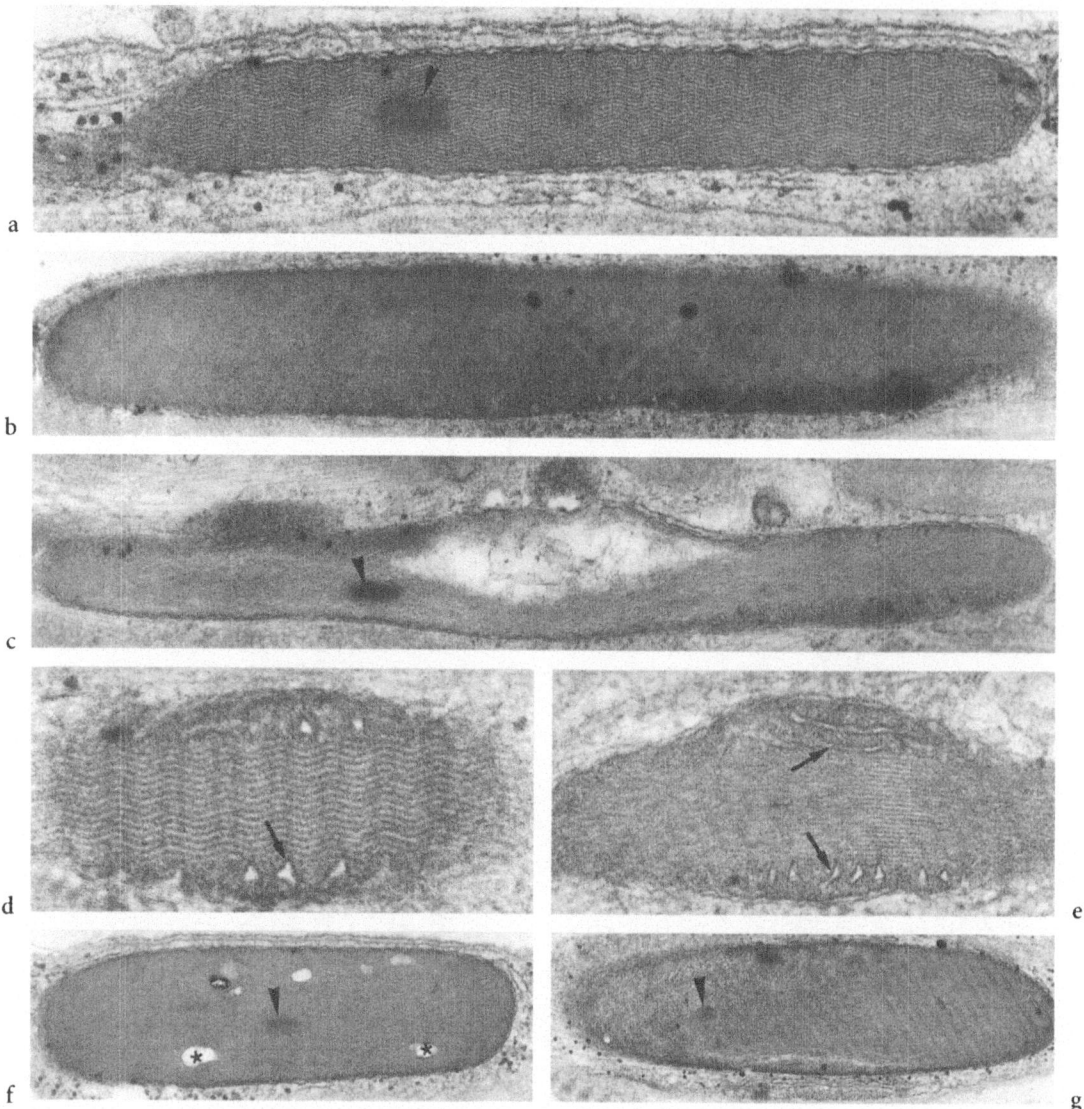

Fig. 168a–g. Different mitochondrial configurations in longitudinally oriented Schwann cells of unmyelinated nerve fibers with zigzag (**a**, **d**), striped (**b**), filamentous (**c**), or amorphic inclusions (**f**, **g**). The *arrows* in **d** and **e** indicate mitochondrial cristae, the *arrowheads* in **a**, **c**, **f**, and **g** amorphous inclusions. **a** 64,600; **b** × 38,000; **c** × 41,600; **d** × 115,000; **e** × 70,000; **f** × 33,000; **g** × 26,700

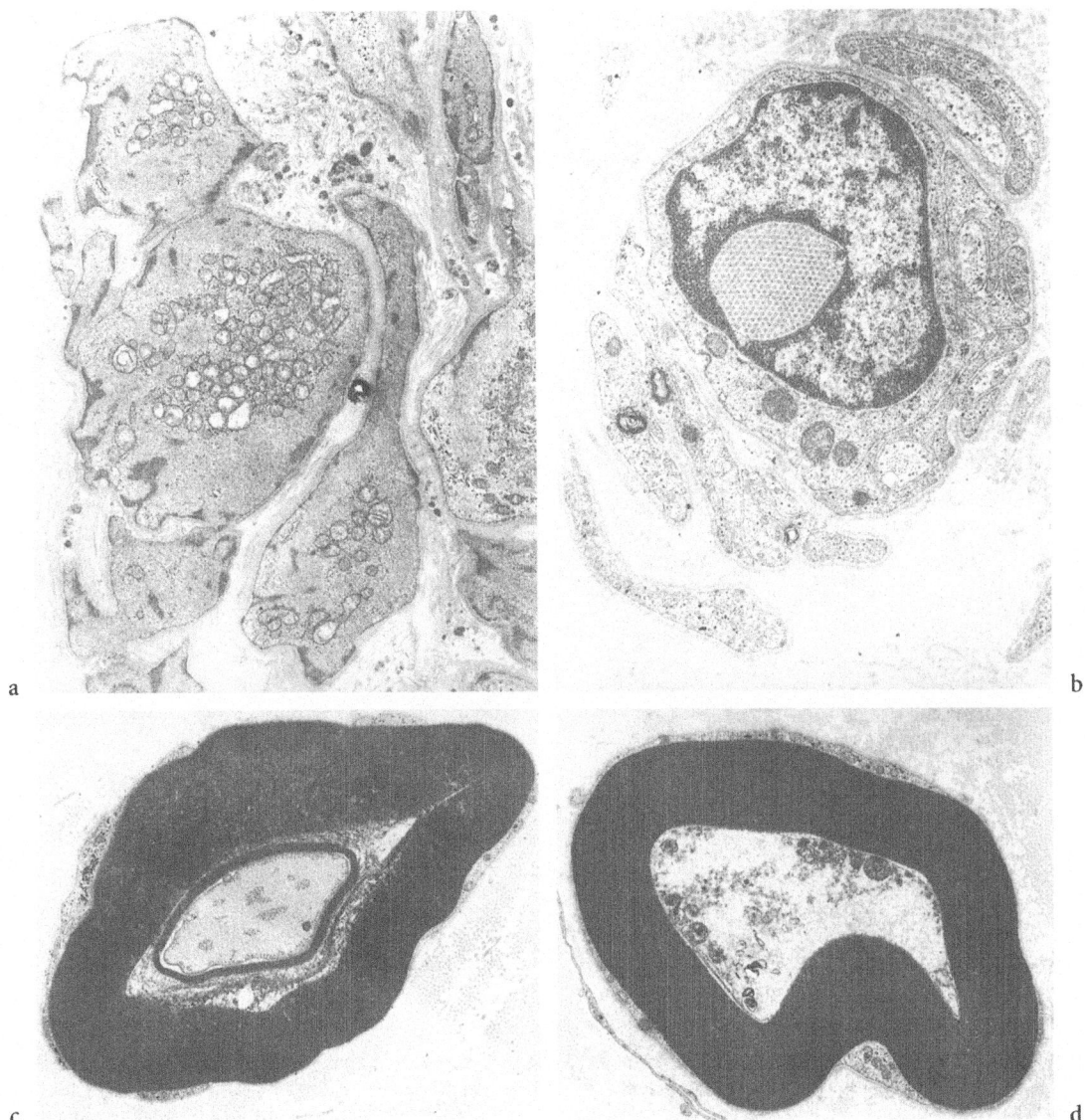

a

b

c

d

Fig. 169 a–d. Mitochondrial myopathy associated with neuropathy due to the typical MELAS mutation (A → G in position 3243 with heteroplasmia over 80%; K. Gerbitz and M. Jaksch, personal communication) and diabetes mellitus type II in a 41-year-old male. **a** In the smooth muscle cells of an epineurial artery, the mitochondria are accumulated without showing paracrystalline inclusions. × 8,800. **b** Unusual nuclear inclusion with paracrystalline arrangement of microtubules (see Fig. 154a) in a cytoplasmic invagination of a Schwann cell with regenerated unmyelinated axons in a band of Büngner. × 18,800. **c** Disproportionately thick myelin sheath around an axon with condensed neurofilaments cut at the level of a Schmidt-Lanterman incisure. × 8,500. **d** Degenerating axon showing loss of neurofilaments and microtubules with focal accumulation of floccular substances and altered organelles while the myelin sheath is still preserved. × 7,100

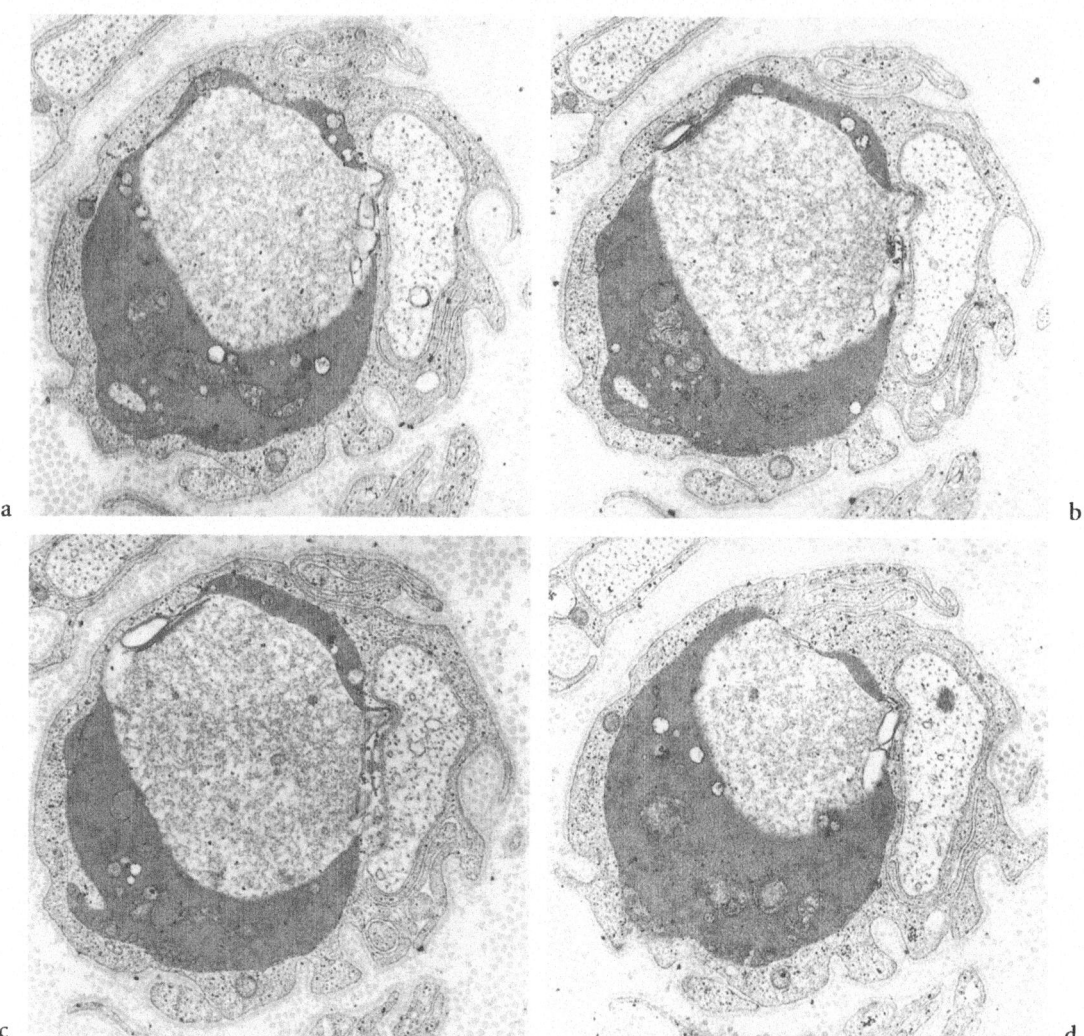

Fig. 170 a – d. Same case as in Fig. 169. Electron microscopic series of four different planes of a section showing an extremely enlarged and altered mitochondrion in a Schwann cell adjacent to an unmyelinated axon. The axon is flattened and focally indented. The inclusion is surrounded by a double membrane and consists of an electron-dense part with degenerating cristae and a dissoluted component with floccular material. **a** × 13,600; **b, c** × 20,800; **d** × 19,800

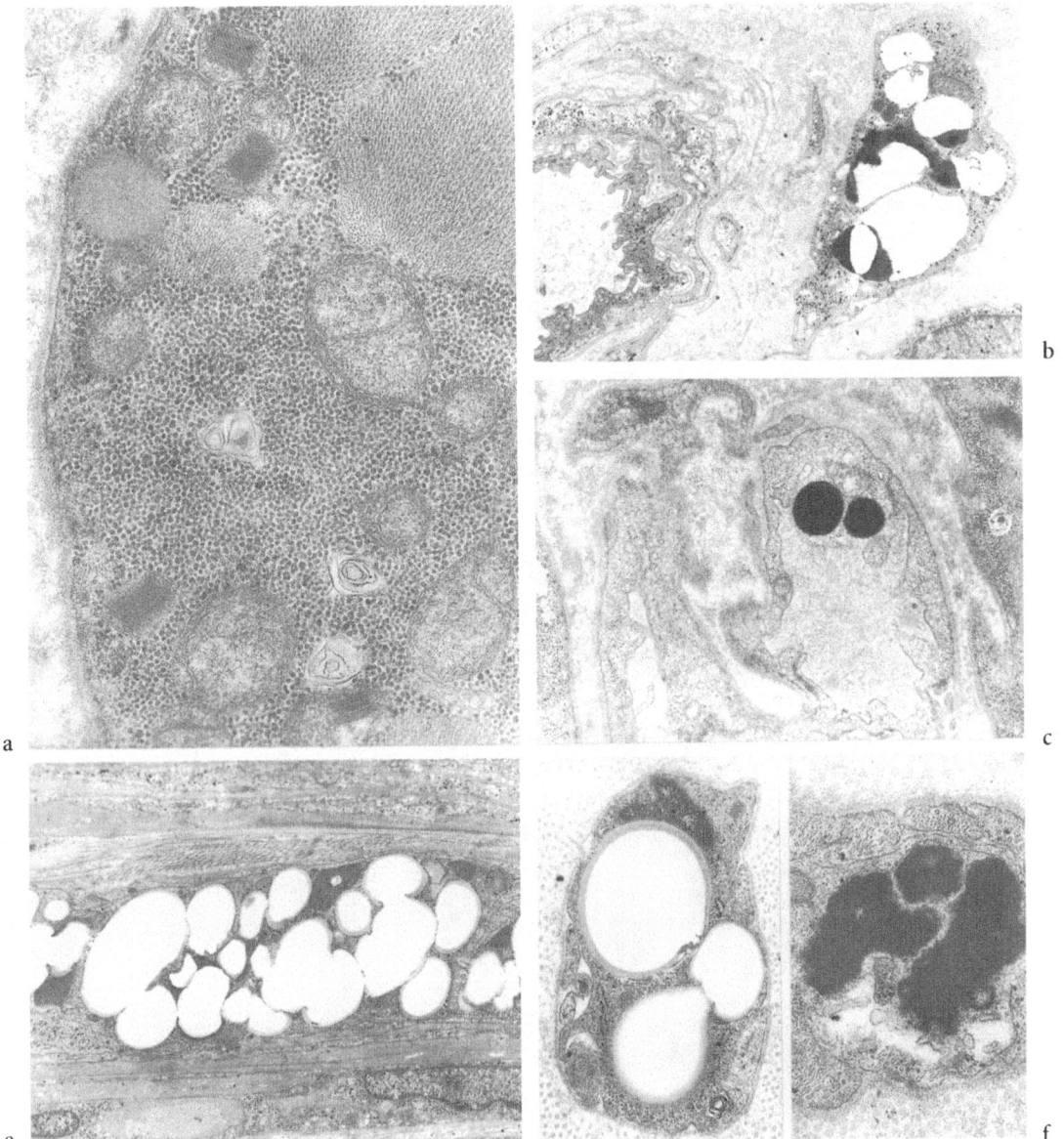

Fig. 171a–f. Polyneuropathy in myo-, neuro-, and gastrointestinal encephalopathy (MNGIE) of a 24-year-old male. The muscle fiber (**a**) shows paracrystalline inclusions in the mitochondria. The nerve contains multiple perivascular vacuoles which are typical for a preceding dextrin application (**b**). Unusual osmiophilic, globoid, melanosome-like inclusions can be seen in the endothelium of endomysial capillaries (**c**). Conspicuous lipid vacuoles are present in the perineurium (**d**) and in Schwann cells (**e**). Severely osmiophilic, non-membrane-bound substances with irregular contours occur in Schwann cells (**f**). **a** × 34,800; **b** × 7,900; **c** × 12,200; **d** × 6,600; **e** × 16,200; **f** × 32,600

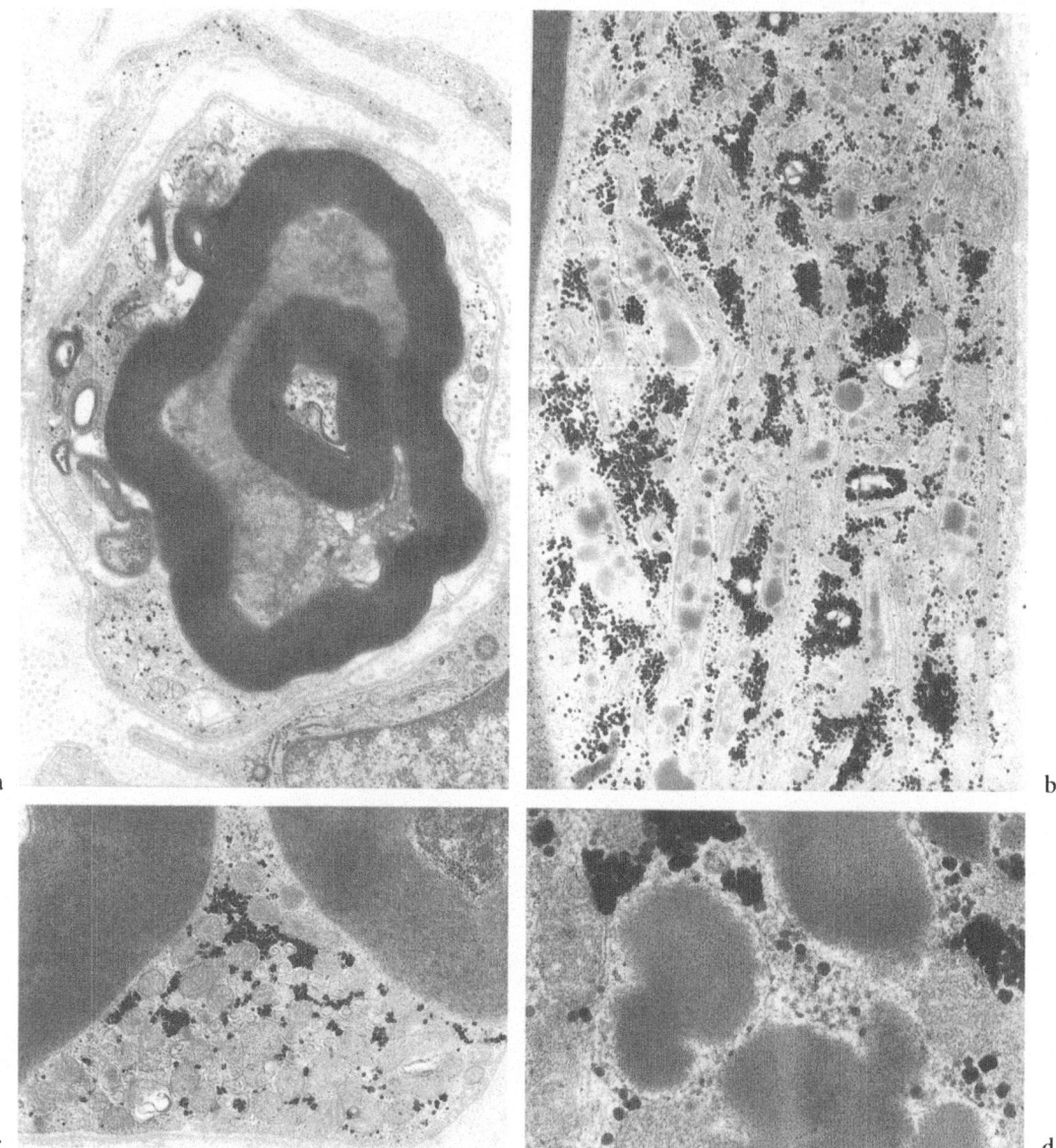

Fig. 172 a–d. Chronic neuropathy of predominantly neuronal type with a demyelinating component in a 21-year-old female with unique lipid-like osmiophilic, round or tubular Schwann cell inclusions (case of [1002]). **a** Acutely degenerating nerve fiber with condensed axoplasm and incipient myelin sheath degradation. Some myelin ovoids can already be seen in the cytoplasm of the focally swollen Schwann cell. × 17,000. **b** Glycogen granules occur in the cytoplasm of the Schwann cell of a myelinated fiber between tubular structures and amorphous osmiophilic lipid-like substances. × 24,000. **c** Accumulation of mitochondria and ring-like structures adjacent to glycogen granules between a myelin sheath and a myelin loop. × 24,000. **d** Lipid-like inclusions which are partially surrounded by a membrane in the cytoplasm of a Schwann cell. × 62,000

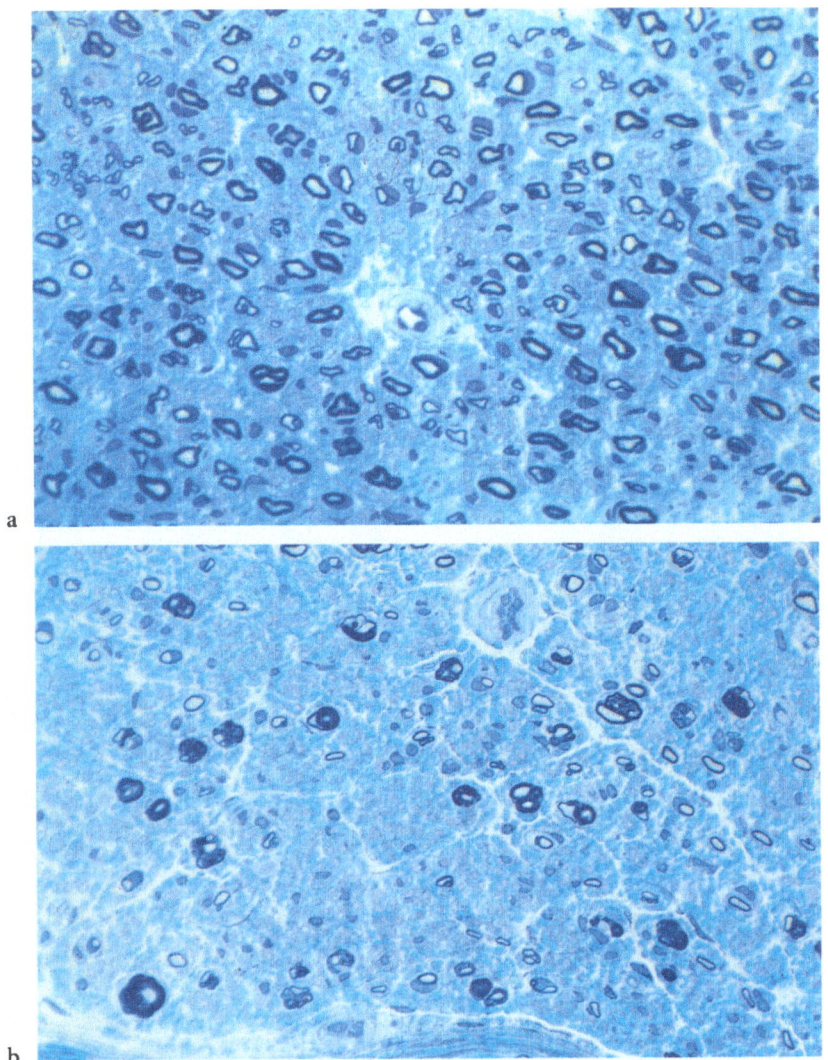

Fig. 173 a–f. Unusual neuropathies. **a** Same case as in Fig. 172. The number of large myelinated fibers is clearly reduced. Instead there are many small atrophic fibers with only occasional axons showing disproportionately thin myelin sheaths and incipient onion bulb formations. Toluidine blue. **b** Hypo-/hypermyelinization neuropathy (neuropathy with focally folded myelin) in an 11-year-old boy (same case as in Fig. 117). Many nerve fibers are lost. There are frequent myelin loops associated with the remaining fibers. Toluidine blue. **c – f** s. p. 194 and 195

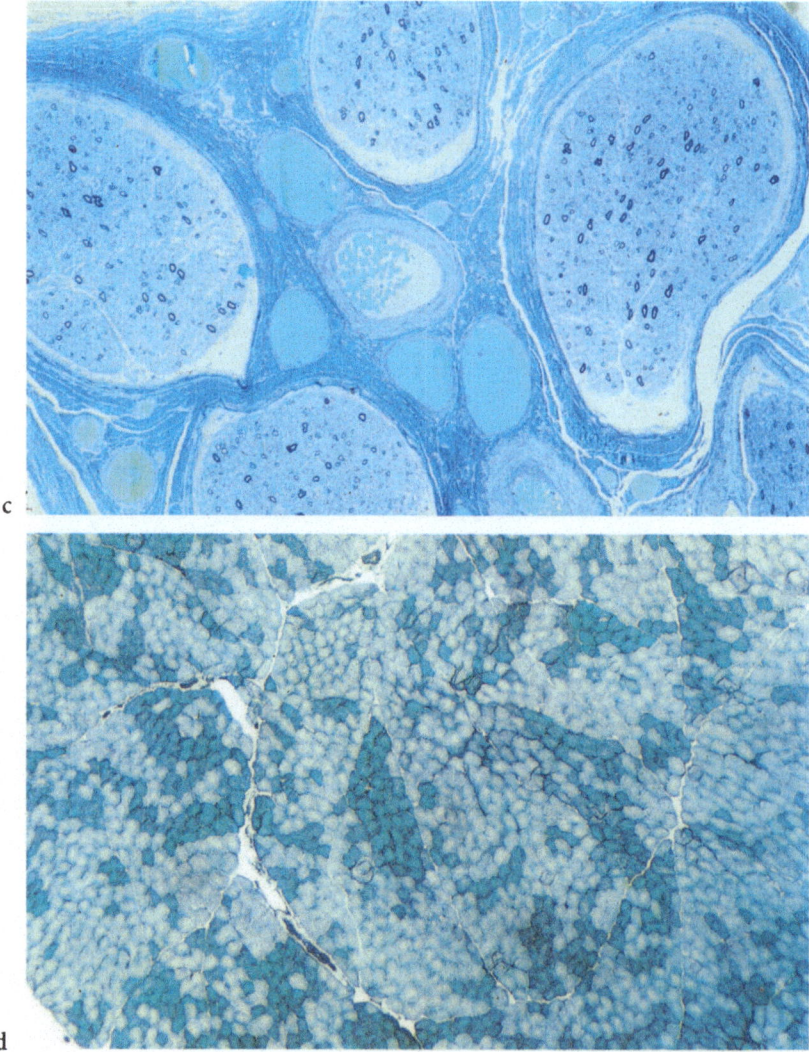

Fig. 173. **c** Severe neuropathy in xeroderma pigmentosum. Toluidine blue. **d** Same case as in **c**. Muscle-fiber-type grouping without significant muscle fiber atrophy indicating that the neuropathy is severely accentuated in the sensory system. NADH. **e, f** s. p. 195

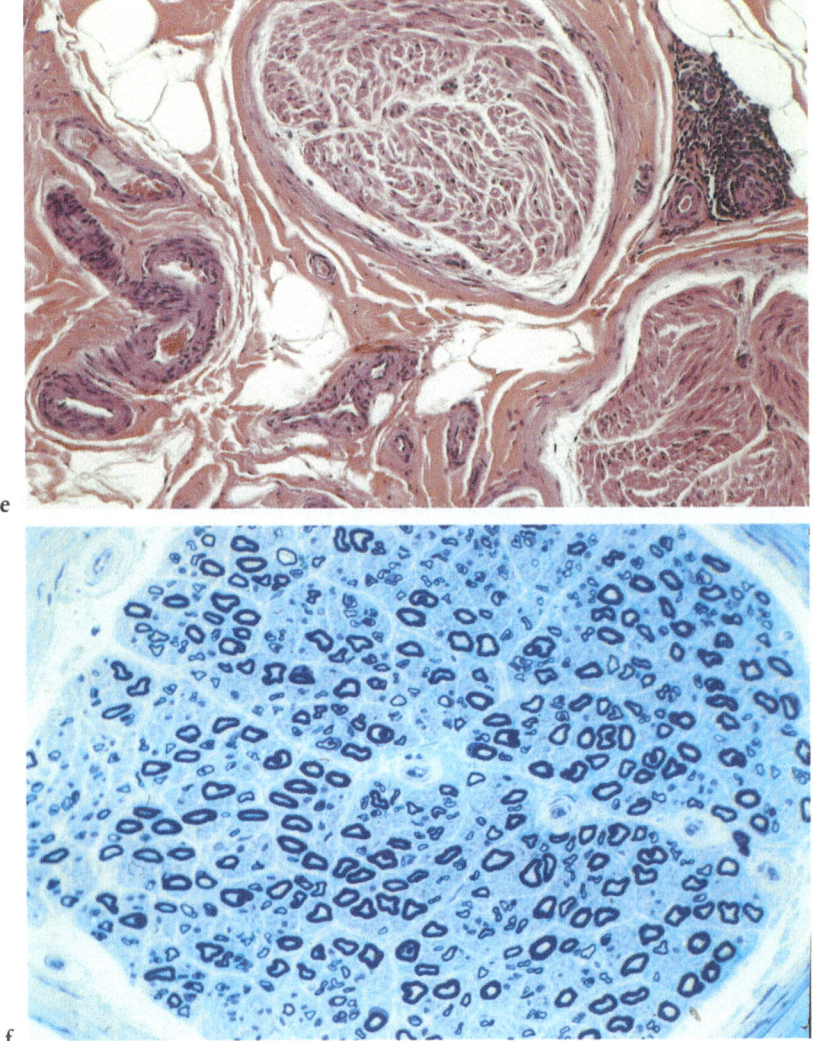

Fig. 173. e, f Autosomal dominant HSAN I with burning feet syndrome. The small myelinated nerve fibers are predominantly affected. In addition, in **e** there is a perivascular cellular infiltrate in the epineurium (case of [1089])

CHAPTER 8

Hereditary Neuropathies with Predominantly Sensory and Autonomous Disturbances

These rare diseases are classified according to the predominant involvement of the sensory and/or autonomous system in connection with the mode of inheritance [251].

Developmental disturbances are characterized by congenital manifestation with no or minimal progression and *no myelin degradation products* in a sural nerve biopsy as in hereditary sensory and autonomous neuropathy type III and IV (HSAN III and IV) (see below). The pathogenesis of some of these diseases may be elucidated by knock-out experiments. E.g., neurotrophin-3 knock-out mice are characterized by a lack of large sensory fibers associated with deficiency of muscle spindles and tendon organs [275]. These experimental animals may allow further studies of transcription, translation, and phenotypic expression.

Hereditary sensory and autonomous neuropathies (HSAN) are usually characterized by slow progression whereas rapid progression with *many myelin degradation products* in a sural nerve biopsy, such as in *acute sensory neuropathy* [1240] (see below), is suggestive of an exogenous or inflammatory disorder.

Autosomal dominant hereditary sensory and autonomous neuropathy type I (*HSAN I*, Thévenard syndrome, hereditary sensory radicular neuropathy [216]), according to the classification of Dyck et al. (1993) [260], is characterized by predominant sensory symptoms with only minor motor signs (Figs. 174a–c). Variants are *sensory atactic neuropathy with autosomal dominant inheritance* [1175], *dominantly inherited congenital indifference to pain* [569], and *autosomal dominant burning feet syndrome* which in one of our cases was associated with perivascular inflammatory infiltrates in the epineurium (Fig. 173e, f) [258,1089].

HSAN II is inherited in an *autosomal recessive* pattern with earlier onset and more severe sensory disturbances. Histopathology reveals fascicular atrophy and severe loss of myelinated fibers whereas the unmyelinated axons are better preserved (Figs. 175–177) [172, 755, 779]. Autosomal recessive hereditary sensory neuropathy with spastic paraplegia is considered as a variant [1132].

An *X-chromosomal recessive sensory and autonomous neuropathy* has also been described [470].

HSAN III (Riley-Day syndrome, familial dysautonomia) is characterized by deficiency or even aplasia of small sensory and autonomous neurons with corresponding lack of unmyelinated and small myelinated nerve fibers in the sural nerve (Fig. 178a–d) [170, 818, 819].

HSAN IV (congenital sensory neuropathy with anhidrosis) is characterized by a rather complete, congenital absence of unmyelinated axons [345, 580, 1097] and reduction of small myelinated fibers although unmyelinated axons may be present in clusters of regenerated fibers [1183]. An acquired form of idiopathic generalized anhidrosis was reported as being caused by a disturbance of the function of sweat glands [711].

Congenital sensory neuropathy with selective loss of small myelinated fibers causes indifference to pain or asymboly for pain [251, 423, 465].

Congenital absence of large myelinated nerve fibers, deafness, and mental retardation [632] appears to represent a nosological entity showing autosomal recessive inheritance [898]. The corresponding areas in the spinal ganglia and anterior horns of the spinal cord also show a lack of large cells (Figs. 108–109) [707] indicating that the motor system is involved at least to some extent. An autosomal dominant form has also been recorded [1251] with a locus on Xq24–26 [850].

Congenital sensory neuropathy with complete or subtotal deficiency of myelinated nerve fibers in the sural nerve with preservation of unmyelinated fibers (Figs. 90, 91) has been reported in cases with arthrogryposis multiplex congenita with absence [1194] or without absence of muscle spindles [303, 979].

A *congenital sensory neuropathy with ichthyosis and anterior chamber cleavage syndrome* [860] was also associated with nearly complete absence of myelinated nerve fibers.

Sporadic noninherited forms of *acute sensory neuropathy* [5, 152, 506, 631, 1083, 1240], *migrating sensory neuropathy* [1293], and a *chronic idiopathic atactic neuropathy (CIAN)* [205, 1042] need to be distinguished from the inherited slowly progressive or nonprogressive forms of sensory neuropathies. An interesting mouse mutant with a deficiency of large sensory neurons and an absence of muscle spindles and tendon organs is the *sprawling mouse* [121] (see also NT-3(-/-) mice, p. 102 and 197).

Further hereditary (or nonhereditary) neuropathies of the peripheral autonomous system include *Hirschsprung syndrome* (Fig. 179 a – c) [831, 1177] with its variants, *Waardenburg syndrome* (iris heterochromasia, dystopic canthus, poliosis, and inner ear deafness), and *Horst syndrome* (Hirschsprung disease, coloboma and cerebral dysgenesis) [263, 495, 831]. In type II Waardenberg syndrome an unusual demyelinating type of the peripheral type of neuropathy was observed [464].

Infantile hypertrophic pyloric stenosis (IHPS) (Figs. 180 – 181) is usually considered to be sporadic, but may also be inherited [153, 226, 230, 274, 474, 976, 1213]. There are numerous changes in axons and smooth muscle cells enabling one to distinguish a neuropathic type from a myopathic type of IHPS [226, 230, 976].

Idiopathic orthostatic hypotension [176, 239] is characterized by progressive disturbances of autonomic function and moderate loss of myelinated nerve fibers in the sural nerve whereas *Shy-Drager syndrome* [1058] shows multiple system atrophy with loss of autonomic function.

Nonhereditary disturbances of the autonomic system comprise *reflex-sympathetic dystrophy (RSD, causalgia, Sudeck's atrophy)* associated with impairment of adrenergic functions [762, 1008].

Disturbance of the *autonomous innervation of blood vessels in the heart* [97, 1087] and *brain* [117, 264, 265, 300, 341, 387, 550, 795, 1277] may be of considerable importance, yet there are very few adequate histopathological studies of the innervation of human cerebral blood vessels under pathological conditions [750]. In cases of Alzheimer's disease, we

were not able to find specific changes or evidence of amyloidosis of intracranial nervi vasorum (Bison, doctoral thesis 1998). There was fiber loss mainly in a case with associated diabetes.

Disturbances of *miction* are frequently due to involvement of autonomic nerves [267]. Studies on pelvic nerves in *fecal incontinence* [162, 1056] have shown pleomorphic changes with degeneration and regeneration, demyelination and remyelination, in one case with severe mitochondrial changes in a muscle specimen, all of which did not allow one to distinguish between primary and secondary changes because of compression of the nerve fascicles by obstipation, perineal prolaps, or insufficiency of the pelvic floor muscles (Schröder and Athanasiadis, unpublished observations).

Erectile function may be disturbed causing sexual impotence by involvement of the pudendal nerve in a variety of neuropathies. Functional disturbances have been studied electrophysiologically (bulbocavernosus reflex latency and SSEP of the pudendal nerve) [1102]. Yet morphological studies do not seem to be available.

Spinal heredoataxias include *Friedreich's ataxia*, which is inherited in an autosomal recessive pattern showing predominant loss of large myelinated nerve fibers (Figs. 17 e, 97 d, 182 – 186) [136, 139, 198, 248, 255, 390, 469, 472, 560, 564, 587, 904, 914, 915, 936, 1093], and *autosomal dominant cerebellar atrophy (ADCA)* of which there are six variants (spinal cerebellar atrophy, SCA 1 – 6) caused by mutations in different genes [249, 277, 290, 378, 424, 531, 797, 813, 1212]. Distinctive changes in sural nerves of cases with Friedreich's ataxia due to different lengths of the underlying CGA repeats and in the various forms of ADCA have not, to the best of my knowledge, been identified thus far.

Autosomal recessive *infantile olivopontocerebellar atrophy* may also show involvement of the peripheral motor system [167].

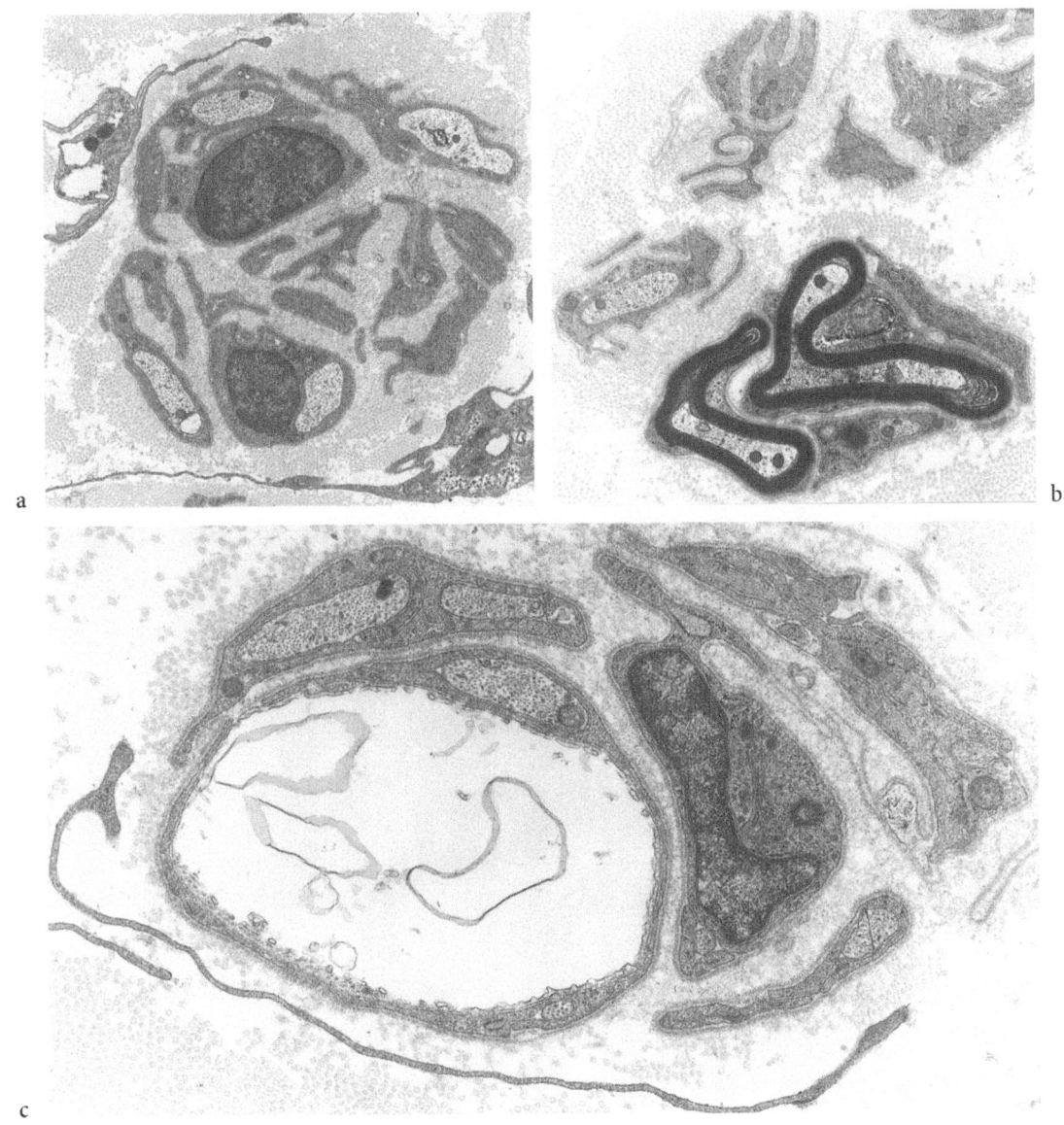

Fig. 174 a – c. HSAN type I in a 43-year-old female suffering from trophic ulcera and showing loss of numerous unmyelinated axons (**a**) among the few preserved, but atrophic small myelinated nerve fibers (**b**) and apparently acute degeneration of some unmyelinated axons (**c**). **a** × 6,800; **b** × 10,200; **c** × 17,000

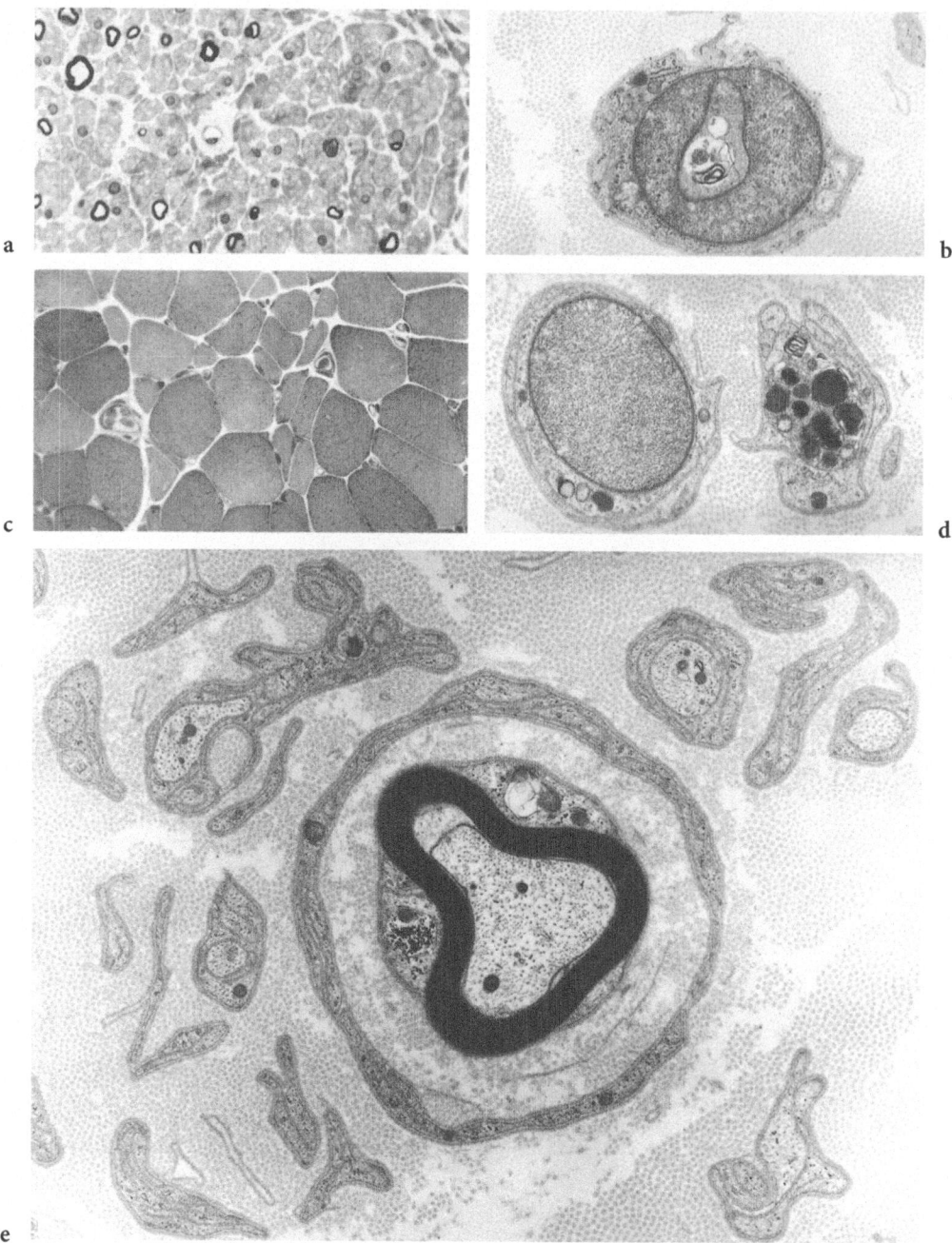

Fig. 175 a–e. Advanced hereditary, autosomal recessive sensory autonomous neuropathy corresponding to the clinically suggested HSAN II with subtotal loss of myelinated nerve fibers in a 9-year-old boy. His brother and maternal aunt (Figs. 176 and 177) are also affected. **a** The number of large and small nerve fibers is severely reduced. × 616. **b, d, e** The unmyelinated axons are also severely reduced. A cytoplasmic nuclear inclusion shown in **b** is associated with degenerative cytoplasmic alterations. In **d** lysosomal structures are accumulated in a cell process. In **e** a myelinated nerve fiber is encircled by empty Schwann cell processes. **b,d** × 10,600; **e** × 9,000. **c** Selected muscle area with relatively numerous atrophic muscle fibers in an otherwise largely inconspicuous muscle indicative of a moderate involvement of the motor system. × 300

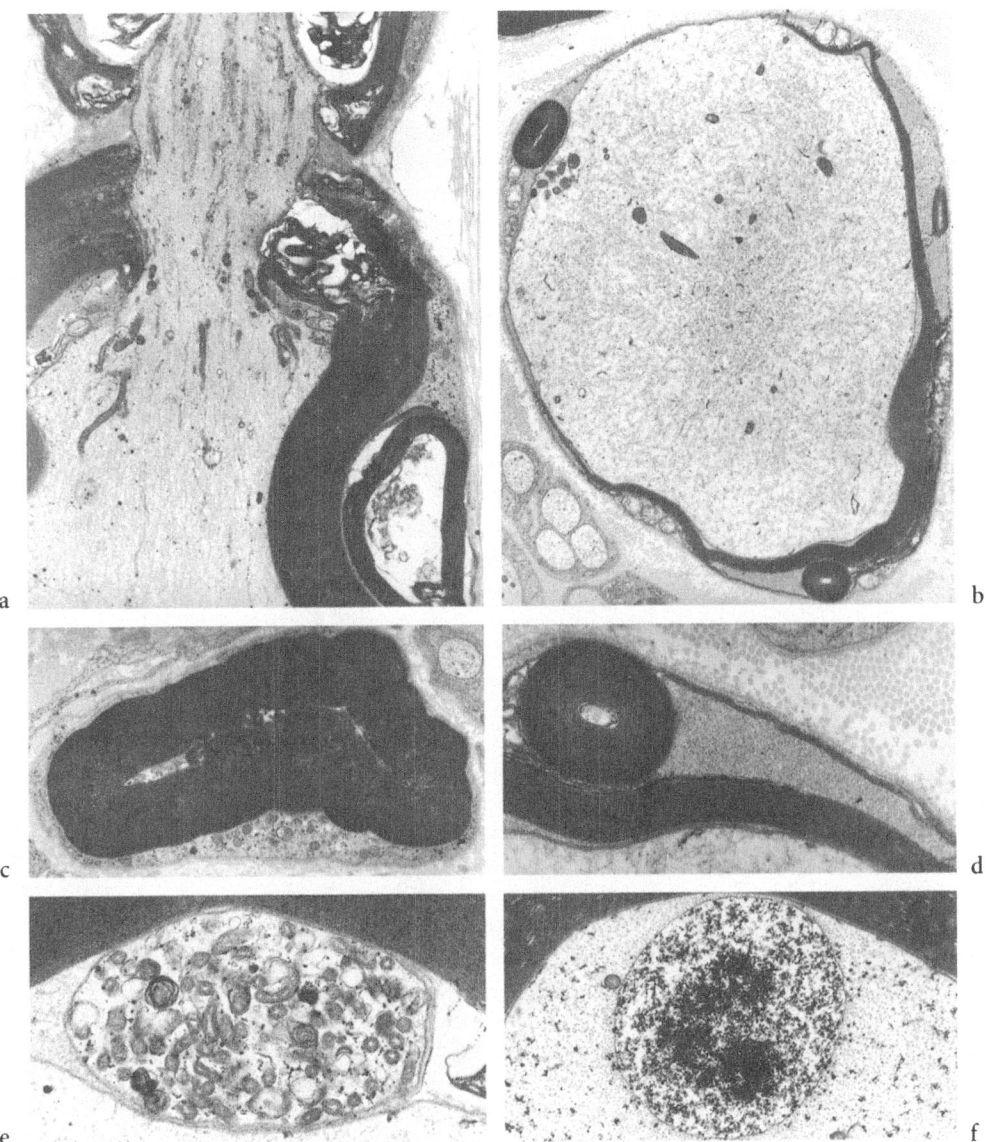

Fig. 176a–f. HSAN II in a 47-year-old female (maternal aunt of the case in Fig. 175). **a** The paranode shows several membranous cytoplasmic inclusions and focal vesicular disintegration. In the adjacent axon-Schwann cell network there are amorphous and membranous deposits. A μ-granule with microvesicular or vacuolar changes can be seen in the *lower right*. × 6,500. **b** Paranodal retraction of myelin lamellae with amorphic inclusions in the abaxonal cytoplasm, but also within the myelin sheath. Several myelin loops are apparent around the distended axon. × 6,200. **c** Acutely degenerating nerve fiber with almost complete degeneration of its axon, but still largely preserved, collapsed myelin sheath. × 8,000. **d** Higher (inverted) magnification of the lower part of the paranodal area with granular inclusions in **b**. In the axon, microtubules and neurofilaments are no longer preserved. × 24,000. **e** Focal accumulation of mitochondria, membranous cytoplasmic bodies, vesicles, and glycogen granules in an axonal process presumably close to the paranodal axon– Schwann cell network. × 16,000. **f** Glycogenosome within the axon of a myelinated nerve fiber. Glycogen-like granules can also be seen in the adjacent axoplasm. × 13,000

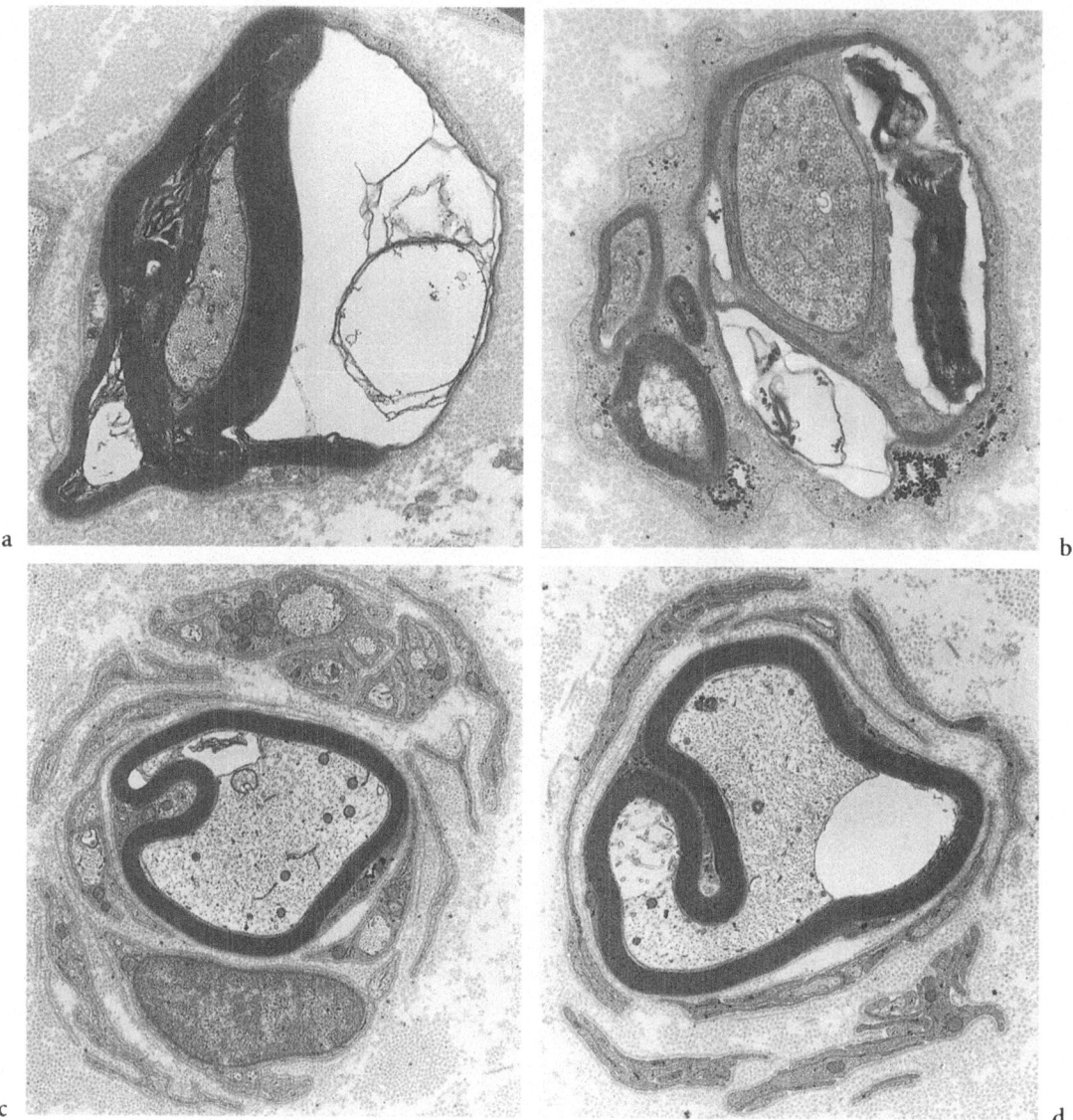

Fig. 177a–d. Same case as in Fig. 176. Vacuolar disintegration of the myelin sheath in **a** and in a paranodal segment in **b** as well as in the adaxonal area of the internode in **c** and **d**. Paranodal myelin loops in **b** are situated within the cytoplasm of the Schwann cell. The myelinated nerve fiber in **c** is surrounded by multiple Schwann cell processes with regenerated unmyelinated axons, whereas the flattened Schwann cell processes in **d** contain less clearly identifiable axons. Both groups in **c** and **d** are indicative of degeneration and regeneration rather than demyelination and remyelination. **a** × 11,500; **b** × 22,000 **c** × 9,500 **d** × 9,700

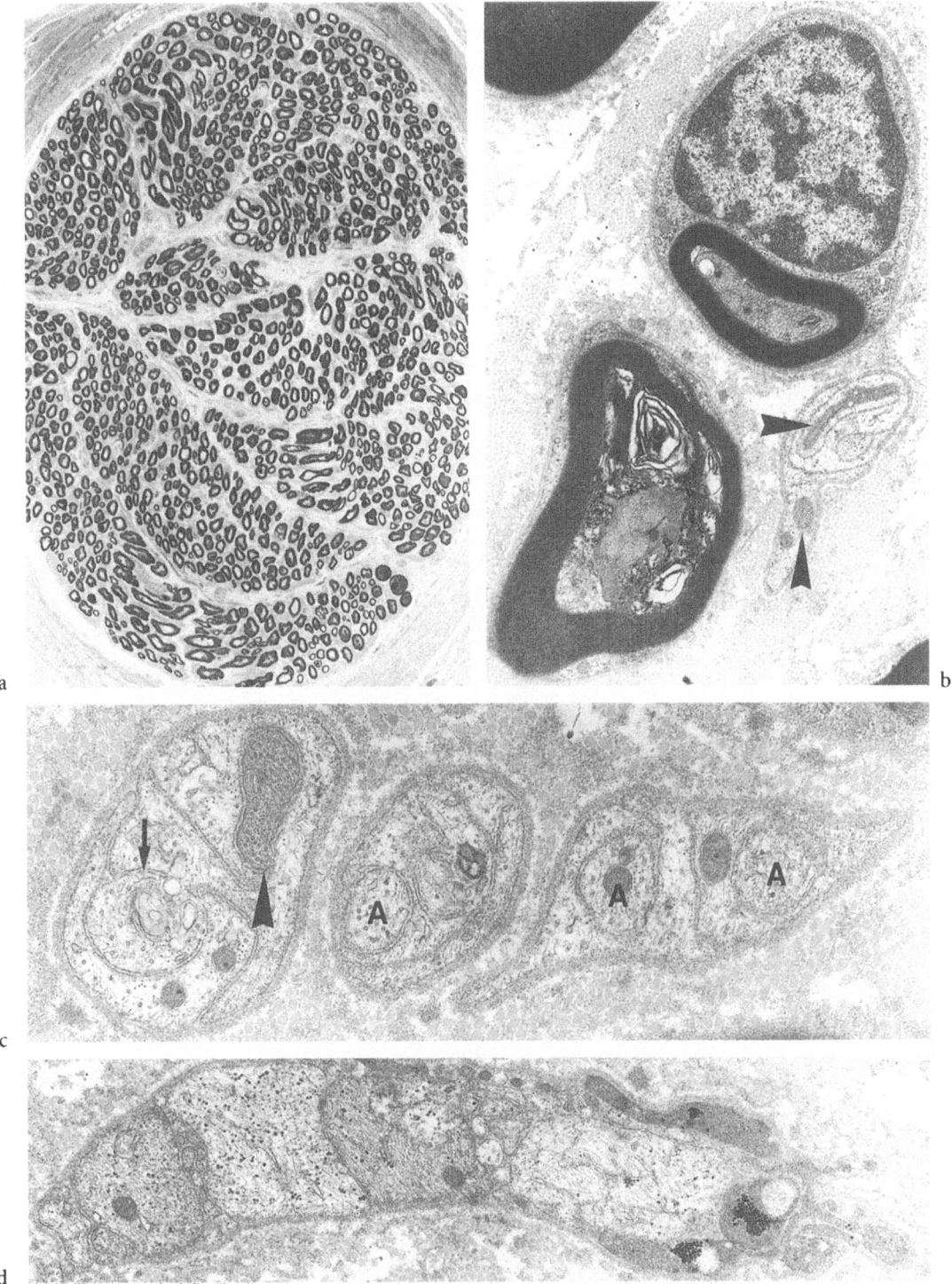

Fig. 178a–d. HSAN III (Riley-Day syndrome) in a 7-year-old boy. **a** The sural nerve contains mainly myelinated nerve fibers and very few unmyelinated ones. × 200. **b** Those few preserved unmyelinated axons are either flattened or atrophic (*arrowheads*). Myelinated nerve fibers may contain membranous inclusions in Schmidt-Lanterman incisures. × 11,500. **c** Rarely inconspicuous unmyelinated axons can be seen (*A*); shrunken (*arrowhead*) or degenerating (*arrow*) axons are more frequent. × 32,000. **d** Bands of Büngner with multiple Schwann cell processes and only ill-defined, single unmyelinated axons may also occur. × 15,000

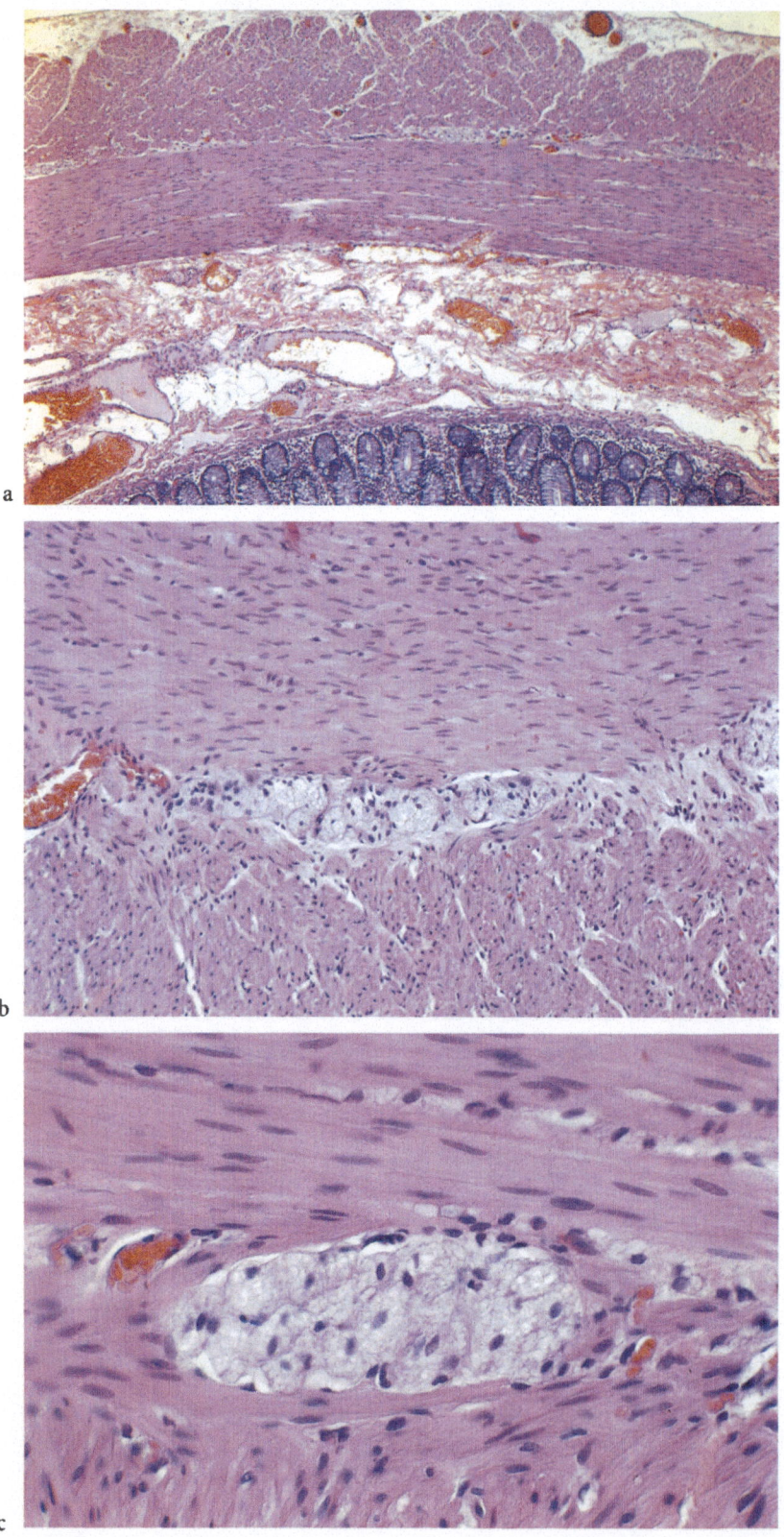

Fig. 179a–c. Hypoganglionosis due to Hirschsprung's syndrome in the colon descendens of an 11-year-old boy. The plexus myentericus contains only unmyelinated nerve fibers with Schwann cells and capsule cells (*aganglionosis*) instead of neurons. Few neurons may still be preserved (*hypoganglionosis*).

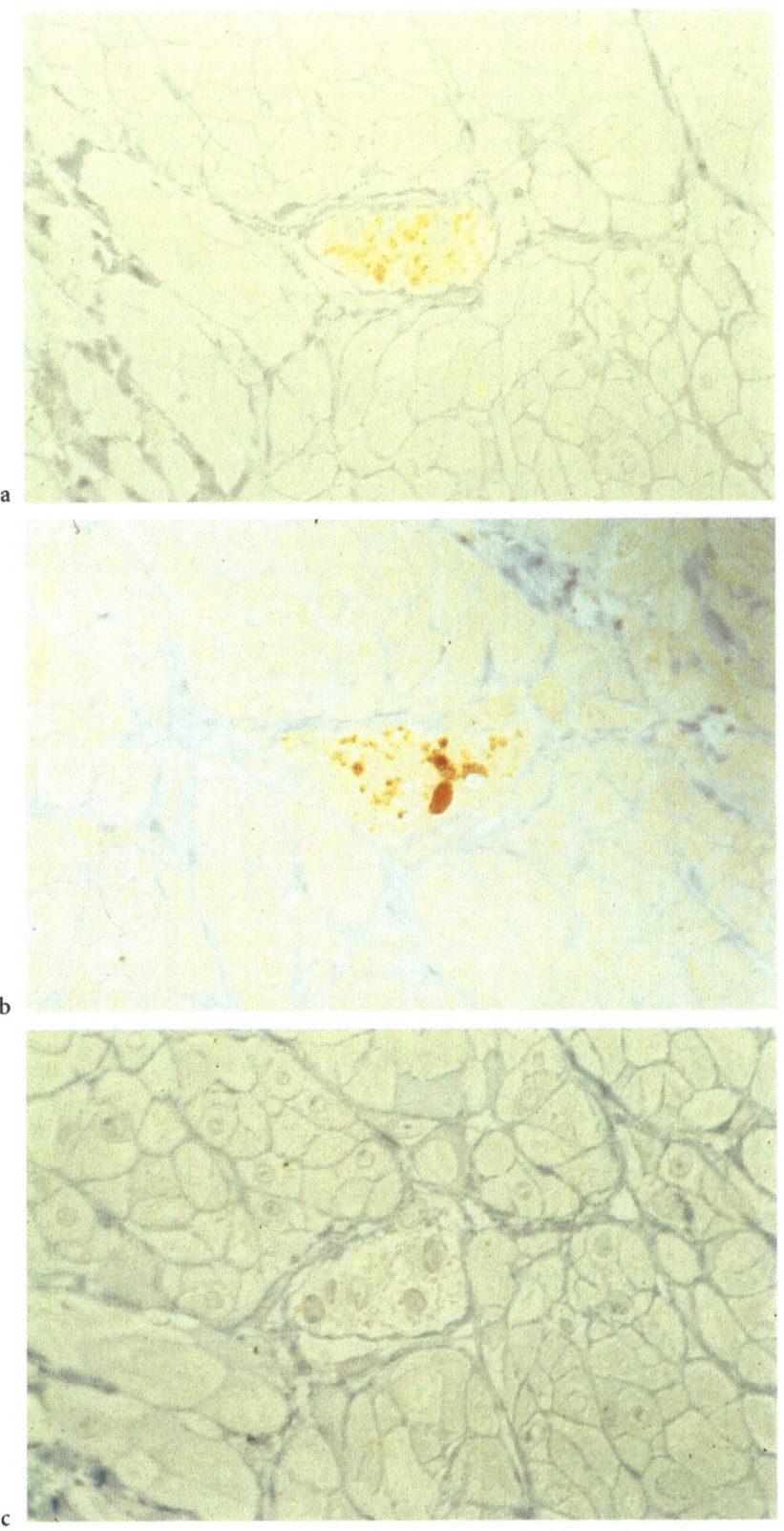

Fig. 180 a–f. Infantile hypertrophic pyloric stenosis. Immunohistochemical reactions reveal intensive immunoreactivity for synaptophysin (**a**) and VIP (**b**), absent (**c**) or focally detectable immunoreactivity for substance P (**d**), uneven immunoreactivity for enkephalin (**e**), and deficient immunoreactivity for calcitonin-gene-regulated peptide (CGRP) (**f**). (Unpublished illustrations to [976]) **d–f.** s. p. 206

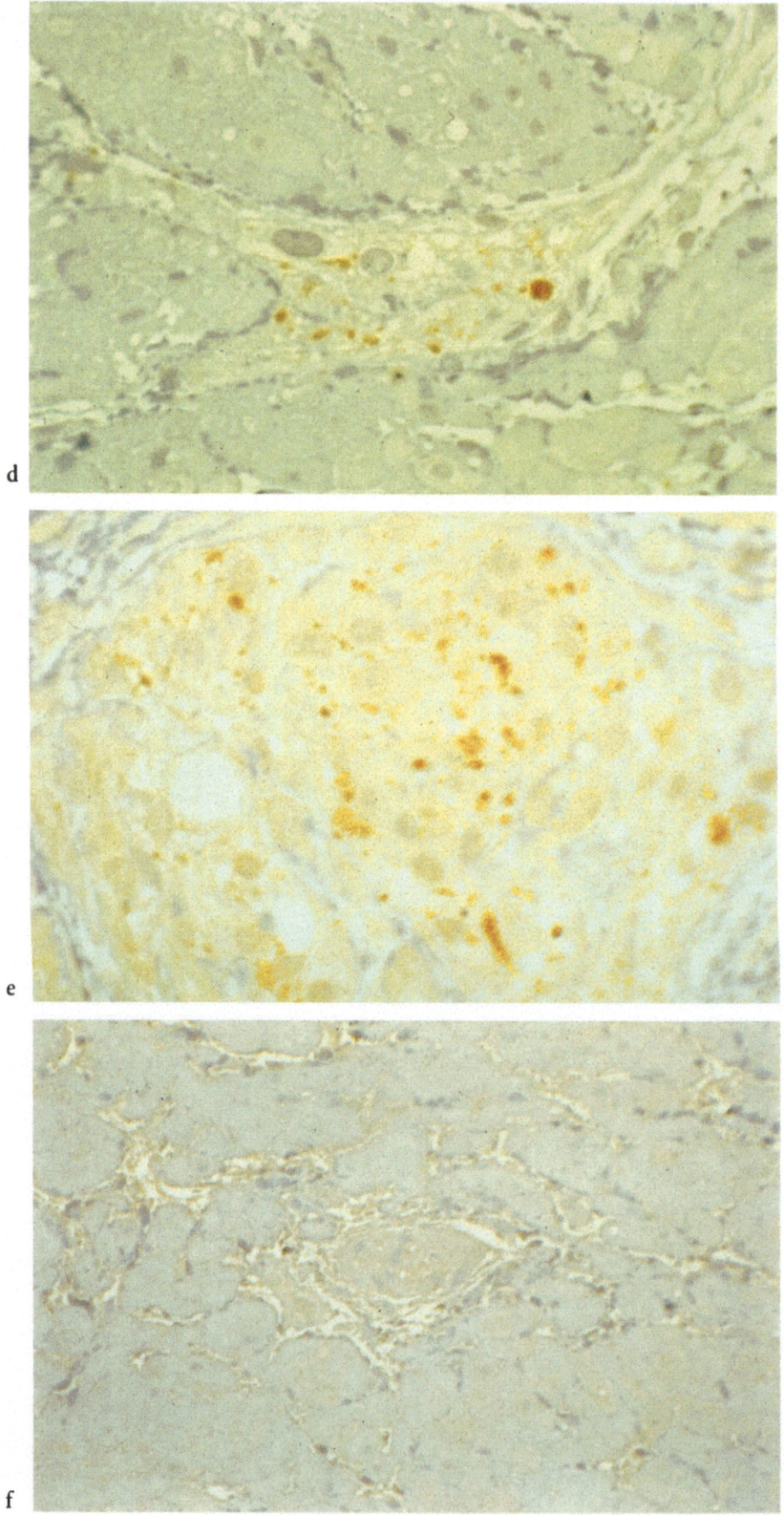

Fig. 180 d–f. Legend s. p. 205

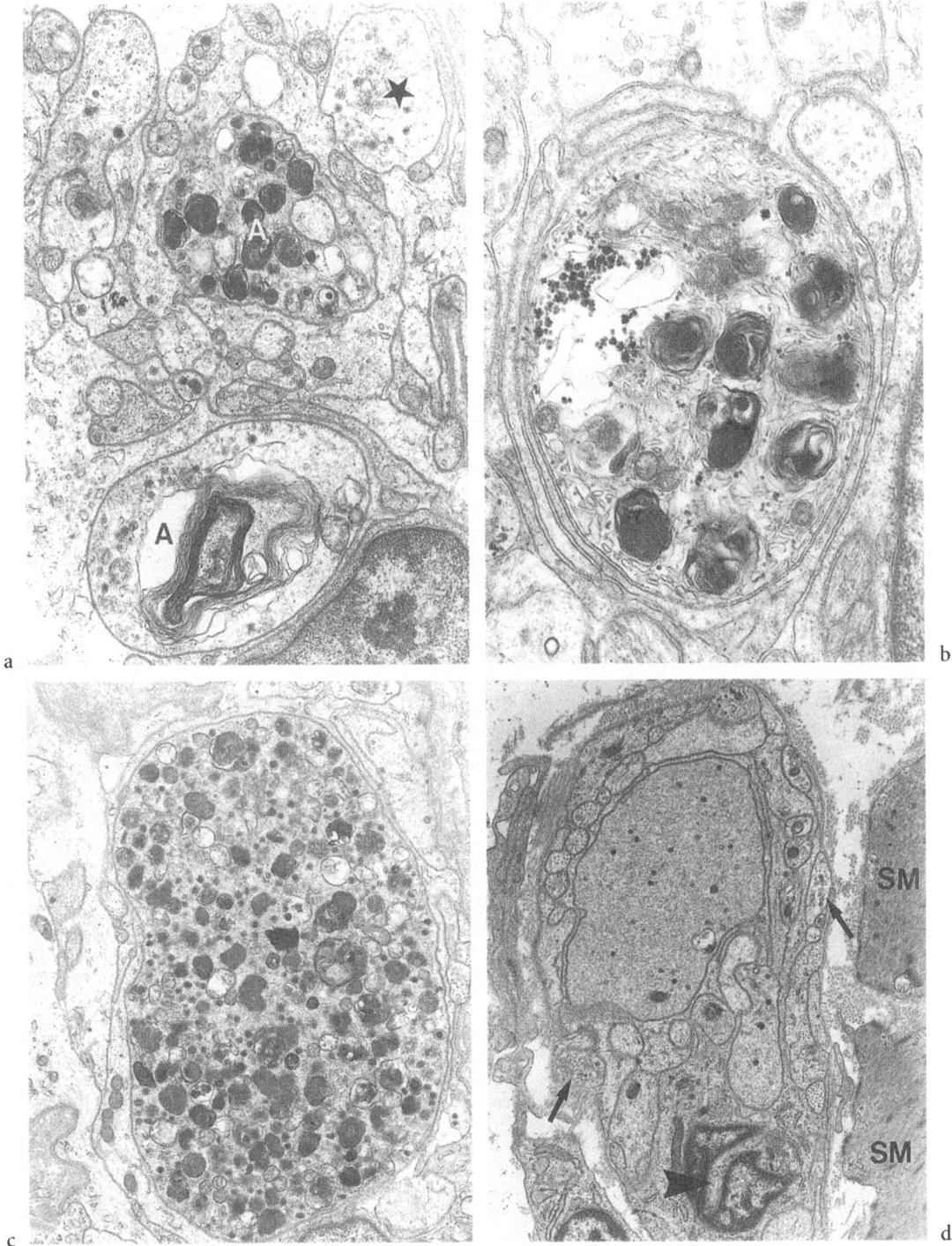

Fig. 181a–d. Neuropathic form of infantile hypertrophic pyloric stenosis (From [226]). The plexus myentericus contains dystrophic axons (**a–c**) with membranous cytoplasmic bodies (*A*), glycogen granules (**b**), and amorphous lysosomal structures (**c**). Enlarged axons with increased filamentous components or neurosecretory granules (*arrows* in **d**) may also occur. The *arrowhead* in **d** indicates a cytoplasmic nuclear inclusion. Adjacent smooth muscle cells of the pylorus are indicated by *SM*.
a × 13,000; **b** × 31,000; **c** × 9,700; **d** × 8,100

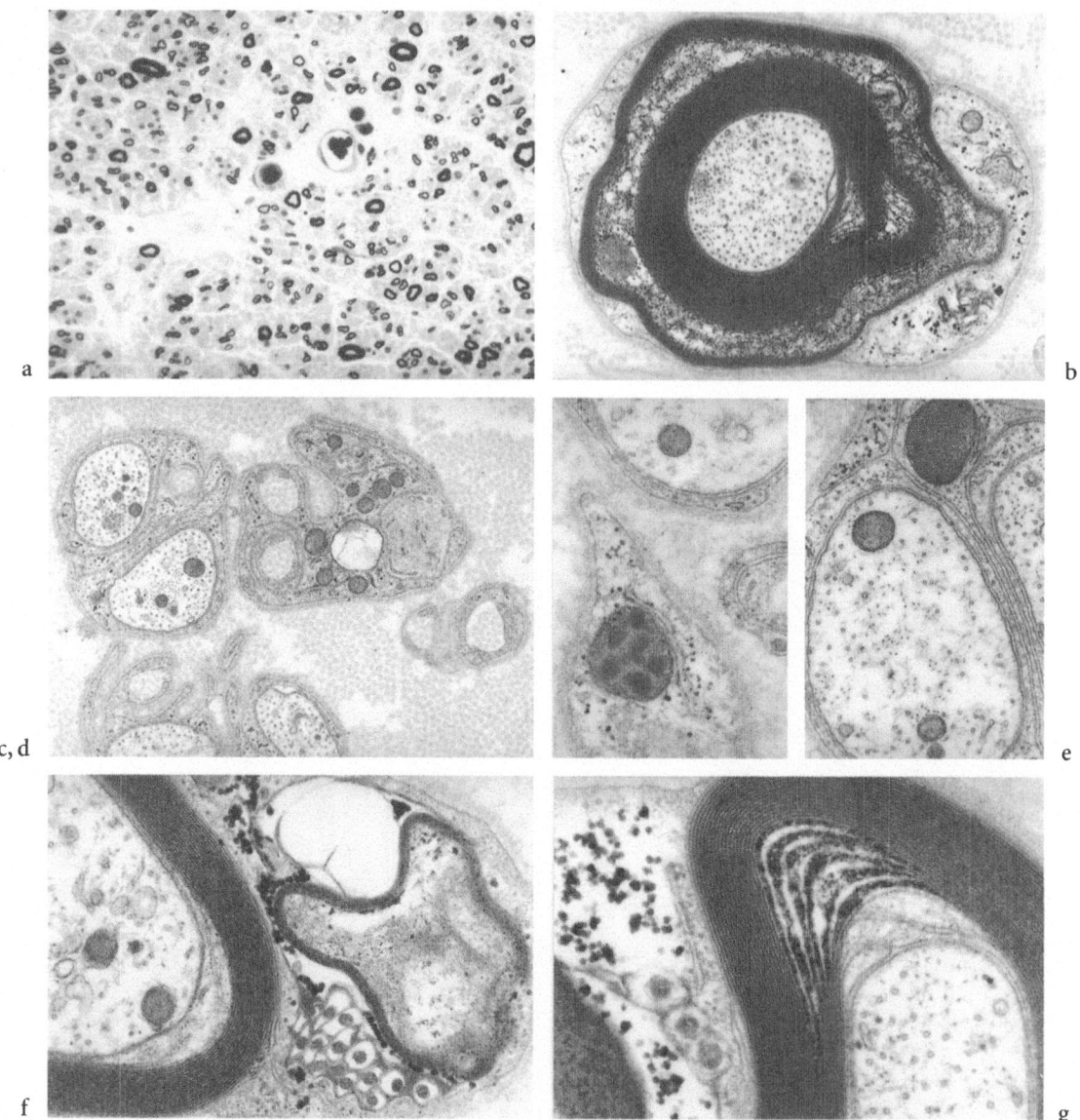

Fig. 182a–g. Friedreich's ataxia in a 60-year-old man. **a** In the sural nerve, the number of large myelinated nerve fibers is severely reduced in contrast to the small ones. Clusters of regenerated fibers are rare. × 310. **b** Preserved small myelinated nerve fiber at the level of several Schmidt-Lanterman incisures with sparse membranous, vesicular inclusions in the abaxonal cytoplasm of the Schwann cell. × 19,000. **c** Degenerated unmyelinated axons are replaced by collagen fibrils (so-called collagen pockets). × 13,500. **d** Unusual mitochondrion in an empty Schwann cell with several osmiophilic homogeneous inclusions in the matrix within a group of unmyelinated axons. × 31,000. **e** Enlarged mitochondrion with granular matrix inclusions in the cytoplasm of a Schwann cell within a group unmyelinated axons. × 26,900. **f** μ-Granule with large vacuole and adjacent smaller vacuoles with an electron-dense center. × 36,400. **g** Higher magnification of the inclusions with osmiophilic center in the cytoplasm of a Schwann cell between the myelin sheath and a myelin loop adjacent to several glycogen granules. × 43,400

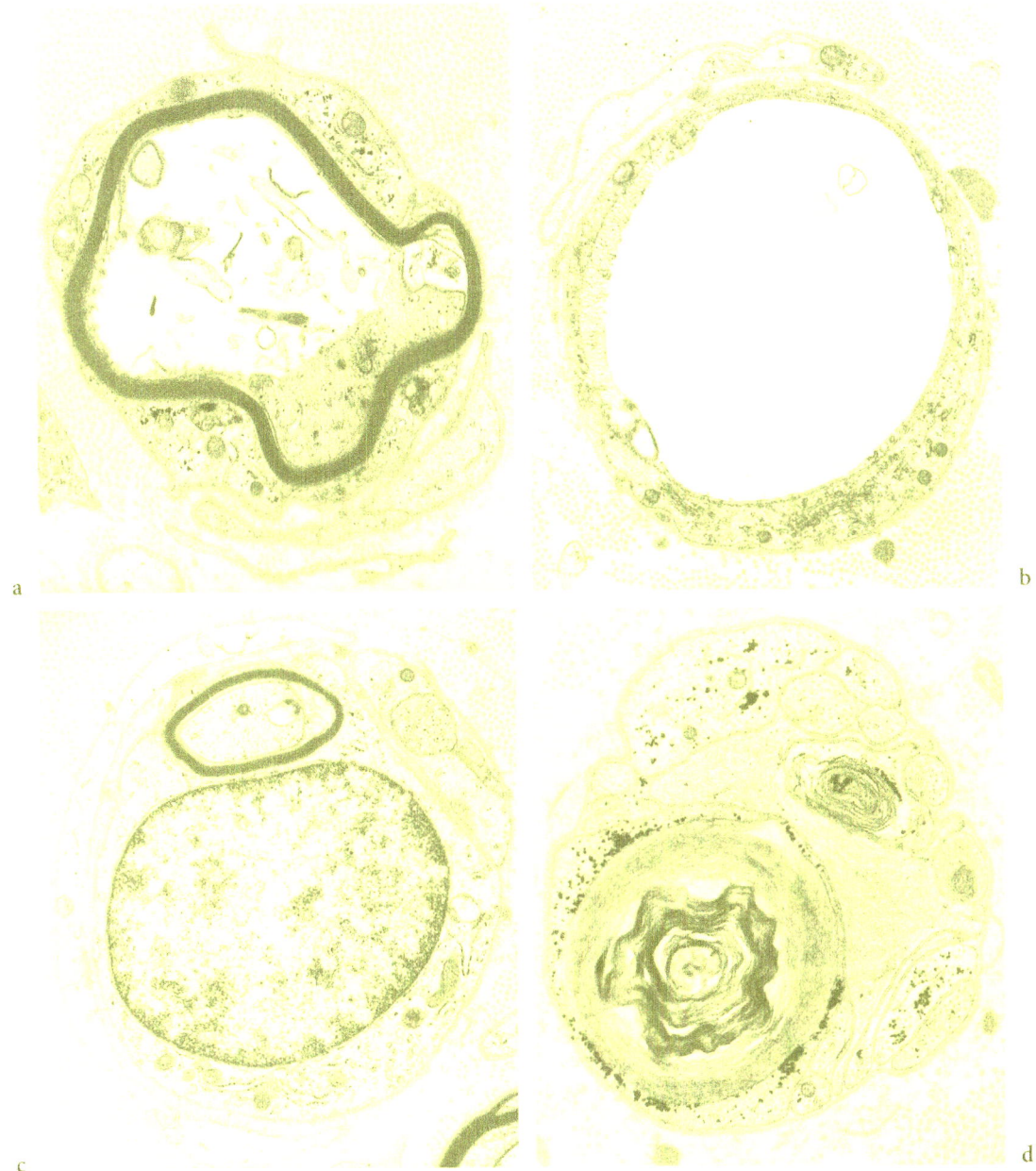

Fig. 183 a – d. Degenerating regenerated myelinated fiber in Friedreich's ataxia (5 ½-year-old girl). **a** This regenerated fiber with a disproportionately thin myelin sheath in a band of Büngner shows a peculiar form of degeneration with vesicles and membranous fragments in a large, electron optically clear space. × 11,700. **b** The large vacuole in an obviously regenerated axon indicates repetitive degeneration and regeneration. × 10,800. **c** Small atrophic, regenerated cluster with one myelinated and one unmyelinated axon. × 11,900. **d** Myelin degradation products in a band of Büngner. × 14,800

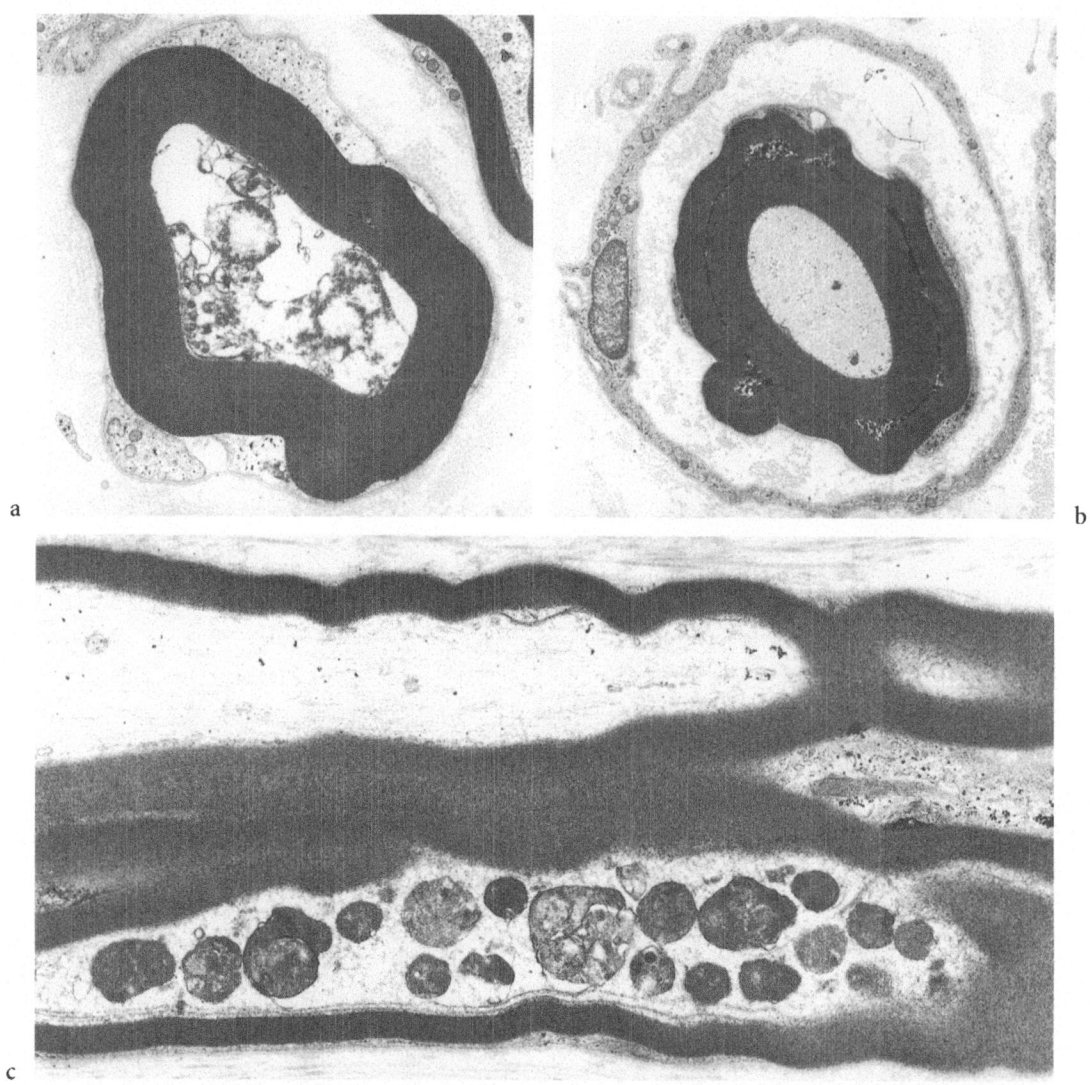

Fig. 184a–c. Friedreich's ataxia in a 20-year-old female. **a** Acutely degenerating large myelinated axon with a still well-preserved myelin sheath. × 8,800. **b** Circularly arranged Schwann cell processes surrounding a large myelinated nerve fiber. The so-called collagen pockets in the *upper left part* of **b** and associated unmyelinated axons indicate preceding degeneration and regeneration. × 6,100. **c** Multiple adaxonal pleomorphic lysosomal inclusions in a longitudinal section of a Schwann cell. × 13,000

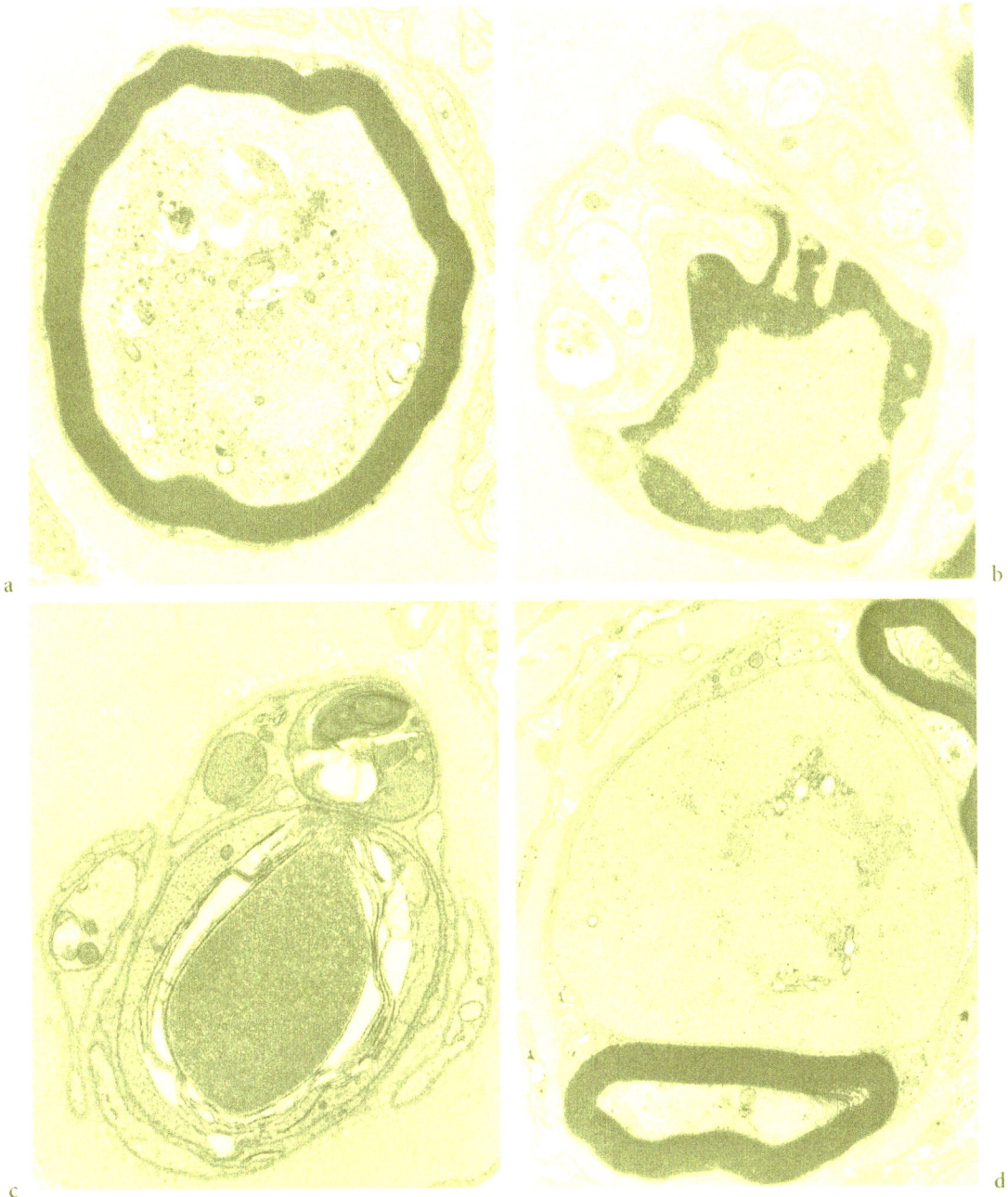

Fig. 185a–d. Unusual aspects in a 7-year-old boy with the clinical diagnosis of Friedreich's ataxia. Dystrophic axonal changes in **a**, abnormal homogeneous nuclear inclusion with marginal condensation of the heterochromatin in a Schwann cell (apoptosis) in **b**, abnormal dystrophic axons with electron cense membranous structures in **c**, and an exceptionally distended axon in a regenerative cluster in **d**. **a** × 10,600; **b** × 15,100; **c** × 11,400; **d** × 8,600

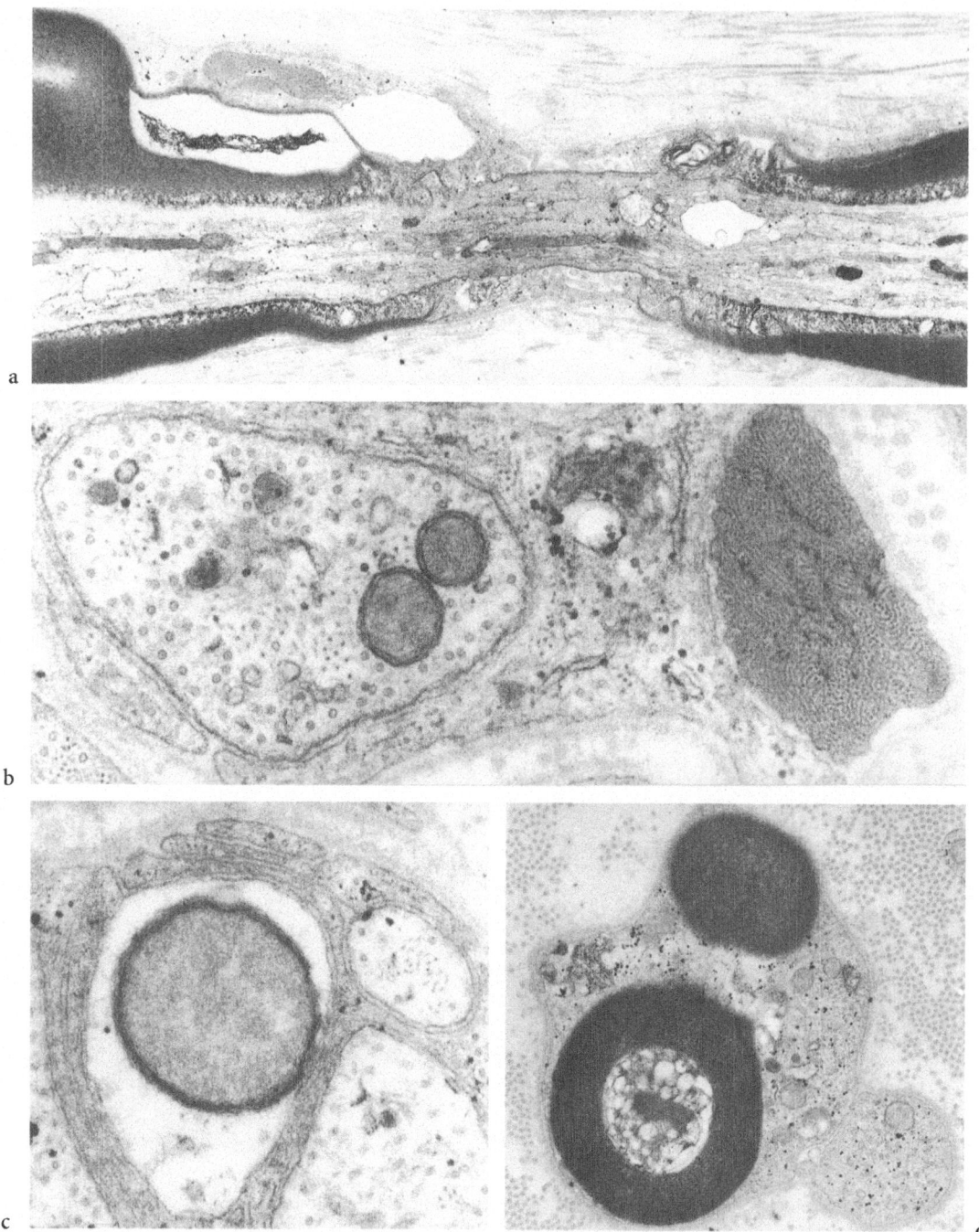

Fig. 186a–d. Further degenerative nerve fiber changes in the same case as in Fig. 185. Vacuolar alterations in an axon and in the paranodal cytoplasm of a Schwann cell as well as in the myelin sheath (**a**), unusual extracellular, not clearly membrane-bound remnant with tubulofilamentous structures, adjacent to an unmyelinated nerve fiber (**b**), abnormal cytosome with homogeneous matrix surrounded by an electron-dense, thickened membrane in an unmyelinated axon(**c**), and an acutely degenerating small nerve fiber still showing a partially preserved myelin sheath and myelin loop (**d**). **a** × 13,000; **b** × 64,000; **c** × 50,000; **d** × 15,100

CHAPTER 9

Further Recessive Disorders Involving Peripheral and Central Neuronal Systems

Neuroaxonal dystrophy is rare and may occur in an *infantile* form (*Seitelberger*) (Figs. 187–189) [4, 328, 343, 507, 863, 1009] and an *adult* form (Fig. 190a–c) (*Hallervorden-Spatz disease*) the molecular genetic basis of which has not been clarified (cf. Waka-hayashi et al. 1999, Neuropathol Appl Neurobiol 25: 363–368). A variant with *spinal neuroaxonal dystrophy and angioneuromatosis* has also been described [637]. *Dystrophic axonal changes* in isolated axons may occur in a variety of neuropathies; these dystrophic changes, however, have not been delineated, e.g., in alpha-*N*-acetylgalactosaminidase deficiency [1247]. Dystrophic axons in typical neuroaxonal dystrophy are nevertheless seen in a small proportion of axons per cross section only (Fig. 187). An experimental model has been described in rabbits [328].

Another rare autosomal recessive disease with typical central and peripheral involvement is *giant axonal neuropathy* (Fig. 191a–e) [26, 66, 95, 297, 301, 509, 526, 537, 699, 896, 1107, 1112, 1113, 1115, 1122, 1144]. Neurons (axons), glial cells, Schwann cells, and endothelial cells may show increased numbers of abnormal intermediate filaments whereas another pathognostic symptom, abnormal hairs with a pathognostic rim (Fig. 191e) may be absent [821].

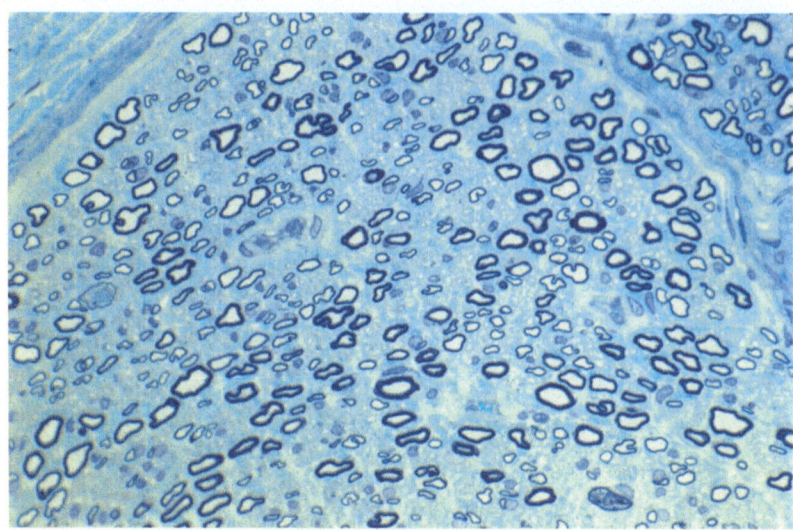

Fig. 187. Neuroaxonal dystrophy in a 3-year-old girl. Only a few myelinated axons are obviously dystrophic. Toluidine blue

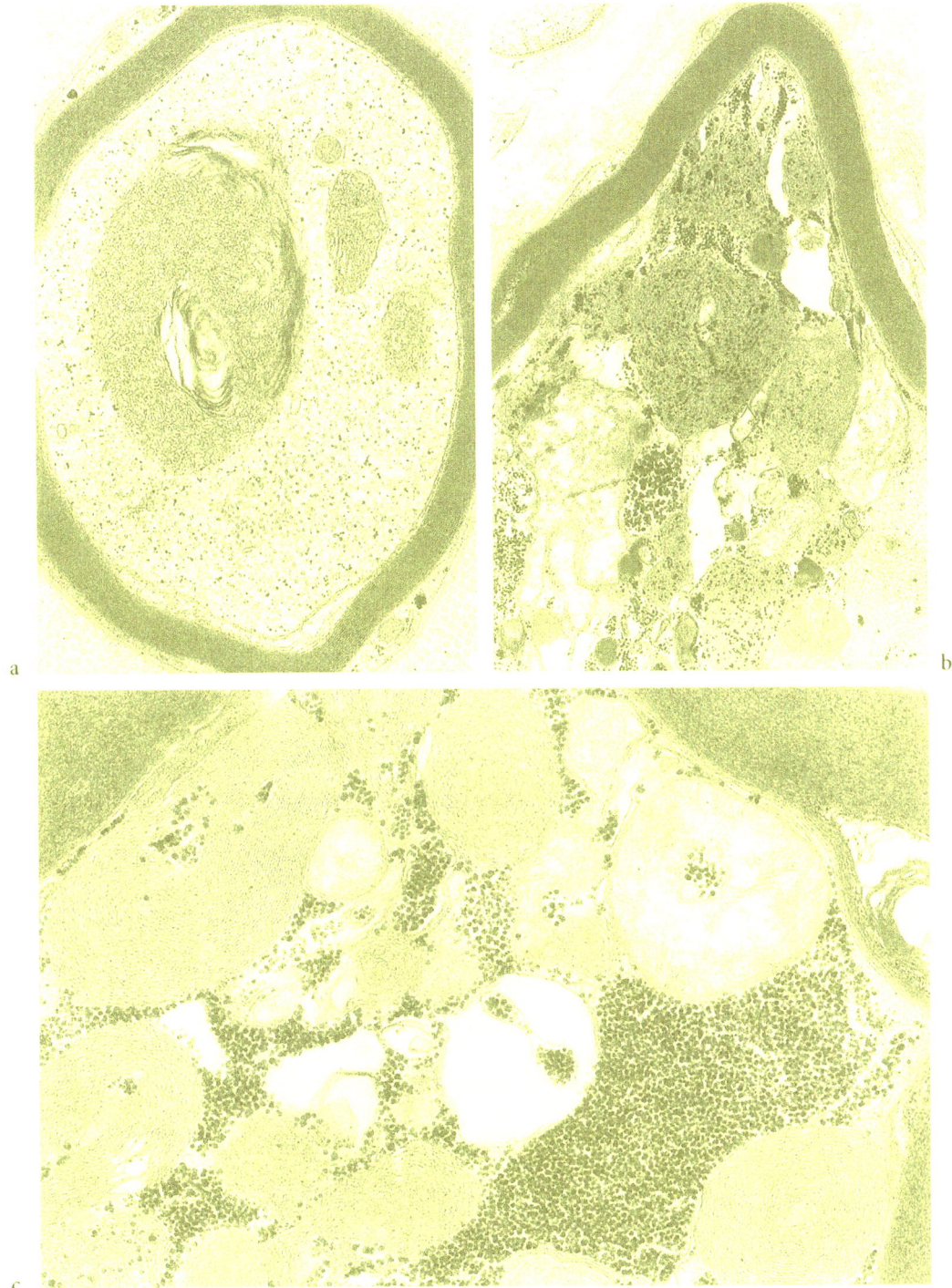

Fig. 188 a – c. Same case as in Fig. 187. **a** Large axon with relatively thin myelin sheath and several tubulovesicular corpuscles of variable size consisting of parallel or concentrically arranged lamellae. × 26,400. **b** Pleomorphic partially vacuolated membranous or granular inclusions with abnormal mitochondria and numerous glycogen granules in an enlarged axon with disproportionately thin myelin sheath. × 21,200. **c** Multiple corpuscles with concentrically arranged membranes and numerous glycogen granules within the axon of a large myelinated fiber. An enlarged mitochondrion includes several glycogen granules in its center. × 40,800

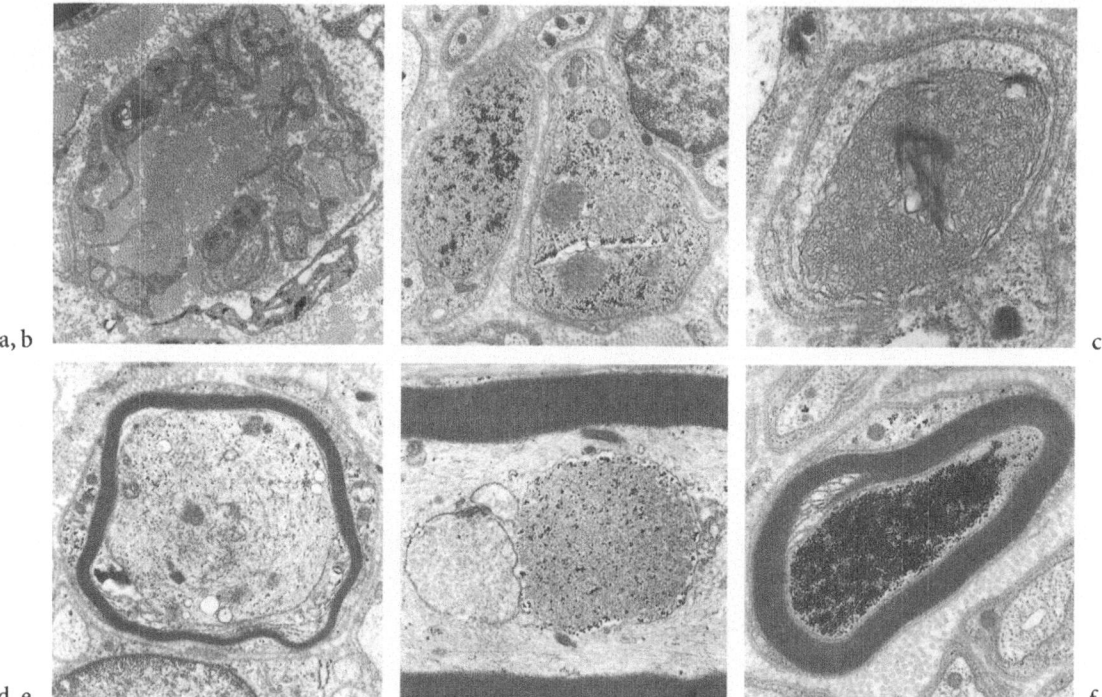

a, b

c

d, e

f

Fig. 189 a–f. Same case as in Fig. 187 and 188. Further axonal abnormalities include loss of unmyelinated axons with replacement by collagen pockets (**a**), distension of axons by glycogen deposits and tubulovesicular inclusions (**b, c, f**), dystrophic distension of an axon of a myelinated fiber (**d**), and membrane-bound axonal inclusions with glycogen or finer granular substances (**e**). **a** × 5,300; **b** × 8,300; **c** × 24,800; **d** and **e** × 9,500; **f** × 17,100

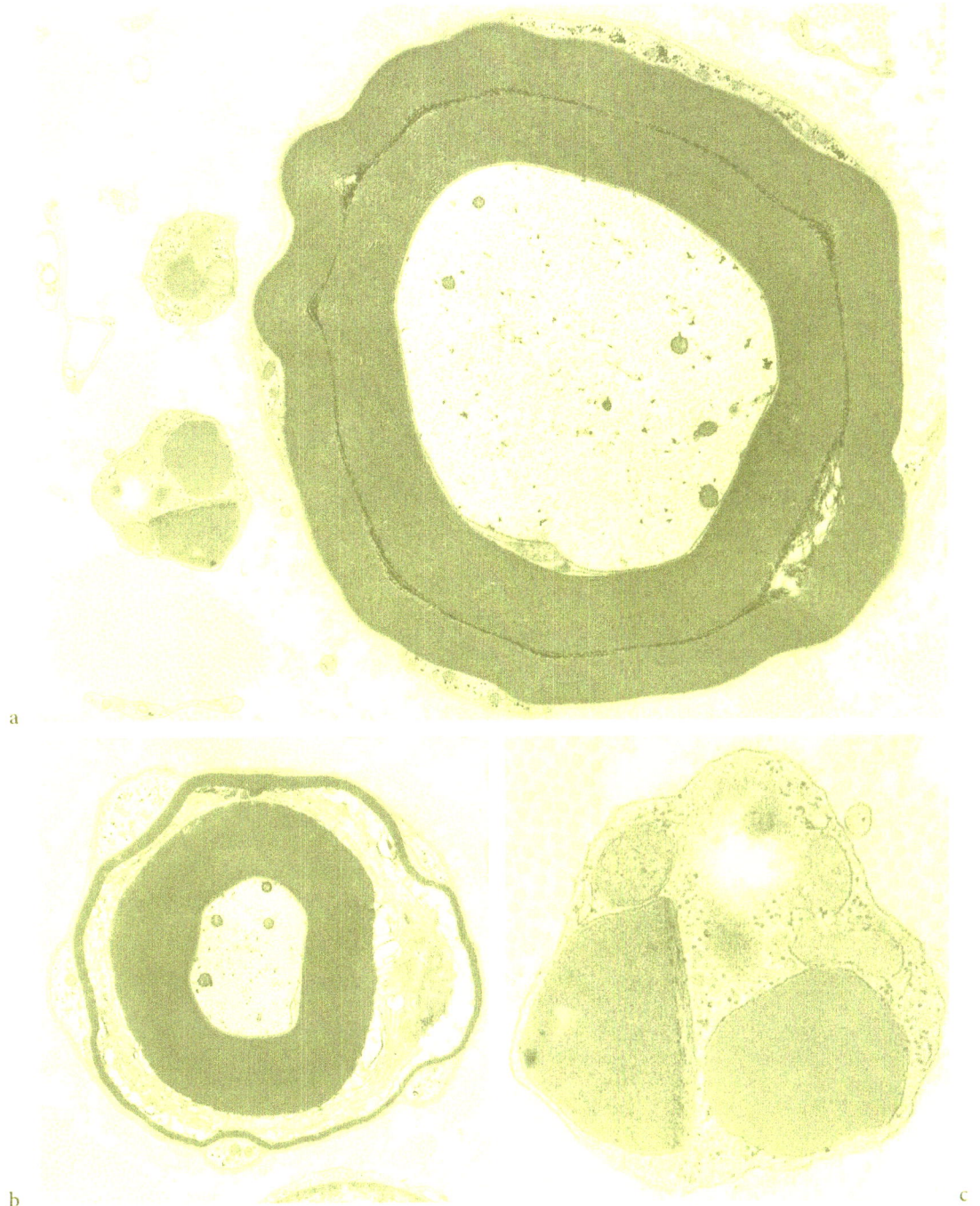

Fig. 190 a – c. Hallervorden-Spatz disease syndrome in a 21-year-old male. Unusual homogeneous lysosome-like inclusions in fibroblasts in **a** and **c**. The Schmidt-Lanterman incisure in **b** is abnormally widened. **a** × 12,600; **b** × 10,200; **c** × 37,000

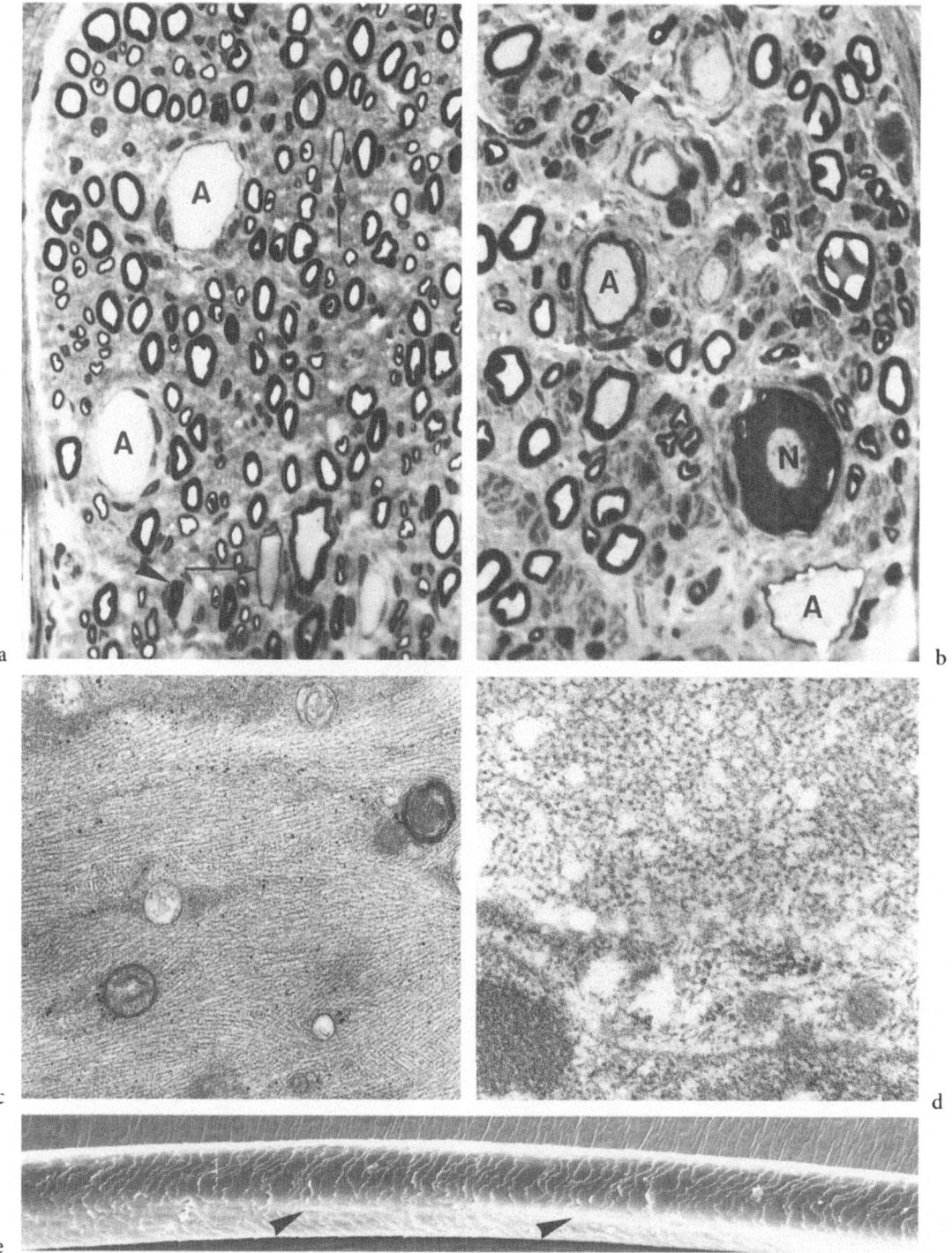

Fig. 191a–e. Giant axonal neuropathy in an 11-month-old girl. Some axons are severely enlarged (*A* in **a** and **b**). Their myelin sheaths may be extremely thin, but there is also a nerve fiber with disproportionately thick myelin sheath (*N* in **b**). **a** × 674; **b** × 1,022. **c** The number of neurofilaments in the giant axons is considerably increased. × 38,200. **d** Microtubules are not preserved between the increased neurofilaments in the area shown. × 81,200. **e** Scanning electron microscopic illustration of a single hair reveals the pathognostic rim which is indicated by *arrowheads*

CHAPTER 10

Hereditary and Sporadic Neuropathies with Special Localization

Diseases of the cranial nerves I–XII are rarely studied by biopsy or at autopsy except for identifying tumors. However, some of the nerves may be rather frequently affected clinically:

- The *optic nerve* (I) [3, 18, 128, 154, 173, 174, 177, 190, 334, 391, 415, 453, 518, 594, 610, 718, 740, 832, 870, 884, 934, 948, 1007, 1030, 1047, 1069, 1091, 1143, 1202, 1220].
- The *olfactory nerve* (II) at the most frequent site (frontobasal) of brain trauma.
- The *oculomotor nerve* (III) [53, 163, 164, 434, 486, 487, 513, 666, 780, 938, 1233, 1286].
- The *trochlear nerve* (IV) [164, 780, 975].
- The *trigeminal nerve* (V) [217, 276, 425, 583, 602, 607, 608, 1170, 1214].
- The *abducens nerve* (VI) by compression.

- The *facial nerve* and nucleus (VII) [88, 217, 354, 447, 458, 717, 769, 833, 861, 931, 975, 1020, 1021, 1082, 1141, 1154].
- The *acoustic/vestibular nerve* (VIII) [10, 58, 72, 131, 134, 188, 191, 287, 386, 390, 429, 447, 453, 464, 482, 499, 551, 629, 632, 708, 742, 831, 850, 884, 898, 1038, 1041, 1057, 1108, 1109, 1135, 1251].
- The *glossopharyngeal nerve* (IX) [107, 1203].
- The *vagal nerve* (X) [176, 303, 698, 918].
- The *accessory nerve* (XI) [107, 146, 356, 574, 982].
- The *hypoglossal nerve* (XII) [25, 33, 107, 217, 356, 397, 574, 721, 782, 836, 1203, 1234].

Many nerves may be affected by *local compression* [709] including rare causes such as the *descending perineum* [671]. An *idiopathic progressive mononeuropathy in young individuals* [272] is of uncertain etiology.

Chapter 11

Inflammatory Neuropathies
(Neuritis, Polyneuritis, Vasculitis, Perineuritis; Sarcoidosis)

This is a frequent group of neuropathies especially important for those involved in examining nerve biopsies because of the *therapeutic implications*. This group of disorders can be treated effectively after being diagnosed microscopically or by other means which may not be as efficient and reliable as a microscopic diagnosis.

Infectious neuropathies include:

- *Herpes zoster virus* infections [60, 195, 276, 280, 336, 376, 500].
- *Herpes simplex virus (HSV)* infections [639, 712].
- *Retrovirus infection in AIDS* [14, 39, 187, 192, 310, 355, 672, 864, 876].
- *Cytomegalovirus* infection as an opportunistic infection in AIDS patients [175].
- *Syphilitic polyradiculopathy*, which is certainly very rare but was nevertheless described in an HIV-positive bisexual man [572].

Peripheral nerve changes may also occur in:

- *HTLV-I-associated myelopathy (HAM, tropical spastic paralysis, TSP, Strachan syndrome)* [79].

Worldwide the most frequent infectious neuropathy is seen in *lepra* caused by mycobacterium leprae [85, 212, 330, 461–463, 900, 901, 1026, 1167], although we have not seen a single case in our series of presently more than 6,000 nerve biopsies.

The following infectious diseases are also not illustrated: *Chagas' disease* [1052], *Lyme borreliosis (Garin-Bujadoux-Bannwarth syndrome)* [385, 539, 659] in which we noted only minor epineurial perivascular cellular infiltrates, and *Epstein-Barr virus-associated autonomous neuropathy* [61]; *Botulism* which has not been noted in our series, but *botulinus toxin* is widely used for the treatment of dystonic states [7, 86, 133, 146, 179, 234, 244, 245, 335, 339, 358, 395, 400, 421, 422, 606, 783, 799, 800, 830, 1078, 1151, 1300]; *papovavirus infection* [78], *diphtheric neuropathy* [41, 853, 854, 1218, 1219 2268], and *tetanus* [41, 296, 911]. It is likely that some of the changes noted in dorsal branches of cervical nerves in spasmodic torticollis may be due to botox injections preceding neurosurgical treatment (see below: Figs. 256–260) [982].

In a sural nerve biopsy from a case with *subacute sclerosing panencephalitis* (SSPE) we could not find the typical nuclear inclusions seen in the central nervous system. In *postpoliomyelitis* cases [206, 337], we examined several muscle biopsies showing evidence of progressive neurogenic muscle atrophy, yet nerve biopsies were not available.

A demyelinating type of neuropathy was described in two patients with *Creutzfeldt-Jakob disease (CJD)* [736]. The only nerve biopsy available in our series of cases with CJD was complicated by diabetes mellitus (Fig. 192 a–c). The spinal ganglion of an experimental animal infected with *scrapie* (provided by H. Budka, Vienna) showed vacuoles in the cytoplasm of neurons similar to those seen in neurons of the central nervous system, but no plaques or filamentous or other unusual deposits (unpublished observations).

Sepsis [802] may be a major cause of critical illness neuropathy (see p. 95).

Immunologically induced, presumably autoaggressive forms of neuropathy are represented much more frequently in our series of nerve biopsies than infectious neuropathies. The main forms among this group of disorders are:

- *Polyraduloneuritis* or *Guillain-Barré syndrome (GBS)* (Figs. 26 c, 193, 198–201) [9, 13, 41, 64, 65, 124, 163, 164, 178, 197, 204, 215, 268, 311, 323, 326, 338, 351, 352, 363–365, 384, 399, 408, 426, 427, 432, 433, 435, 441, 442, 456, 485, 490, 491, 504, 512, 553, 555, 567, 619, 655, 705, 718, 747, 764, 789, 790, 804, 810, 834, 844, 848, 849, 865, 868, 880, 888, 895, 920, 937, 1024, 1025, 1044, 1060, 1062, 1099, 1168, 1173, 1182, 1200, 1233, 1270, 1271, 1273–1276, 1296].
- *Experimental allergic neuritis (EAN)* (Figs. 194–197) [23, 124, 246, 346, 347, 380, 381, 510, 565, 576, 596, 597, 625, 654, 846, 882, 1084, 1199, 1284, 1289].
- *Chronic inflammatory demyelinating polyneuropathy (CIDP)* (Figs. 20 e, 203–209) [103, 186, 284, 645, 1049, 1086, 1158].
- An *axonal variant of GBS* (Fig. 202 a–d) [197, 311, 364, 432, 441, 555, 1060, 1270, 1276].
- *Miller-Fisher syndrome* [164, 308, 444, 720], a local variant of GBS involving the cranial nerves.

- *Bell's palsy* (facial nerve) [717, 833, 1082].
- *Hypertrophic brachial plexus neuritis* [202, 280, 620].
- *Localized hypertrophic neuropathy of the index finger and the thumb* [1301].
- *Idiopathic lumbosacral neuropathy* [414].
- *Multifocal neuropathy* (Fig. 209) [189, 329, 467, 480, 571, 756, 760, 770, 771, 811, 919, 1159, 1217].
- *Acute pandysautonomia* (autonomic ganglionitis) (Figs. 210, 211) [585, 959].

The cause of occasional, presumably autoimmune disorders of peripheral nerves remains unidentified (e. g., Fig. 21).

Involvement of peripheral nerves in other well defined autoimmune disorders may also occur, for example, in:

- *Multiple sclerosis* [11, 222, 338, 842].
- *Bronchial asthma* in respect to local nerve terminals [69], and critical illness neuropathy.
- *Crohn's disease* [733].
- *Myasthenia gravis* [161, 224, 1257].
- *Inclusion body myositis* and *polymyositis* (Figs. 212–214) [991], whereas dermatomyositis is usually not combined with peripheral neuropathy.
- *Vasculitis* in a special form specifically affecting the peripheral nervous system [151, 210, 515] is said to occur although no autopsy studies have been performed, proving that peripheral nerves only were affected. *Systemic forms of vasculitis* are certainly more common (Figs. 32 c, 215 a – d, 216; 236; 245, 246, 248–254) [71, 105, 141, 151, 169, 252, 266, 325, 477, 515, 803, 878, 903, 1186, 1269]. There are 20 primary and 24 secondary varieties of vasculitis that may be distinguished [825]. *False negative* nerve biopsies not revealing vasculitis were noted in 43% of our series of combined nerve and muscle biopsy cases with vasculitis [969]. An increase in the thickness of the basal laminae may be an indirect although rather nonspecific sign of vasculitis. Neuropathies are frequently associated with connective tissue diseases.
- *Eosinophilic fasciitis* [919, 952] may also affect the peripheral nervous system.
- *Eosinophilia myalgia syndrome* [238] needs to be distinguished form *eosinophilic fasciitis*.

Perineuritis [528, 1040, 1073] appears to be an entity of its own although it may be mimicked by vasculitis of vessels passing the perineurium, lepra, cryoglobinuria, Spanish toxic oil syndrome, and Boeck's sarcoidosis. Since perineuritis may simultaneously affect the sural nerve and intramuscular nerve fascicles (Figs. 217–220), it is obviously not confined to sensory nerves as originally suggested [26]. Severe perineuritis was also seen 2–4 weeks after heterotopic subcutaneous implantation of heterologous nerves (Figs. 42 a – d, 43).

Boeck's sarcoidosis (Figs. 221–223) [609, 781, 1012], on the other hand, is etiologically not defined, whether it is infectious, inflammatory for other reasons, or neoplastic.

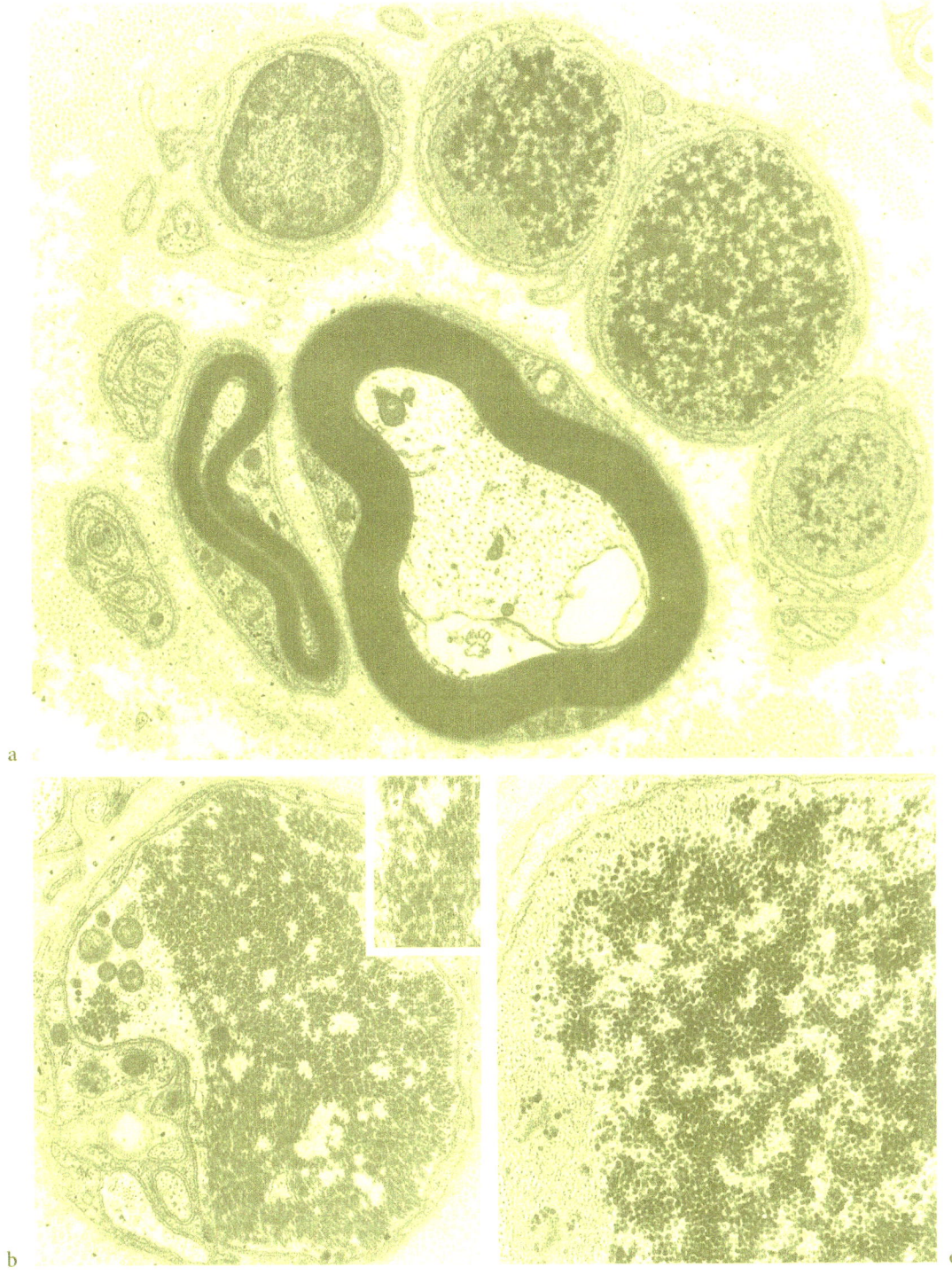

Fig. 192a–c. Creutzfeldt-Jakob disease combined with diabetes mellitus in a 61-year-old man. There are masses of glycogen granules in the distended, regenerated axons in **a** and **c**. These must be distinguished from the paracrystalline filaments in the axon in **b**. **a** × 15,200; **b** × 23,800; inset × 48,200; **c** × 53,600

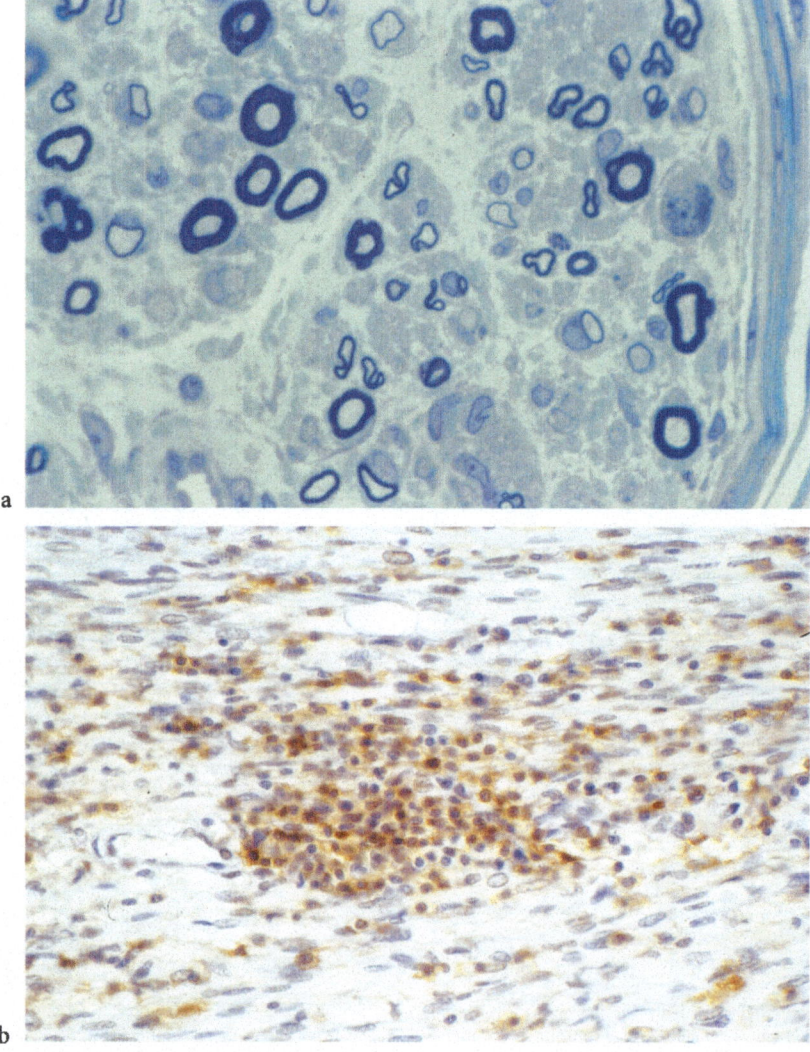

Fig. 193 a – d. Guillain-Barré syndrome in different cases. Inflammatory cellular infiltrates in the endoneurium with focally accentuated demyelination of myelinated nerve fibers. In semithin sections, there are usually only a few mononuclear cellular infiltrates detectable (**a**), whereas these are considerably more numerous in the thicker cryostat and paraffin sections (**b – d**). **b – d** Autopsy cases which succumbed to Landry's paralysis. **c, d** s. p. 225

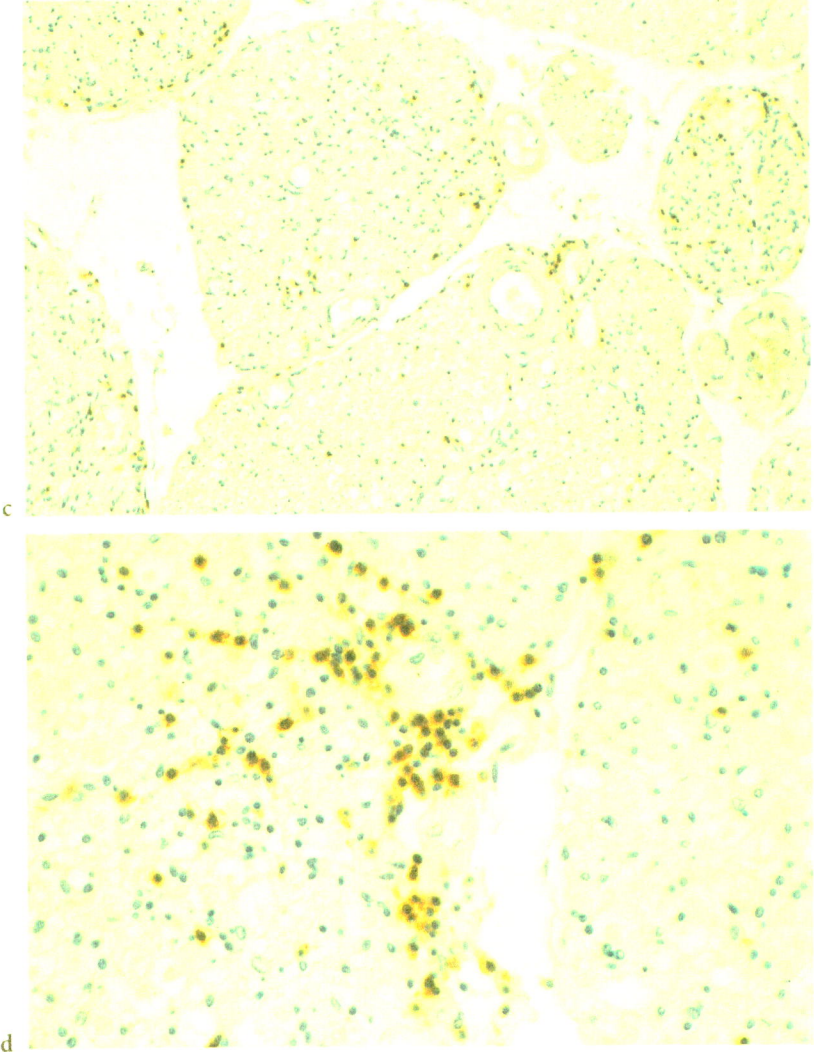

Fig. 193 c, d. Legend s. p. 224

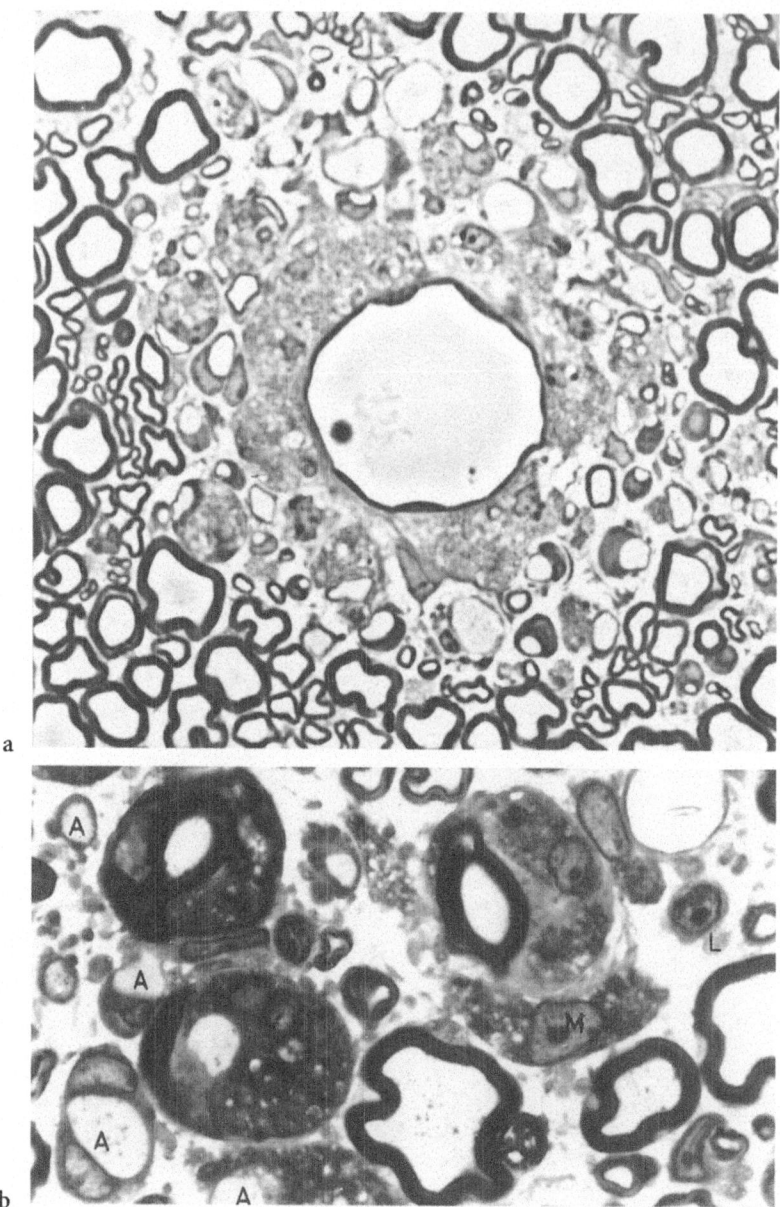

Fig. 194 a, b. Experimental allergic neuritis. **a** Perivascular area of infiltration and demyelination 21 days after the last injection of the antigenic emulsion. Numerous nerve fibers around a centrally located vein are completely demyelinated. Many macrophages are located close to the blood vessel. × 880. **b** Florid demyelination of three different nerve fibers is seen adjacent to a blood vessel (in the *upper right corner*) and already demyelinated axons (*A*) on the left. Close to the blood vessel a lymphocyte with narrow cytoplasm is indicated by *L* and a macrophage by *M*. The latter contains many myelin degradation products. × 1,480. (From [986])

Fig. 195 a–k. Sequelae of axon and myelin sheath changes in experimental allergic neuritis (EAN). **a–i** Cross-sectional series of a group of segmentally demyelinated nerve fibers in a perivascular focus of demyelination. One axon (*x*) shows a prolapse-like deformation with prominent myelin changes, which in another nerve fiber (*o*) are even more pronounced. Other demyelinated axons show alterations of the contour and the diameter with severe Schwann cell changes. × 800. **j** Perivascular focus of demyelination in the sciatic nerve of a rabbit with numerous cells and cell processes arranged in an onion-bulb-like pattern around remyelinated nerve fibers with disproportionately thin myelin sheaths 7 and 11 months after two injections of the antigen emulsion. **k** Perivascular focus of demyelination and remyelination in a dorsal root 2 years after EAN. The myelin sheaths remain disproportionately thin, the axon diameters appear to be reduced. Supernumerary Schwann cells and other cell processes around the remyelinated nerve fibers are extremely thin or have disappeared. **j, k** × 650. (Figs. 195 and 196 from [949])

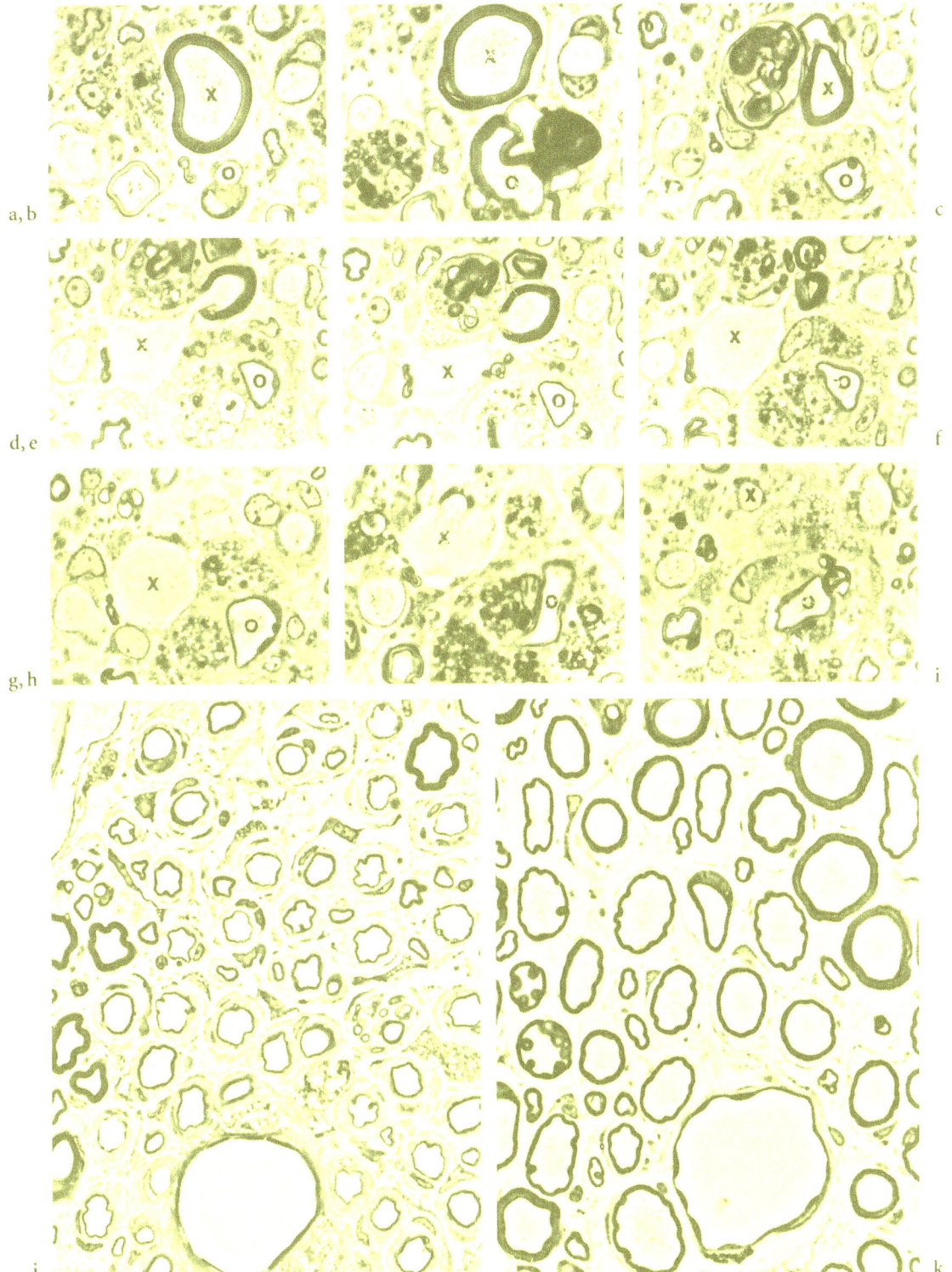

Fig. 195a–k. Legend s. p. 226

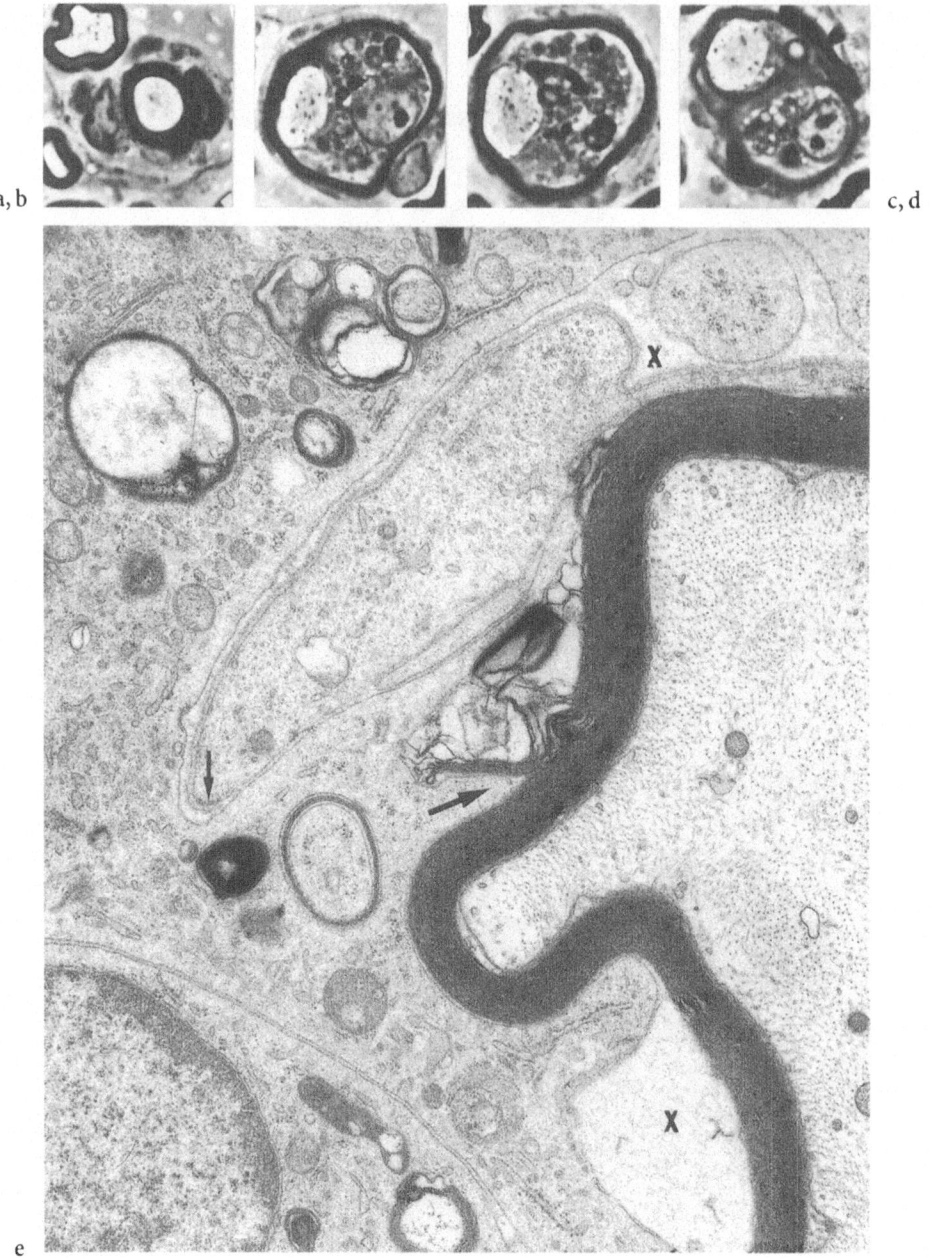

a, b

c, d

e

Fig. 196 a–d. Four different section planes of the same nerve fiber indicate various aspects of myelin sheath degradation. In **a** the nerve fiber appears to be still intact; a macrophage is noted on the *left* adjacent to the paranode. In **b** a macrophage filled with myelin degradation products is seen between the axon and the myelin sheath. In this section plane as well as in the next (**c**), the outer contour of the myelin sheath is still preserved although distended. In **d** another macrophage is seen inside the damaged myelin sheath. × 1,200. In **e** an infiltrating cell penetrates the basal lamina of a nerve fiber (*small arrow*). The myelin sheath in a circumscribed area is in immediate contact with the invading cell which apparently induces vacuolar disintegration and delamination of the penetrated myelin lamellae (*large arrow*). At another site, a finely floccular substance (*x*) is seen between the myelin sheath and the infiltrating cell corresponding to the extracellular space outside the basal lamina in the endoneurium (*x*). The nucleus in the *lower left* belongs to another infiltrating cell in close contact with the other one. Myelin degradation products are seen in the cytoplasm of both infiltrating cells (presumably macrophages). × 17,500

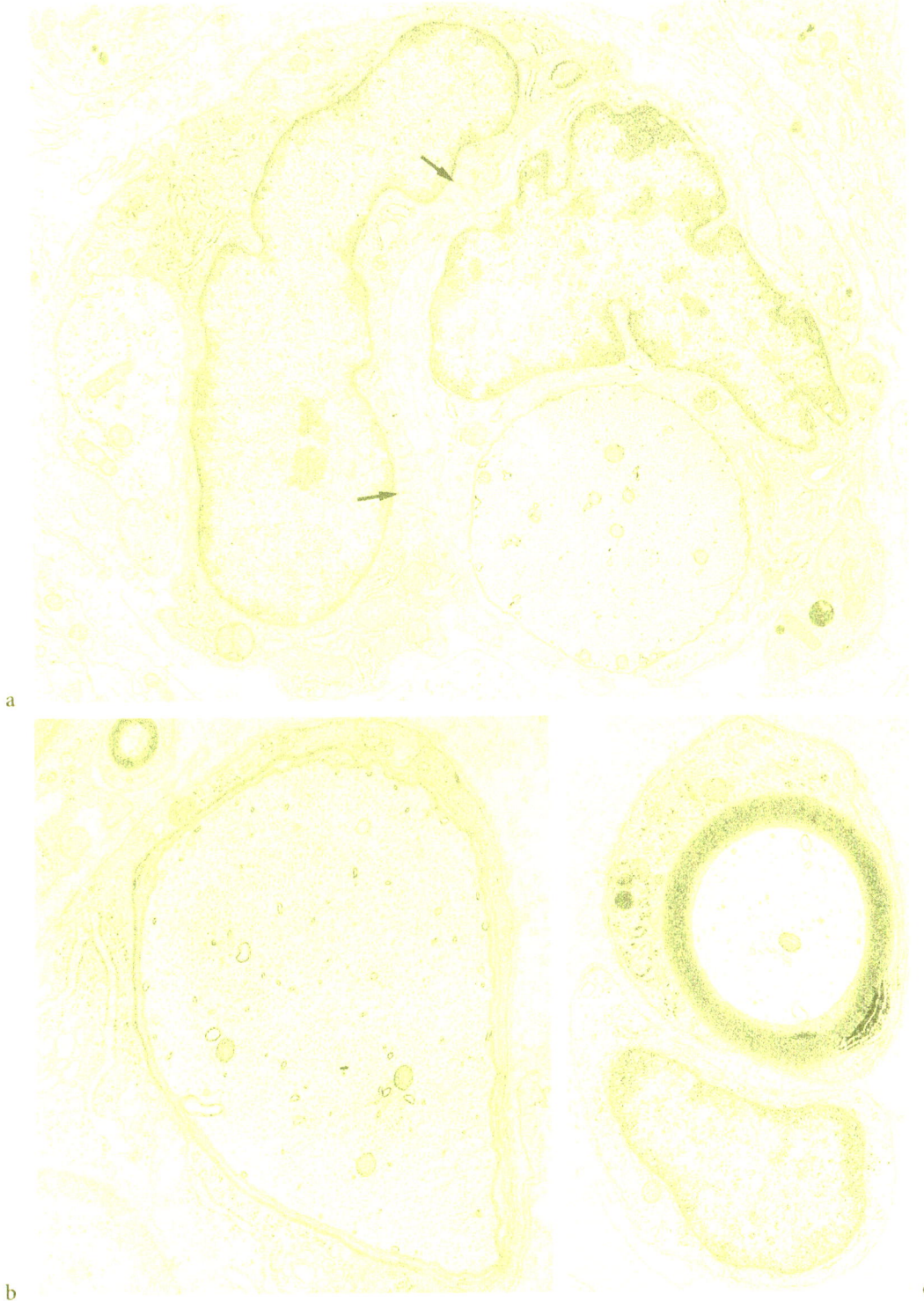

Fig. 197. a Demyelinated axon with two Schwann cells cut at the level of their nucleus. One of the Schwann cells encloses the axon completely, the other one is separated from the axon, and its nucleus is irregularly indented. The *arrows* indicate leptomer fibrils, 7 and 11 weeks after two injections of the antigen. × 18,200. b A relatively large demyelinated axon is surrounded by a Schwann cell process in three spirals, one of which has partially fused to form a major dense line. × 19,000. c A supernumerary Schwann cell shows an incipient onion-bulb-like arrangement adjacent to a remyelinated nerve fiber. × 17,200. (From [942])

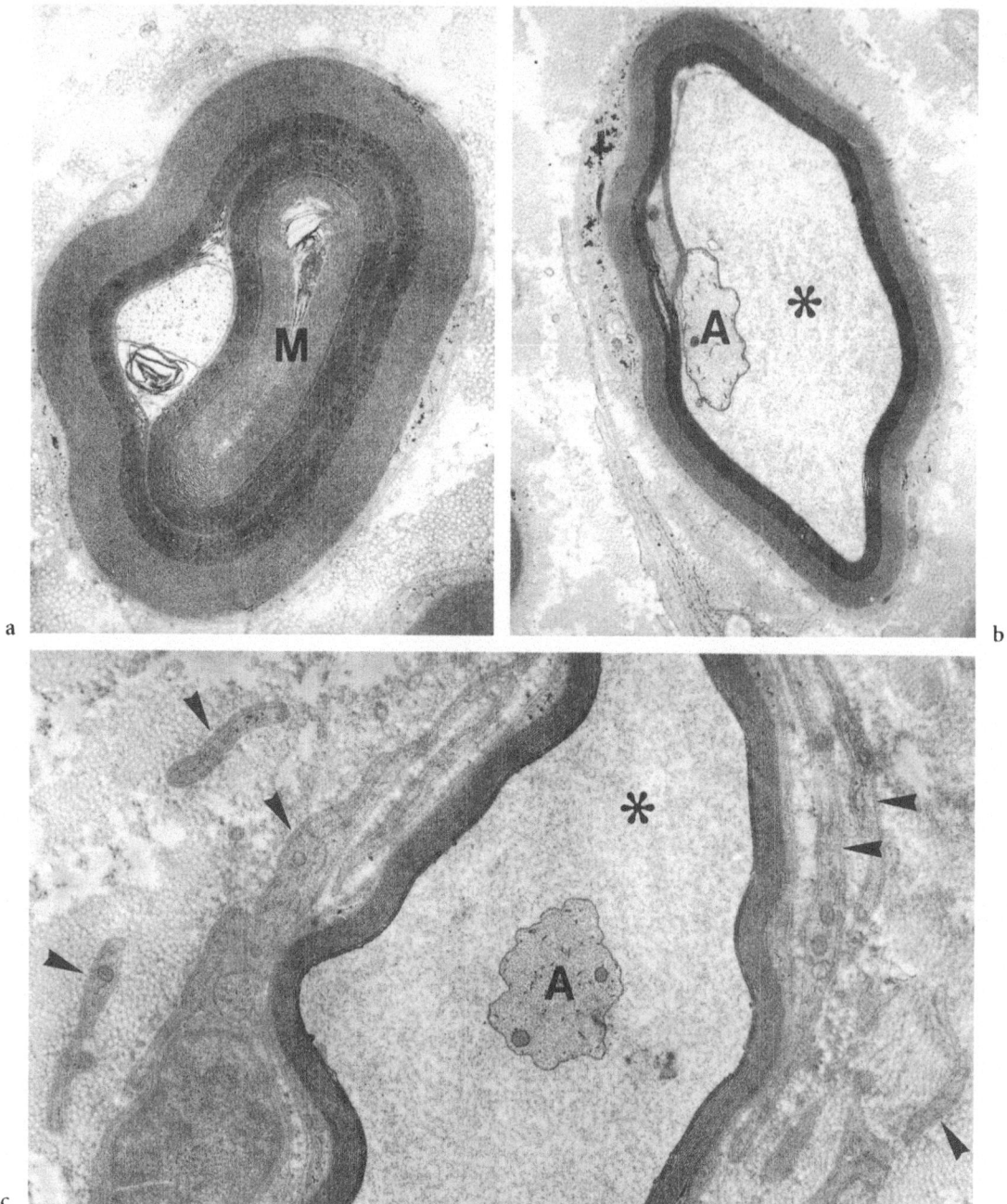

Fig. 198a–c. Recurrent polyradiculoneuropathy (with relapses after 2 and 6 years) in a 32-year-old female (without dysglobulinemia). **a–c** Altered periodicity of the outer myelin sheath with loose lamellae where the intraperiod lines are twice as wide
(approximately 26 nm) as in the inner, normally compacted myelin sheath (where the distance between the major dense lines
measures roughly 13 nm as determined at approximately × 100,000 magnification). There is an extraordinarily wide, nonartifi-
cial enlargement of the adaxonal extracellular space in **b** and **c** between the axon (*A*) and the myelin sheath filled with a finely
floccular, evenly distributed plasma-like material (*). An inner, presumably paranodal myelin loop (*M*) is apparent in **a**, several
concentric layers of Schwann cell processes as evidence of recurrent demyelination and remyelination in **c** causing onion bulb
formation (*arrowheads*). – Electroneurographically no sensory or motor potentials were elicitable. **a** × 10,800; **b** × 8,200;
c × 11,900. (From [955])

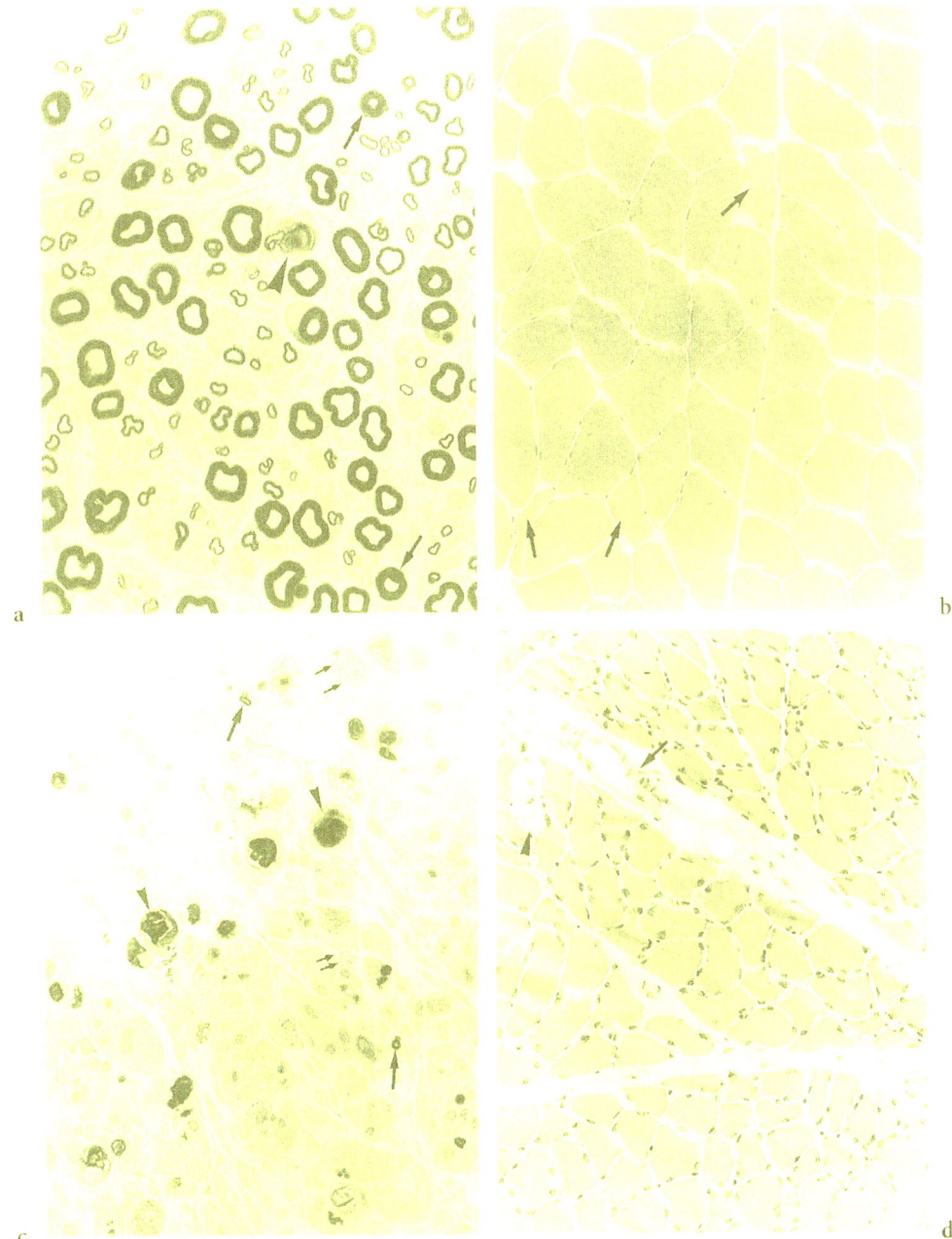

Fig. 199 a–d. Immune mediated neuropathy and myopathy in a 22-year-old man with complete flaccid tetraparesis and immune complex induced rapid progressive glomerulonephritis after an infection with group A streptococci (same case as in Fig. 88, from [1070]). **a** Sural nerve at the time if the first biopsy, 4 weeks after onset of the disorder. The number of myelinated fibers is moderately decreased. Some axons are slightly atrophic (*arrows*), and myelin degradation products (*arrowhead*) are only occasionally seen. × 590. **b** Cryostat section of the muscle biopsy specimen (H & E stain). Only a few muscle fibers are atrophic (*arrows*). × 380. **c** Contralateral sural nerve at the time of the second biopsy 14 weeks after onset of the symptoms. Only very few myelinated nerve fibers are preserved (*arrows*). Myelin degradation products (*arrowheads*) and lipid-laden macrophages (*small arrows*) are apparent in large numbers. × 570. **d** Peroneal muscle at the time of the second biopsy. Most muscle fibers are atrophic. The walls of the capillaries (*arrow*) and the basal laminae (*arrowhead*) are increased in thickness. Paraffin section: H & E, × 370

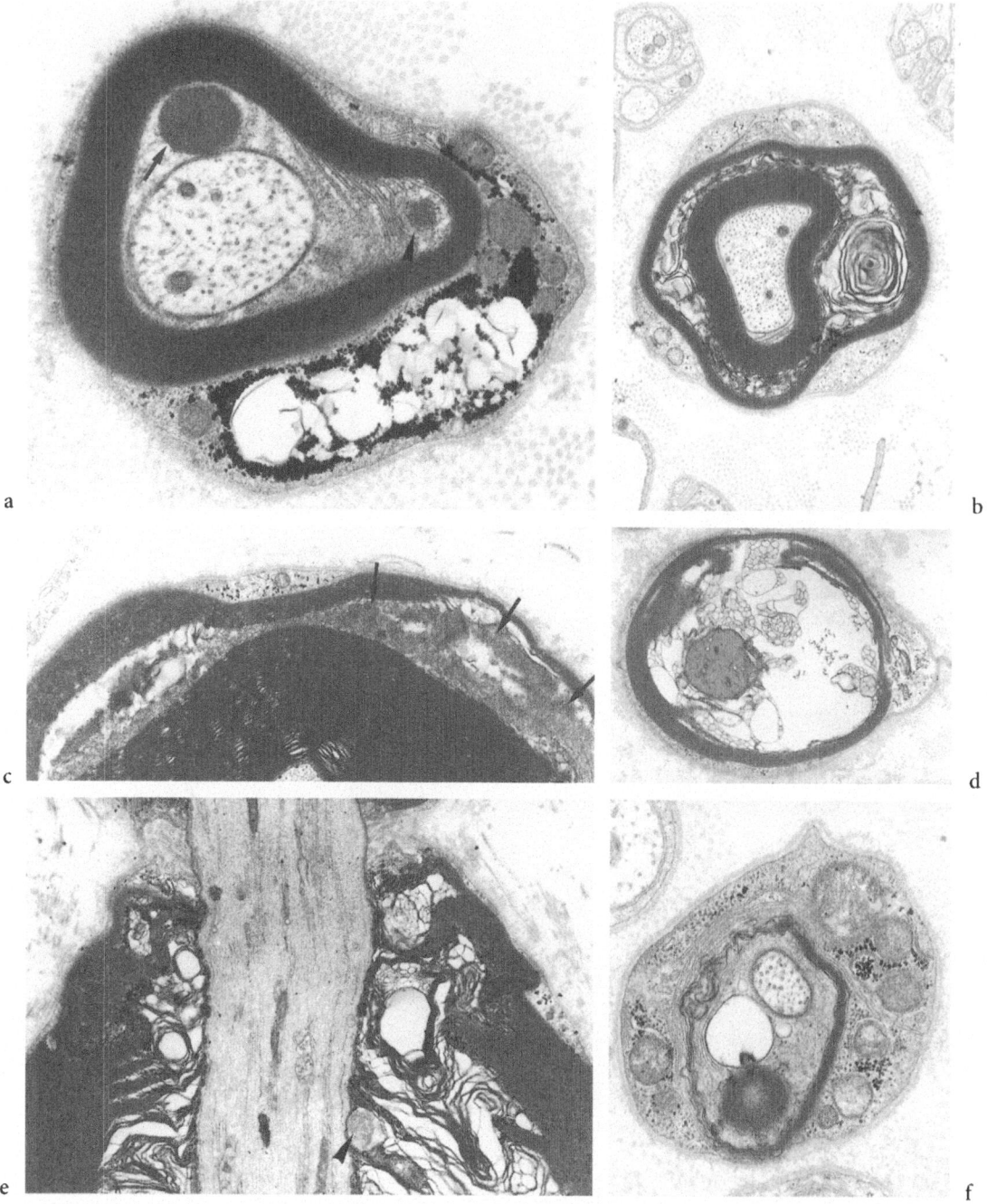

Fig. 200 a–f. Same case as in Fig. 199. Electron microscopic images of the sural nerve at the time of the first biopsy. **a** Lysosome-like bodies are apparent in paranodal, adaxonal spirals of the innermost Schwann cell layers of the myelin sheath (*arrow*) and between some of the inner myelin lamellae (*arrowhead*). × 26,000. **b** Membranous cytoplasmic body within a Schmidt-Lanterman incisure. × 10,000. **c** An amorphous substance (*arrows*) is seen between the inner and outer layers of the myelin sheath. × 10,000. **d** Paranodal vesicular degeneration of myelin lamellae. × 5,000. **e** Incipient paranodal vesicular and vacuolar disintegration of the myelin sheath. The *arrowhead* indicates deposition of amorphic material in the paranode. × 24,000. **f** Cross section of a paranode with incipient vacuolar myelin degradation. × 9,500

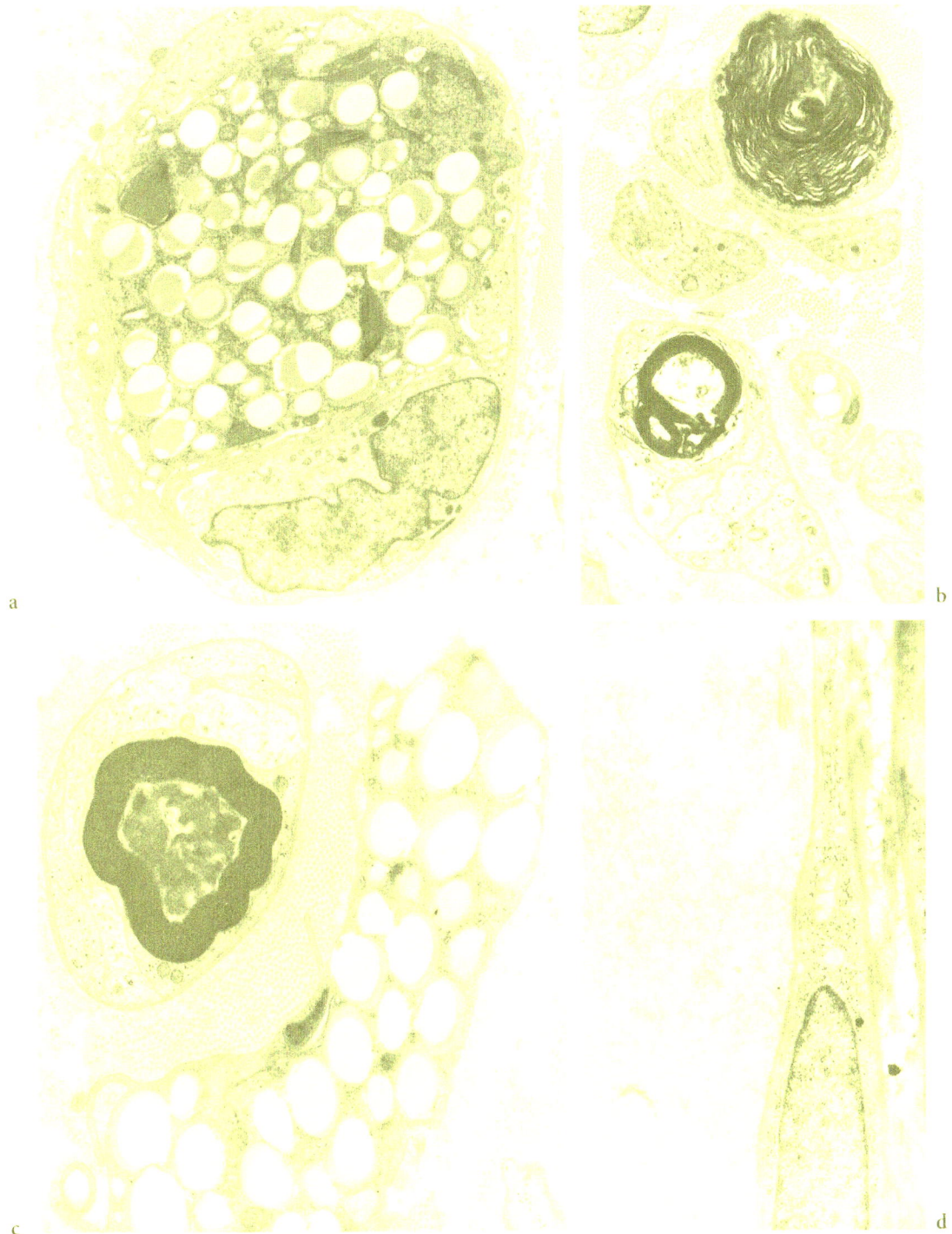

Fig. 201 a–d. Same case as in Figs. 199 and 200: sural nerve at the time of the second biopsy. **a** A lipid-laden macrophage is surrounded by Schwann cell processes and a persistent basal lamina. × 7,000. **b** Myelin degradation products are present in bands of Büngner. × 8,000. **c** A degenerated axon is surrounded by a relatively well-preserved myelin sheath lying within a band of Büngner adjacent to a macrophage. The latter is overloaded with lipid droplets which are partially eluted due to the preparative procedure. × 11,000. **d** The subperineurial space is filled with a plasma exsudate. × 12,000

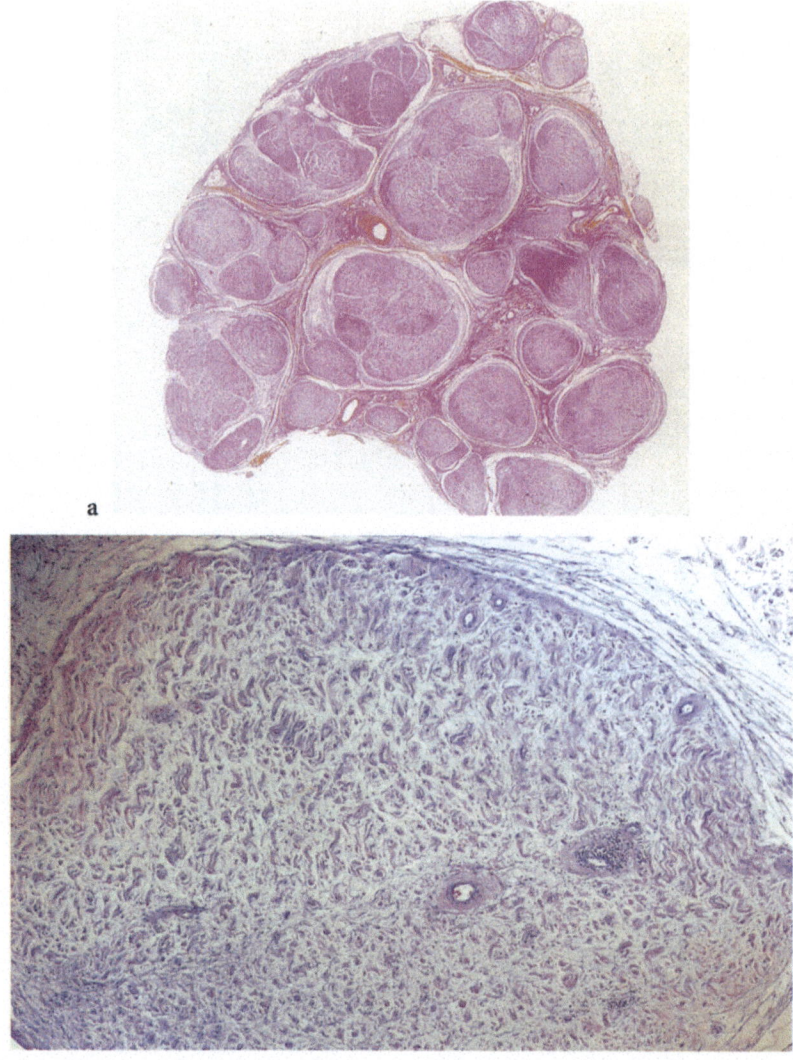

Fig. 202a–d. Axonal variant of GBS/CIDP with nearly a complete loss of nerve fibers and only a few onion bulb formations, but still apparent inflammatory cellular infiltrates in the endoneurium and epineurium of the femoral nerve from a 63-year-old man

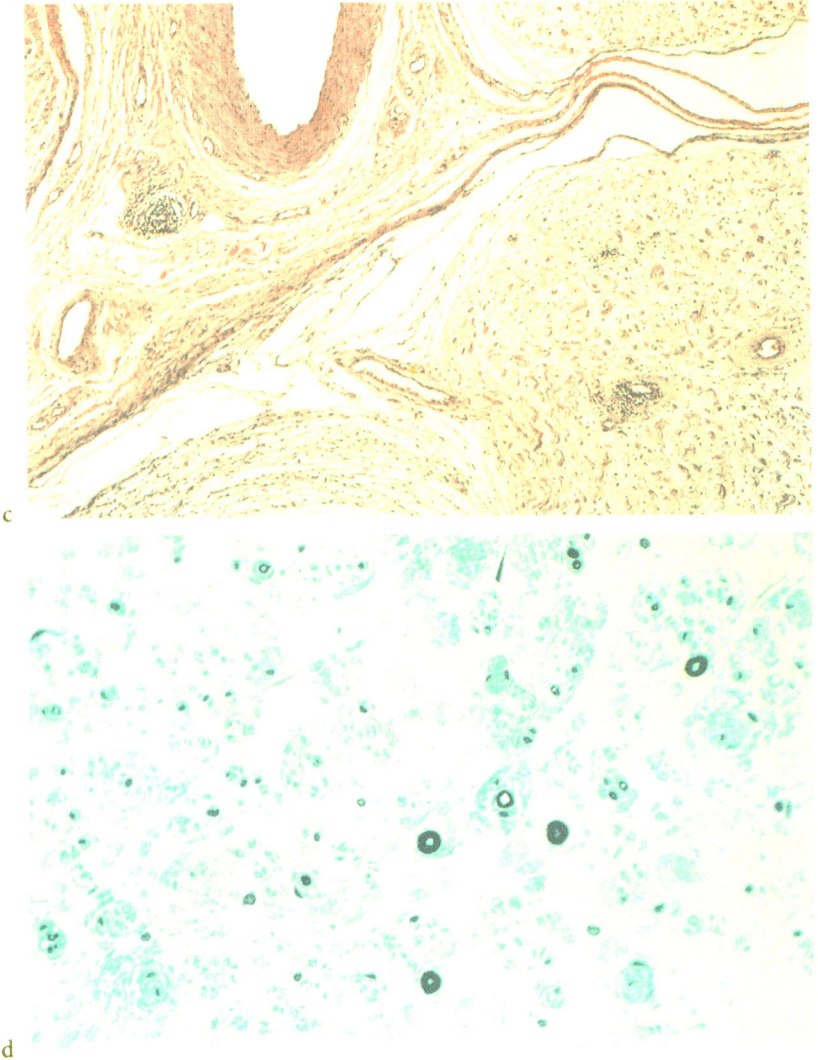

Fig. 202 c, d. Legend s. p. 234

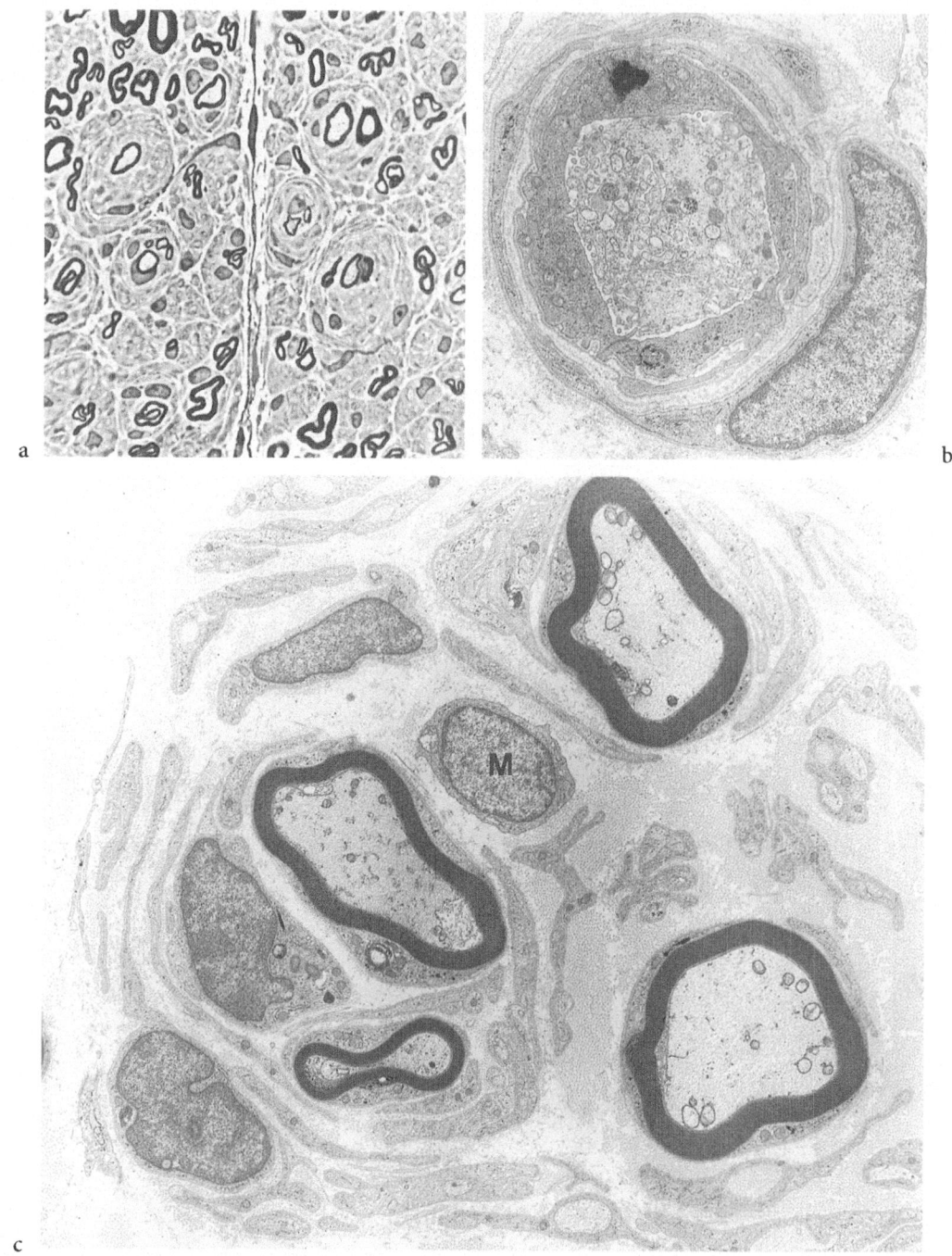

Fig. 203 a–c. Chronic inflammatory demyelinating polyneuropathy (CIDP) in a 51-year-old female. **a** There are onion bulb formations seen around several thinly myelinated nerve fibers with or without a nucleus in the section plane. Some onion bulbs include a cluster of two or more regenerated myelinated fibers indicating preceding axonal degeneration and regeneration. × 880. **b** An endoneurial blood vessel is filled with and apparently occluded by thrombocytes. × 8,600. **c** Complex group of demyelinated and remyelinated or degenerated and regenerated myelinated nerve fibers; these nerve fibers are surrounded by numerous flattened and interdigitating processes of supernumerary Schwann cells. A mononuclear cell, presumably not a resting macrophage (*M*) but a lymphocyte, is also seen. × 7,700

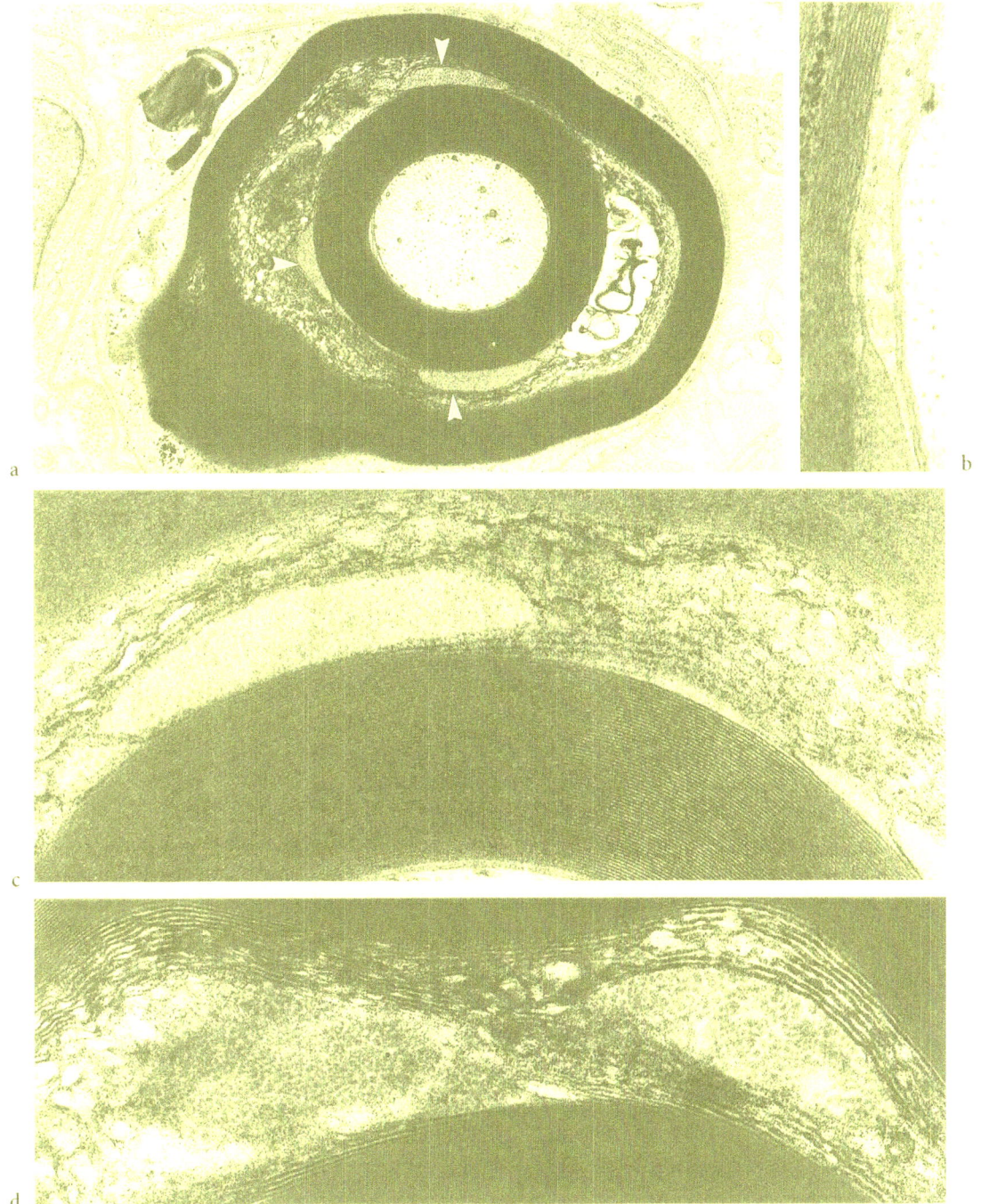

Fig. 204 a – d. Dilatation of the intraperiod lines at Schmidt-Lanterman incisures with inclusion of grossly granular structures (size of the particles approximately 5 – 25 nm) in a case with chronic inflammatory demyelinating polyneuropathy (**a, c, d**) and vasculitis (**b**). **a** Granular deposits within a Schmidt-Lanterman incisure in addition to membranous structures at different sites (*arrowheads*). × 10,400. **b** The granular structures are deposited between Schwann cell processes at the site of the intraperiod line or the mesaxon. × 60,000. **c** Higher magnification of **a**. The granular material with particles of different size is located between the major dense lines. × 44,000. **d** The granular depositions are limited by adjacent loose myelin lamellae. × 40,000. (From [980])

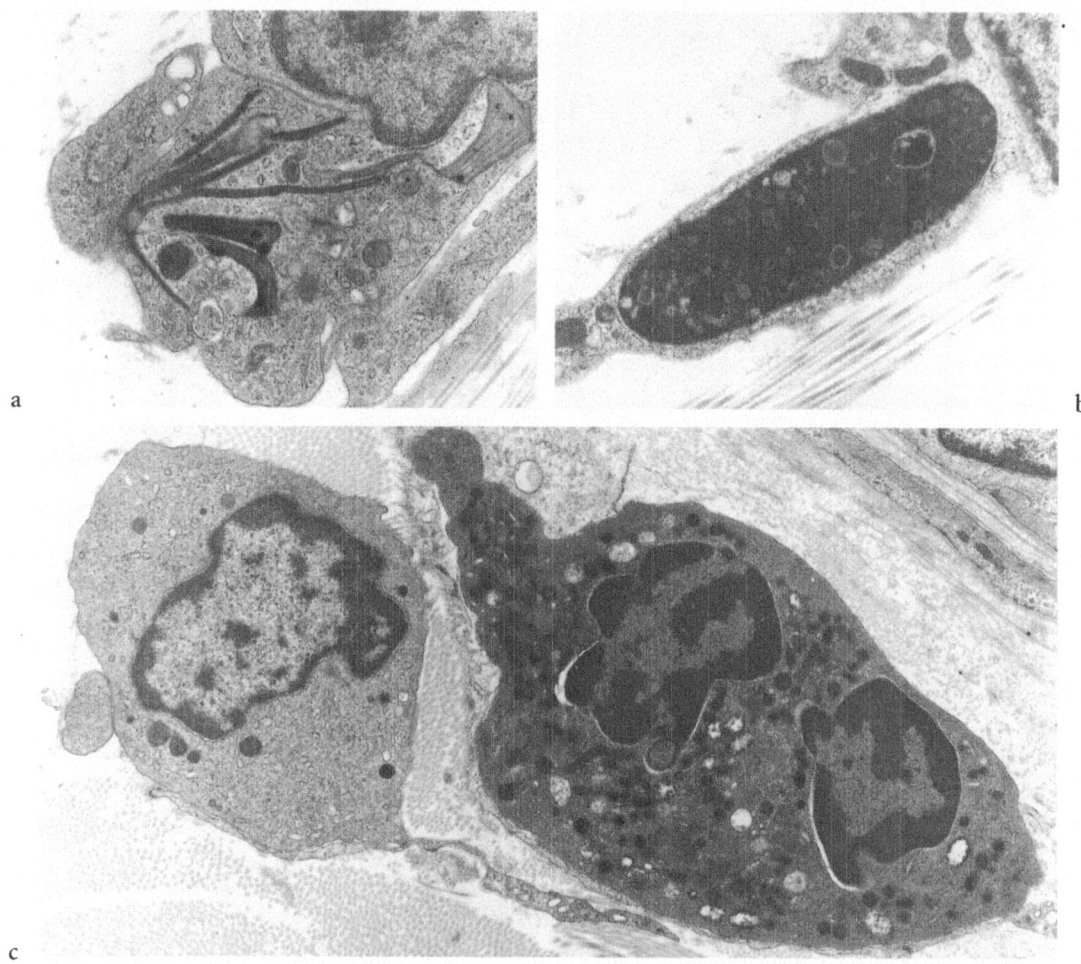

Fig. 205a–c. Chronic inflammatory demyelinating polyneuropathy in a 70-year-old female. **a** In a mononuclear cell there are lamellated bodies of different size and form. × 14,000. **b** An unusual condensed cytoplasmic inclusion in an endoneurial fibroblast; its nucleus is seen in the *upper right corner*. The cytoplasmic inclusion resembles so-called reducing bodies in reducing body myopathy. × 11,300. **c** Mononuclear cell, presumably a macrophage, in contact with an endoneurial fibroblastic process adjacent to a granulocyte close to an epineurial blood vessel. × 10,000

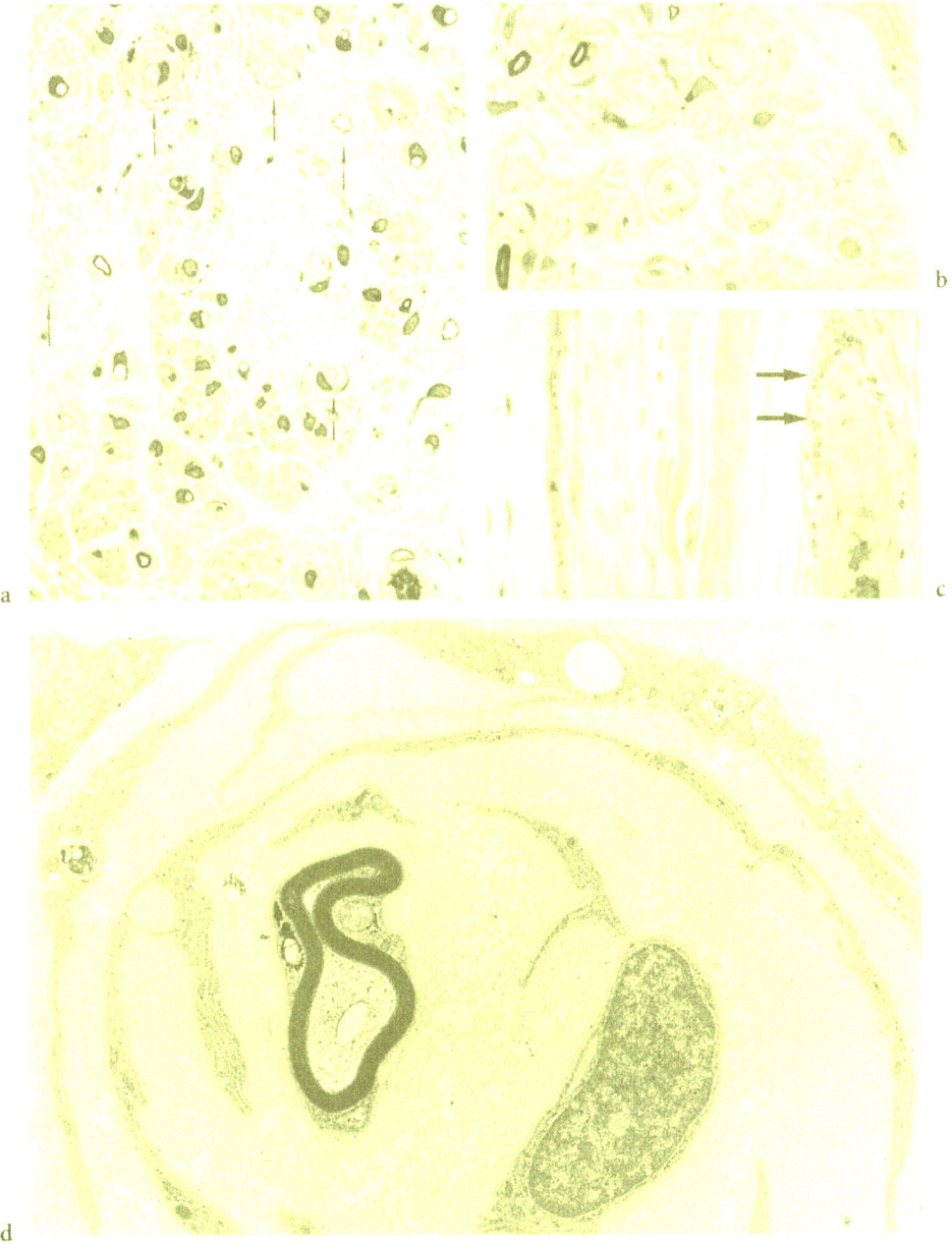

Fig. 206 a–d. Comparison between HMSN III and CIDP. **a** Hypomyelination in a 16-year-old girl with hypertrophic neuropathy of the Dejerine-Sottas type and extremely reduced NCV (2.5 m/s) (cf. Fig. 98c). There are numerous onion bulb formations around demyelinated or thinly remyelinated axons (*arrows*). The endoneurial connective tissue is increased. × 688. **b–d** Hypertrophic neuropathy in chronic recurrent polyradiculoneuritis (33-year-old female with a history of 21 years of disease). **b** Prominent onion bulb formations with or without central myelinated nerve fibers and with severely increased endoneurial connective tissue. × 896. **c** Perivascular mononuclear cellular infiltrates in the epineurium (*arrows*); the endoneurium and perineurium are seen on the *left*. × 260. **d** Onion bulb formation with multiple interdigitating, concentrically arranged flattened Schwann cell processes, which are surrounded by a common basal lamina. In its center is a thinly myelinated nerve fiber. The collagen fibrils are densely packed and increased in number (pseudohypertrophy). × 9,000. (From [958])

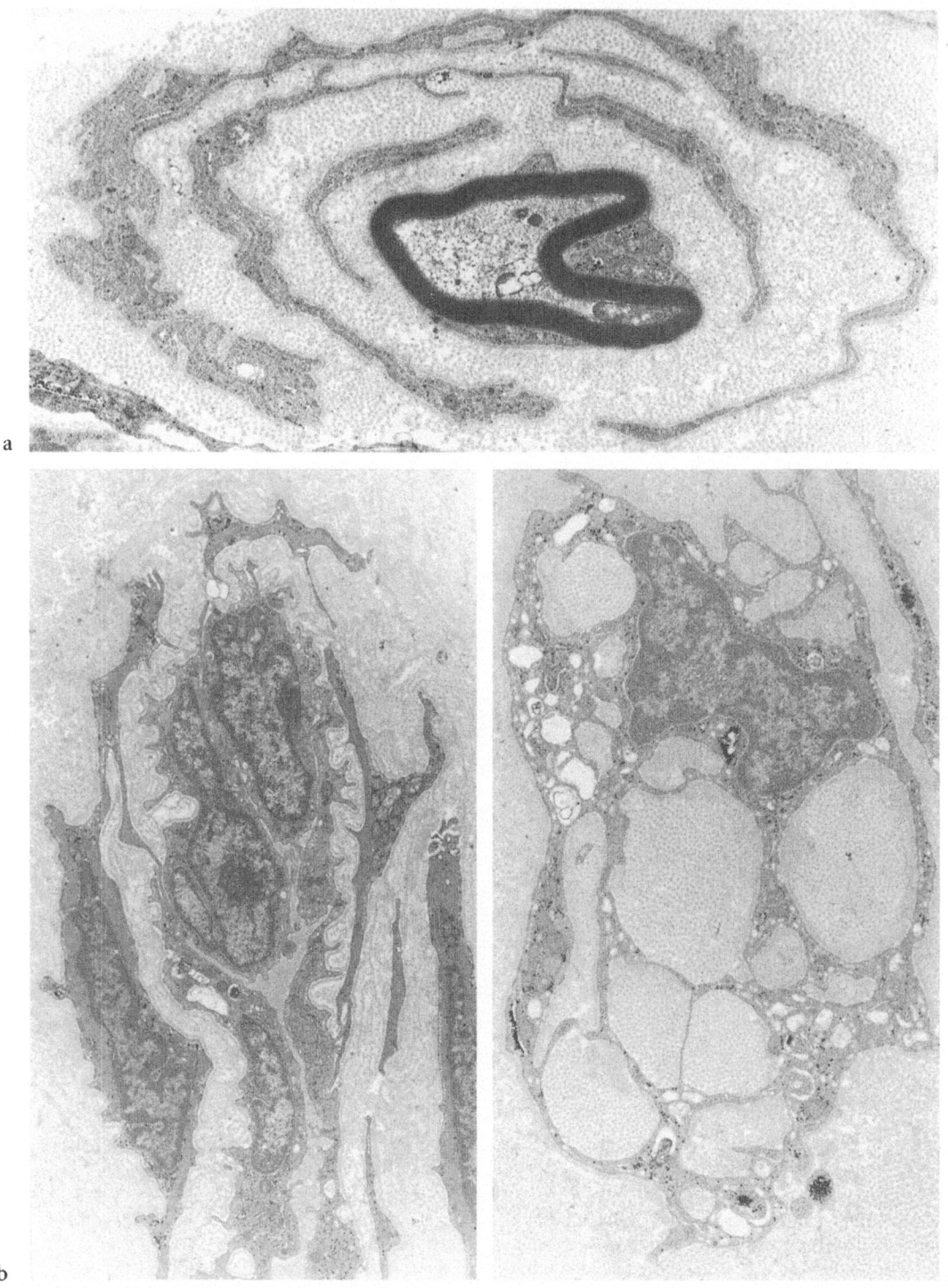

Fig. 207a – c. Same case as in Fig. 206 b – d. **a** Typical onion bulb formation with concentrically arranged Schwann cell processes. × 12,200. **b** Endoneurial blood vessel with small protrusions at the surface of the endothelial and the smooth muscle cells as a sign of intravital shrinkage. × 7,400. **c** Subperineurial cell which encloses numerous collagen fiber bundles and focally also oxytalan fibrils. It is surrounded at its surface and within the cavities by a basal lamina. It may be derived from a perineurial cell. × 12,200

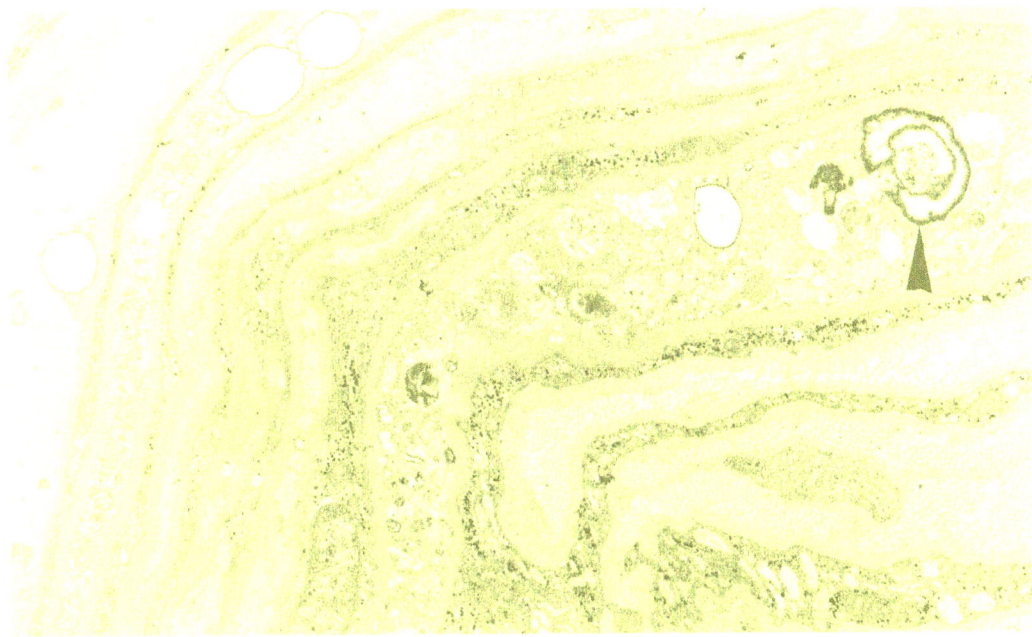

Fig. 208. Same case as in Fig. 207. Nonspecific degenerative changes in the perineurium with cellular debris, vacuoles, and calcospherites (*arrowhead*). The basal lamina is focally increased in thickness. × 13,300

Fig. 209. Major auricular nerve of a 50-year-old female with multifocal hypertrophic neuropathy due to CIDP with a history of more than 20 years of disease. Several layers of interdigitating Schwann cell processes are concentrically arranged around a small myelinated nerve fiber separated by a large number of collagen fibrils. × 13,500. (Modified from [940, 1217])

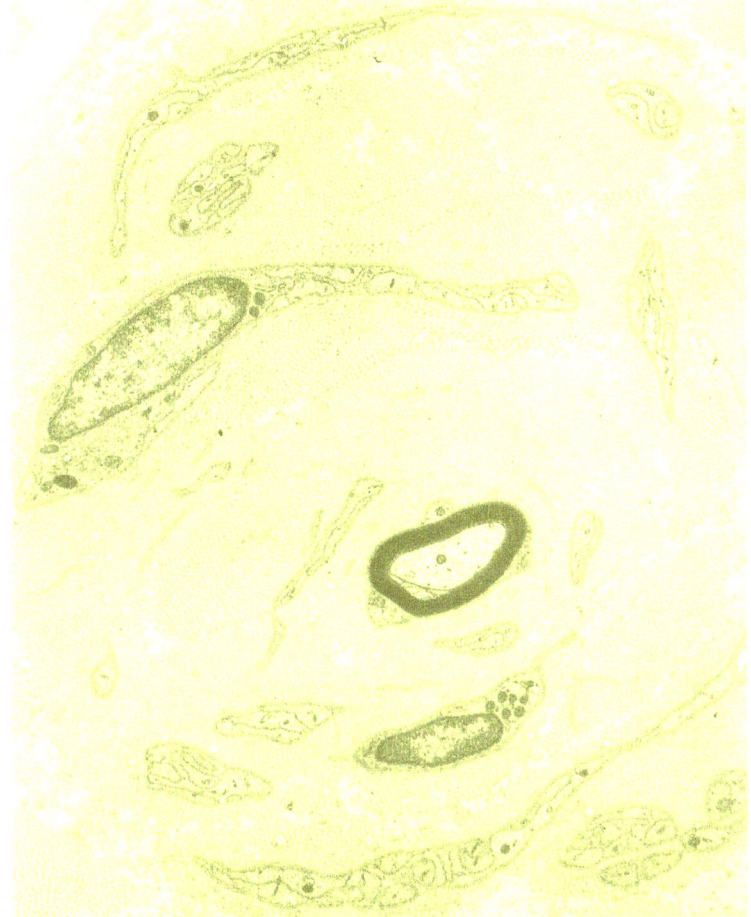

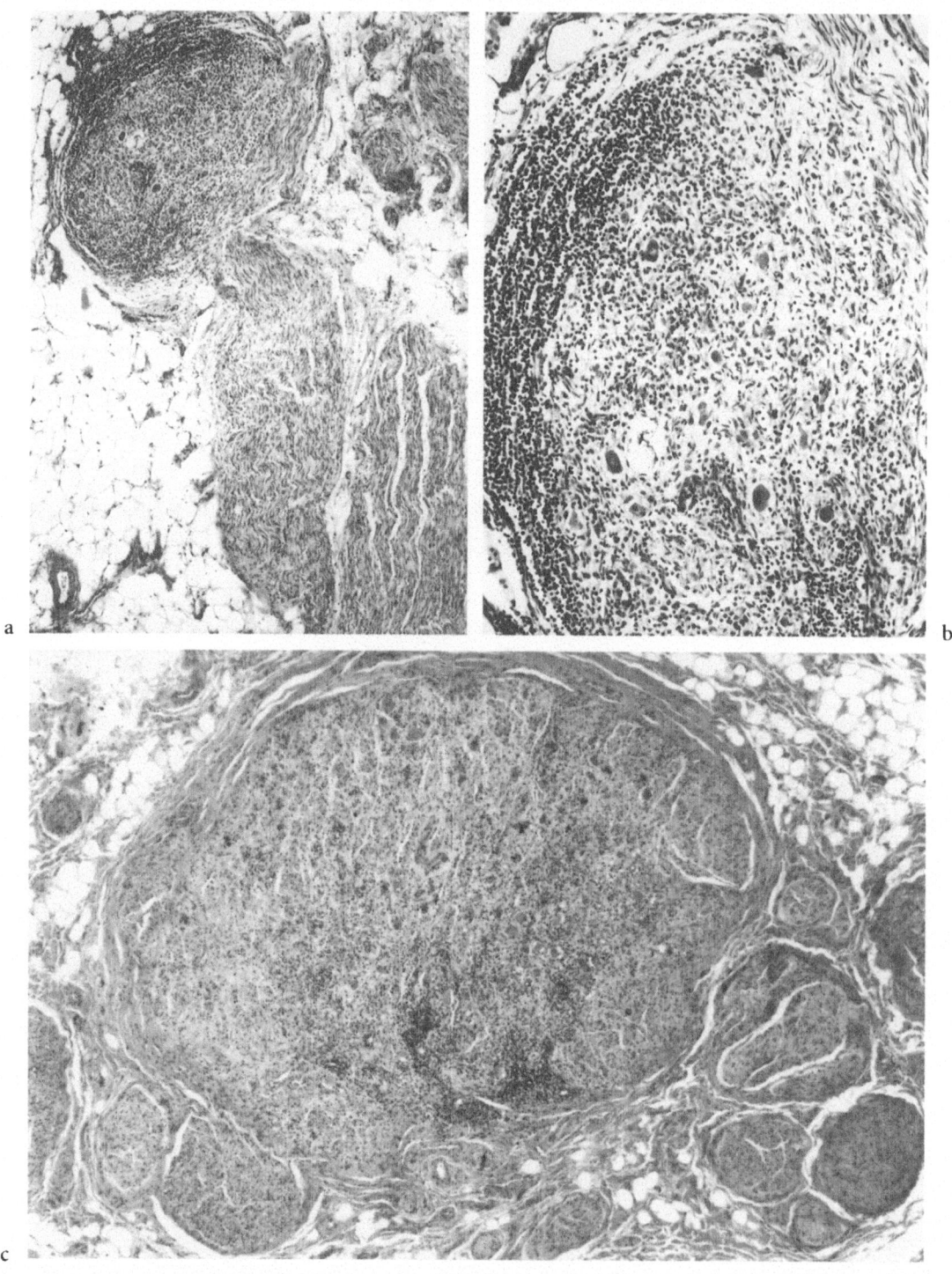

Fig. 210. a, b Spinal ganglion with extensive mononuclear cellular infiltrates focally involving the covering connective tissue in Guillain-Barré syndrome with involvement of cranial nerves (Miller-Fisher syndrome) in a 50-year-old female (autopsy case). **c** Acute dysautonomia in a 57-year-old patient. Solar plexus with mononuclear cellular infiltrates mainly in the area of the autonomous neurons, but not in the adjacent nerve fascicles. Paraffin: H & E. **a** × 62; **b** × 156; **c** × 58. (From [958])

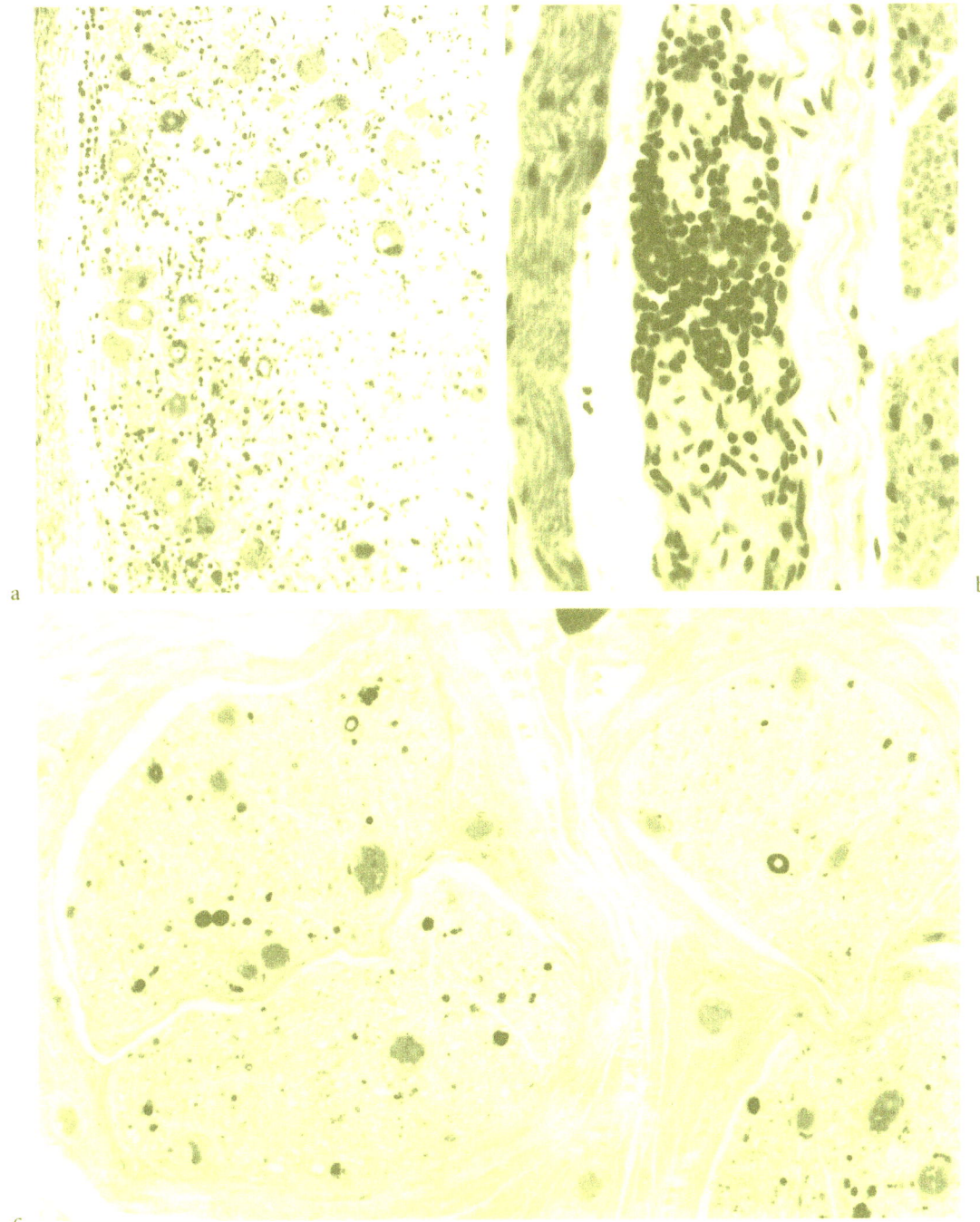

Fig. 211a–c. Same case as in Fig. 210 c. **a** Mononuclear cellular infiltrates around neurons of the solar plexus and **b** around neurons in Auerbach's plexus. **c** In the sural nerve nearly all myelinated nerve fibers are lost, indicating that the somatosensory system is also involved. Inflammatory cellular infiltrates are not found in the peripheral sensorimotor nerve fascicles studied. The inflammatory process appears to be limited to the spinal and autonomous ganglia. **a, b** Paraffin: H & E. **a** × 180; **b** × 410; **c** × 248. (From [958])

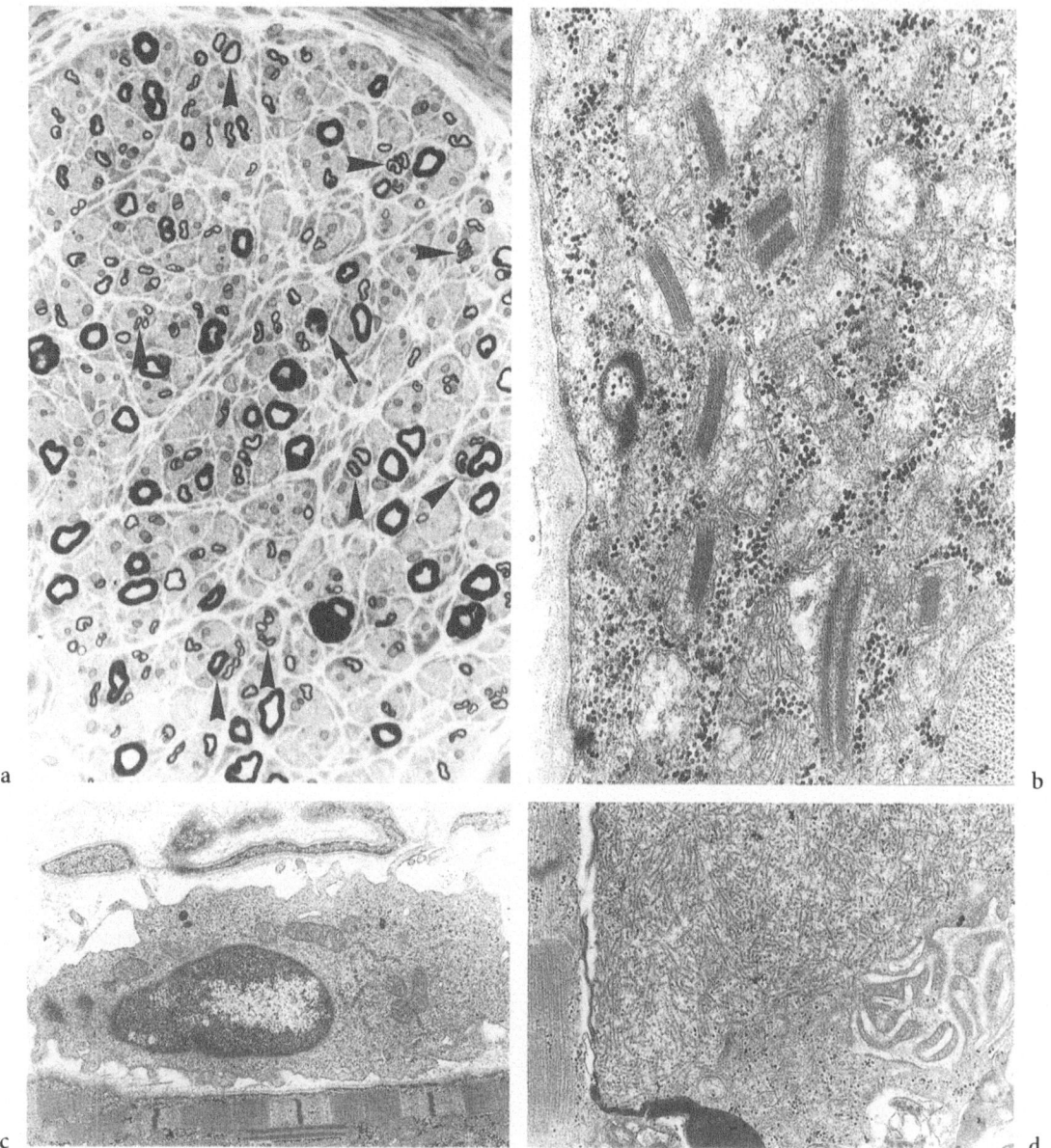

Fig. 212a–d. Prominent neuropathy in a 78-year-old female with inclusion body myositis. **a** The sural nerve shows numerical reduction of the large myelinated nerve fibers. The *arrow* indicates a myelin degradation product, the *arrowheads* indicate groups of regenerated nerve fibers. **b** In this muscle fiber there are numerous mitochondria with paracrystalline inclusions. **c** An infiltrating mononuclear cell can be seen adjacent to a muscle fiber. **d** The tubulofilamentous inclusions characteristic for inclusion body myositis are seen in a muscle fiber but were not found in peripheral nerves. **a** × 780; **b** × 37,200; **c** × 31,200; **d** × 23,000. (Modified from [991])

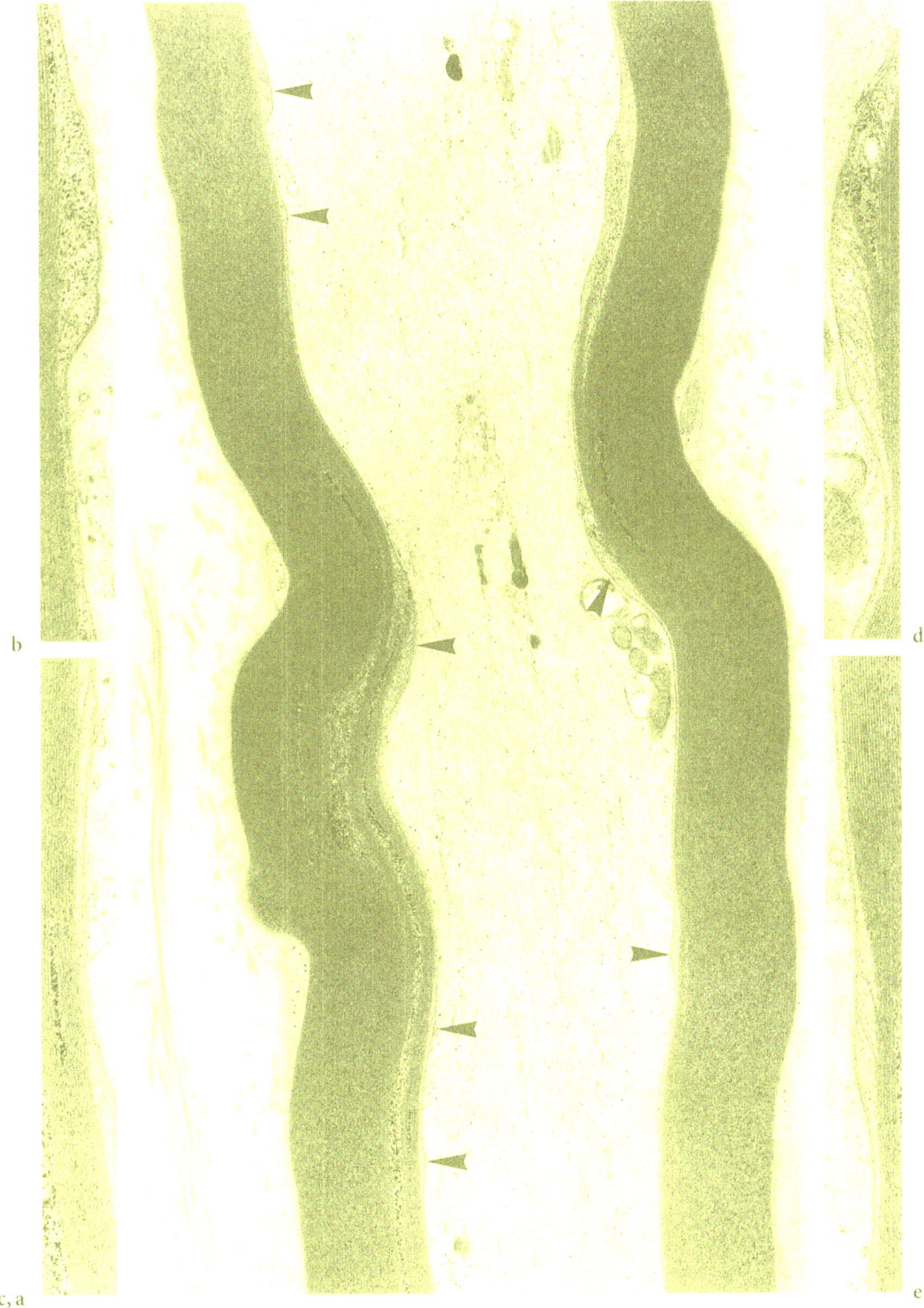

Fig. 213a–e. Peripheral neuropathy in a 38-year-old man with inclusion body myositis and lymphoma. The terminal myelin loops adhere discontinuously to different sites of the axons (*arrowheads*). Some of them are illustrated at higher magnification in parts **b–e**. Otherwise, the myelin sheath appears normally structured although the Schmidt-Lanterman incisures are somewhat unevenly distributed. **a** × 13,000; **b** × 48,500; **c, d** × 40,000; **e** × 42,000. (Modified from [966])

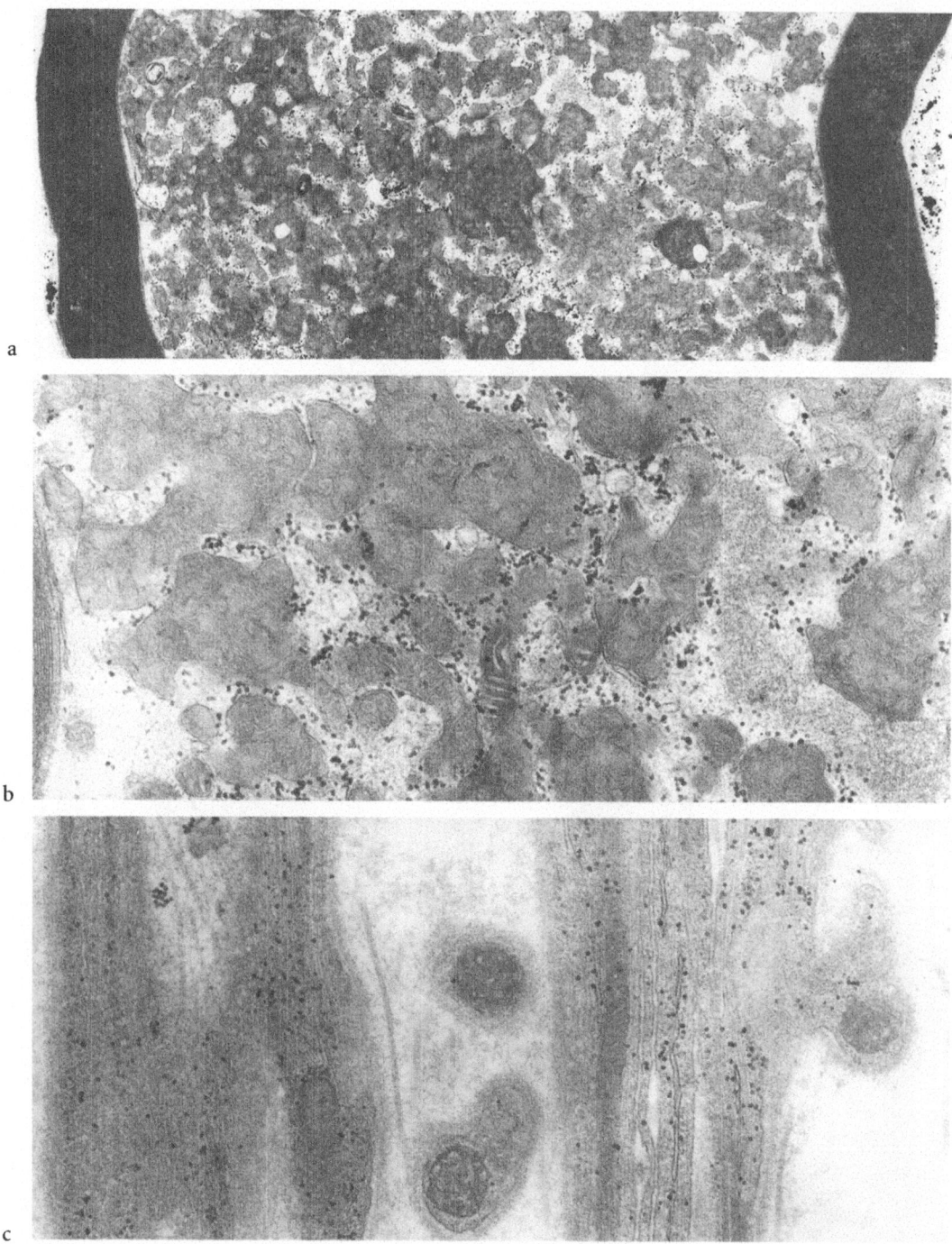

Fig. 214a–c. Unusual curvilinear axoplasmic inclusions presumably of lysosomal origin (a, b) in a 55-year-old man with polymyositis. The perineurial cells in **c** show nonspecific budlike protrusions each with a lysosome-like inclusion. **a** × 12,200; **b** × 45,500; **c** × 40,300

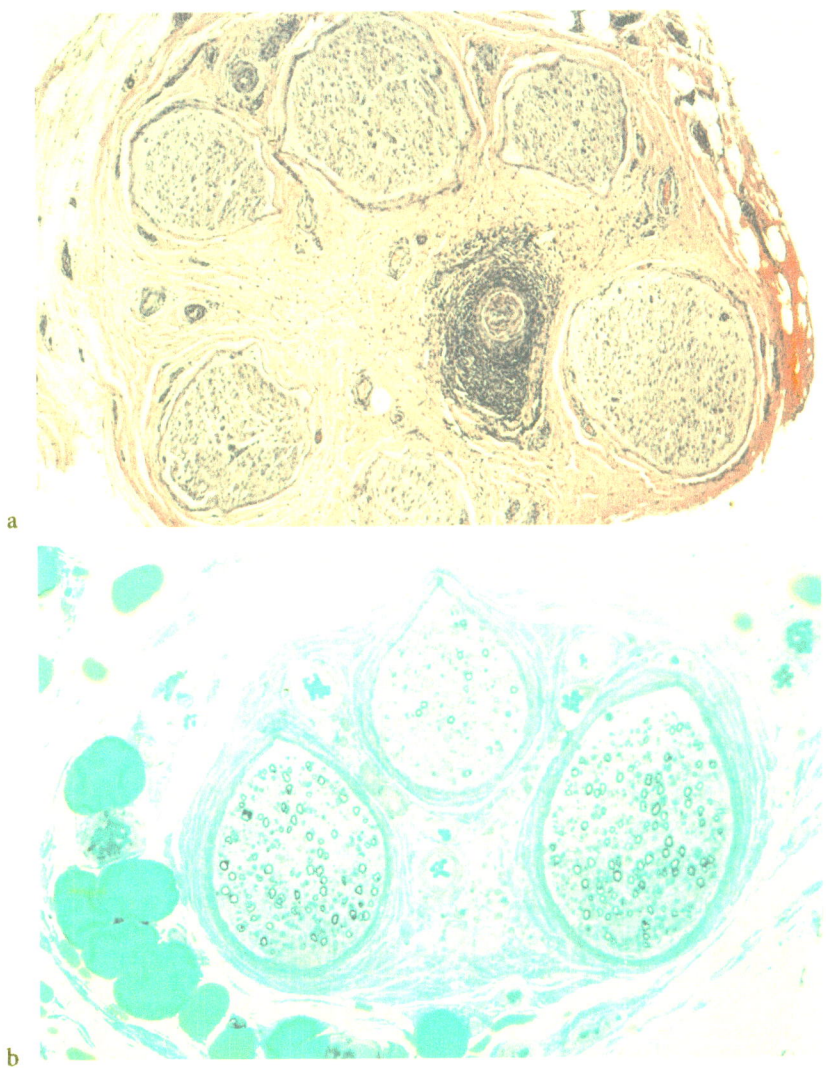

Fig. 215. a Necrotizing, obliterative vasculitis in the epineurium of the sural nerve in a 69-year-old female with lupus erythematodes. The other blood vessels in the epineurium show an increase in cellularity. The connective tissue in the epineurium is clearly increased (sclerosis of the epineurium internum). **b** The unequal loss of myelinated nerve fibers in the different fascicles indicates a multiplex type of neuropathy in a 70-year-old female with autoimmunethyreoiditis and diabetes mellitus, while there are only sparse epineurial mononuclear cell infiltrates, especially plasmacellular infiltrates associated with a clear increase of the number of epineurial capillaries. **c, d** s. p. 248

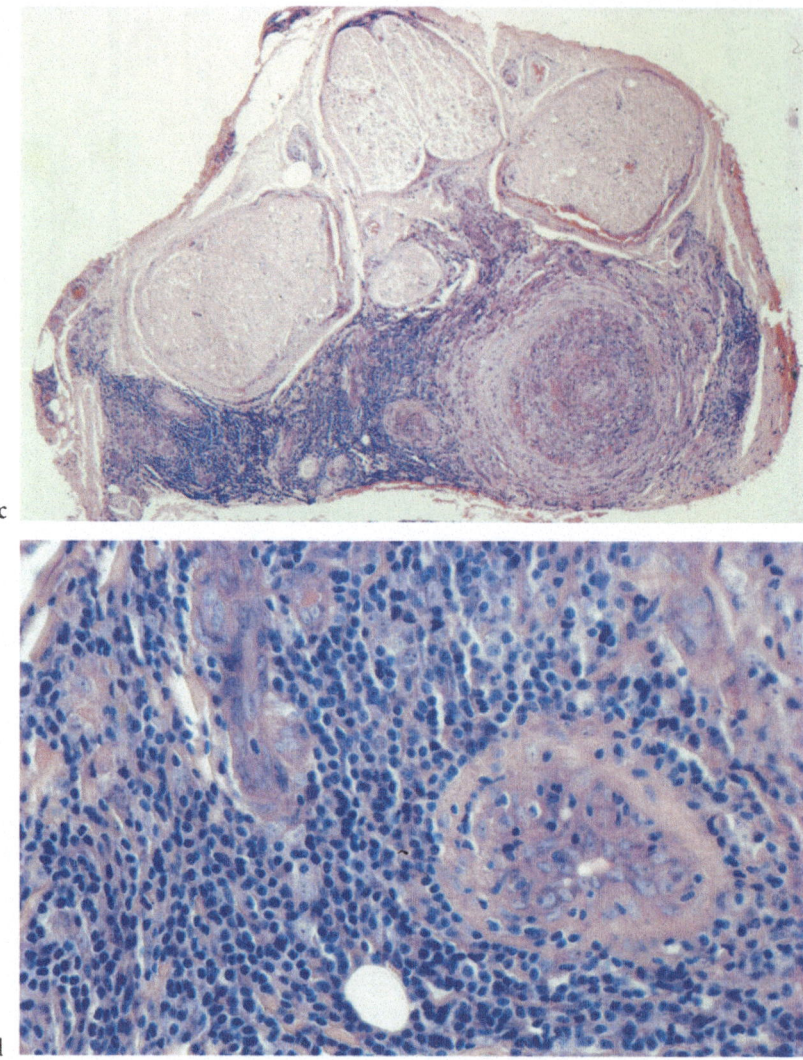

Fig. 215 *(continued).* **c** Extensive epineurial cellular infiltration in a 58-year-old man with chronic lymphatic lymphoma. This lymphoma has obviously induced a necrotizing vasculitis with obliteration of the major epineurial blood vessels. **d** Higher magnification of the infiltrating cells in **c** with obliterative endothelial cell proliferation in a small epineurial blood vessel. **c, d** Paraffin: Giemsa. (From [963])

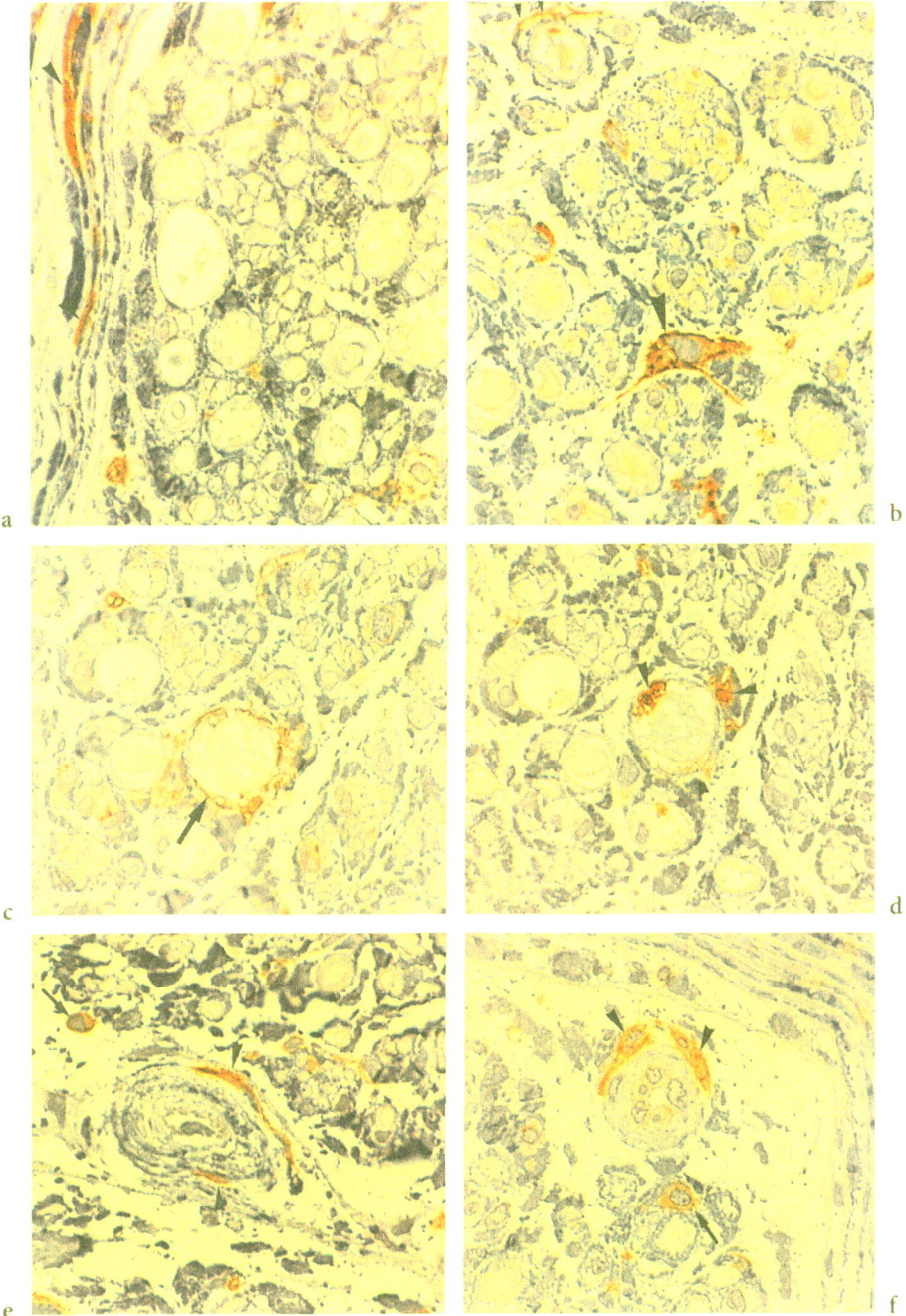

Fig. 216a–f. HLA-DR- and CD68-immunoreactive cells in vasculitis (**a, f**), panarteritis nodosa (**b**), IgG-kappa-gammopathy (**c, d**) and HMSN II (**e**). (From [1304]). **a** HLA-DR-immunoreactive perineurial cells (*arrowheads*). **b** HLA-DR-immunoreactive fibroblast (*large arrowhead*) and fibroblastic cell process immediately adjacent to a myelinated nerve fiber (*small arrowheads*). **c** HLA-DR-immunoreactive processes surrounding a degenerating nerve fiber (*arrow*). **d** Serial section stained with CD68-antibodies identifies some of the processes as belonging to a macrophage (*arrowheads*). **e** HLA-DR-immunoreactive fibroblastic processes surround a blood vessel (*arrowheads*). A separate, clearly stained cell is indicated by an *arrow*. **f** HLA-DR-immunoreactive fibroblasts adjacent to a blood vessel (*arrowheads*) and other mononuclear cells in the area (*arrow*) are labeled in this 61-year-old patient with vasculitis. **a–f** × 600

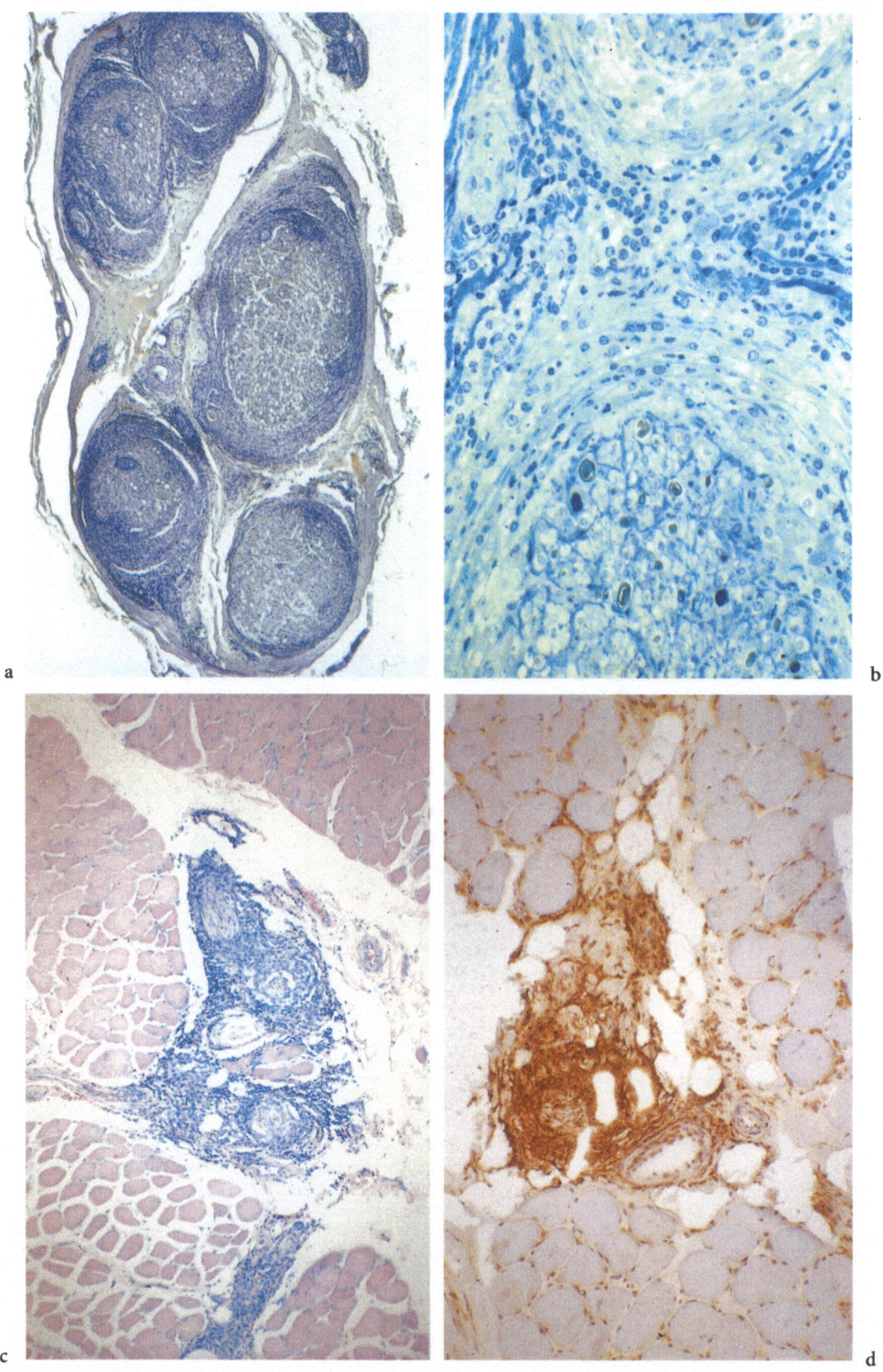

Fig. 217. Legend s. p. 251

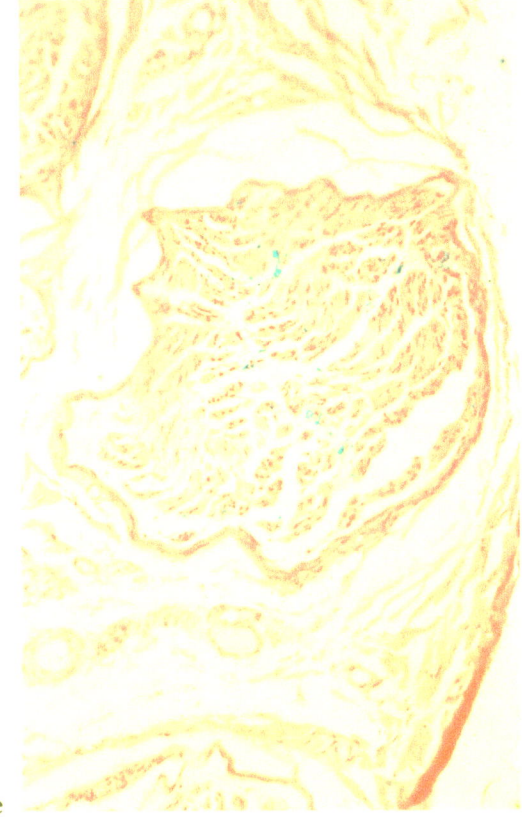

e

Fig. 217. a, b, d, e Severe perineuritis in a 29-year-old man. **a** Infiltration and thickening of the perineurium around several nerve fascicles in a sural nerve. Antibody reaction against interleukin 6 (1:100). **b** Semithin section, stained with toluidine blue, showing infiltration of the perineurium and loss of numerous myelinated nerve fibers in the endoneurium. **c** Intramuscular nerve fascicle with severe perineuritis. Giemsa stain. **d** T-cell reaction. **e** Perivascular hemosiderin deposits in the endoneurium of the sural nerve in a 42-year-old female with Sharp syndrome. (From [963])

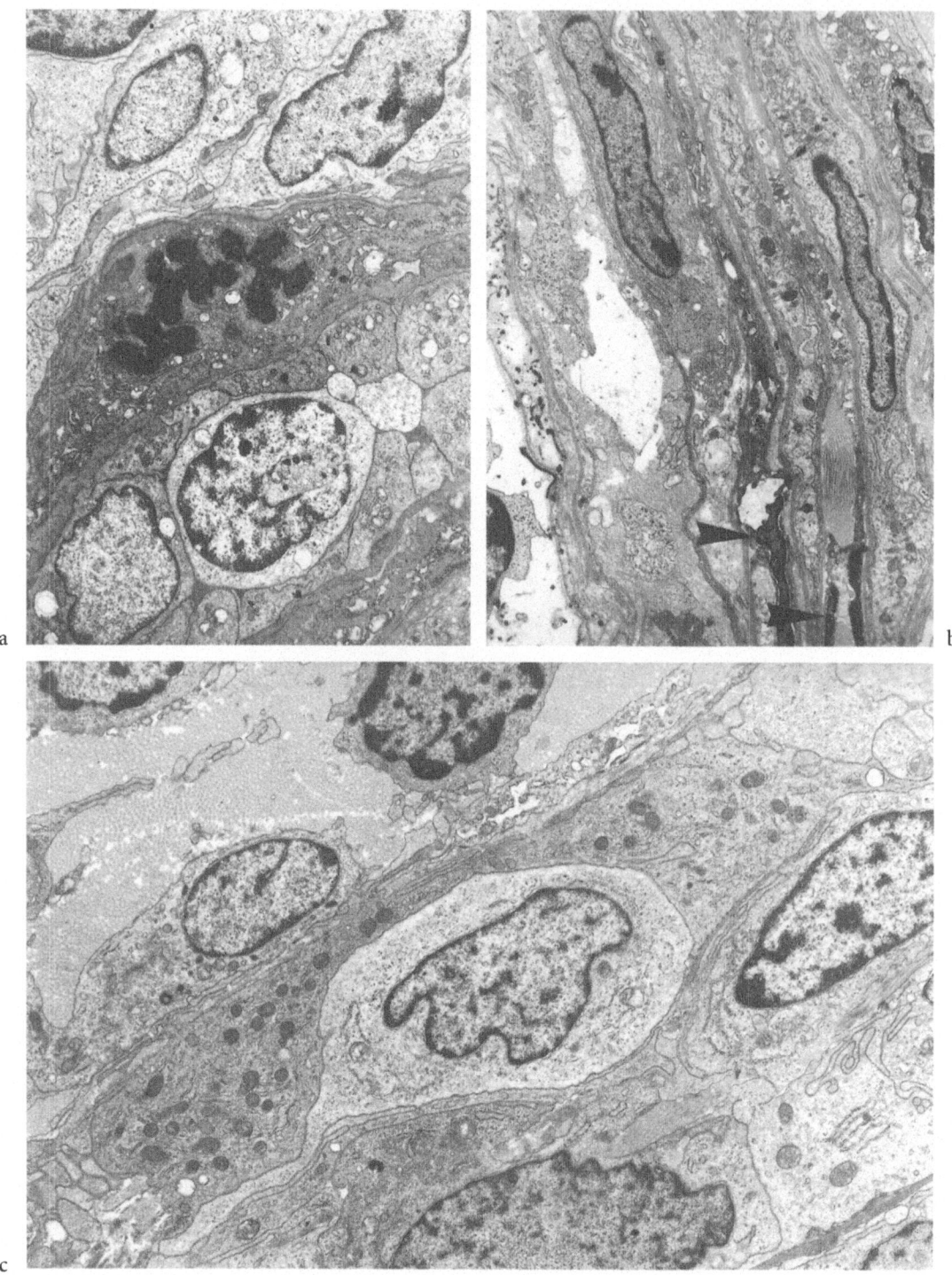

Fig. 218 a–c. Same case as in Fig. 217 a–d. **a** Among the cellular infiltrates in the perineurium one cell is seen in mitosis. × 6,700. **b** The architecture of the perineurium is disturbed. An infiltrating cell can be seen at the *lower left*. Degenerating cells are pycnotic and indicated by *arrowheads*. Some cell processes are vacuolated. × 4,900. **c** Dense mononuclear cell infiltrate at the border to the epineurium which is also infiltrated by cells. × 6,700

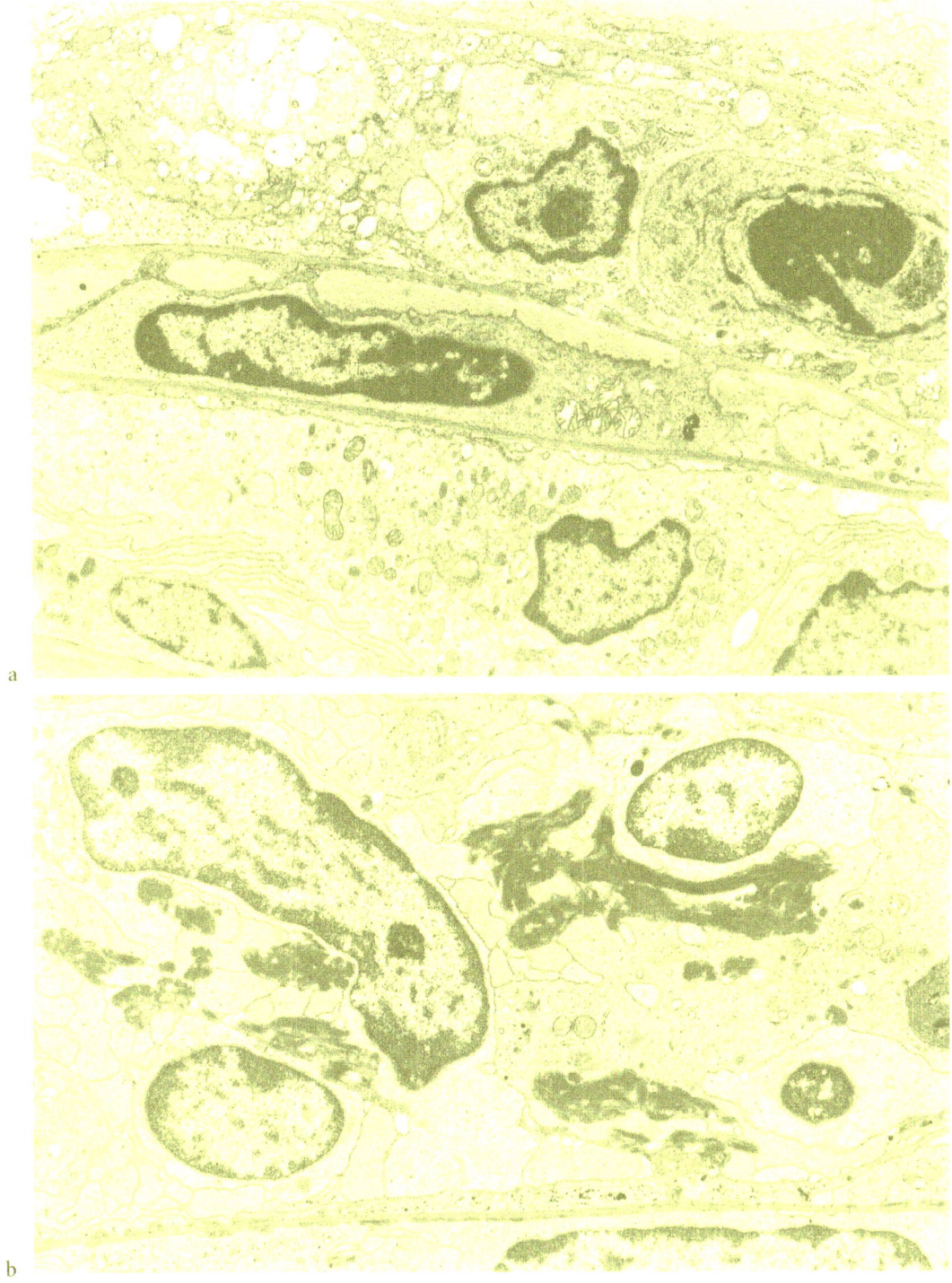

Fig. 219 a, b. Same case as in Fig. 218. **a** Infiltrating cells with or without regressive changes can be seen between the preserved basal laminae of the perineurial cells. Below is a cell with multiple interdigitating processes which presumably represents an unusual macrophage. **b** Fibrin precipitates between the infiltrating cells in the epineurium. **a, b** × 7,100

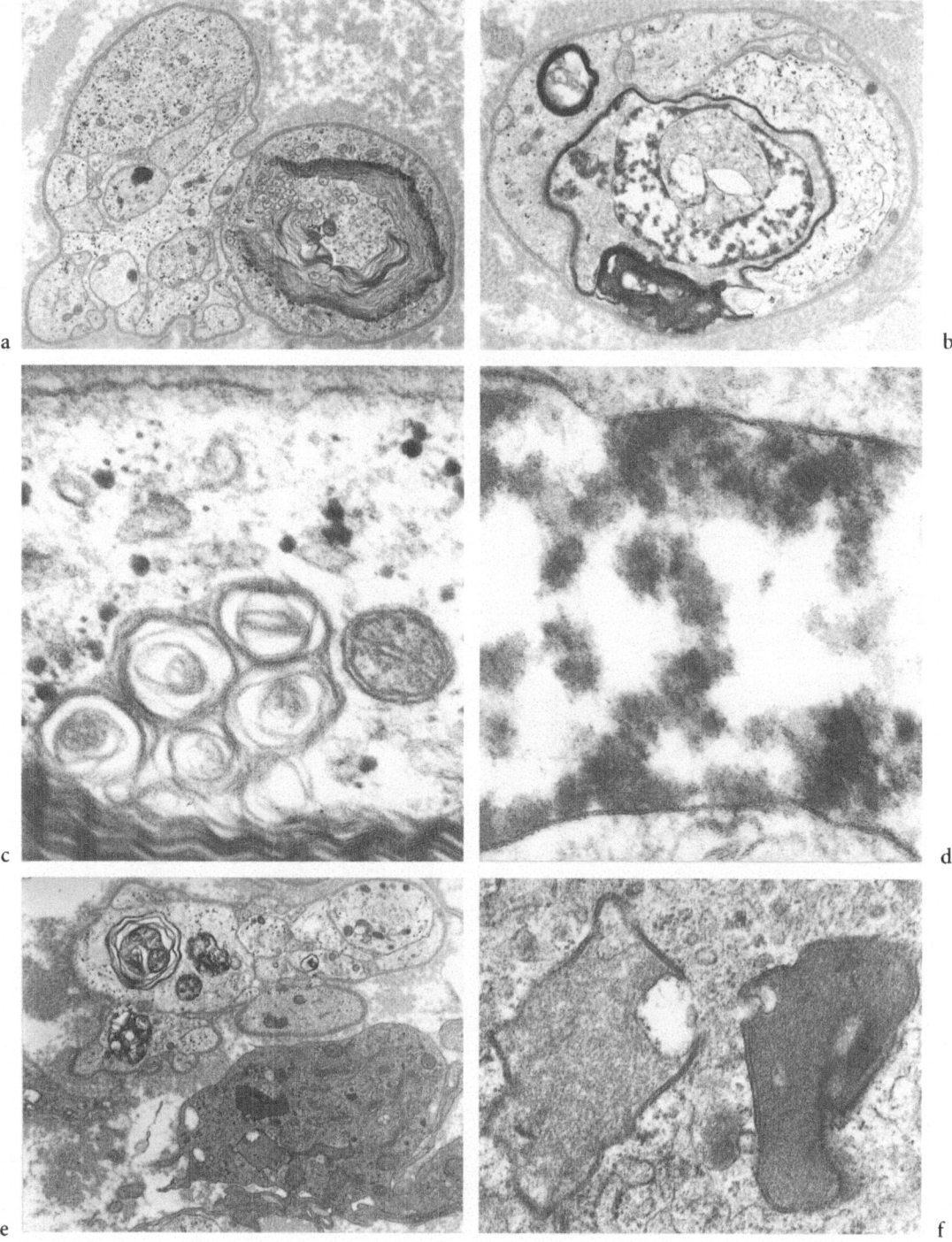

Fig. 220a–f. Unusual aspects in the same case as in Fig. 219. **a** Büngner-band with advanced myelin degradation. The ring-like lamellated structures at the site of the destructed myelin lamellae are illustrated in **c** at higher magnification. × 7,500. **b** Myelin sheath degradation in a band of Büngner with unusual osmiophilic floccular precipitates which are limited by a membrane and shown at higher magnification in **d**. **b** × 10,600; **c** × 103,000; **d** × 95,000. **e** Bands of Büngner with advanced myelin degradation and an adjacent macrophage. The unusual cytosomes therein are shown at higher magnification in **f**. **e** × 7,700; **f** × 42,000

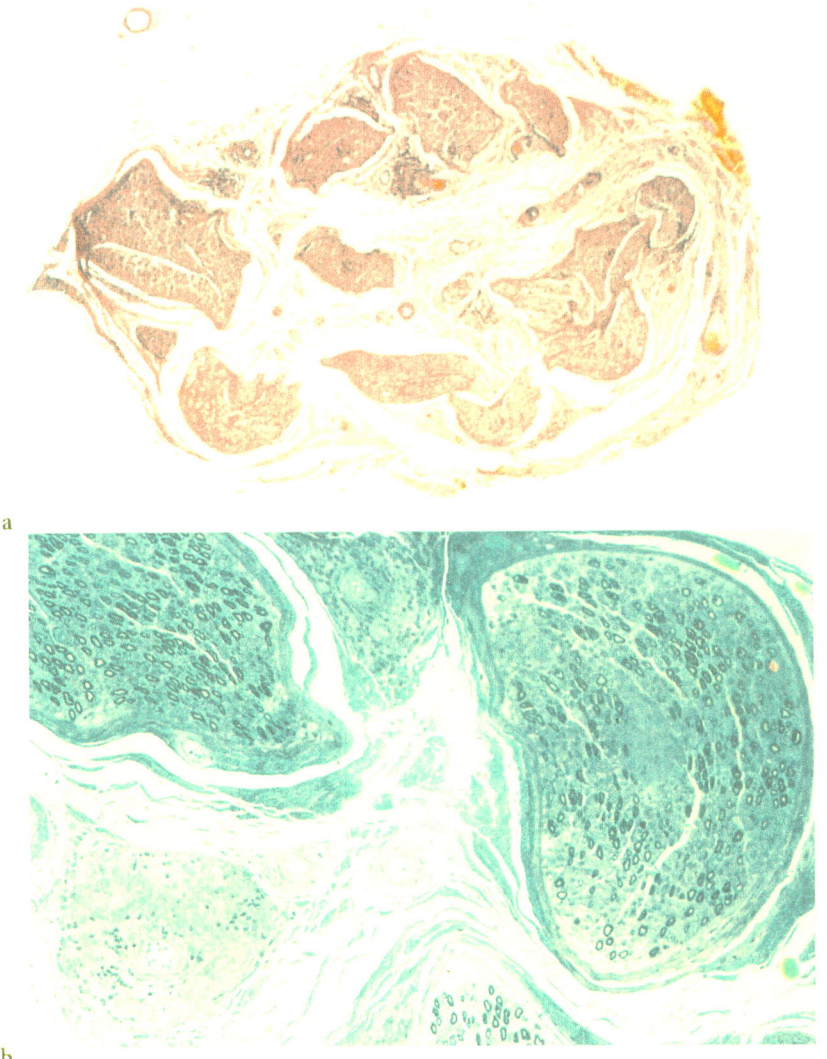

a

b

Fig. 221a, b. Severe neuropathy in neurosarcoidosis (Boeck's disease) in a 51-year-old female

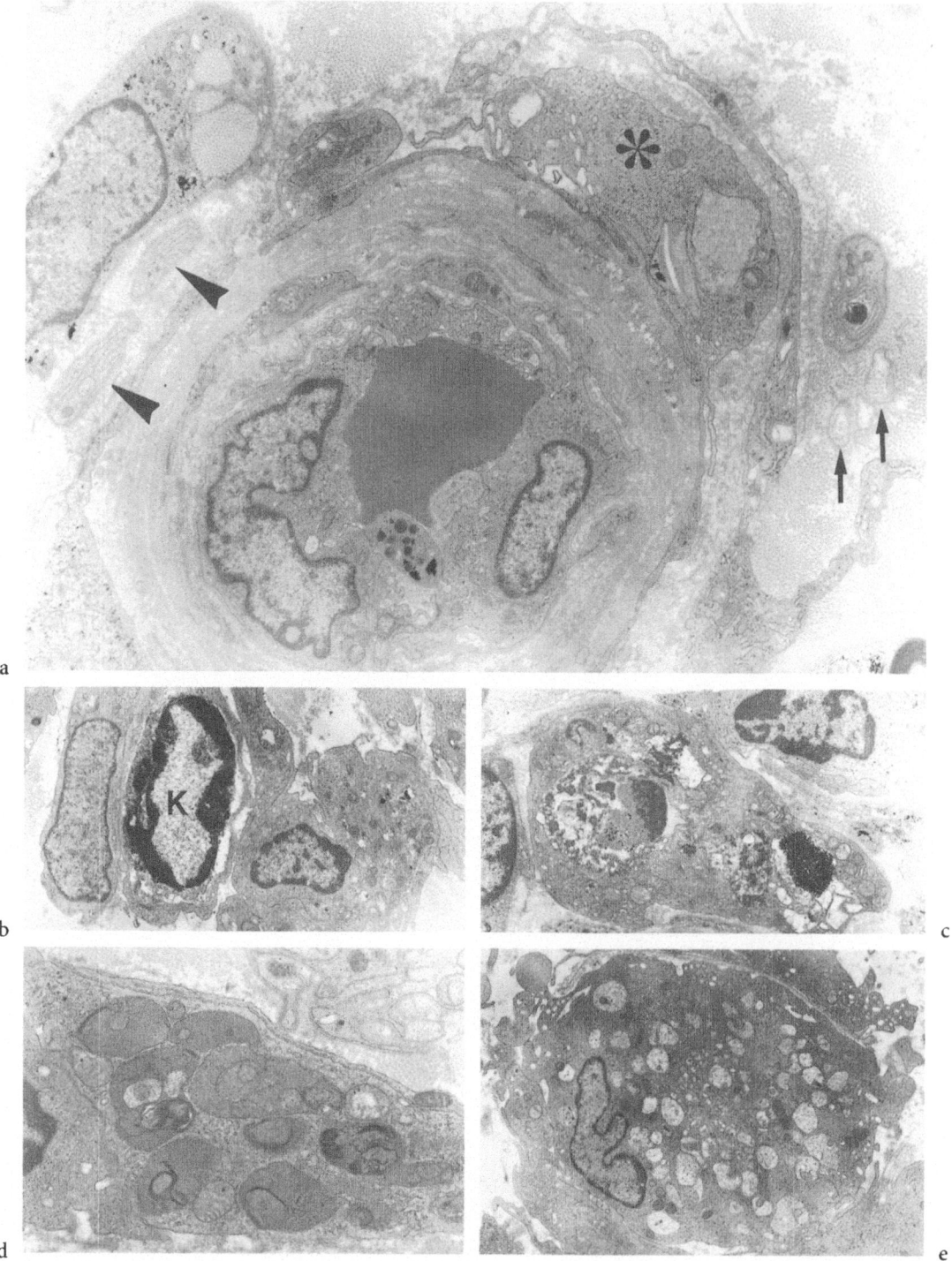

Fig. 222 a–e. Same case as in Fig. 221. **a** Abnormal cells surround a reactively altered endoneurial blood vessel; its basal lamina is increased in number as well as in thickness. The cell with abnormal polygonal inclusions is indicated by an *asterisk*. One of these inclusions shows a small cleft. The cell in the *upper left* encloses three bundles of collagen fibrils and is surrounded by a basal lamina, beside the perineurium, so that it can tentatively be identified as a Schwann cell. Adjacent, lies a group of Schwann cell processes (*arrowheads*). Empty basal laminae are also present in this area (*arrows*). × 8,300. **b** Closely apposed epitheloid cells may show regular cell organelles, but also one apoptotic cell (*K*). × 4,900. **c** Degenerating epitheloid cell with various degradation products which are of uneven osmiophilia and are surrounded by vacuoles. × 5,400. **d** Cytoplasmic inclusions in an epitheloid cell resembling those in **a**. These lysosome-like inclusions are membrane-bound showing different lamellar and vacuolar components. The matrix appears mainly homogeneous. × 12.000. **e** Epitheloid cell with numerous, largely uniform vacuoles of uneven size and a nucleus with cytoplasmic invaginations and irregular superficial protrusions in an obviously condensed cytoplasm. × 4,900

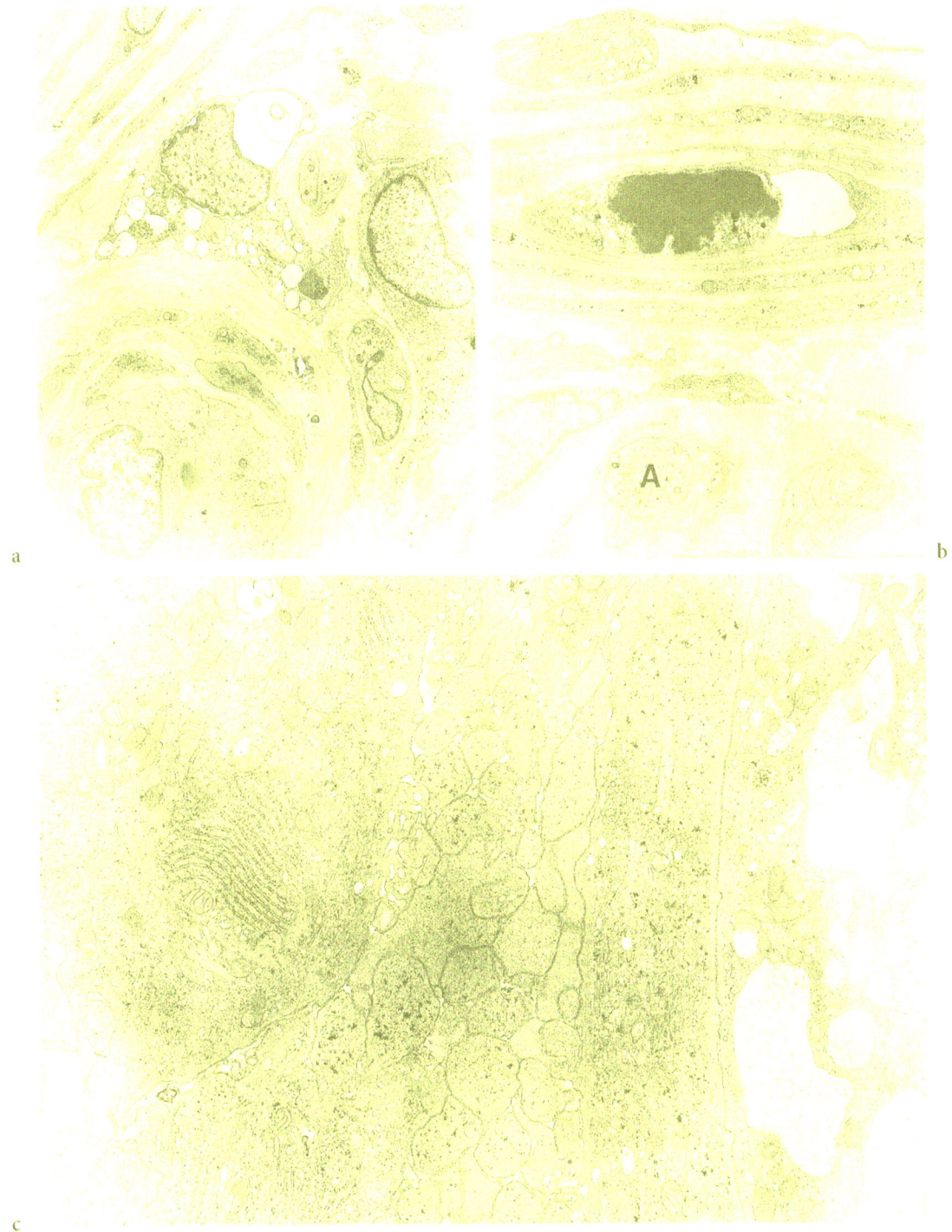

Fig. 223a–c. Same case as in Figs. 221 and 222. **a** Increased number of perivascular basal laminae with an adjacent macrophage which contains multiple vacuoles, one of which is caused by dilatation of the outer nuclear membrane. Some empty Schwann cell processes and perineurial cells are also apparent. × 5,400. **b** Degenerating cell with a homogeneous inclusion and an electron optically empty vacuole within the perineurium. In the endoneurium a dystrophic enlarged unmyelinated axon is indicated by *A*. × 8,300. **c** Multiple closely packed cell processes between unusual cells showing a prominent ergastoplasma. Another cell includes numerous of vacuoles which are filled with finely floccular substances. × 9,000

CHAPTER 12

Paraneoplastic Syndromes

Paraneoplastic neuropathies may occur in association with carcinomas, especially:

- *Small cell carcinomas of the lung* (Fig. 224a–d) or other carcinomas (Figs. 18, 19, 225a–d) [17, 20, 241, 266, 312, 366–368, 438, 689, 772, 851, 1180, 1207], which many also cause *Lambert-Eaton syndrome* [180, 242, 406, 1114].
- *Lymphoreticular diseases, especially lymphomas* (Fig. 227a–c) [243, 324, 443, 536, 549, 591, 1193, 1207], *lymphatic leukemia* (Fig. 215c, d) [1124], and *myeloma (plasmocytoma)* (Figs. 17a, 228a–d), which should be distinguished from direct infiltration of the peripheral nervous system by neoplasmic carcinomatous or lymphoid cells (Figs. 215c, d, 226a–d).
- A syndrome with polyneuropathy, organomegaly, endocrinopathy in association with increased monoclonal (M)-protein, and skin lesions, called *POEMS* [723], or *Crow-Fukase syndrome* (polyneuropathy, anasarka, pigmentation, endocrinopathy, dysglobulinemia, and organomegaly) [905, 1155, 1192].
- *Thymoma* [319].
- *Polycythemia* [1263].
- Further neuropathies associated with *dysproteinemias* (disturbances of the quantitative composition of immunoglobulins in blood plasma) and *paraproteinemias* (disturbances of the qualitative composition) (Figs. 229–235) [1165] may occur in *B-cell lymphomas* and *plasmocytomas* or Waldenström's disease [1187].
  - If not (yet) associated with lymphoma or plasmocytoma these types of dysglobulinemia are designated as *benign monoclonal gammopathies of unknown significance (MGUS)* (Fig. 24c–e, 234, 235) [181, 182, 237, 489, 498, 514, 579, 696, 1039, 1050, 1094, 1166, 1184].

- Most frequently, *IgM antibodies* are involved in causing neuropathy (Figs. 229–230)[40, 92, 113, 181, 359, 404, 457, 460, 489, 498, 554, 557, 578, 615, 660, 662, 667, 678, 692, 725, 748, 749, 823, 851, 867, 871, 907, 916, 1036, 1053, 1067, 1079, 1080, 1094, 1104, 1123, 1165, 1185, 1187, 1189, 1267, 1272].
- *IgG* gammopathy (Fig. 231a–d) is the next disease, in terms of frequency, to be considered as a cause of dysglobulinemic neuropathy [409, 530, 555, 734, 768, 789, 1065, 1094, 1173, 1273, 1275].
- *IgA* is less frequently involved (Figs. 233a–c) [735, 1039].

Immunoglobulin titers may be raised without significant correlation to the development of a neuropathy [223, 1079, 1165, 1198, 1238]. Lymphocytes and plasma cells in the nerve may play an additional role in the pathogenesis of neuropathy [1065]. They may occur as isolated subperineurial or perivascular cells. Mast cells tend to be increased in numbers in all cases of immunological disorders in the peripheral nervous system, particularly vasculitis (Fig. 236).

Plasmocytomas can induce *amyloidosis* of the light chain type (AL type; see above) (Figs. 24a, 124–126; 128a–c, 238f) [558, 928].

Essential and secondary cryoglobulinemias (Figs. 17h, 237, 240b, 245c) may also cause peripheral neuropathies [145, 505, 528, 599, 666, 1123, 1191], some of which are characterized by immunotactoid precipitates in the wall or the lumen of blood vessels [696, 851].

Myelomonoblastic leukemia may also be associated with neuropathy showing leukemic cells in the endoneurium [1188].

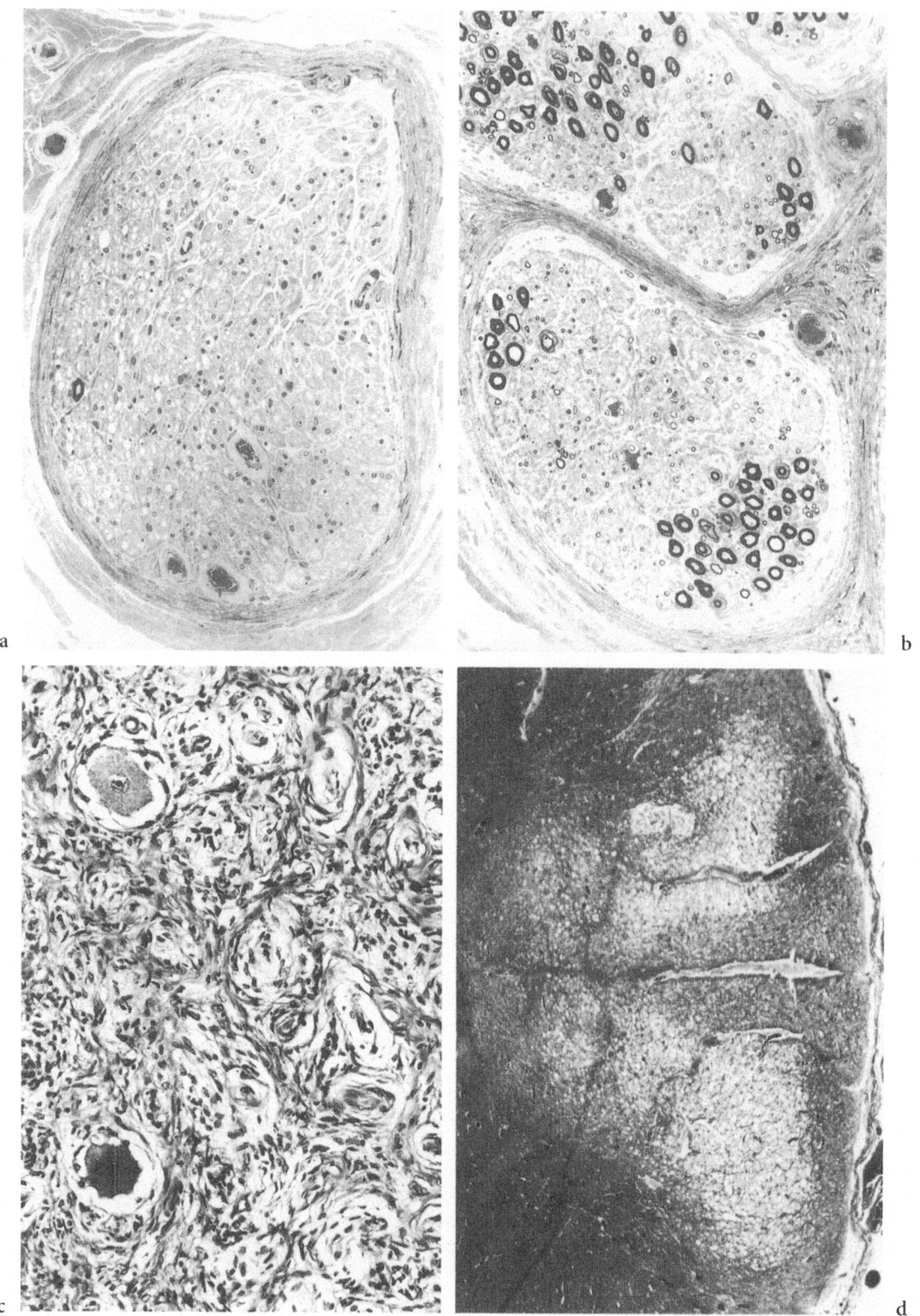

Fig. 224a–d. Paraneoplastic neuropathy in bronchial carcinoma with loss mainly of the sensory nerve fibers in the sural nerve (**a**), loss of numerous spinal ganglia neurons (**c**) and degeneration of the posterior tracts in the spinal cord (**d**), but better preservation of the presumably motor nerve fibers in the sciatic nerve (**b**). **a–c** × 215; **d** × 30. (From [1207])

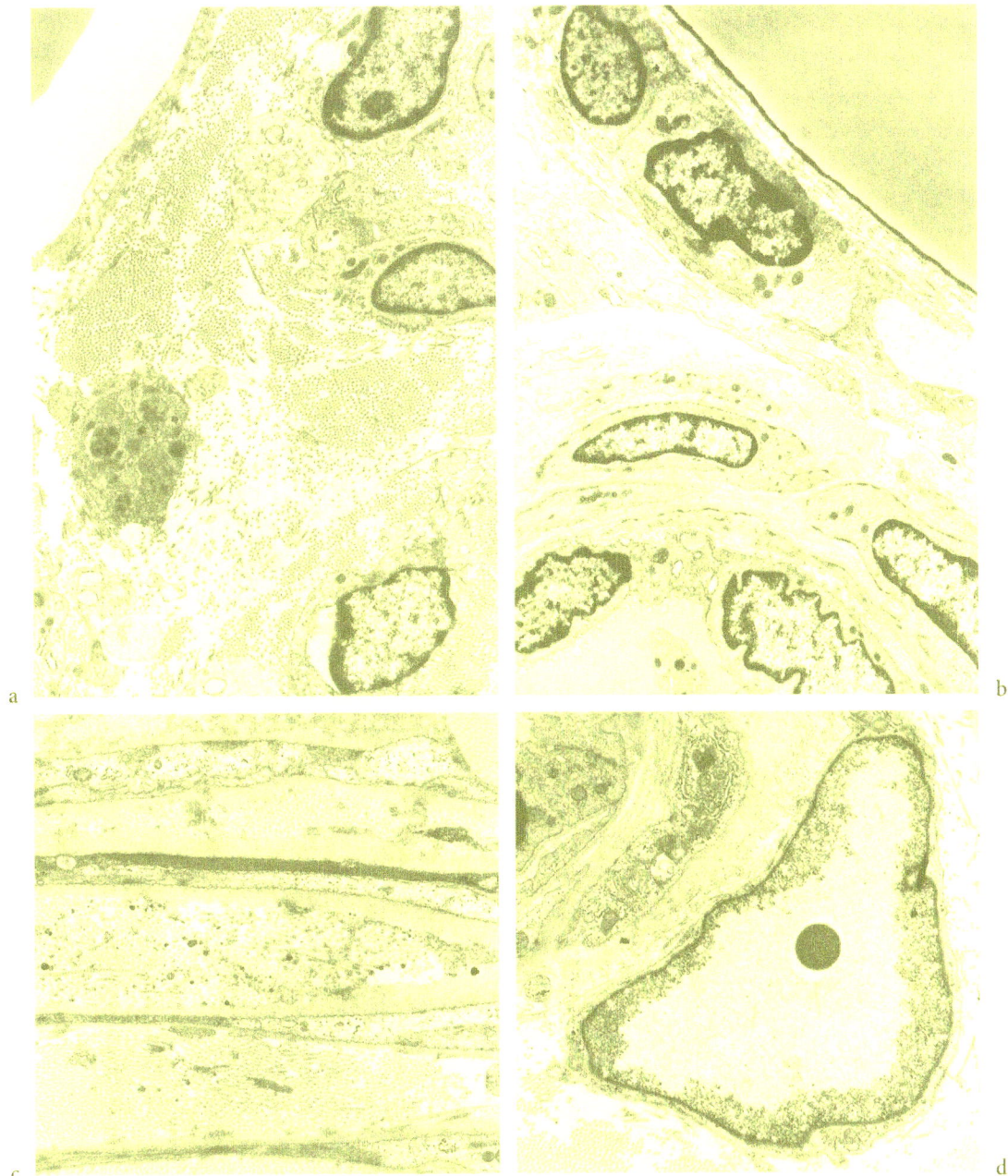

Fig. 225 a–d. Neuropathy in prostatic carcinoma. **a,b** Cellular infiltrates in the epineurium adjacent to a vein (**a**) and between a fat cell and an epineurial artery (**b**). **a** × 2,700; **b** × 5,900. **c** Numerous non-specific extracellular matrix granules are seen in the perineurium between collagen fibrils and elastic fibers. One perineurial cell is pycnotic. The thickness of the basal laminae is focally increased. × 9,700. **d** Unusual homogeneous osmiophilic nuclear inclusion in a perivascular cell detected in the epineurium. The nuclear inclusion is surrounded by a loose caryoplasm in the center; the peripheral nuclear chromatin appears to be preserved. × 9,400

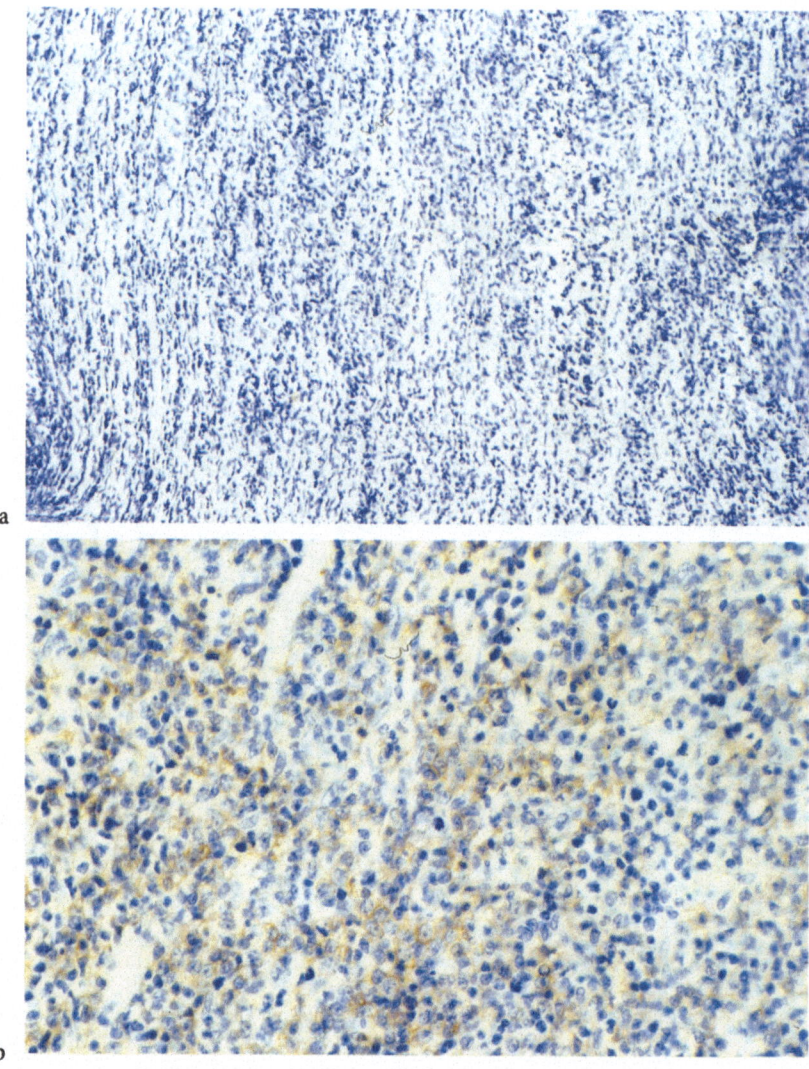

Fig. 226. a, b Infiltration of the median nerve in a 63-year-old male with a malignant lymphoma of the B-cell type with low malignancy (immunocytoma) which was known for 5 years. **c, d** s. p. 263

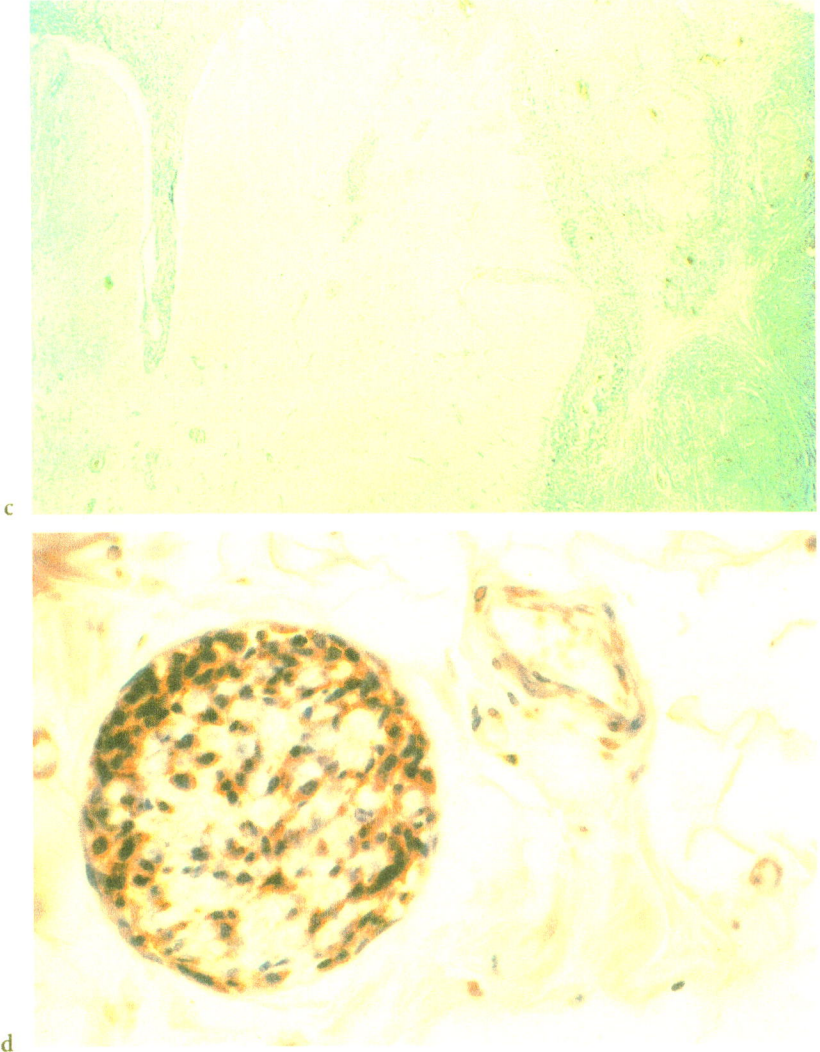

Fig. 226. c T-cell lymphoma with infiltration of the spinal canal and peripheral nerve fascicles. d T-cell reaction

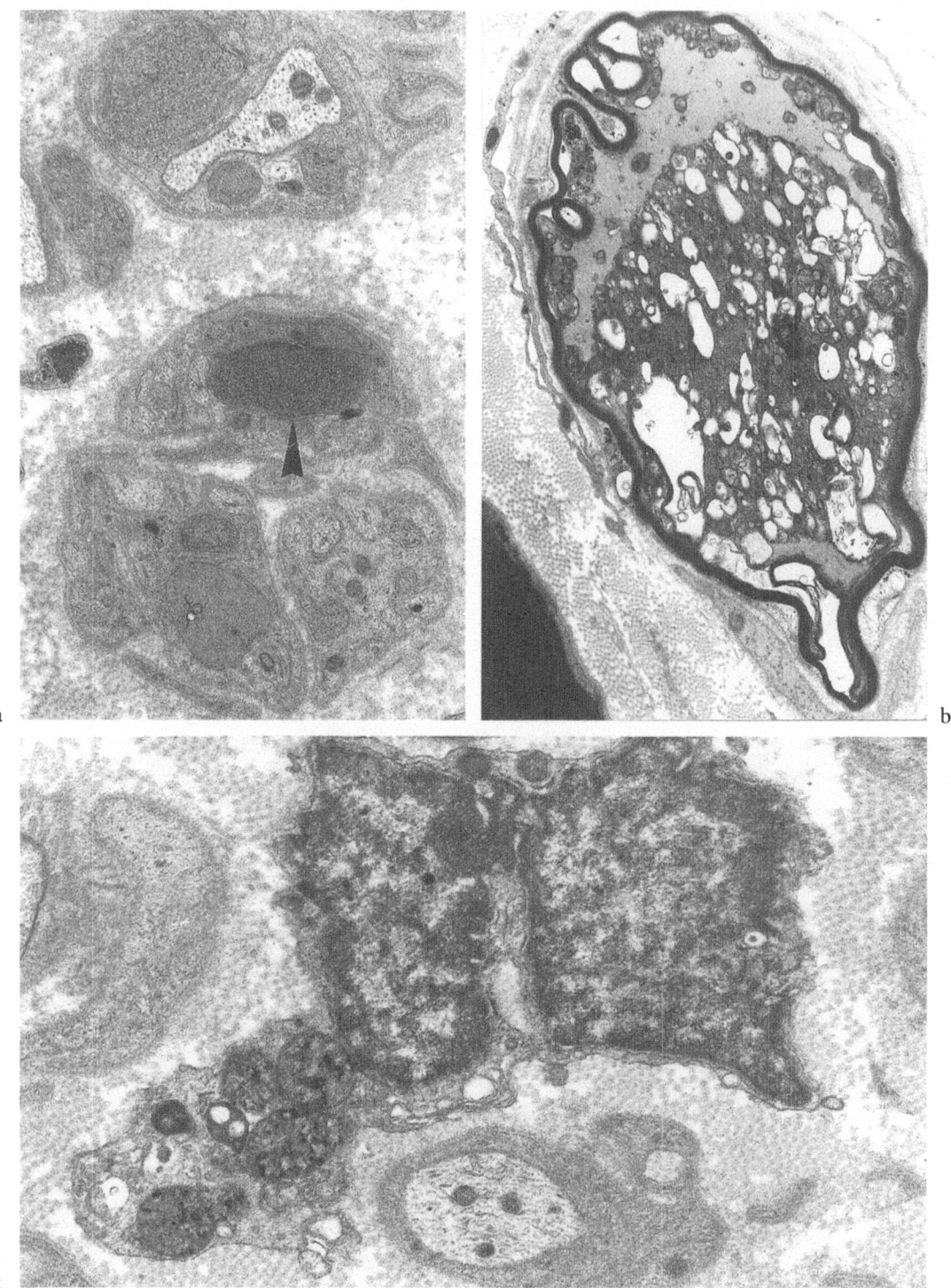

Fig. 227a–c. Malignant lymphoma associated with inclusion body myositis and peripheral neuropathy (same case as in Fig. 213). **a** Tubuloreticular inclusion (*arrowhead*) in a Schwann cell. × 14,800. **b** Large autophagolysosome with multiple vesicles in a thinly remyelinated axon. × 9,200. **c** Degenerating endoneurial fibroblast with presumptive calcium precipitates in the mitochondria. × 19,100

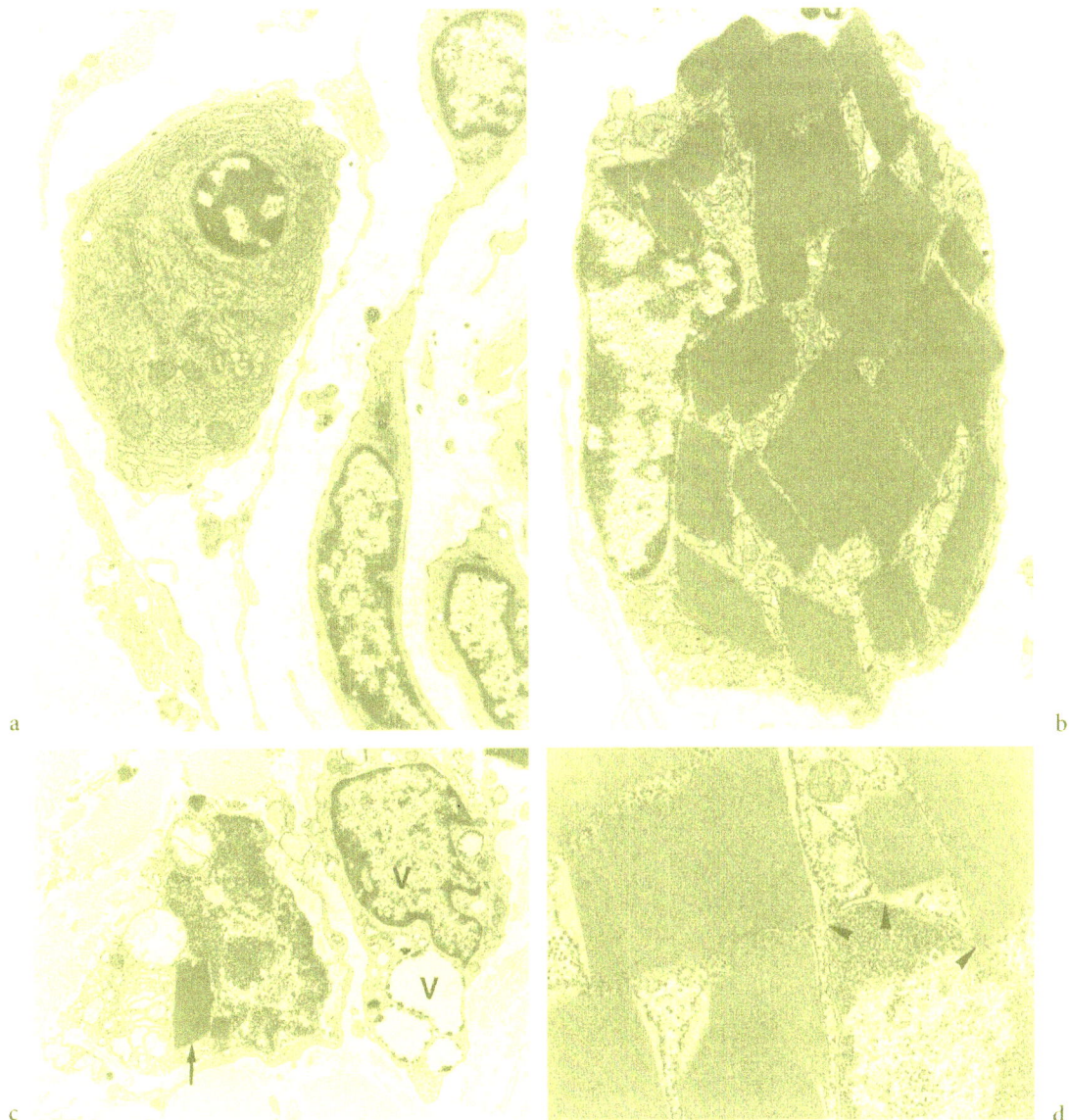

Fig. 228a–d. Paracrystalline inclusions in an epineurial plasma cell of a 66-year-old female patient with vasculitis and dysproteinemia. **a** Perivascular plasma cell adjacent to fibroblasts and smooth muscle cells without paracrystalline inclusions. × 8,000. **b** Higher magnification of a neighboring plasma cell. There are large numbers of partly rhombic, partly rectangular, partly polygonal paracrystalline inclusions in the ergastoplasma of this cell. × 9,300. **c** Isolated paracrystalline inclusion (*arrow*) in a regressively altered plasma cell adjacent to another cell with presumably dextrin-like substances containing vacuoles (*V*). × 5,900. **d** Higher magnification of the paracrystalline inclusions in a plasma cell. The inclusions are located in the granular endoplasmic reticulum which is enlarged, containing at its margin amorphous or finely granulated substances. The ergastoplasma is connected at three sites with the outer nuclear membrane (*arrowheads*). × 34,000

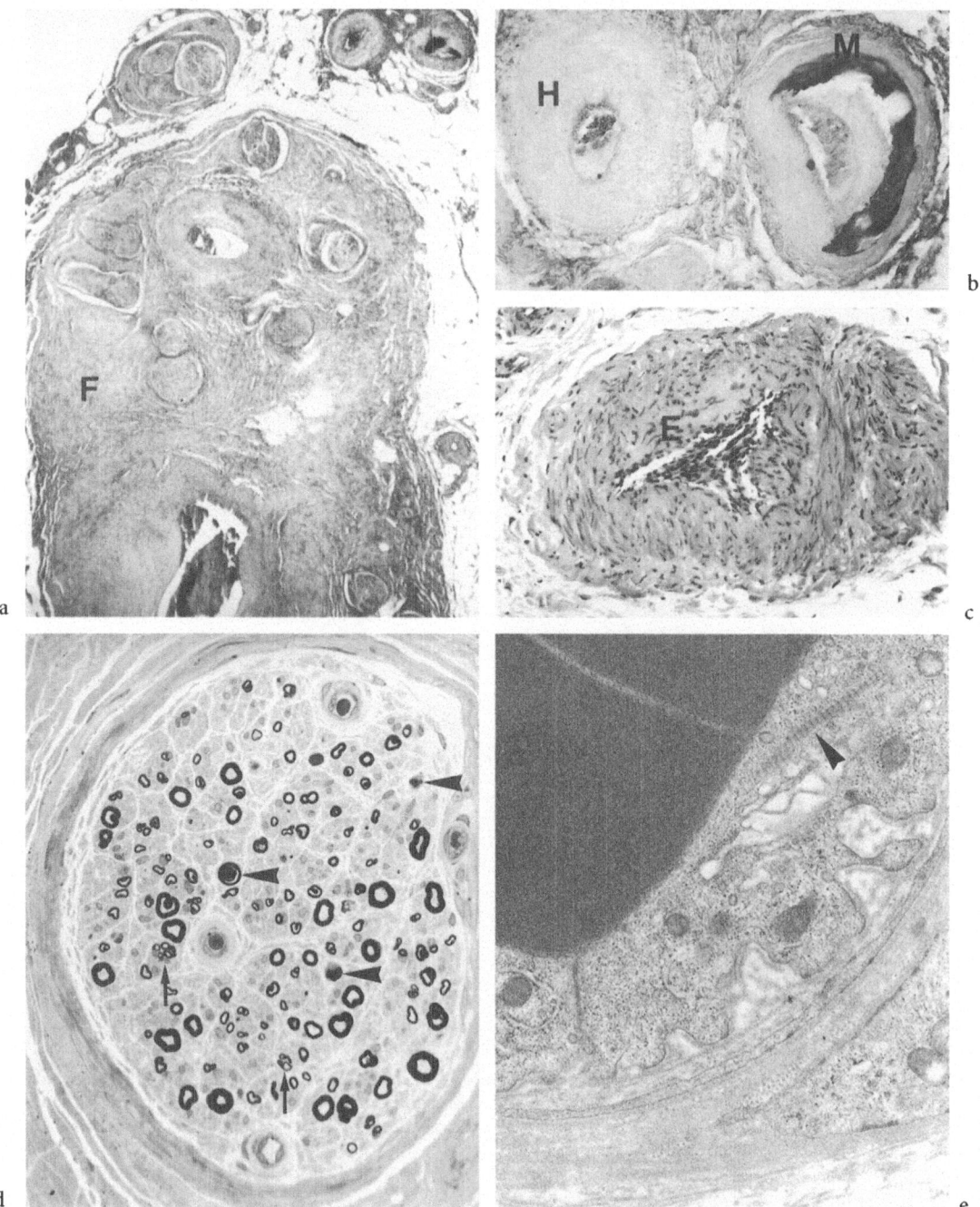

Fig. 229a–e. Extraordinary severe angiopathy. *F*, fibrosis of the epineurium in **a**; *H*, hyalinization of a blood vessel wall in **b**; *M*, Mönckeberg's media calcification; *E*, endothelial cell proliferation and blood vessel obliteration in **c** in a case with IgM-gam-mopathy, clinically thought to represent selective motor neuropathy (same case as in [725]), but with morphologically clear signs of a rapidly progressive neuropathy also in the sensory system. The *arrowheads* in **d** indicate acutely degenerating nerve fibers, the *arrows* on typical groups show where regenerating nerve fibers sprouted at the site of degenerated nerve fibers. In **e** a leptomer fibril in an endothelial cell is indicated by an *arrowhead*. **a–c** H & E; **d** Semithin section: toluidine blue; **e** electron microscopic illustration, × 15,000. (From [961])

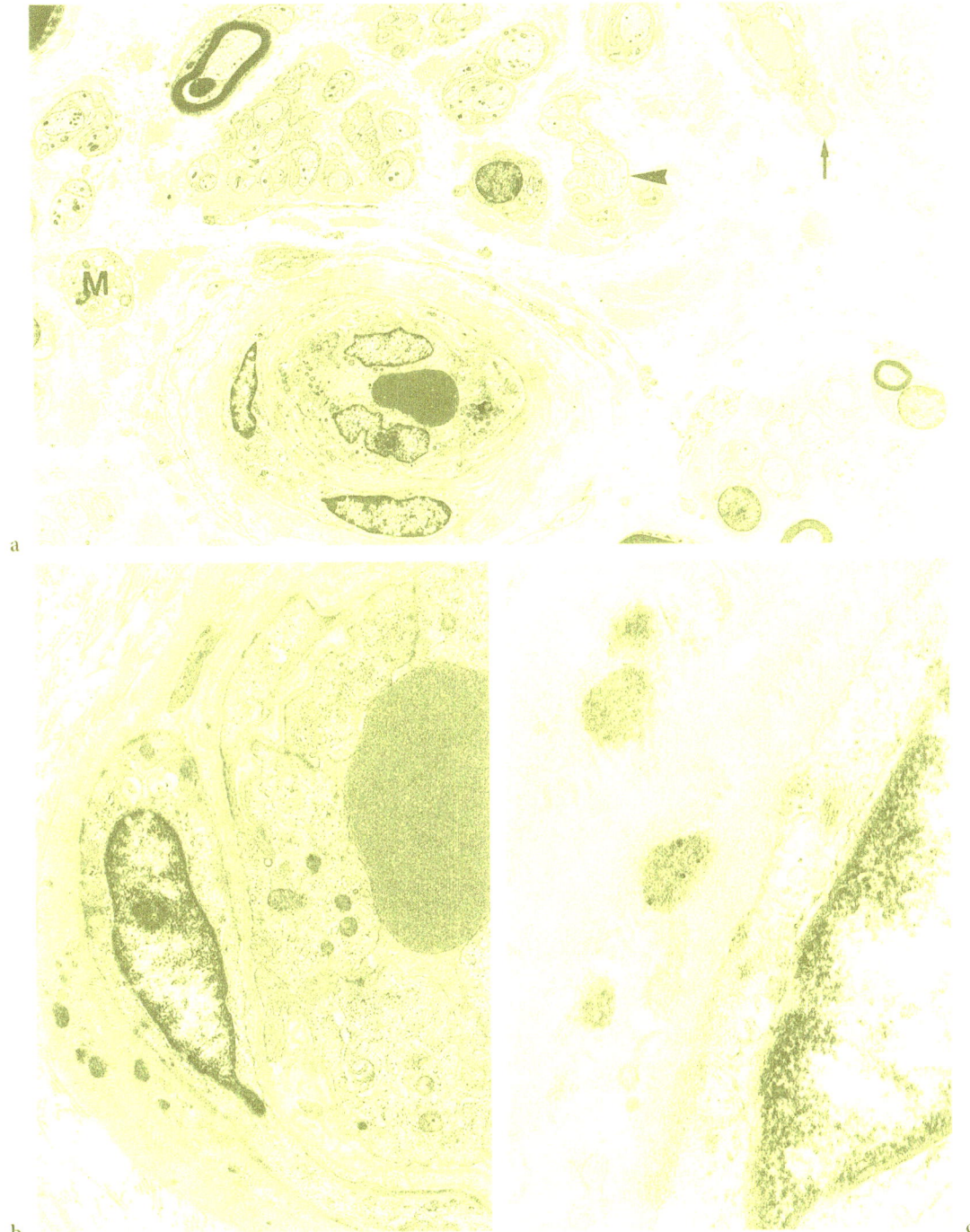

Fig. 230 a–c. Same case as in Fig. 229. **a** There is considerable endoneurial edema. Beside a blood vessel with an erythrocyte in its lumen are several bands of Büngner of myelinated (*arrowhead*) and unmyelinated nerve fibers in addition to a macrophage (*M*) and a Schwann cell which encloses large bundles of collagen fibers (*arrow*). × 2,800. **b** Endoneurial blood vessel with perivascular electron dense granular deposits resembling immune complexes. These are illustrated in **c** at higher magnification. **b** × 11,300; **c** × 47,000

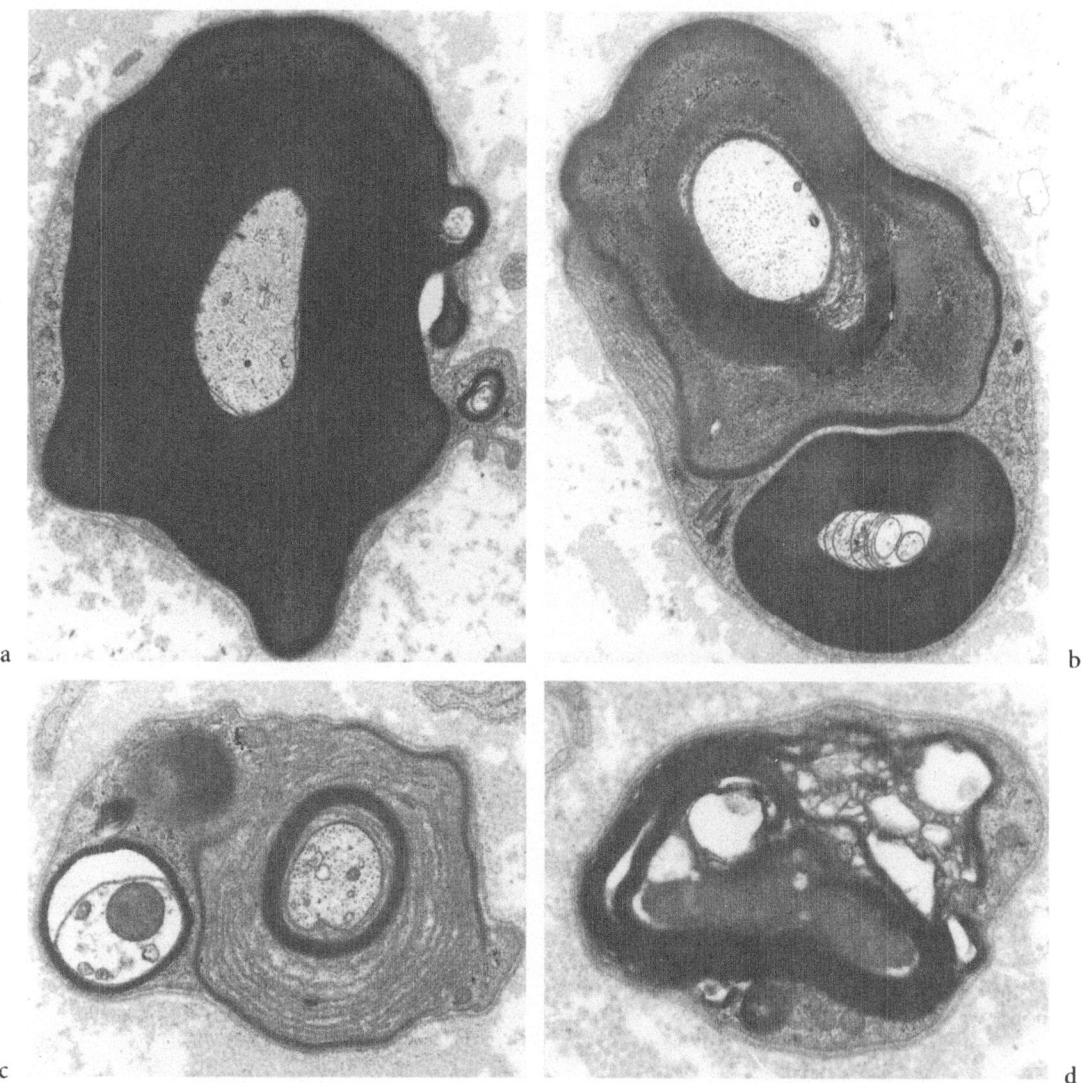

Fig. 231a–d. Atrophic nerve fiber changes in a 49-year-old patient with IgG-gammopathy. **a** Dense finely granulated substances within a compact Schmidt-Lanterman incisure at the site of small projections of the myelin sheath. **b** Finely distributed granular substances in the enlarged cytoplasm of a Schmidt-Lanterman incisure adjacent to a compact myelin loop. **a, b** × 8,600. **c** Uncompacted myelin lamellae in a Schmidt-Lanterman incisure which communicates with the abaxonal Schwann cell cytoplasm adjacent to two myelin loops, one of which is cut tangentially. × 14,700. **d** Splitting and vesicular or vacuolar degeneration in a myelin sheath of a nerve fiber which appears to be in an early stage of Wallerian degeneration. The axoplasm is severely condensed. × 19,000. (From [980])

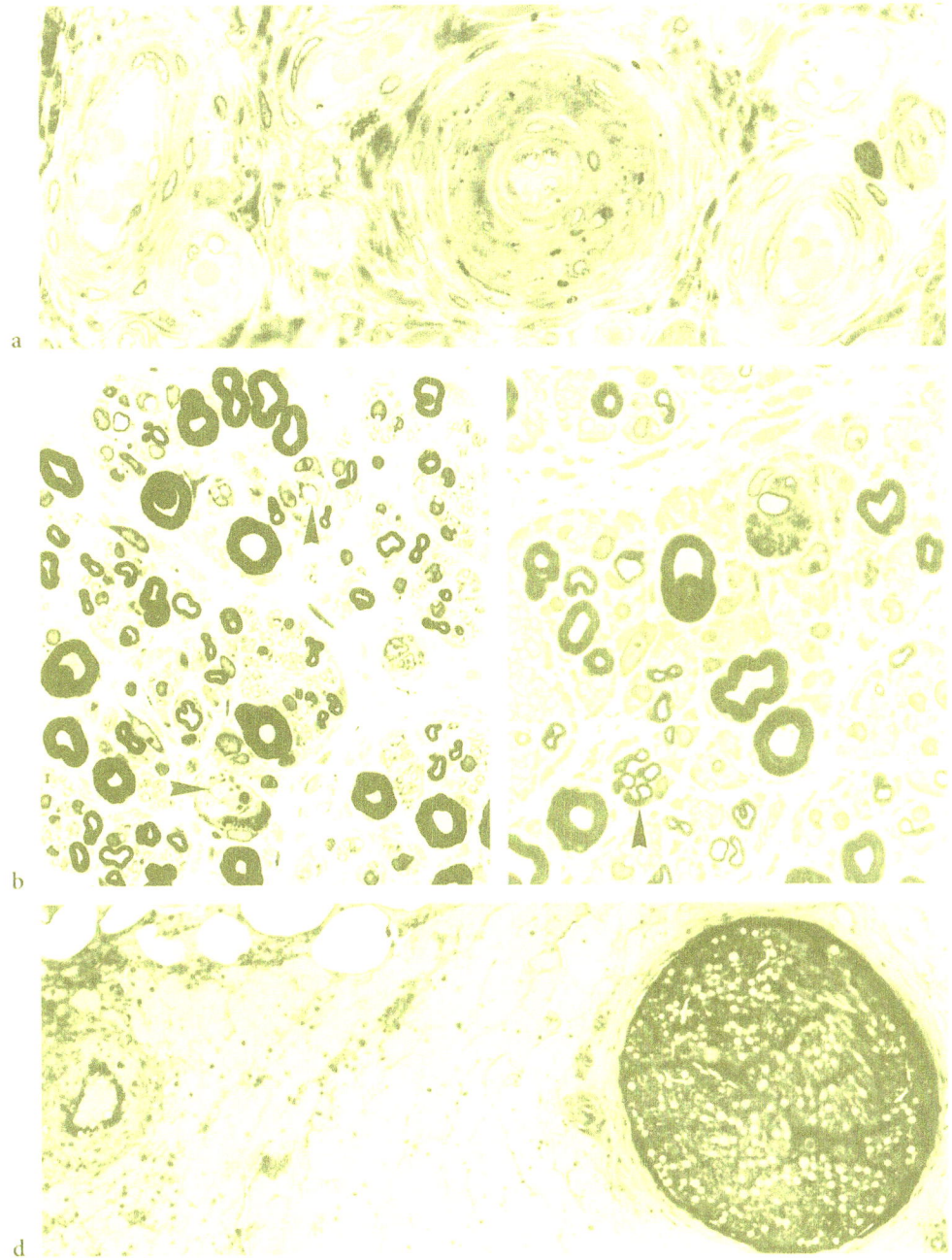

Fig. 232 a–d. Chronic, mainly demyelinating neuropathy in monoclonal gammopathy of the kappa light chain type in a 70-year-old man. **a** The number of the epineurial blood vessels is focally considerably increased without detectable inflammatory cellular infiltrates. × 750. **b** The number of large myelinated nerve fibers is clearly reduced. Demyelinated axons are repeatedly seen circumferentially surrounded by supernumerary Schwann cells or macrophages (*arrowheads*). × 736. **c** In addition to disproportionately thinly remyelinated nerve fibers there are occasional clusters of regenerated fibers with small myelinated nerve fibers indicating previous axonal degeneration (*arrowheads*). × 1,250. **d** Immunoreaction for kappa light chains (at a concentration of 1:500). The endoneurium of the nerve fascicle is intensely stained, indicating accumulation of kappa light chains, whereas the surrounding perineurium, the fat cells, and several blood vessels remain unstained. × 152

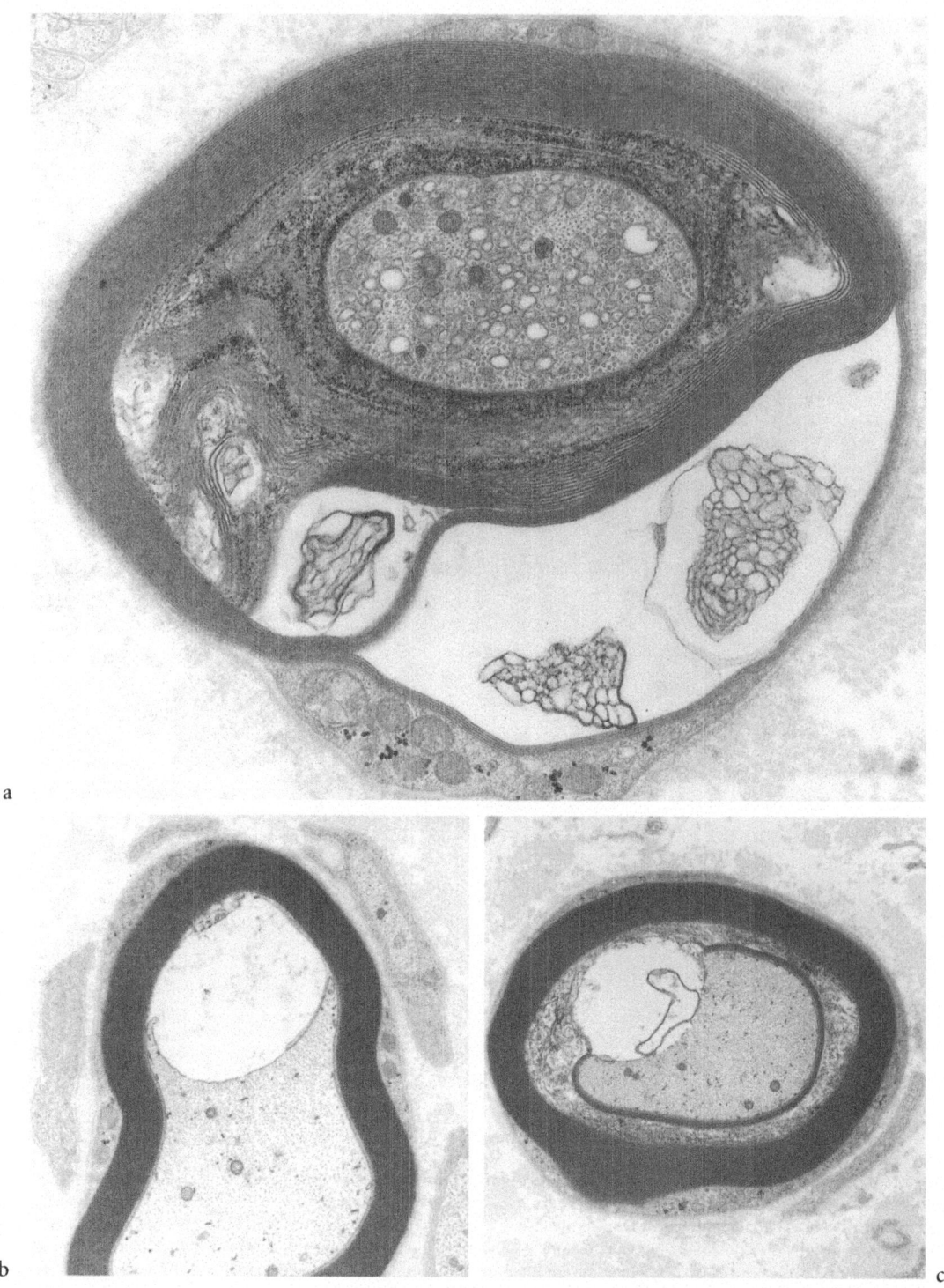

Fig. 233 a–c. Demyelinating neuropathy in gammopathy of the IgA-type in an 80-year-old female. **a** Paranodal myelin segment showing vesicular and vacuolar lysis of myelin lamellae. × 32,700. **b** Adaxonal vacuole in a degenerated and regenerated nerve fiber within a cluster with associated empty Schwann cell processes and unmyelinated axons. × 14,200. **c** Adaxonal vesicular lysis of myelin lamellae in a demyelinated and remyelinated nerve fiber with a single circumferentially arranged Schwann cell process in the periphery. × 9,500

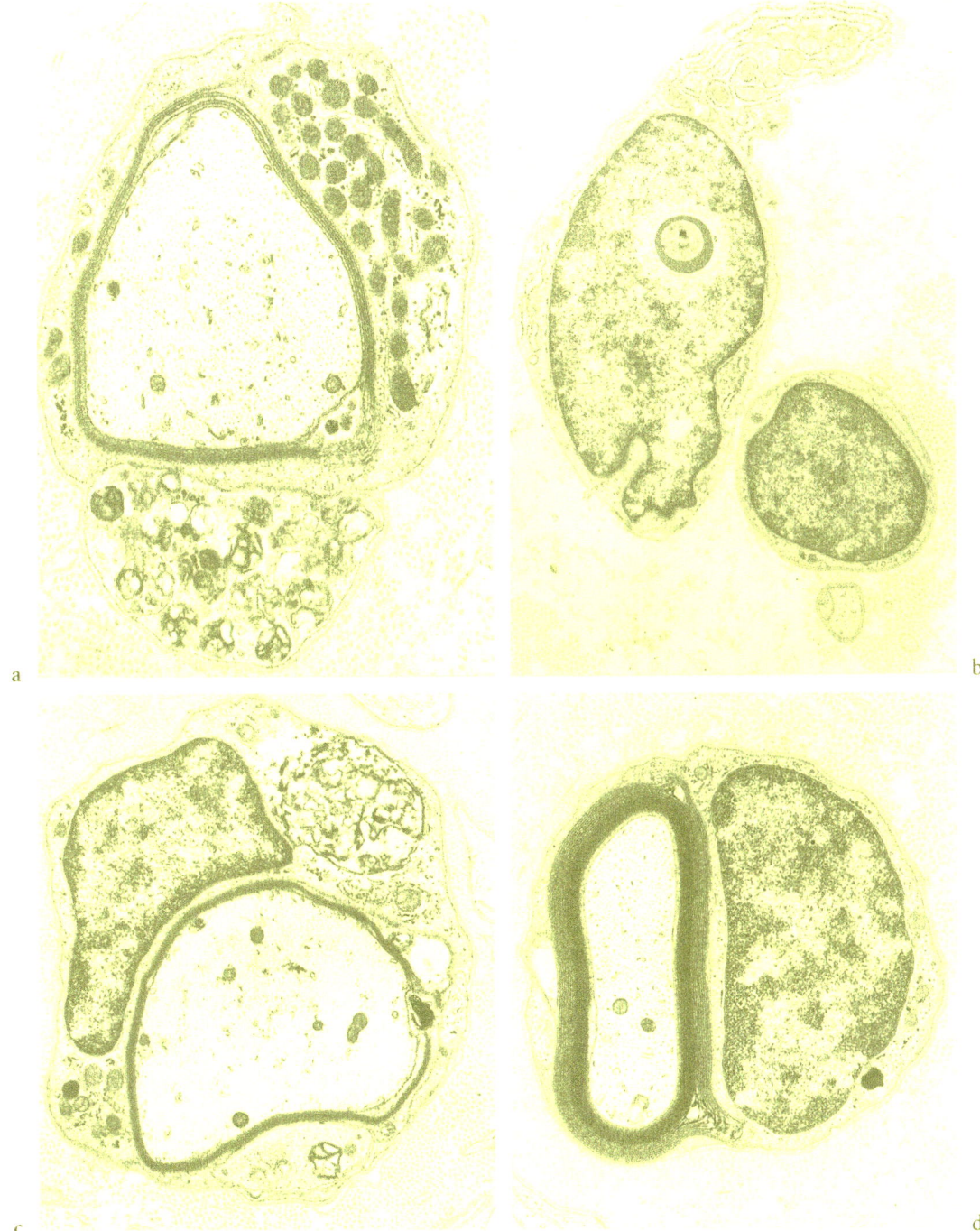

Fig. 234a–d. Demyelinating neuropathy in a monoclonal gammopathy of unknown significance (MGUS) in a 70-year-old female. Thinly remyelinated nerve fiber with myelin degradation products in the same (**c**) or a neighboring (**a**) Schwann cell. **a** × 21,200; **c** × 13,700. **b** Endoneurial fibroblast adjacent to an "empty" Schwann cell without axons. The fibroblast shows an unusual ring-like nuclear inclusion. × 11,500. **d** Loose peripheral myelin lamellae around compact myelin lamellae in a small nerve fiber. × 16,200

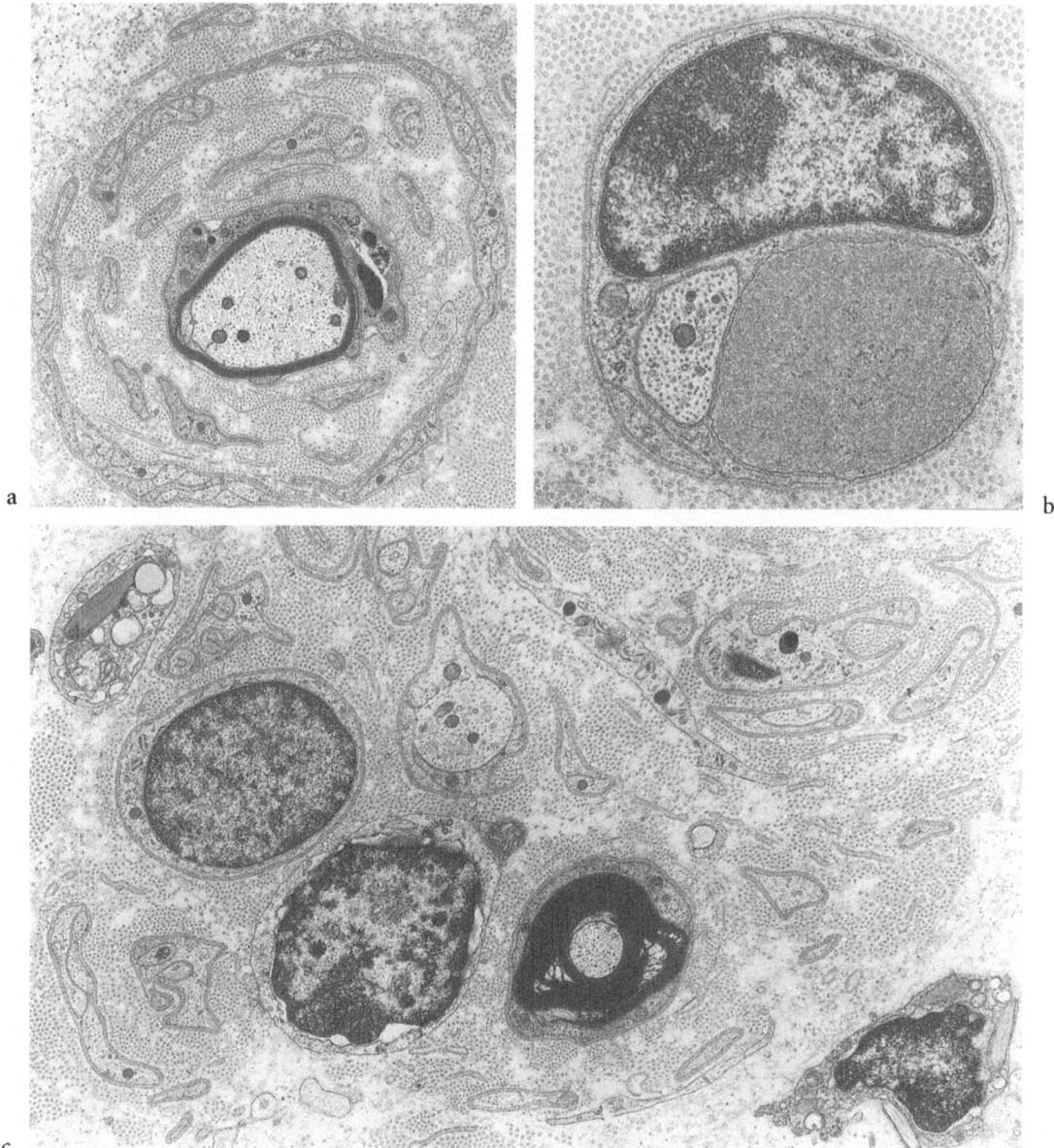

Fig. 235 a–c. Same case as in Fig. 234. **a** Onion bulb formation with numerous concentrically arranged Schwann cell processes forming a nearly complete ring around a central, disproportionately thinly remyelinated nerve fiber. The collagen fibrils are somewhat thinner than in surrounding endoneurium. × 9,760. **b** Abnormal unmyelinated axon adjacent to a regular axon. The abnormal axon is severely dilated and filled with amorphic or finely granulated substances. × 21,000. **c** In the vicinity of an atrophic myelinated nerve fiber are numerous empty Schwann cell processes associated with rare unmyelinated axons. There are also mononuclear cells containing π-granule-like structures. The cell in the center resembles a lymphocyte with focally distended outer nuclear membrane. × 10,300

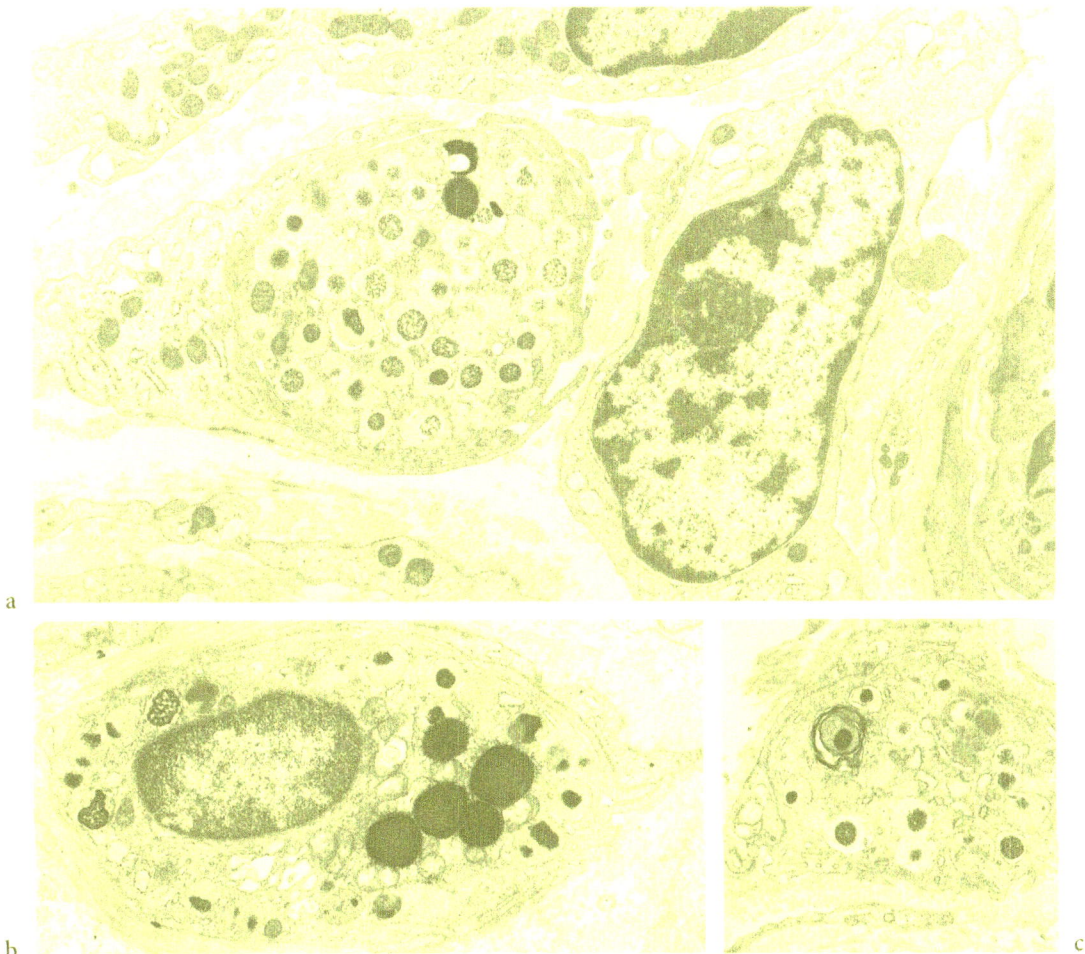

Fig. 236 a – c. Vasculitis in a 40-year-old female. **a** Incompletely degranulated mast cell attached to an epineurial fibroblast adjacent to a perivascular infiltrating inflammatory cell. × 10,400. **b** Unusual mast cell with several highly osmiophilic cytosomes and two finely granulated corpuscles on the other side of the nucleus. × 13,000. **c** Largely degranulated mast cell with a granule that is surrounded by several membranes. × 11,100

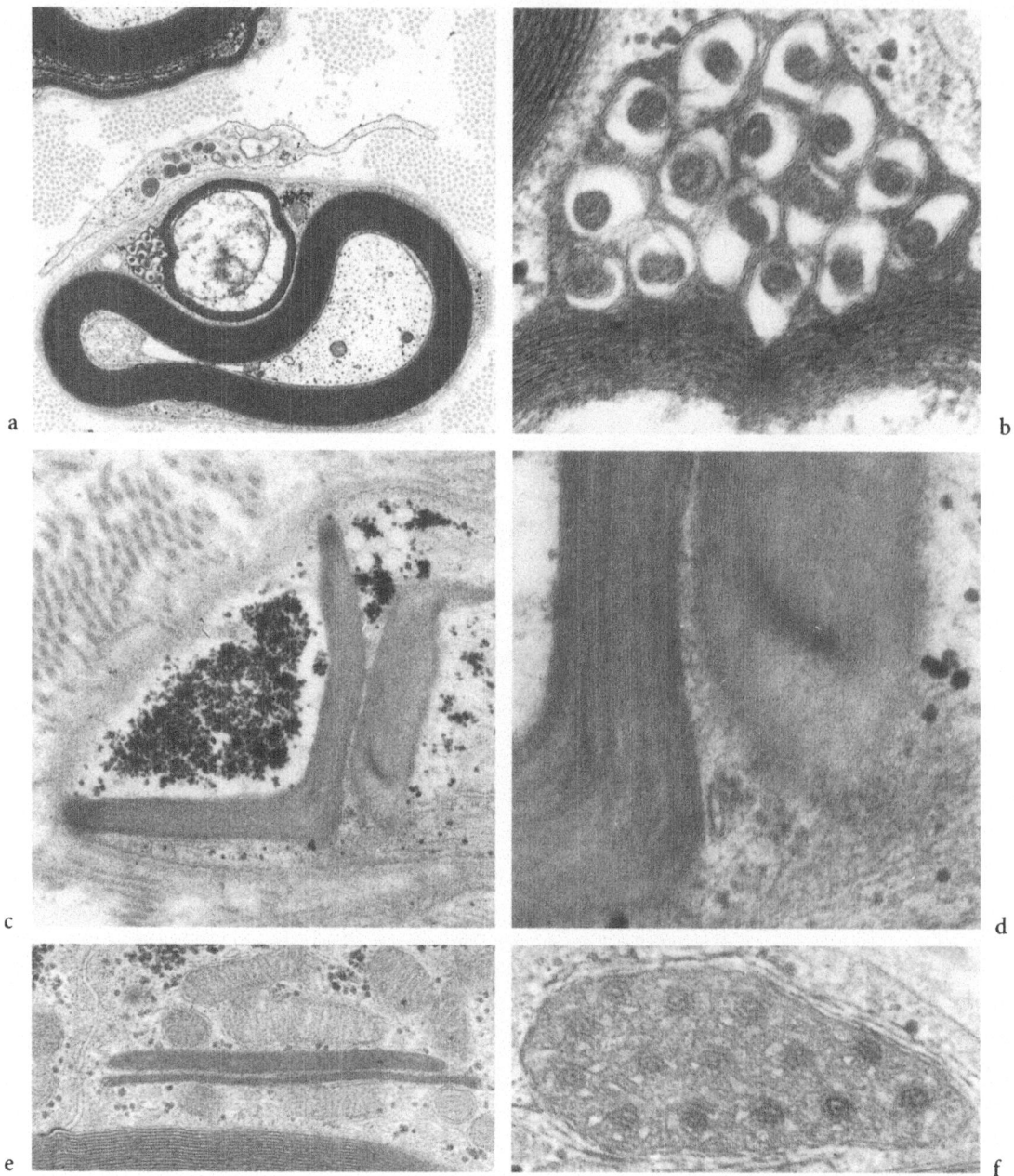

Fig. 237 a – f. Cryoglobulinemia in a 67-year-old female. **a, b** Frequent pattern of lysis of myelin ovoids (μ-granule of Elzholz) adjacent to a preserved myelin sheath. The pattern of lysis is illustrated in **b** at higher magnification. In the center of each ring-like structure is a globoid or lamellated spherical structure surrounded by a light halo; the lamellae have a reduced periodicity compared to that of the myelin lamellae. **a** × 12,600; **b** × 104,000. **c, d** Unusual forms of π-granules adjacent to glycogen granules in the cytoplasm of a Schwann cell in a case with progressive neuropathy. **c** × 23,400; **d** × 90,000. **e** Flat and lengthy forms of π-granules between mitochondria. × 38,400. **f** Abnormal mitochondrion with numerous matrix granule-like condensations and irregularly arranged mitochondrial cristae. × 38,400

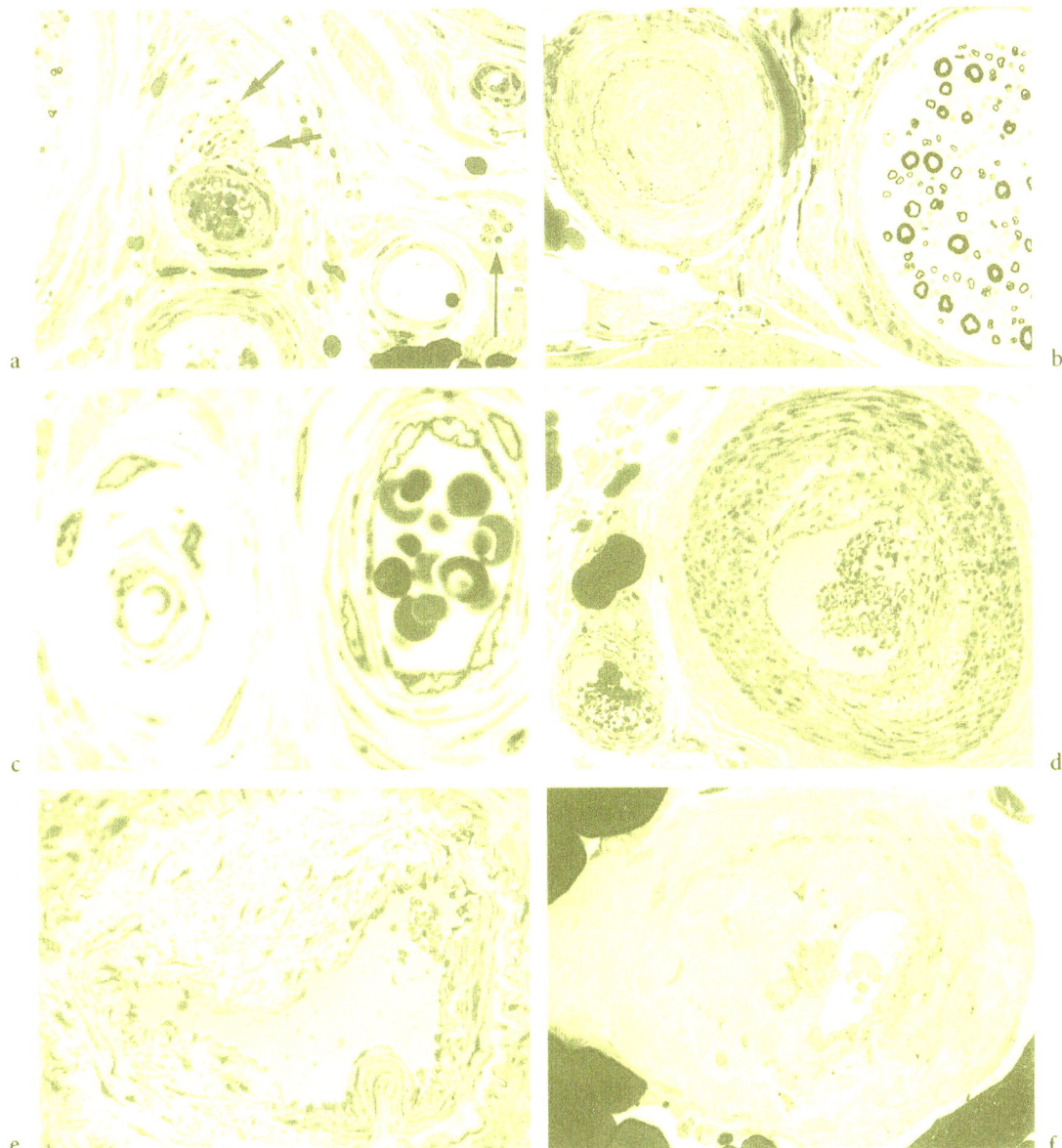

Fig. 238. **a** Immune complex vasculitis in a 68-year-old female. Some smooth muscle cells of an epineurial blood vessel are dissociated from the vessel wall in a sector-like area (*short arrows*) and surrounded by excentrically increased collagenous connective tissue (higher magnification: see **g – h**). Isolated smooth muscle cells are indicated by a *long arrow*. × 290. **b** Stenosing angiopathy in clinically assumed familial dementia of the Alzheimer-type in a 61-year-old male. The intima of an epineurial artery inside the elastica interna is increased in thickness and severely altered, similar to what is seen in arteriosclerosis, by immigrated and proliferated smooth muscle cells. The lumen is severely stenosed. The neuropathy is of an axonal type and of intermediate severity. × 280. **c** Prominent microangiopathy associated with circulating immune complexes in a 59-year-old male. Some of the pericapillary basal laminae in the epineurium are severely increased in thickness without apparent inflammatory cell infiltrates. × 1,200. **d** Epineurial blood vessel changes in scleroderma (see Fig. 245 d). **e** Same case as in **d**. Severe enlargement of the intima with an increase in cells and connective tissue (sclerosis) in an epineurial vein. × 1,650. **f** Amyloidosis with prominent amyloid deposits in the wall of a vein in a 91-year-old male. × 360 (From [958]).

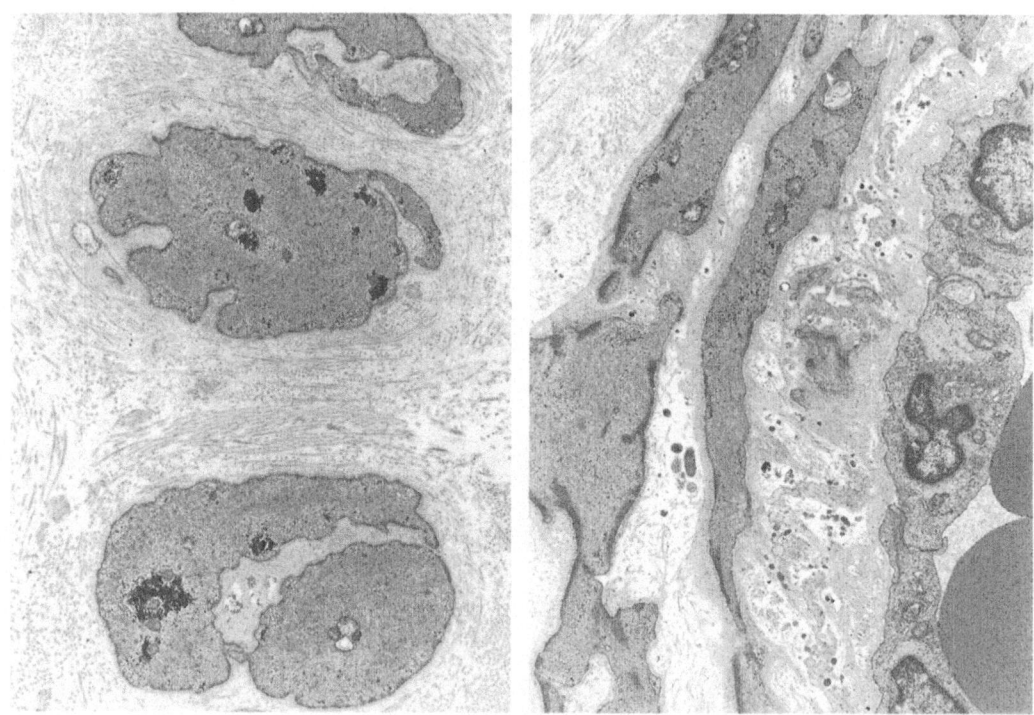

g   h

Fig. 238 *(continued).* **g** Higher magnification of the changes shown in **a** illustrating the dissociated (**g**) and still regularly arranged smooth muscle cells (**h**). Between the endothelium and the smooth muscle cells are numerous matrix granules in the extracellular space. The basal laminae are unevenly increased in thickness. The collagen fibrils are arranged in variable directions. Erythrocytes are seen in the lumen. **g** × 8,300; **h** × 7,200. (From [957])

CHAPTER 13

Angiopathic Neuropathies and Hypoxidosis

Peripheral nerves are luxuriously vascularized resulting in a high safety margin. Counts revealed 32–72 (mean: 57) blood vessels with one arteria nutritia in the epineurium of human sural nerves (Fig. 239) [1006]. These, as well as the endoneurial blood vessels (the endoneurium contains mainly capillaries), show numerous pathognostic or nonspecific changes (angiopathies) which may or may not cause neuropathy due to ischemia or inflammation.

Ischemia may result from:

- *Stenosis* or *occlusion* (Fig. 238b) of large or small arteries, arterioles, and capillaries in *arteriosclerosis* [759], *amyloidosis* (Fig. 238f) (see above), *embolism* (Fig. 247a–d) [57], and *vasculitides* (Figs. 245a, b, 246, 248–254) (references see above).
- *Compression* (trauma, tumors, tourniquets etc.) (Figs. 244a–d) [751–754, 756–758].
- *Compartment syndromes* [612], e.g., tibialis anterior syndrome.

One of the most frequent vascular alterations seen is an increase in the number of *perivascular basal laminae* or *thickening of the basal laminae* (Figs. 238c, 240) [54, 109, 508, 847, 952]. *Calcification* of an epineurial blood vessel (mainly the arteria nutritia) is only rarely seen (Fig. 229b) whereas *extracellular matrix granules* are a frequent, nonspecific finding (Fig. 238h) usually indicating *arteriosclerosis* when occurring with an increase in the basal laminae, the number of ingrown or proliferated smooth muscle cells (myofibroblasts) in the intima, and collagen fibrils. *Proliferation of epineurial capillaries* occurs as a compensatory process following occlusion of epineurial arterioles (Fig. 245c). *Proliferation of adventitial smooth muscle cells* (Figs. 238a, g, h, 245d) is a nonspecific change indicating angiopathy and should not be mistaken for perivascular inflammatory cellular infiltrates [957]. *Erythrodiapedesis* (Fig. 75) and *hemorrhage* (Fig. 241) with subsequent epineurial *siderosis* (Fig. 30) indicates severe angiopathy if not caused by traumatic lesions, especially fresh excision trauma. Dysplastic veins (Figs. 242a–c) may be associated with *varicosis* or *phlebectasia* [203]. Other, exceptional perivascular endoneurial findings of unknown etiology in old age are illustrated in Fig. 243a–c.

Hypoxia is also considered as a cause of neuropathy [50, 62, 135, 250, 253, 752, 759, 763, 843, 857, 1088, 1259, 1297]. *Hyperventilation*, on the other hand, differs from *ischemia* in causing ectopic discharges leading more rapidly to paresthesia than to fasciculations, presumably because of its rather selective effect on threshold channels [687].

Lymphatic vessels are absent in the endoneurium but do occur in variable sizes and numbers in the epineurium. Accumulation of lymphocytes in their lumen does not appear to be associated with vasculitis or polyneuritis if restricted to the lumen (Fig. 255a, b). No references were found for this.

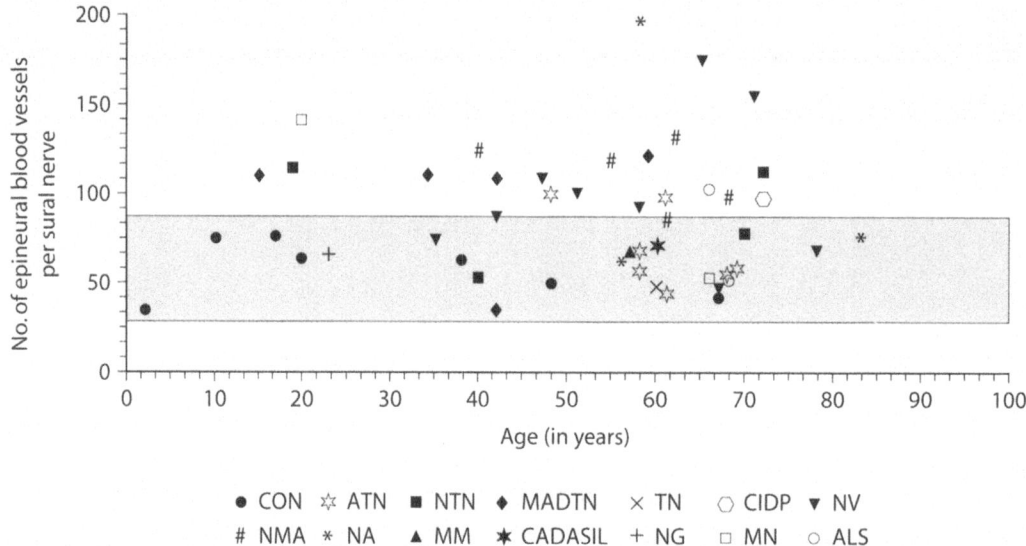

Fig. 239. Number of epineurial blood vessels (*y-axis*) in relation to the age of the patients studied (*x-axis*). The control cases are indicated by dots; they are located within the grayish area (*CON*), which corresponds to twice the standard deviation of the control values. Further abbreviations: *ATN*, axonal type of neuropathy; *NTN*, neuronal type of neuropathy; *MADTN*, mixed axonal and demyelinating type of neuropathy; *TN*, tomaculous neuropathy; *CIDP*, chronic inflammatory demyelinating polyneuropathy; *NV*, neuropathy with vasculitis; *NMA*, neuropathy with microangiopathy; *NA*, neuropathy with angiopathy of large blood vessels; *NM*, Mönckeberg's media calcification; *CADASIL*, cerebral autosomal dominant arteriopathy with subcortical infarcts and leukoencephalopathy; *NG*, neuropathy in gammopathies; *MN*, motor neuropathy; *ALS*, amyotrophic lateralsclerosis. (Modified from [1006])

Fig. 240 a–f. Increased thickness of the basal lamina of endoneurial blood vessels (Inaugural dissertation of W. Beinborn, Aachen, 1991). **a** Forty-six-year-old female with diabetic microangiopathy. The basal laminae of the endoneurial blood vessels are considerably increased in thickness (*thin arrows*). A large pericyte at a blood vessel is indicated by a *thick arrow*, endoneurial fibroblasts by *arrowheads*. The number of myelinated and unmyelinated nerve fibers is reduced. There is considerable endoneurial edema. **b** Fifty-seven-year-old male with cryoglobulinemia. Two endoneurial blood vessels with prominent endothelial cells and pericytes showing only moderate increase of their basal laminae are surrounded by fibroblasts or perineurial cells. Some bundles of collagen fibers can be seen adjacent to the blood vessels. **c** Microangiopathy of unidentified etiology in a 63-year-old male. **d** Sixty-nine-year-old male with diabetic microangiopathy. One endoneurial blood vessel shows prominent thickening of the basal lamina (*arrowhead*). Another blood vessel is characterized by an increase in the number of endothelial cells. **e** Same case as in **c**. The blood vessel with a severe increase in the thickness of the basal lamina (*arrowhead*) shows large endothelial cells and a pycnotic pericyte (*arrow*). A fibroblast (*F*) is circularly arranged around the blood vessel. **f** Microangiopathy in hypertonia. There is no detectable lumen in the endoneurial capillary which, however, may also be due to collapse because of excision under anemic conditions at surgery. The nuclei of the proliferated endothelial cells and the fibroblast (*arrow*) are indented. **a–f** × 1,000

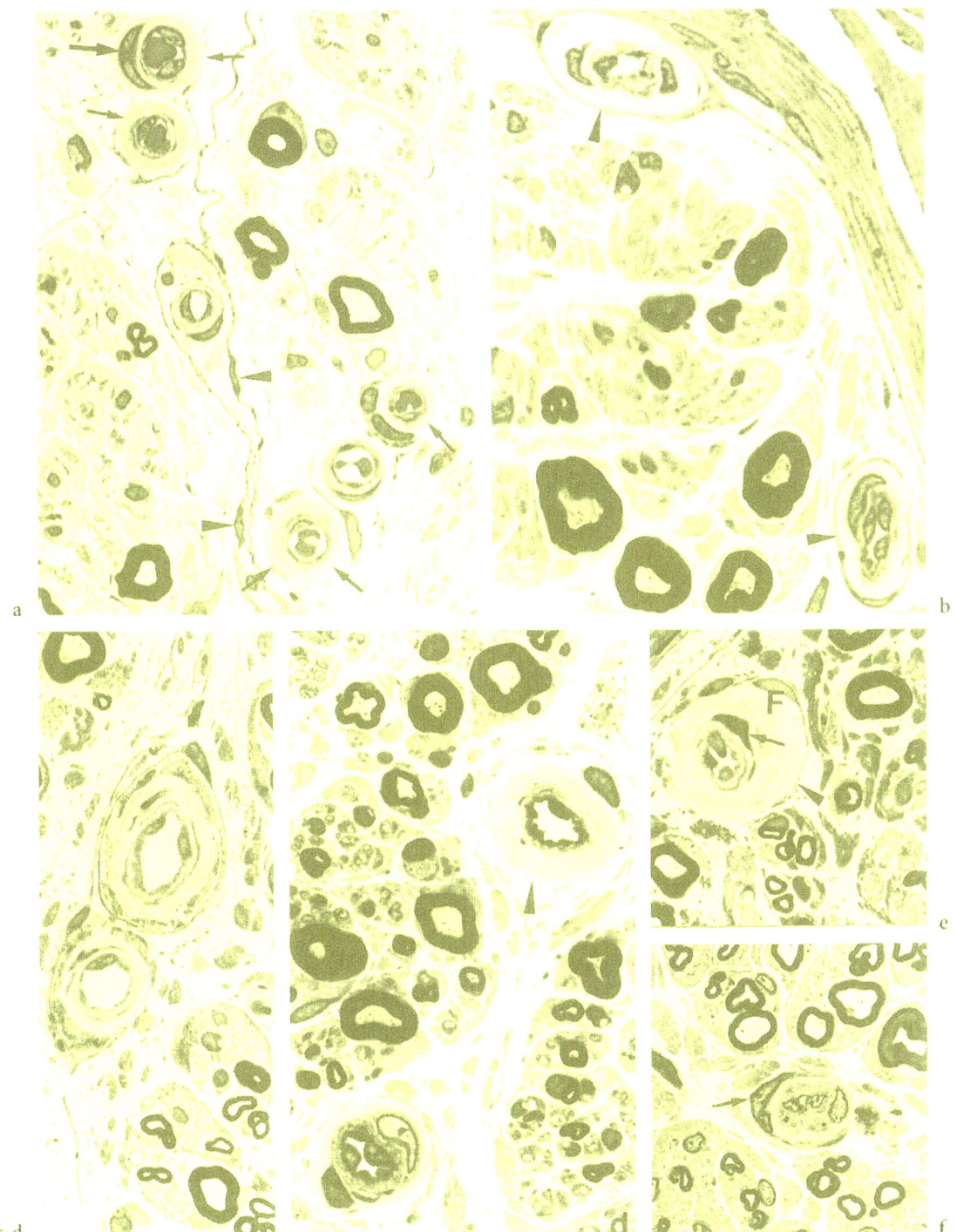

Fig. 240 a–f. Legend s. p. 278

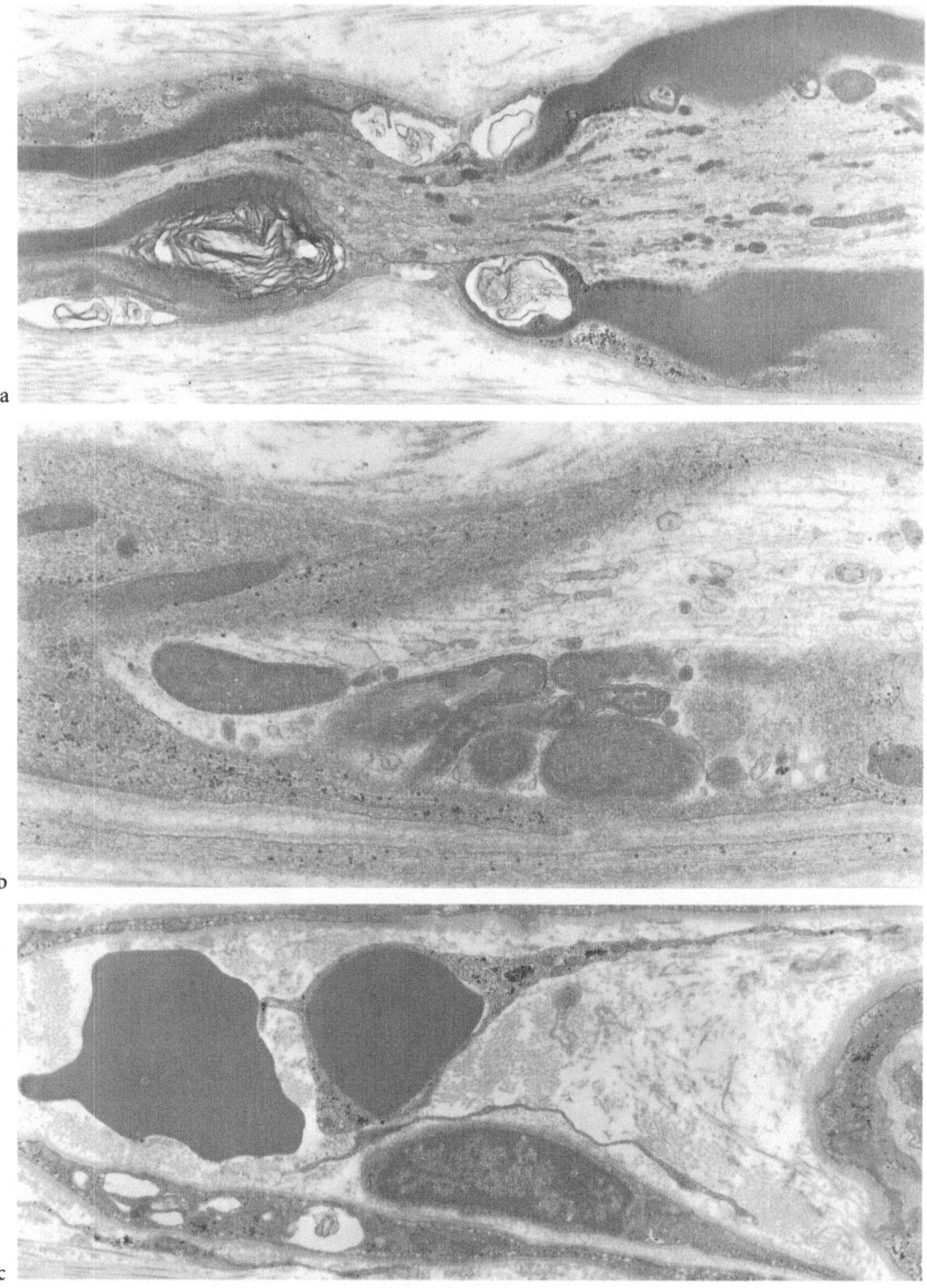

Fig. 241a–c. Thirty-eight-year-old male showing erythrodiapedesis after previous intoxication. **a** Paranodal vacuolar and vesicular disintegration of the myelin lamellae with focal multilamellar structures. × 11,000. **b** Focal accumulation of large mitochondria in an axon within a bundle of unmyelinated nerve fibers. × 29,000. **c** Perivascular erythrocytes one of which has already been phagocytosed. × 9,400

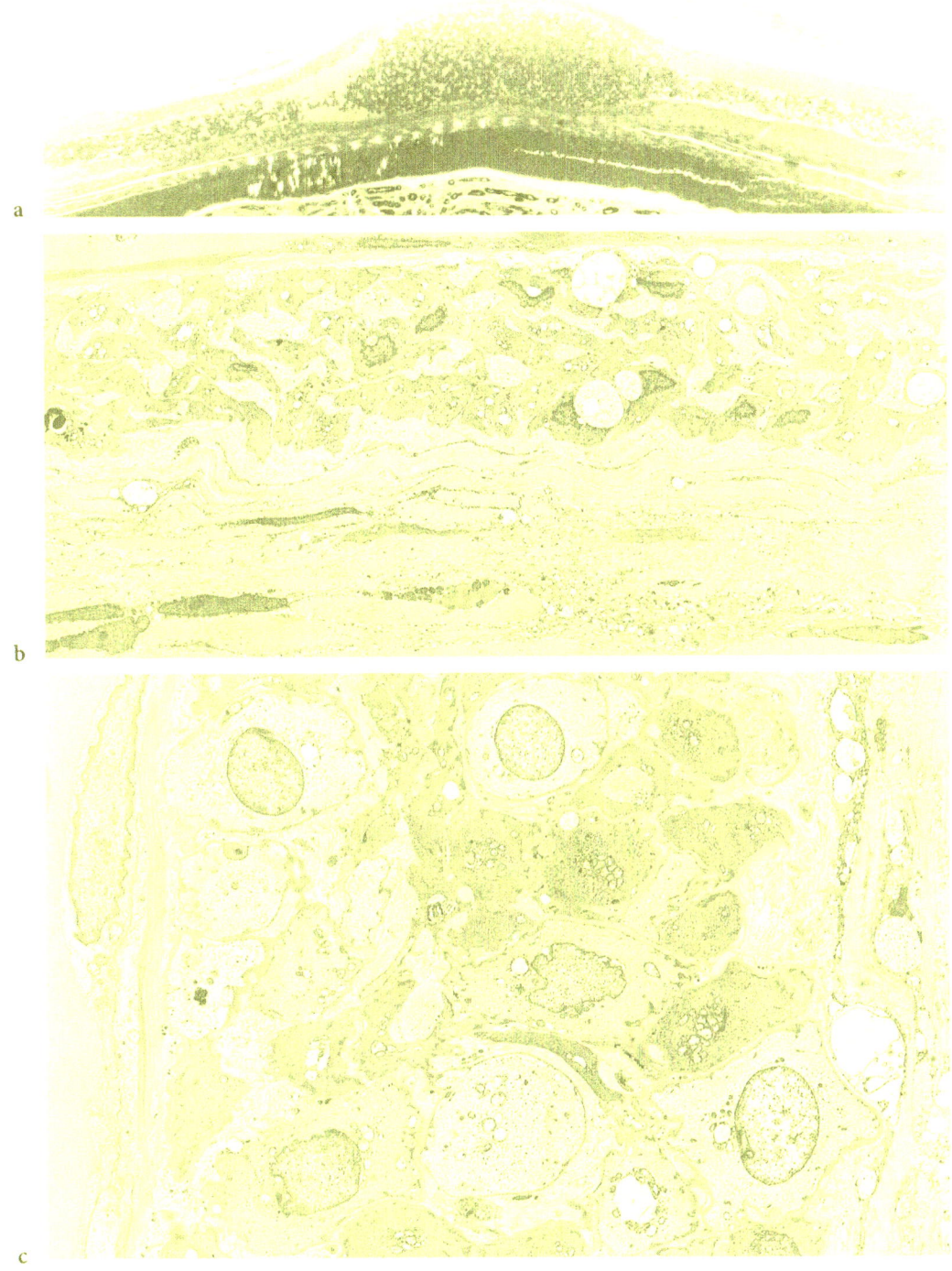

Fig. 242. **a** Focal varicosity with accumulation of erythrocytes inside an epineurial vein which shows a dilated and attenuated wall in the sural nerve of a 35-year-old man with chronic neuropathy of an axonal type. × 84. **b** Electron microscopic view of the wall of the varicose vein illustrated in **a**. The smooth muscle cells are dissociated and include many vacuoles of uneven size containing more or less numerous granular substances. Numerous matrix granules and fine vesicles between the collagen fibrils are accumulated in the extracellular space of the adjacent adventitia. × 2,000. **c** Many smooth muscle cells at the transitional zone between the varicose and the normal wall are pycnotic and show accumulated mitochondria in their center. Vacuoles predominate in the adventitia. × 3,800

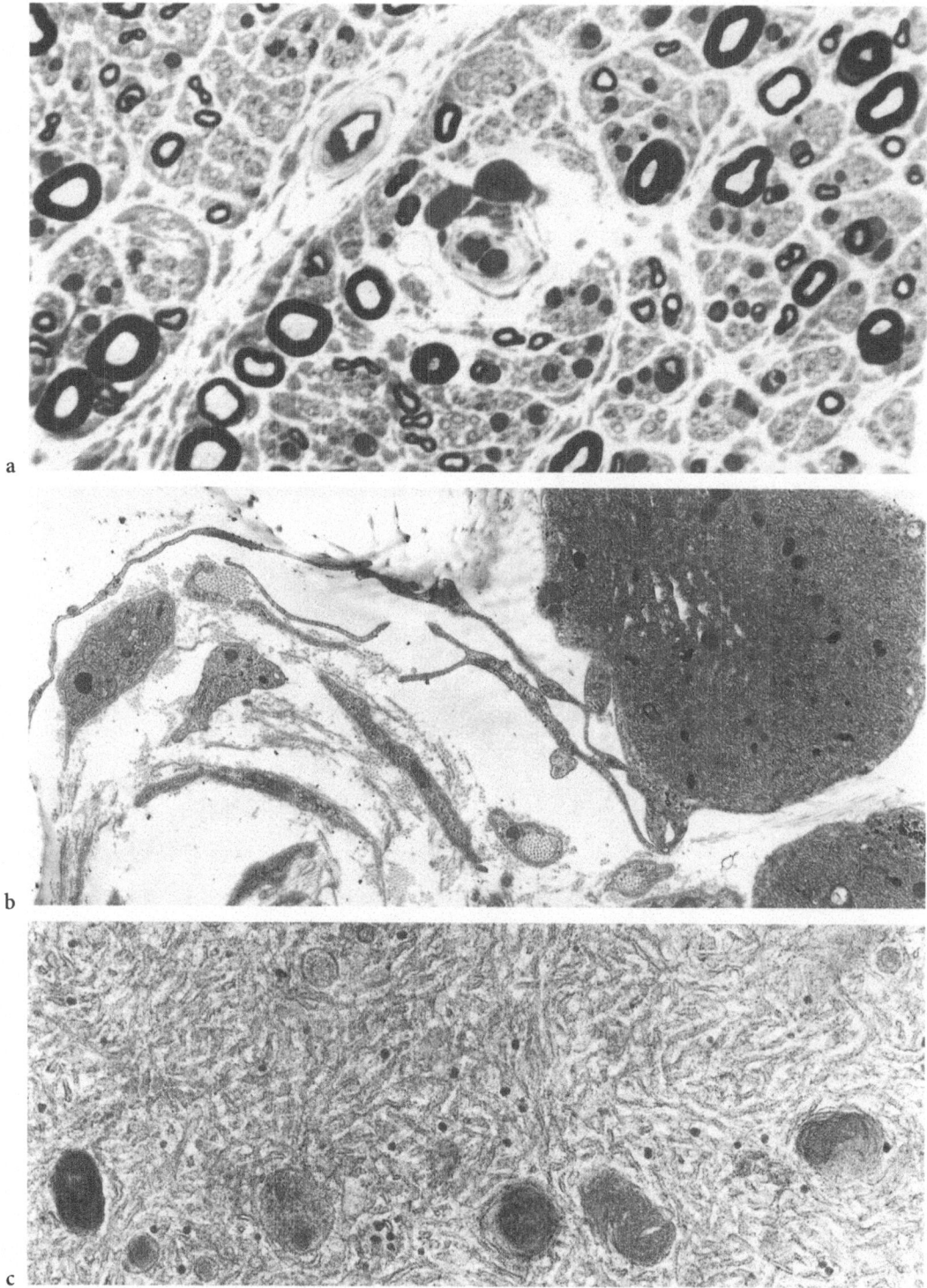

Fig. 243 a – c. Unusual perivascular endoneurial cells with masses of tubulovesicular structures in a 78-year-old patient with neuropathy of an axonal/neuronal type of uncertain etiology. **a** × 10,000; **b** × 8,700; **c** × 53,000

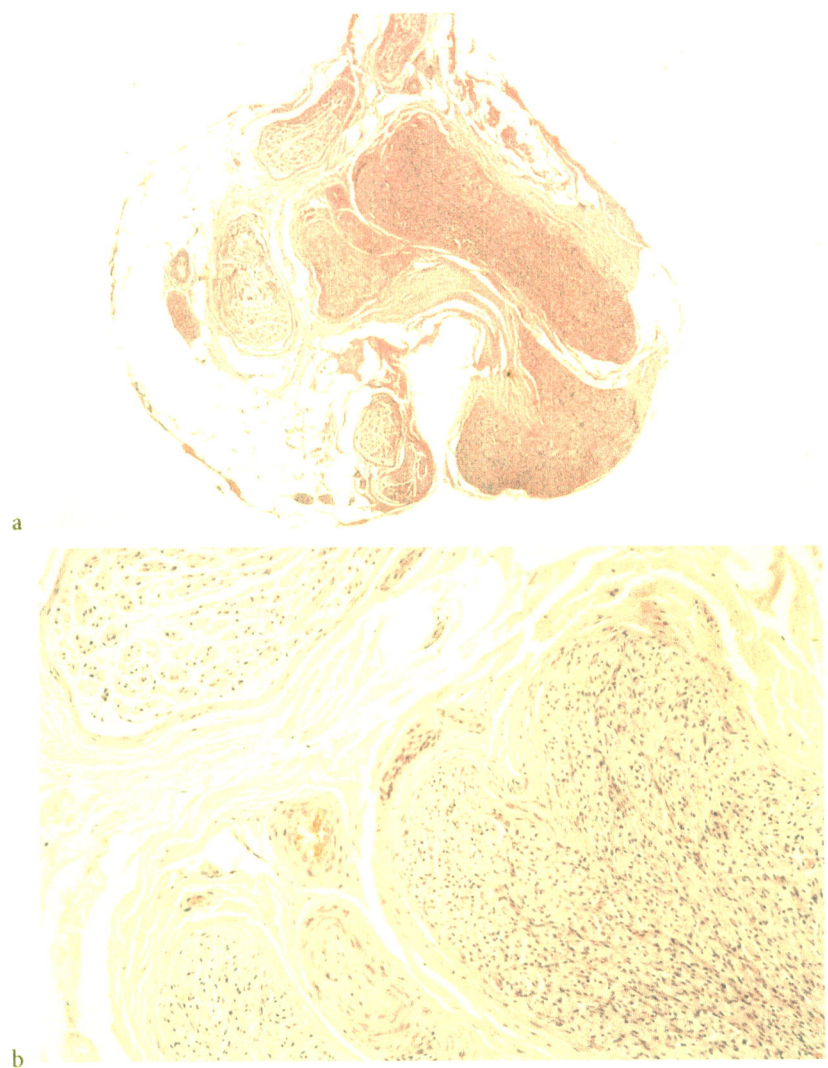

a

b

Fig. 244a–d. Traumatic and/or ischemic lesion of reinnervated, partially fibrotic nerve fascicles adjacent to nearly normal fascicles. **a** and **b** Paraffin: H & E; **c, d** s. p. 284

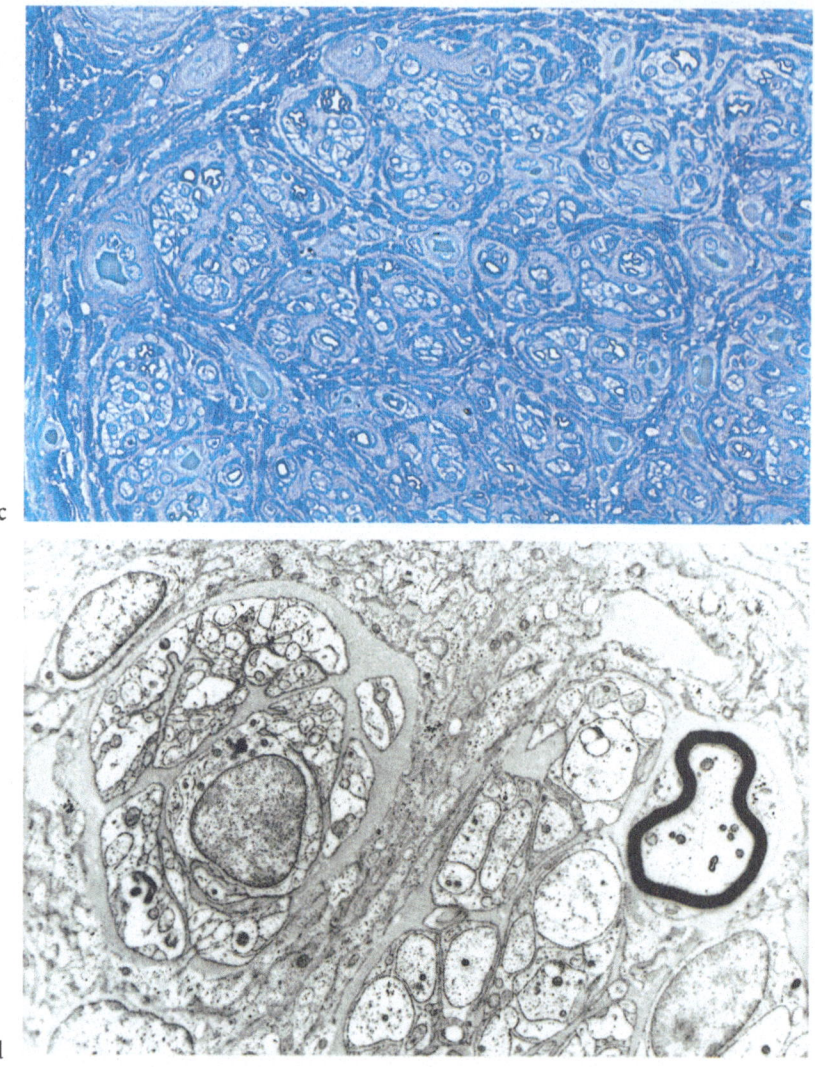

Fig. 244c, d. c Semithin section, toluidine blue; **d** electron microscopic illustration of minifascicle formation which must be distinguished from the growth pattern in a perineurioma (see Figs. 275–276)

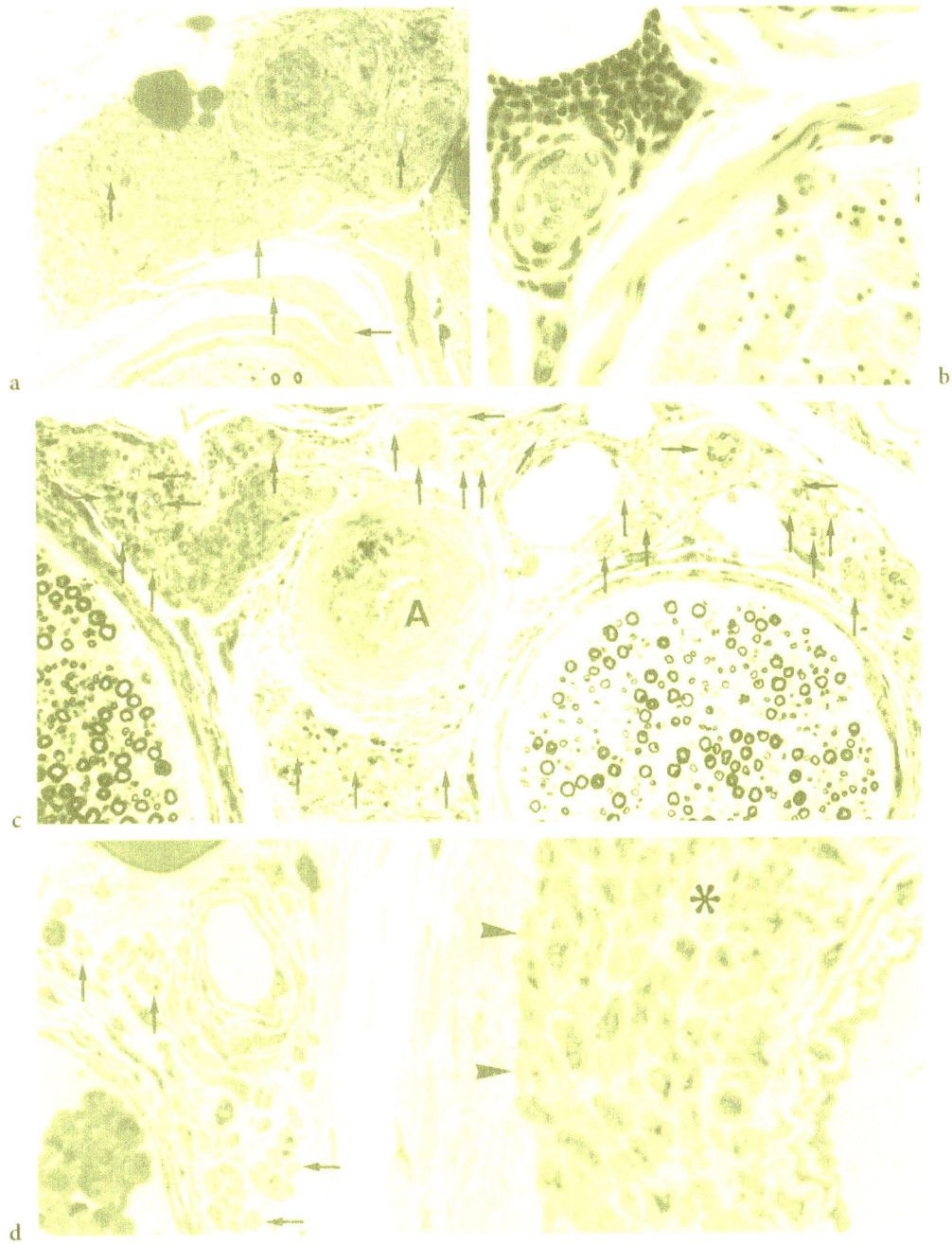

Fig. 245. a Chronic rheumatoid arthritis in a 65-year-old female. Chronic microvasculitis in the epineurium with considerable proliferation of capillaries (*arrows*) and regressively altered infiltrating cells following auro-detoxin therapy. Advanced neuropathy of a neuronal type. × 196. **b** Circumscribed epineurial microvasculitis of uncertain cause with neuropathy mainly axonal in type. Paraffin: H & E. × 430. **c** Chronic vasculitis in cryoglobulinemia (41-year-old female). In the epineurium there are inflammatory mononuclear cellular infiltrates. The number of the capillaries is considerably increased (*arrows*). The neuropathy is of a neuronal type and of moderate severity. × 1,368. **d** Scleroderma in a 67-year-old female (same case as in Fig. 238 d). The epineurial blood vessels show disintegration and sclerosis of the wall with focal separation of smooth muscle cells from the wall (*arrows*) which should not be mistaken for inflammatory cellular infiltrates. The *arrowheads* indicate an adjacent, relatively intact venous wall (*asterisk*). × 640. (From [958])

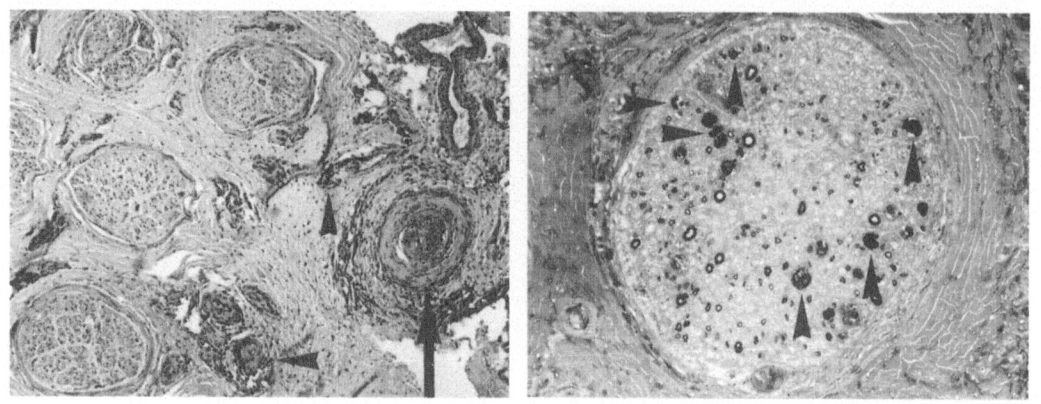

Fig. 246 a, b. Sural nerve biopsy of a 74-year-old man in panarteritis nodosa. **a** Characteristic involvement of several small (*arrowheads*) and large (*thick arrow*) epineurial blood vessels. Paraffin: H & E × 67. **b** The number of myelinated nerve fibers is reduced to less than 10 %. Multiple myelin degradation products (*arrowheads*) indicate an advanced stage of rapidly progressive axonal damage followed by Wallerian degeneration. × 190

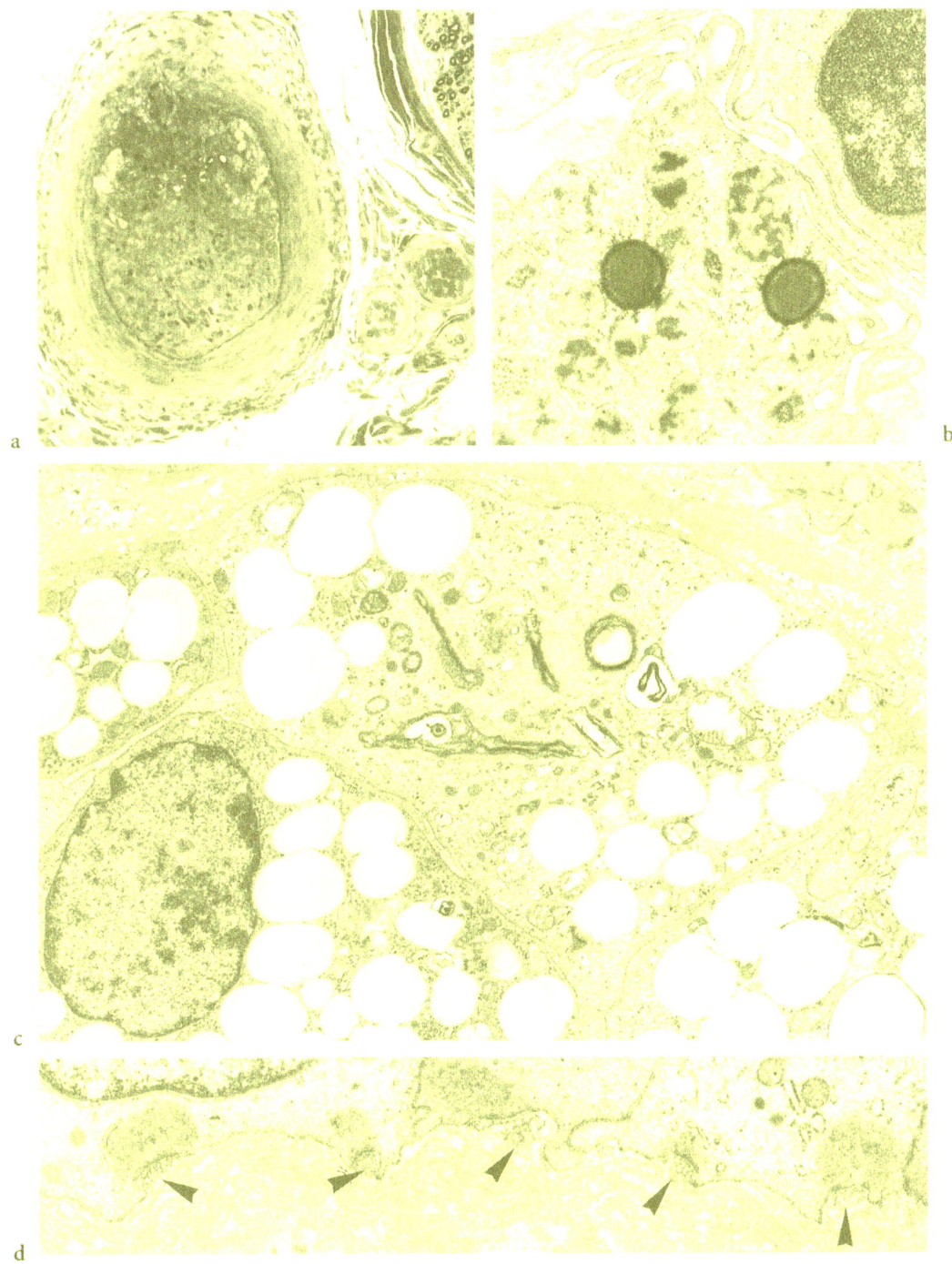

Fig. 247a–d. Epineurial artery obliterated by a cholesterol embolus in a 41-year-old female. **a** The artery is completely occluded. × 168. **b** A partially degranulated mast cell with two calcospherites and an adjacent mononuclear cell show finger-like processes at their surface. × 18,400. **c** Multiple lipid droplets and some membranous structures are apparent within the four adjacent macrophages (foam cells). × 9,800. **d** At the border between the basal lamina, which is irregularly structured, and the underlying endothelial cells there are focal extracellular granular deposits engulfed in small indentations of the surface membrane. Granular or microfilamentous structures are apparent on the adjacent intracellular side (*arrowheads*). × 18,500

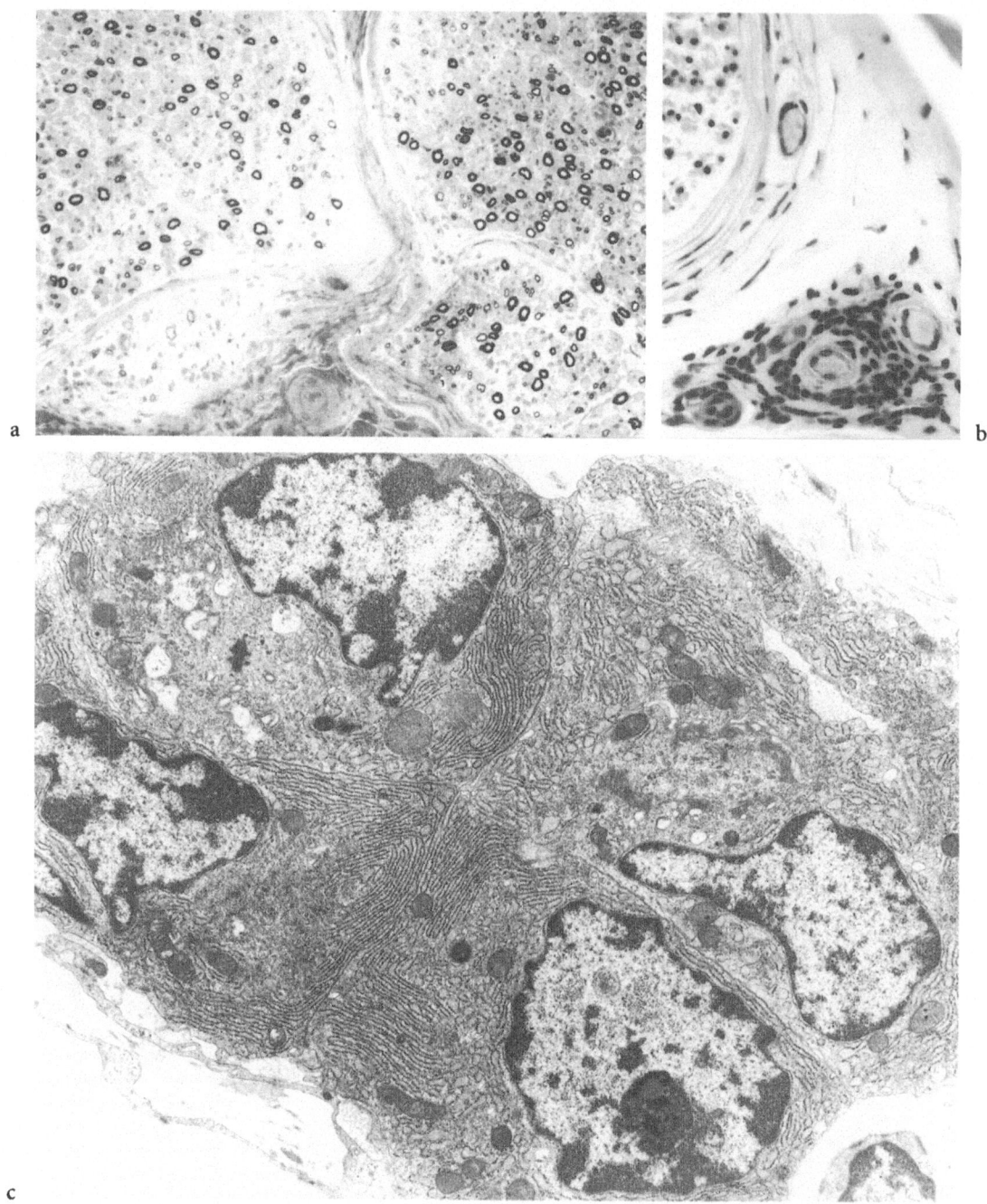

Fig. 248a–c. Epineurial perivascular cellular infiltrates indicating microvasculitis (**b**) associated with chronic neuropathy (**a**) and an unusual cluster of four plasma cells closely attached to each other (**c**) in a 75-year-old female. **a** × 190; **b** × 380; **c** × 8,000

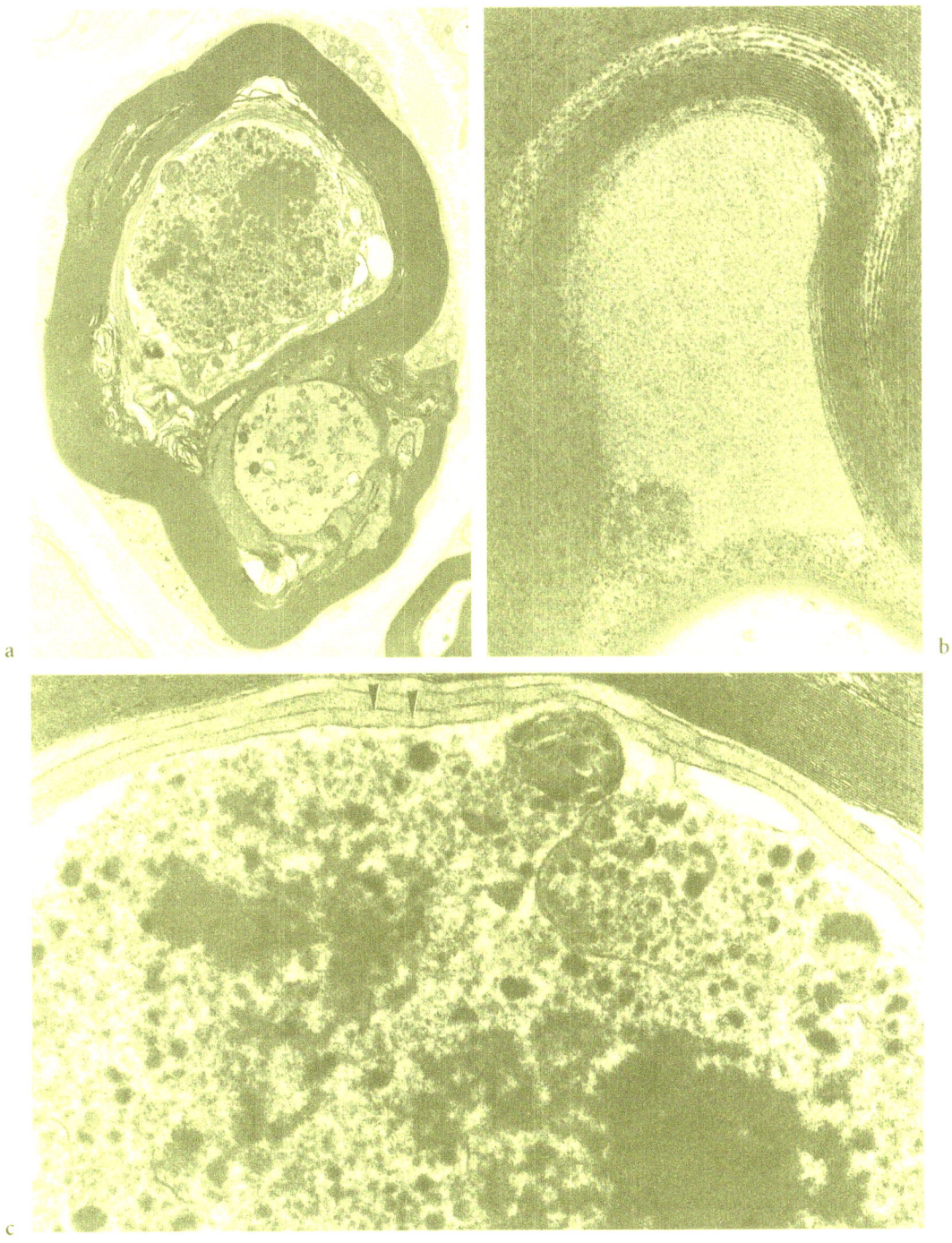

Fig. 249a–c. Exceptionally prominent granular inclusions in the myelin sheaths of a 73-year-old patient with vasculitis. **a** Accumulation of heterogeneous dense granular substances of uneven size at the site of the intraperiod line adjacent to loosely structured myelin lamellae. × 6,800. **b** Homogeneous granular particles which clearly differ from the normal finely granulated substances in Schmidt-Lanterman incisures (see adjacent lamellae). × 44,000. **c** Higher magnification of an area in **a**. The granular substances show diameters between 5 and 1,000 nm. They are of different electron density adjacent to loose myelin lamellae. Between the major dense lines the loose myelin lamellae are subdivided by three to four thinner lines (*arrowheads*). × 34,000. (From [980])

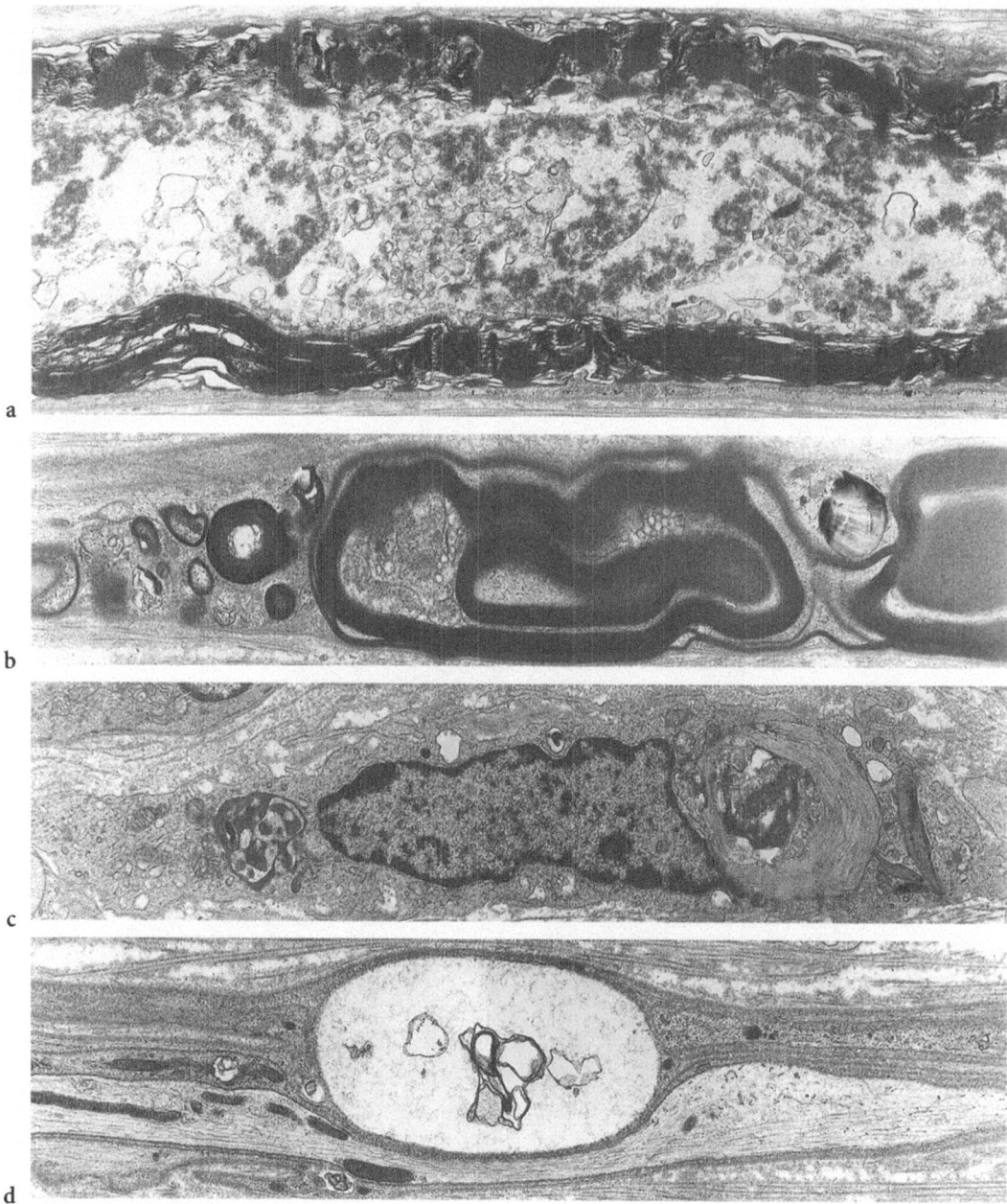

Fig. 250 a – d. Vasculitic neuropathy in a 69-year-old female. **a** Acutely degenerating nerve fiber with focal homogenization of the myelin lamellae and disintegration of the axon, which shows vesicular and amorphic components. × 9,700. **b** Typical pattern of Wallerian degeneration with ovoid formation by the degenerating myelin sheath. × 9,400. **c** Longitudinally oriented macrophage with unevenly large, old myelin degradation products, π-granule-like deposits and a pleomorphic, vacuolated or indented cytosome with a homogeneous matrix adjacent to the nucleus. × 7,300. **d** A large vacuole, presumably derived from a degraded unmyelinated axon, with some vesicular membranous components, has obviously indented a neighboring unmyelinated axon. The mitochondria and small vesicles are accumulating in the axoplasm on one (the proximal?) side, some glycogen granules, microtubules, and amorphous substances on the other. × 9,400

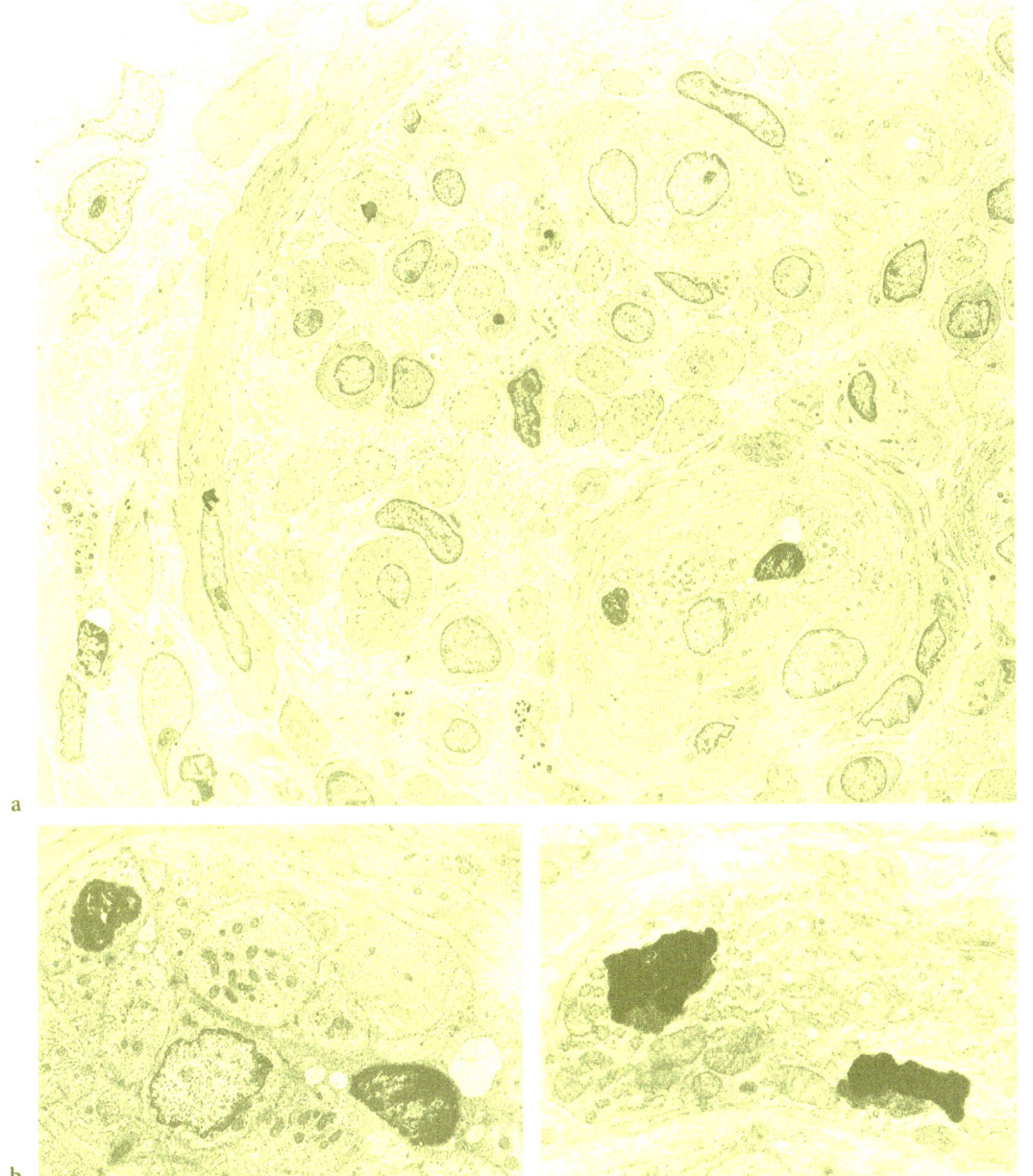

Fig. 251a–c. Obliterated epineurial blood vessels in giant cell arteritis. **a** Numerous smooth muscle cells, most of them in a circular shape, lie at the site of an obliterated artery which is recanalized by three newly formed arterioles. A circularly arranged group of smooth muscle cells still indicates the previous contour of the obliterated blood vessel. × 2,120. **b** Higher magnification of an area in **a**. A myelin-like body is included in an endothelial cell. A pycnotic, karyorrhectic nucleus (apoptosis) can be seen on the *lower right*. × 4,500. **c** Irregular osmiophilic bodies are apparent in a perivascular cell which is rich in components of the ergastoplasma, mitochondria, and Golgi complexes. × 12,400

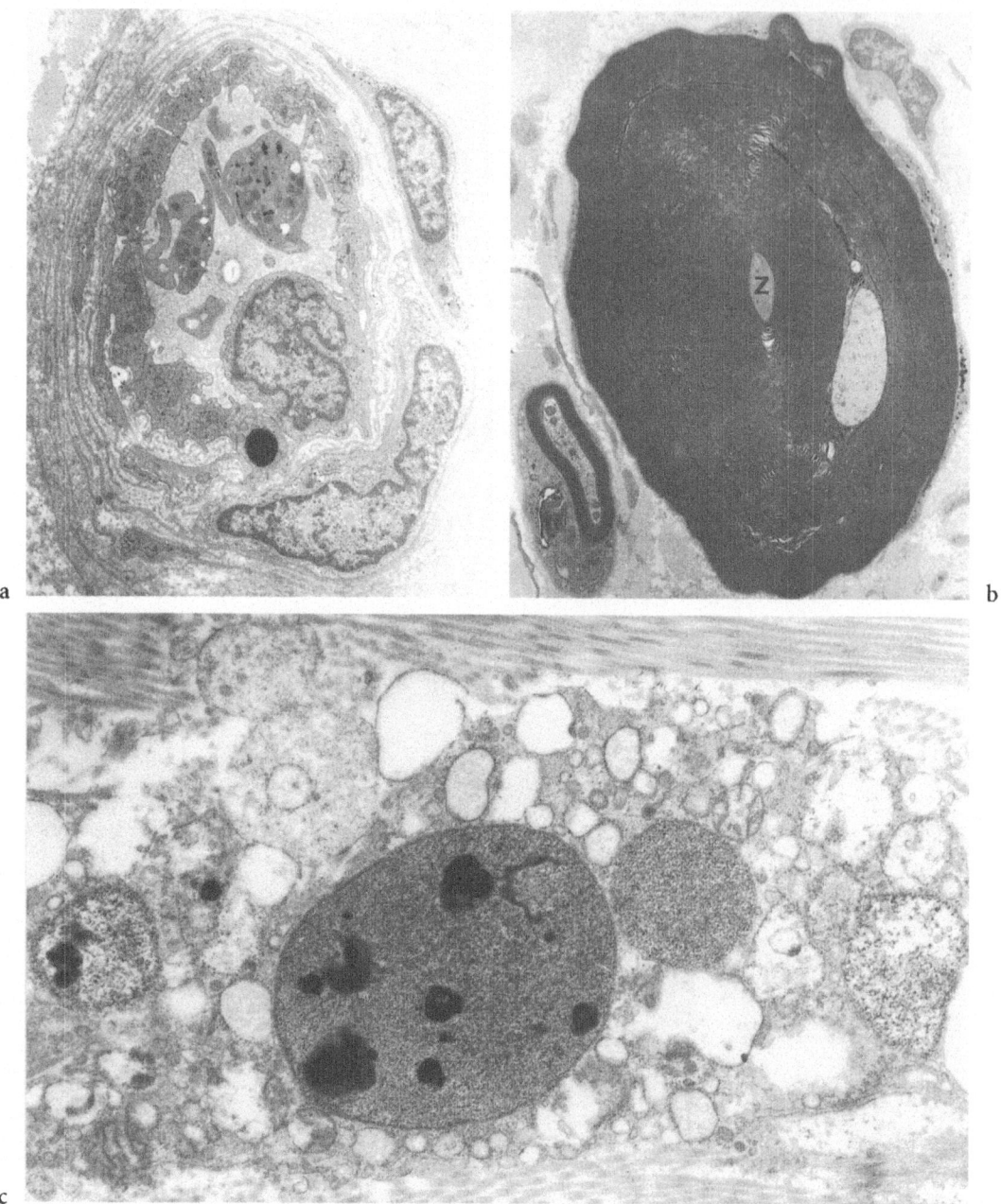

Fig. 252 a – c. Blood vessel and nerve fiber changes in vasculitis with Raynaud's syndrome in a 48-year-old male. Previous mercury exposure was recorded. **a** The number of basal laminae between endothelial cells and smooth muscle cells as well as in the immediate surroundings is increased, but there is no increase in thickness. A large pigment granule is seen in an endothelial cell close to the lower lumen. **b** The center of a large inner myelin loop is indicated by a *Z* adjacent to an atrophic axon. A small myelinated nerve fiber can be seen in the *lower left corner*; its Schwann cell cytoplasm includes a pleomorphic cytosome. A mononuclear cell, presumably a quiescent endoneurial macrophage, is illustrated in the *upper right corner*. **a, b** × 6,500. **c** Degenerating endoneurial fibroblast in a 66-year-old male with vasculitis and psoriasis after administration of corticoids (according to clinical data). A lysosome-like cytosome is characterized by several osmiophilic inclusions. An adjacent cytosome shows a granular substructure; swollen components of the ergastoplasma are also apparent. The surface membrane is focally interrupted. × 15,700

Fig. 253. a Same case as in Fig. 252a, b. Normal structure of unmyelinated axons with a typical glutaraldehyde-related swelling artifact (*arrowhead*) of a longitudinally oriented mitochondrion. The unmyelinated axons are moderately indented at several sites of their surface. × 12,200. **b** Same case as in Fig. 252c. Here the unmyelinated axons show multiple lysosomal and vacuolar inclusions in addition to vesicular and neurosecretory vesicles and glycogen granules. Several asteroid crystalline calcium precipitates can be seen in a Schwann cell process on the *upper right*. × 2,600

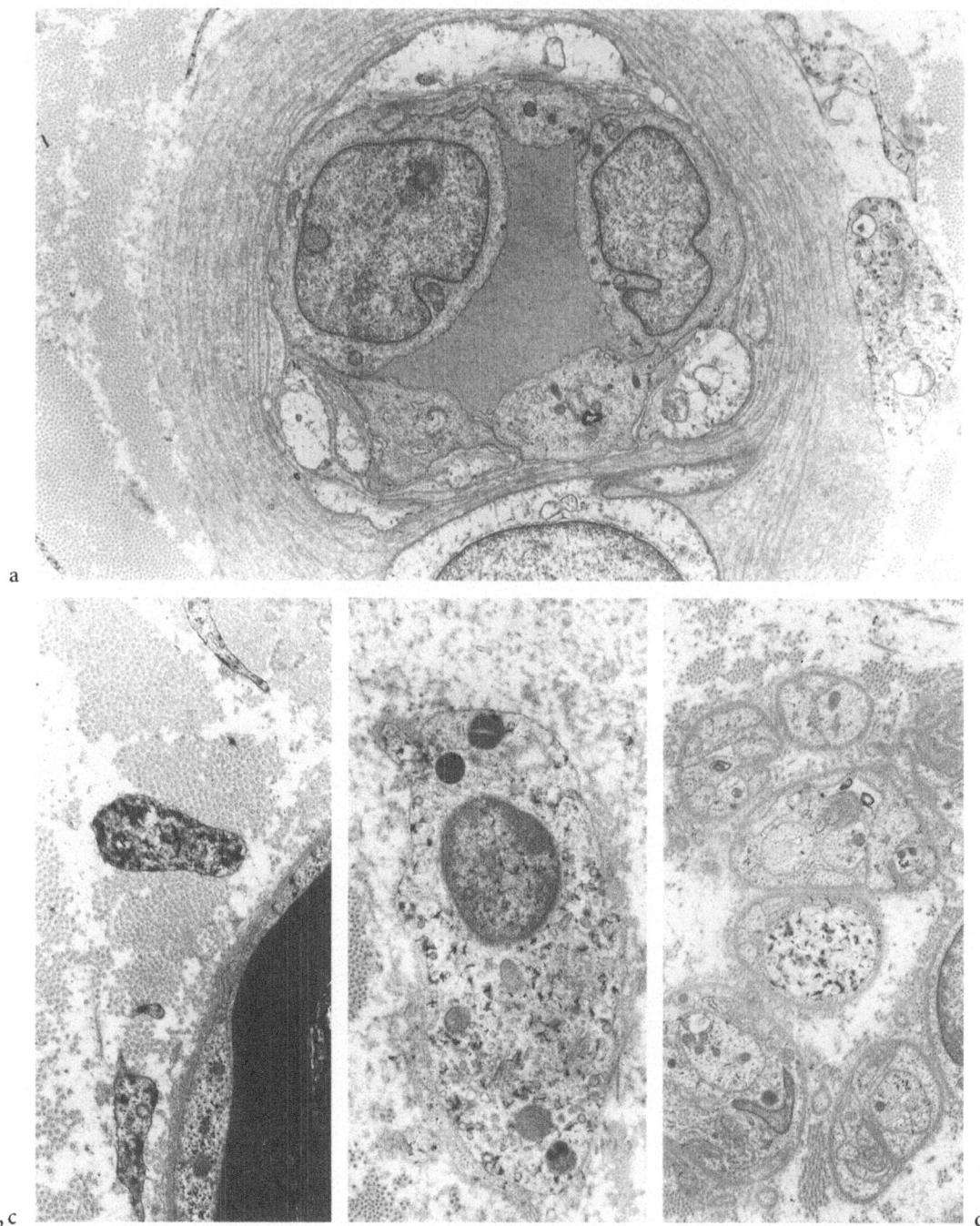

Fig. 254 a–d. Same case as in Figs. 252 c and 253 b. **a** The number of pericapillary basal laminae is considerably increased although not thickened. Multiple asteroid calcium precipitates are seen in the perivascular fibroblasts. × 7,400. **b–d** There are multiple asteroid calcium precipitates in other endoneurial fibroblasts also (**b** and **c**) and in an unidentified cell process in the center of **d**. **b** × 12,200; **c** × 9,700; **d** × 8,300

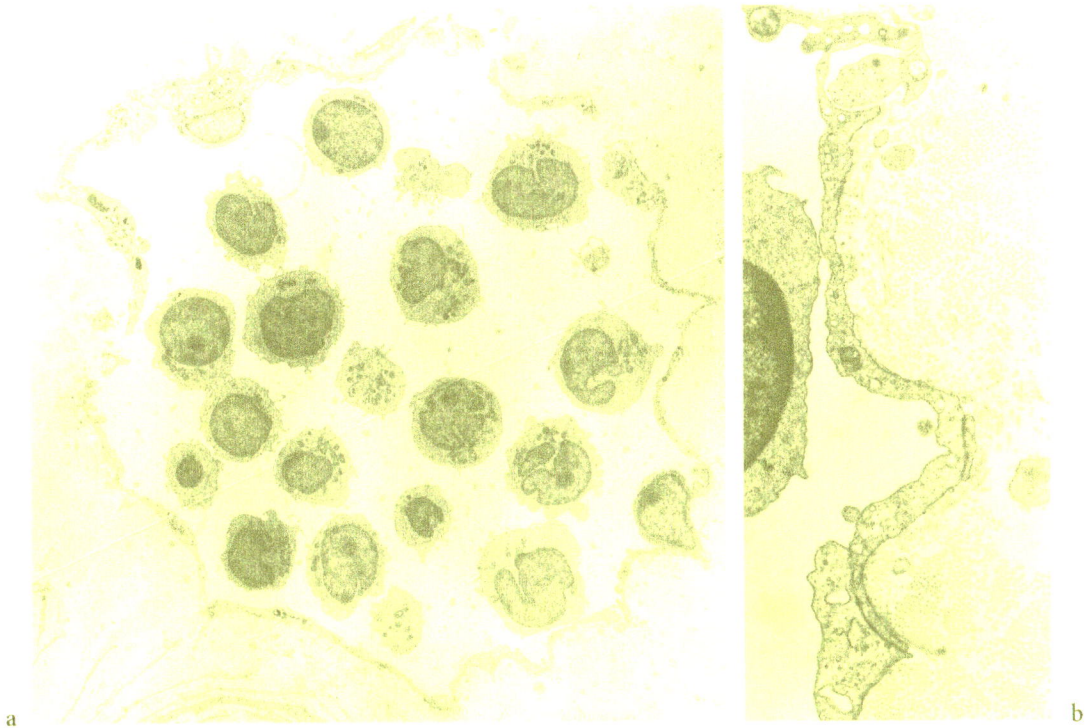

Fig. 255. a Accumulation of lymphocytes in an epineurial lymphatic capillary of a 73-year-old male with polyneuropathy and epineurial vasculitis. × 2,000. **b** Higher magnification of the wall of the lymph vessel in **a**. The endothelial cells of the lymph capillary are connected to each other by special contacts. Epineurial collagen filaments can be seen on the *right*, a lymphocyte on the *left*. × 8,800

Association of Neuropathy with Predominating Diseases of the Central Nervous System

Numerous diseases of the central nervous system are associated with disorders of the peripheral nervous system and vice versa. On the other hand, *amyotrophic lateral sclerosis* (ALS) or *motor neuron disease* (MND), for example, may be erroneously diagnosed instead of demyelinating neuropathy with conduction block or tomaculous neuropathy [278]. Therefore these and other diseases or disorders need to be regarded in this context.

Spinal muscular atrophy (SMA) usually affects proximal muscles (Fig. 34 a, b) [167, 168, 200, 369, 372, 393, 529, 603, 721, 727, 787, 852, 1206, 1282, 1283]. Its distal form [392, 393, 817] is classified by some authors as *distal hereditary motor neuropathy (HMN)* [1136, 1137]. The diseases exclusively or predominantly affecting the motor system are usually diagnosed by muscle biopsies if necessary, without a nerve biopsy. Motor nerve biopsies are rarely performed [185]. Therefore pathomorphologic studies of motor nerves are usually restricted to autopsy material concerning the peripheral nervous system.

ALS is the most frequent disorder affecting the pyramidal system [6, 12, 32, 33, 55, 104, 171, 217, 219, 220, 240, 269, 278, 321, 397, 405, 454, 455, 488, 492, 503, 552, 561, 644, 646, 647, 670, 685, 706, 710, 713 – 715, 780, 786 – 788, 792, 793, 796, 808, 855, 881, 889, 913, 916, 938, 1003, 1037, 1058, 1059, 1103, 1106, 1118, 1147 – 1149, 1153, 1230, 1266].

The *sensory system* in ALS is involved to a minor extent (Fig. 97 e, f) [56, 405, 452, 496]. Usually there are only some fibers with disproportionately thin myelin sheaths presumably indicating preceding demyelination and remyelination. But we often have difficulties in deciding: (1) whether a considerable loss of nerve fibers indicates polyneuropathy and excludes ALS, (2) whether this is still within the limits of a side effect of ALS, or (3) whether there is a chance association of ALS with a neuropathy of a different etiology. Because of this difficulty and because of the heterogeneity of ALS (e.g., sporadic and inherited forms; references see above), no such changes are illustrated in the present atlas.

The spinocerebellar system is involved in *Friedreich's disease* and *dominant cerebellar atrophy (ADCA)*; these diseases are discussed in the chapter on hereditary neuropathies (see above).

Dystonic disorders may involve the peripheral nervous system, such as in *spasmodic torticollis* (Figs. 17 b, 256 – 260) [76, 115, 179, 221, 358, 769, 982, 1300] or *writer's cramp* [133, 146, 479, 765, 1151]. There is increasing evidence that dystonia may be induced by lesions of peripheral nerves [299, 982], especially IA afferents of muscle spindles [371].

Sudden infant death syndrome (SIDS) may be associated with minor changes in the hypoglossal nucleus [782] or in the phrenic nerve [1227], although these changes represent only minor aspects, if any, of the many reasons causing SIDS.

In *Joseph* or *Machado-Joseph disease*, the peripheral nervous system may be involved [291, 378, 466, 486, 513, 517, 527, 544, 641, 642, 813, 906, 1111]. The disease is now considered to be identical with spinocerebellar ataxia type III (SCA3) (see above).

In *granular nuclear inclusion body disease* with central, spinal, and neuromuscular symptoms, characteristic nuclear changes were seen in the muscle and nerve biopsy (Fig. 261 a – d) [952, 985].

Pathognostic granular deposits on the surface of smooth muscle cells are apparent in *cerebral autosomal dominant angiopathy with cortical infarcts and leukoencephalopathy (CADASIL)* affecting not only the intracerebral blood vessels but also smooth muscle cells of arterioles in the sural nerve, muscle (Figs. 262, 263), skin, and the other organs investigated [225, 344, 436, 475, 522, 563, 891, 995].

Unidentified syndromes with changes in the central and peripheral nervous system, such as the one illustrated in Fig. 264 showing peculiar extracellular deposits and lysosomal structures similar to those seen in Kuf's disease, are more frequent in our series than usually indicated in textbooks (unclassified disorders, and diseases waiting for a name).

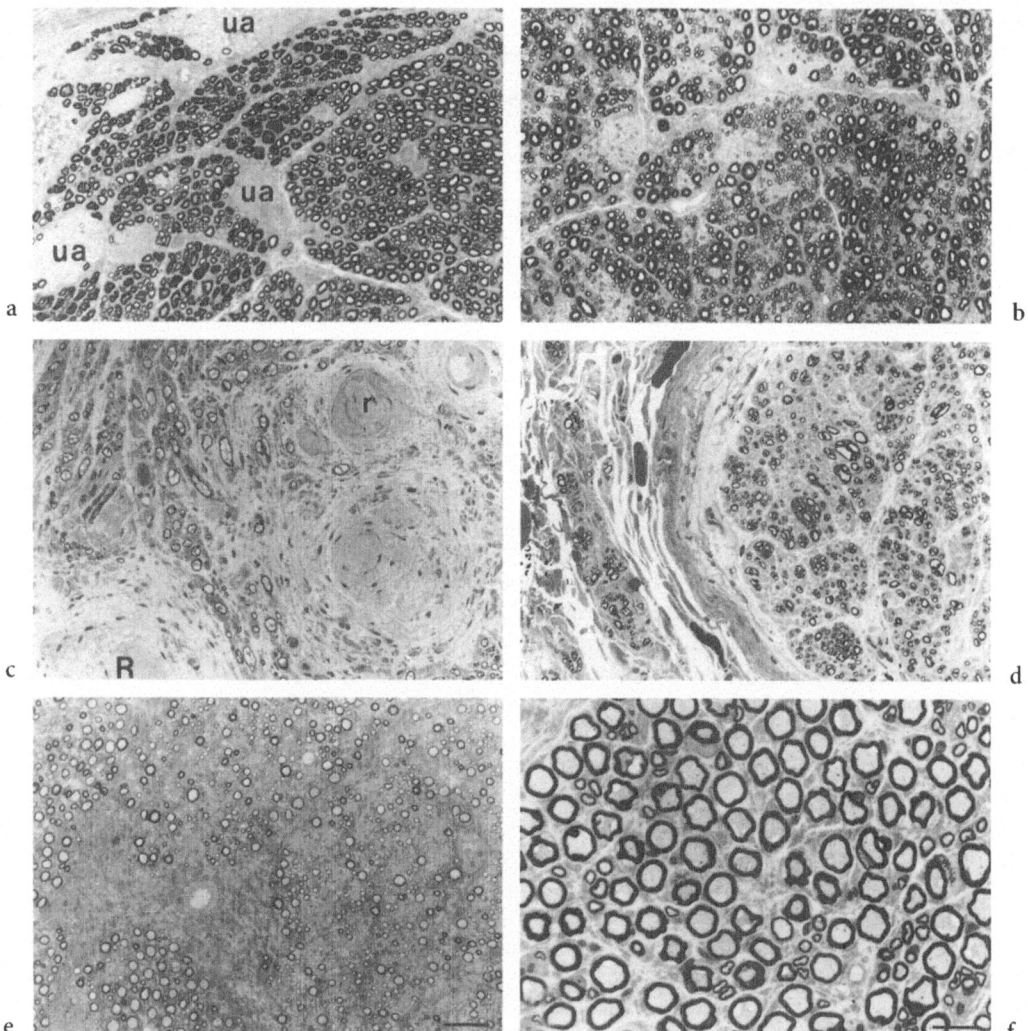

Fig. 256 a–f. Dorsal branches of cervical nerve C1 (**f**) and C2 (**a–e**) in cases with spasmodic torticollis. (From [982]). **a** Normal, large groups of unmyelinated axons (*ua*) are seen between largely preserved myelinated nerve fibers as well as in the subperineurial area of a 46-year-old man whose other studied nerve roots (C3–6) showed only some Renaut bodies but were otherwise inconspicuous. **b** Most nerve fibers in this fascicle appeared to be normal although nerve fibers with relatively thin myelin sheaths were repeatedly seen in this 39-year-old female. **c** Large and small Renaut bodies with adjacent nerve fibers showing abnormally thin myelin sheaths in this 63-year-old female. **d** Same case and same nerve as in **b**, 22 months after the excision of a 1.0 cm-long segment of this nerve revealing spontaneous reinnervation. Numerous unevenly distributed regenerated nerve fibers are found in the preexisting fascicle and in some newly formed epineurial minifascicles (neuromatous type of the reinnervation) in the adjacent connective tissue. The axons are usually small, and the myelin sheaths relatively thinner than in the first surgical specimen (morphometric evaluation: see Fig. 257). **e** Most axons are relatively large, but their myelin sheaths are disproportionately thin in comparison to the nerves in **a** and **b**. Only a few groups of small regenerated nerve fibers are apparent. The endoneurial connective tissue is considerably increased. Onion bulb formations are not apparent (ramus dorsalis of C2 in a 59-year-old female). **f** The myelinated nerve fibers in this dorsal branch of the C1 root are (as usual at this site in the 34 cases studied) inconspicuous, except for isolated fibers with disproportionately thin myelin sheaths and an occasional cluster of regenerated fibers. **a–e** × 168; **f** × 420

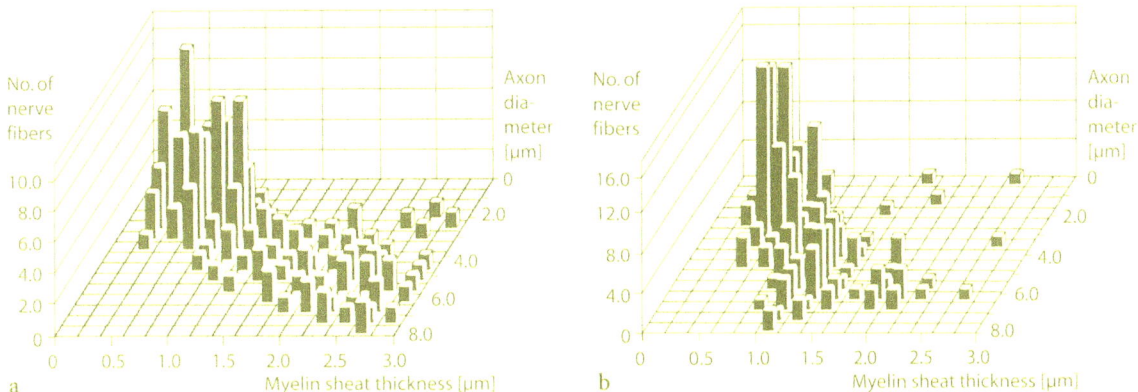

Fig. 257 a, b. Three-dimensional diagram of the relation between axon diameter, myelin sheath thickness, and the number of nerve fibers in the dorsal branch of cervical nerve no. 2 in a 49-year-old female with spasmodic torticollis. **a** At the time of the first operation (same case as in Fig. 256 b). **b** At the time of the second operation: result of reinnervation 22 months after excision of a nerve segment, approximately 11 mm in length. There are considerably more small and thinly myelinated nerve fibers as in the normal nerve (**a**); the number of large, thickly myelinated nerve fibers is clearly reduced. (Modified from [114])

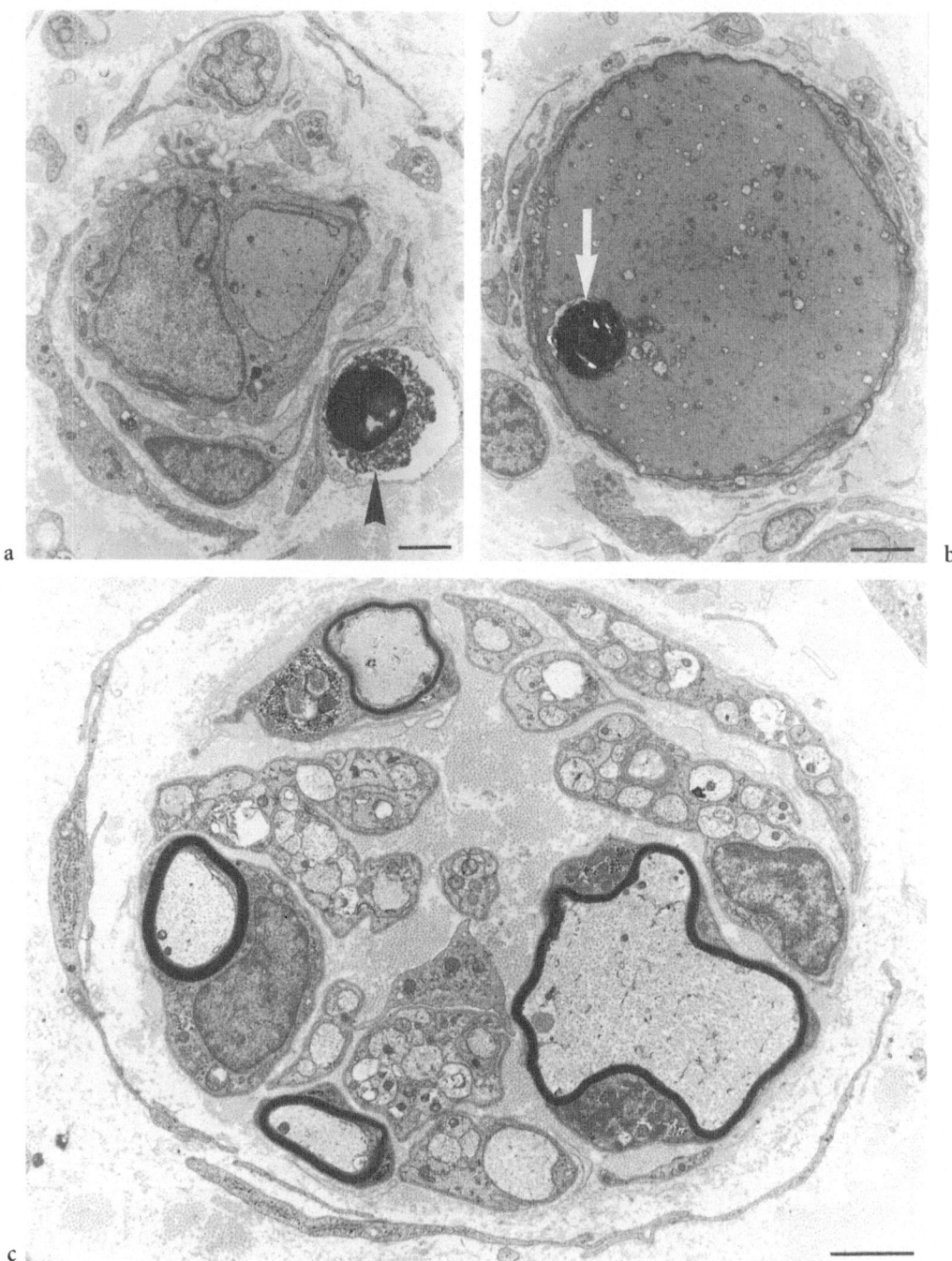

Fig. 258a–c. Dorsal branch of C2 in a 59-year-old female with spasmodic torticollis. **a, b** Thinly remyelinated, condensed axons with numerous densely packed neurofilaments. Several circularly arranged processes of Schwann cells and fibroblasts can be seen in the surrounding area. A degenerated cell (apoptotic body, *arrowhead*) is obviously phagocytosed by another cell (presumably a macrophage). Bar = 3 μm. **b** A large axon with an increased number of neurofilaments contains at major membranous cytoplasmic body as a sign of a nonspecific focal degradation (*arrow*). Bar = 2 μm. **c** A group of thinly myelinated and unmyelinated regenerated axons is almost completely surrounded by endoneurial fibroblastic processes, presumably as a sign of incipient minifascicle formation (compartmentalization). (From [982]).

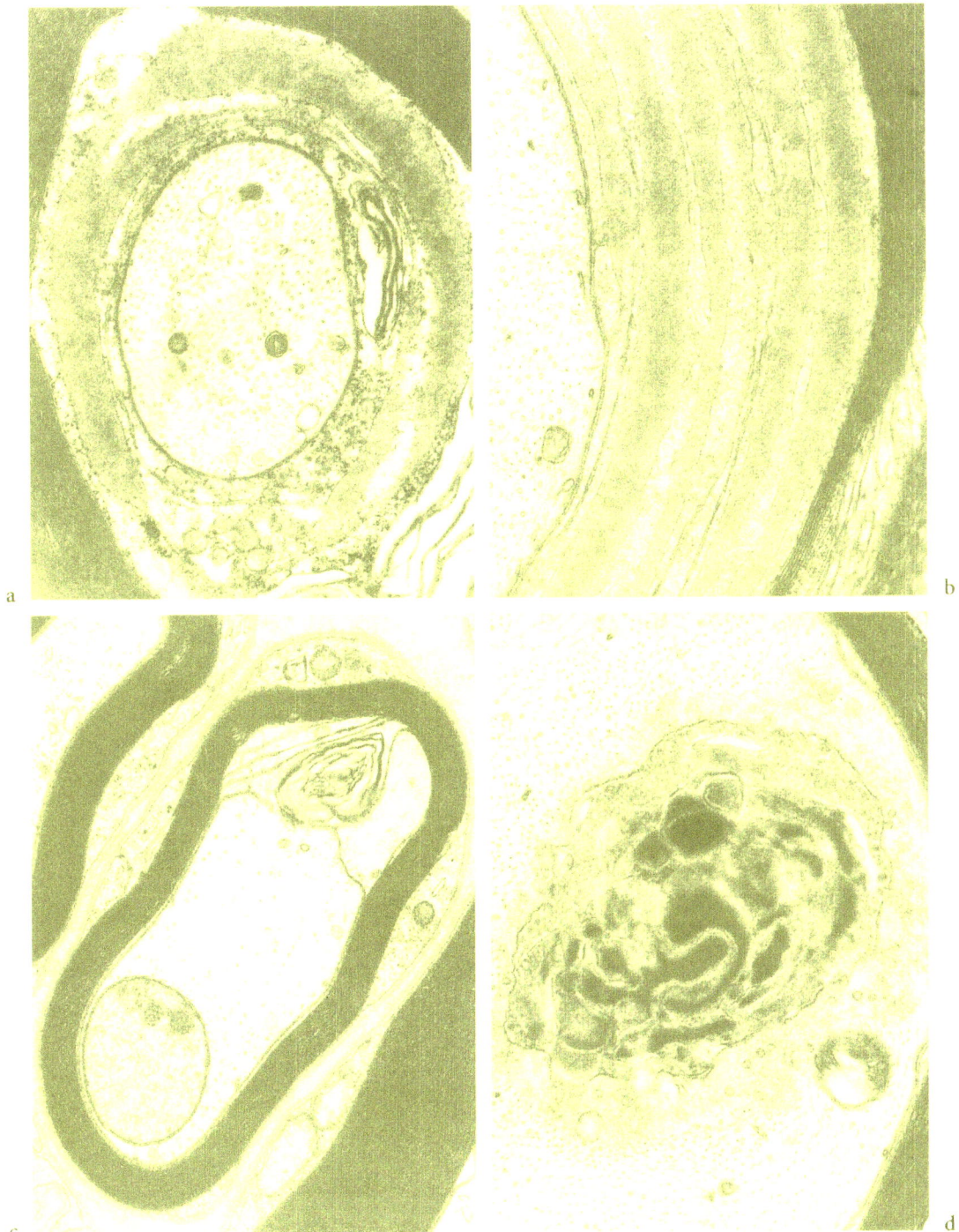

Fig. 259 a – d. Spasmodic torticollis in a 66-year-old man. **a, b** Amorphous or finely granulated masses resembling deposits of immunoglobulins can be seen in the extracellular space between axon and inner, noncompacted myelin lamellae. **a** × 31,000; **b** × 40,000. **c** Unusually large mitochondrion with abnormal, irregularly arranged tubular structures in a regenerated myelinated nerve fiber. × 24,000. **d** Abnormal membrane-limited axonal inclusion with partly granular, partly osmiophilic amorphous components and adjacent fine vesicular components. × 34,000

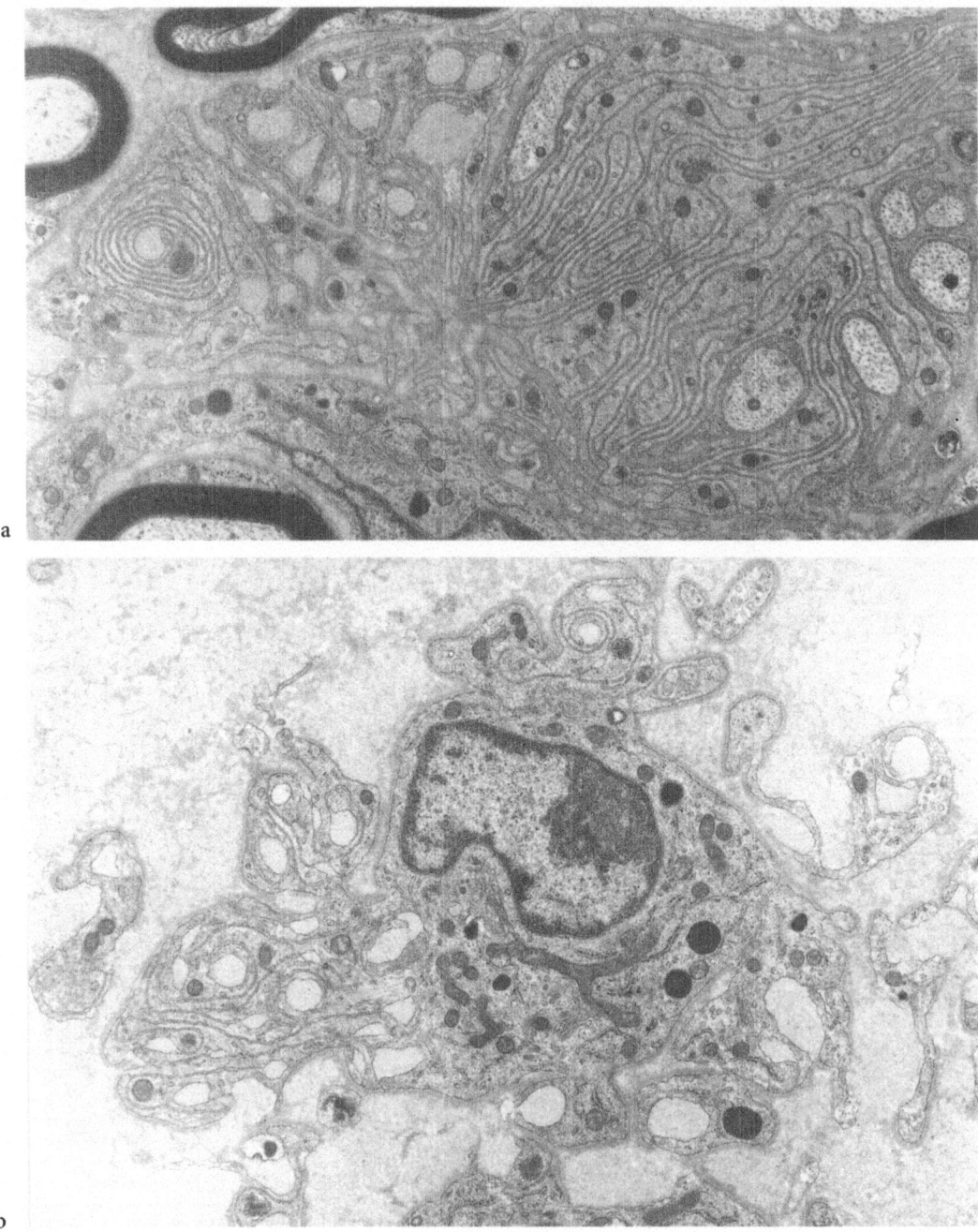

Fig. 260 a, b. Same case as in Fig. 259. **a** Complex interdigitating Schwann cell processes (as seen in neurinomas) with unmyelinated axons on the *right side* and so-called collagen pockets on the *left side*, focally with five noncompacted Schwann cell lamellae around a bundle of collagen fibrils. × 12,200. **b** Schwann cell with multiple processes and numerous collagen pockets at the site of presumably degenerated unmyelinated axons. × 13,300

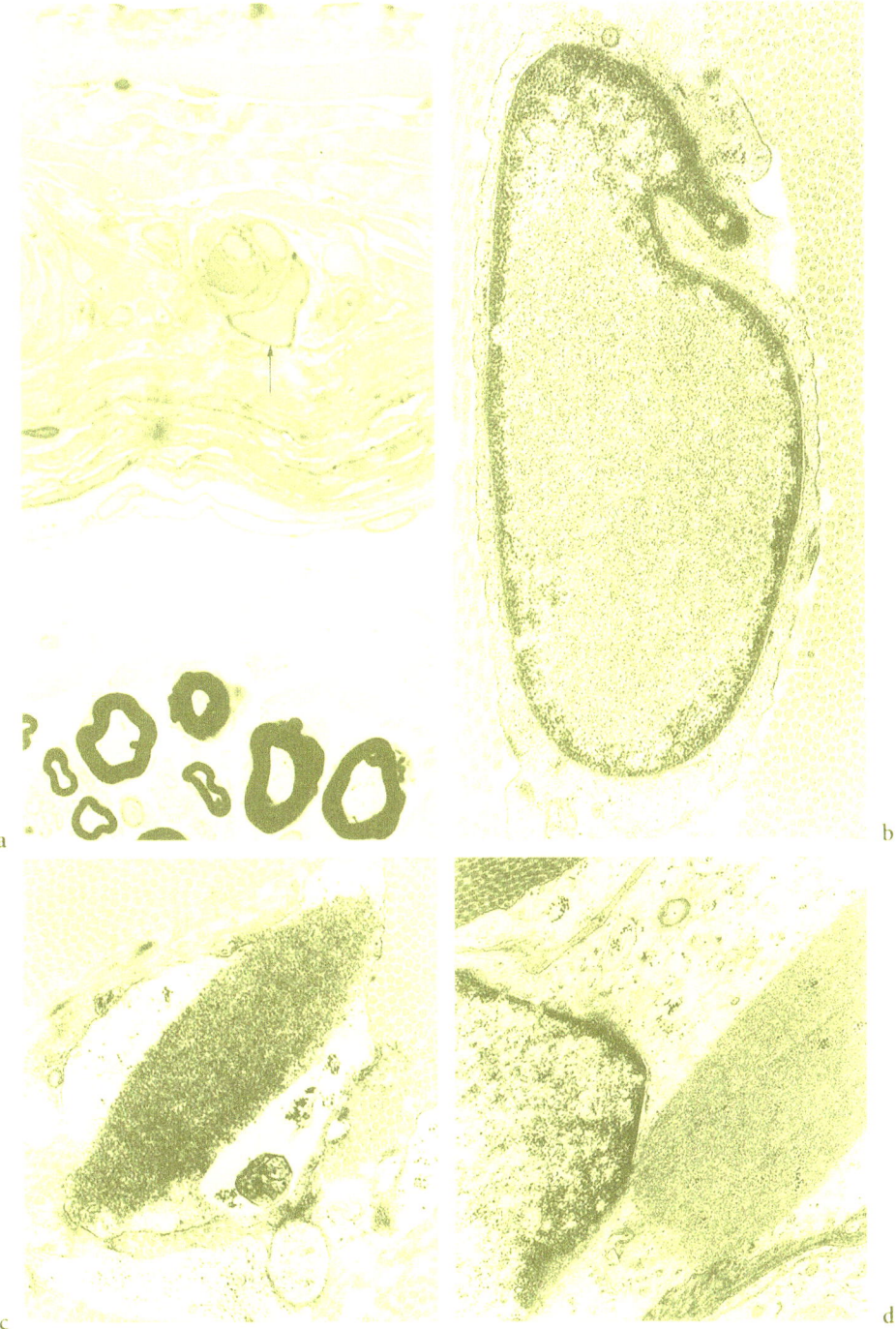

Fig. 261a–d. Granular nuclear inclusion body disease in a 32-year-old female. (From [985]). **a** An enlarged nucleus of a fibroblast is seen adjacent to an epineurial blood vessel showing an intranuclear hyaline inclusion body (*arrow*). The perineurial and endoneurial cells did not contain such nuclear inclusions. × 710. **b** Epineurial fibroblast with a hyaline granular nuclear inclusion body. The cytoplasm is narrow and undifferentiated. × 38,000. **c** Abnormal granular cytoplasmic inclusion without a surrounding nuclear membrane in a swollen fibroblastic process showing some adjacent glycogen granules and a considerable degree of cytoplasmic swelling. × 21.000. **d** Finely granulated, non-membrane-bound cytoplasmic inclusion in contact with a nucleus in an epineurial fibroblast. Some glycogen granules can be seen between the finely granulated substances. × 19,700

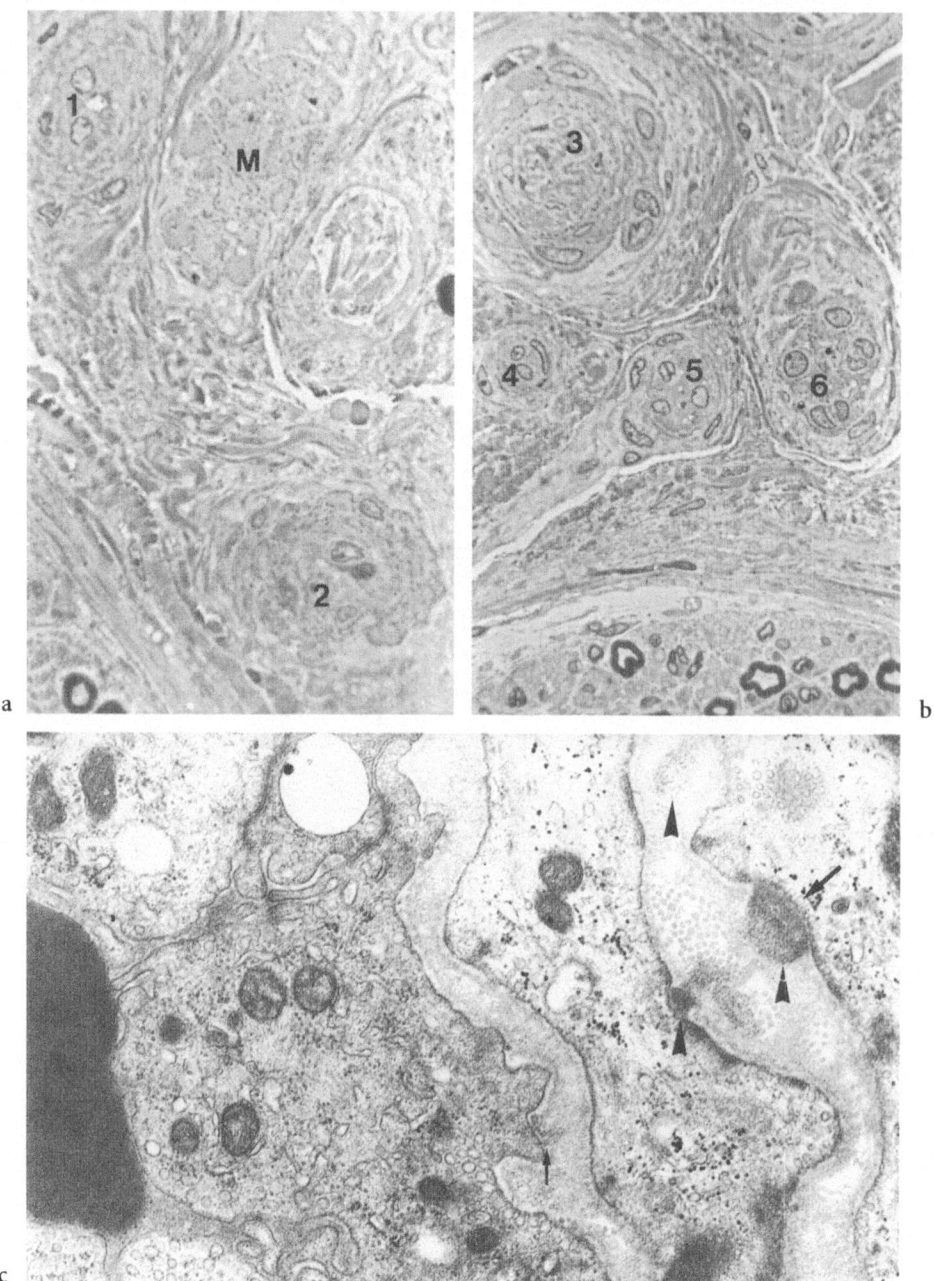

Fig. 262. a, b Thickened epineurial blood vessels in a sural nerve biopsy of a 60-year-old female with cerebral autosomal dominant arteriopathy with subcortical infarcts and leukoencephalopathy (CADASIL). (From [995]). **a** A group of proliferated smooth muscle cells (*M*) is seen adjacent to blood vessel no. 1 in **a**. Three smooth muscle cells appear to be separating from arteriole no. 3 in **b**. The number of cells are increased according to counts of the nuclei in blood vessels no. 1 and 4–6. The lumina of the blood vessels appear to be occluded or collapsed, presumably because of ischemia during excision of the nerve. **c** Electron microscopically, there is a characteristic granular osmiophilic material (GOM) in the extracellular space (*arrowheads*). These precipitates are usually connected to the surface membrane of smooth muscle cells. On the inside, there may be numerous pinocytotic vesicles attached to this site (*arrow*). An accumulation of vesicles of similar size can be seen immediately above this area in the cytoplasm. The basal lamina is interrupted by the GOM. Other GOMs are apparent between collagen fibrils. A very small precipitate appears to be connected to an endothelial cell (*small arrow*). An erythrocyte is seen in the lumen of the blood vessel. **a** × 940; **b** × 750; **c** × 34,000

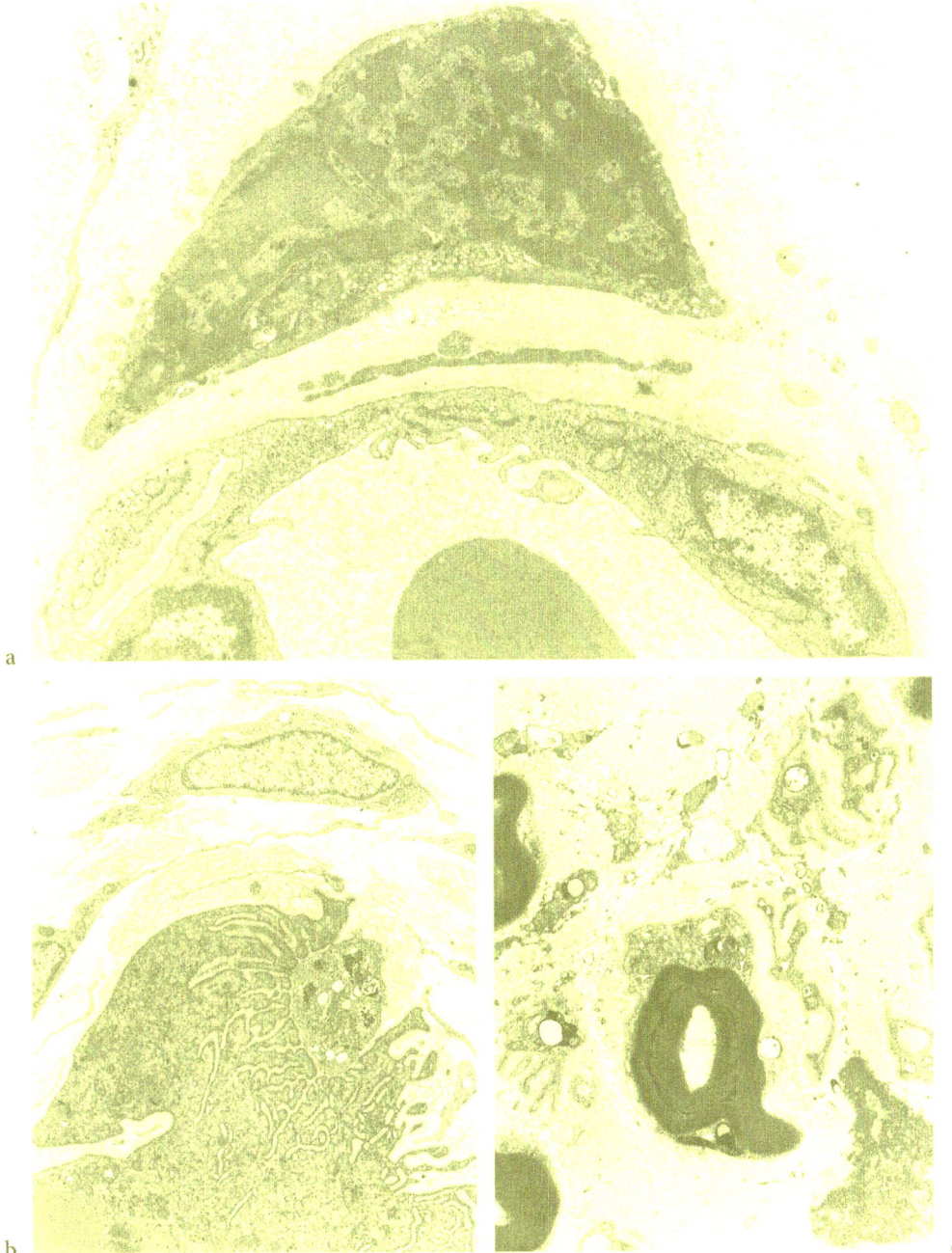

Fig. 263 a–c. Muscle biopsy of a 57-year-old man with CADASIL. **a** CADASIL-specific depositions (GOMs) are apparent in the vicinity of perivascular condensed cells which are likely to be degenerating smooth muscle cells. × 12,600. **b** Motor end plate with increased basal lamina remnants, an altered terminal axon with increased glycogen deposits, and other organelles as well as abnormally branched synaptic folds in a partly atrophic muscle fiber. CADASIL-specific deposits (GOMs) do not occur at this site. × 8,600. **c** This intramuscular nerve fascicle shows regressive alterations including empty Schwann cell processes which appear to be shrunken, a degenerating endoneurial fibroblast which has lost most of its cytoplasm (*lower right*), and an atrophic axon with a shrunken myelin sheath showing a myelin loop at the level of a Schmidt-Lanterman incisure. In the vicinity are numerous cell degradation products in the form of vacuoles, granules, and remnants of thin processes. × 7,200

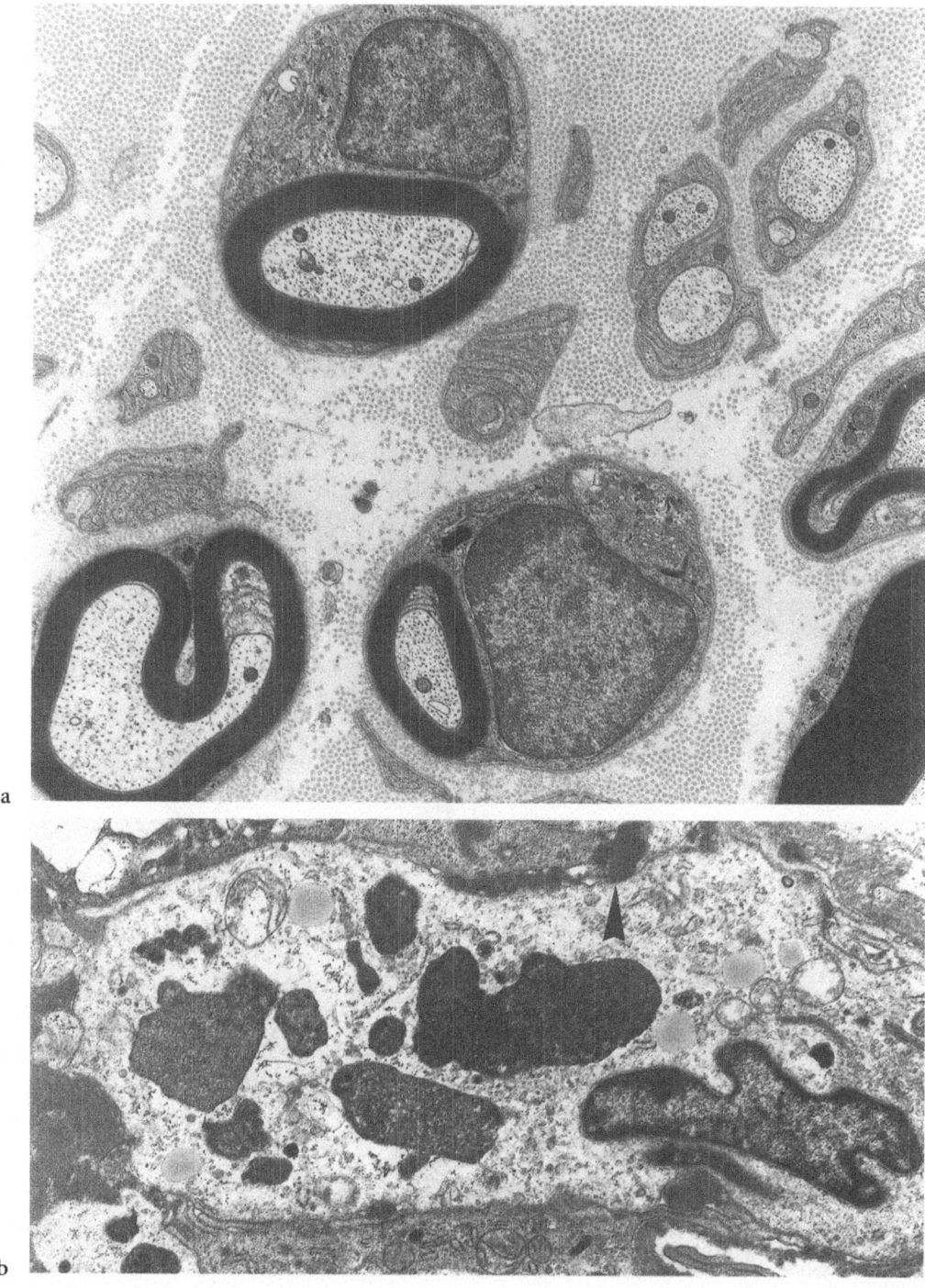

Fig. 264 a, b. Fourty-two-year-old female with unidentified myopathy, polyneuropathy, cardiomyopathy, alterations of the white substance, and mental retardation. **a** Groups of empty Schwann cell processes in the endoneurium indicate previous degeneration mainly of unmyelinated axons, whereas the myelinated fibers shown here appear to be rather inconspicuous. × 13,000. **b** Abnormal lysosomes with focally suggestive curvilinear substructure, similar to those seen in Kuf's disease (adult variant of ceroidlipofuscinosis), are seen in a cell within a myophagic reaction. The conspicuous electron dense, homogeneous deposits in the adjacent extracellular space (*arrowhead*) are of unknown nature and origin

CHAPTER 15

Tumors of the Peripheral Nervous System

Detailed information about tumors of the peripheral nervous system with molecular genetic data is nowadays available [519, 520, 927], although some classic monographs mainly on histopathological aspects are also recommended [80, 273, 394, 534, 541].

The most frequent nerve sheath tumors are benign with isolated occurrence. If multifocal, they are associated with *neurofibromatosis type 1 (NF1)* (Figs. 269–272) [374, 605, 634, 1196], or *neurofibromatosis type 2 (NF2)* [81, 618, 621, 894, 1010, 1011, 1081]. These are:

- *Neurinomas (Schwannomas)* (Figs. 265–267) [10, 34, 43, 58, 81, 137, 140, 165, 218, 304, 417, 648, 649, 778, 815, 935, 1057, 1081, 1108, 1231, 1242, 1249, 1262].
- *Neurofibromas* (Figs. 268–272) [16, 43, 63, 194, 214, 288, 374, 540, 618, 621, 634, 649, 816, 866, 894, 899, 933, 935, 1010, 1011, 1034, 1054, 1061, 1072, 1129, 1196, 1211, 1261].

Malignant peripheral nerve sheath tumors (MPNSTs) are much less frequent (roughly 1.6% of nerve sheath tumors in our series) (Figs. 273, 274) [193, 307, 410, 411, 575, 877, 921, 933, 1035].

Other rare tumors of the peripheral nervous system include *neurothekeomas* (nerve sheath myxomas) [814], *perineuriomas* (localized hypertrophic neuropathy) (Figs. 275, 276) [82, 166, 581, 680, 682, 822, 1150], *psammomatous melanotic neurinomas, fibrolipomatous hamartomas,* and *neuromuscular hamartomas (triton tumors)* [36, 77, 122, 386, 1248] occurring in a benign form (*benign triton tumor,* neuromuscular hamartoma, neuromuscular choristoma) and in a *malignant form (malignant triton tumor,* MPNST with rhabdomyoblastic differentiation).

Myxomatous cysts (neuropathia pseudocystica) derived from adjacent synovial components are most frequently seen in the peroneal nerve at the caput fibulae (Figs. 277, 278) [541].

Benign granular cell tumors and *alveolar soft tissue sarcoma* (malignant alveolar cell tumor) may originate from peripheral nerves and other tissues (see Figs. 150 a, b, 151 a – e in [952]). *Hemangiomas* are also not specific for peripheral nerves. *Fibromas,* on the other hand, may focally develop in nerve fascicles.

Neuromas (Fig. 44 a) are not neoplasmas or blastomas, but reactive enlargements of peripheral nerves at the site of transection and regeneration with or without achieving contact to the peripheral nerve stump (see above).

Tumors of peripheral neurons include those of the *sympathic system,* namely:

- *Ganglioneuromas* (Fig. 269 f) [1265].
- *Ganglioneuroblastomas* (Figs. 279 a, b, 281 a – d, 282) and *neuroblastomas* (Fig. 280 a, b) [233, 370, 476, 493, 532, 1029, 1146, 1244].
- *Phaeochromocytomas* [119, 214, 588, 885, 1265].
- Sympathic *paragangliomas* of extra-adrenal chromaffine cells innervated by the sympathicus.

Tumors of the *parasympathic system* include parasympathic *paragangliomas* (chemodectomas) of chemoreceptors innervated by the parasympathicus [119, 214, 1071].

Tumors of *paraneurons* [309] include some of those belonging to the *amine precursor uptake and decarboxylation (APUD) system,* so-called *Askin tumors* [31] corresponding to supraclavicular metastases of small cell bronchial carcinomas, *mucosa neuromas* in *multiple endocrine neoplasia (MEN) type IIb* [214, 420, 588, 1177], and others such as *Merkel cell tumors* (see [573]), which are more appropriately described and illustrated in articles or monographs on skin and other tumors.

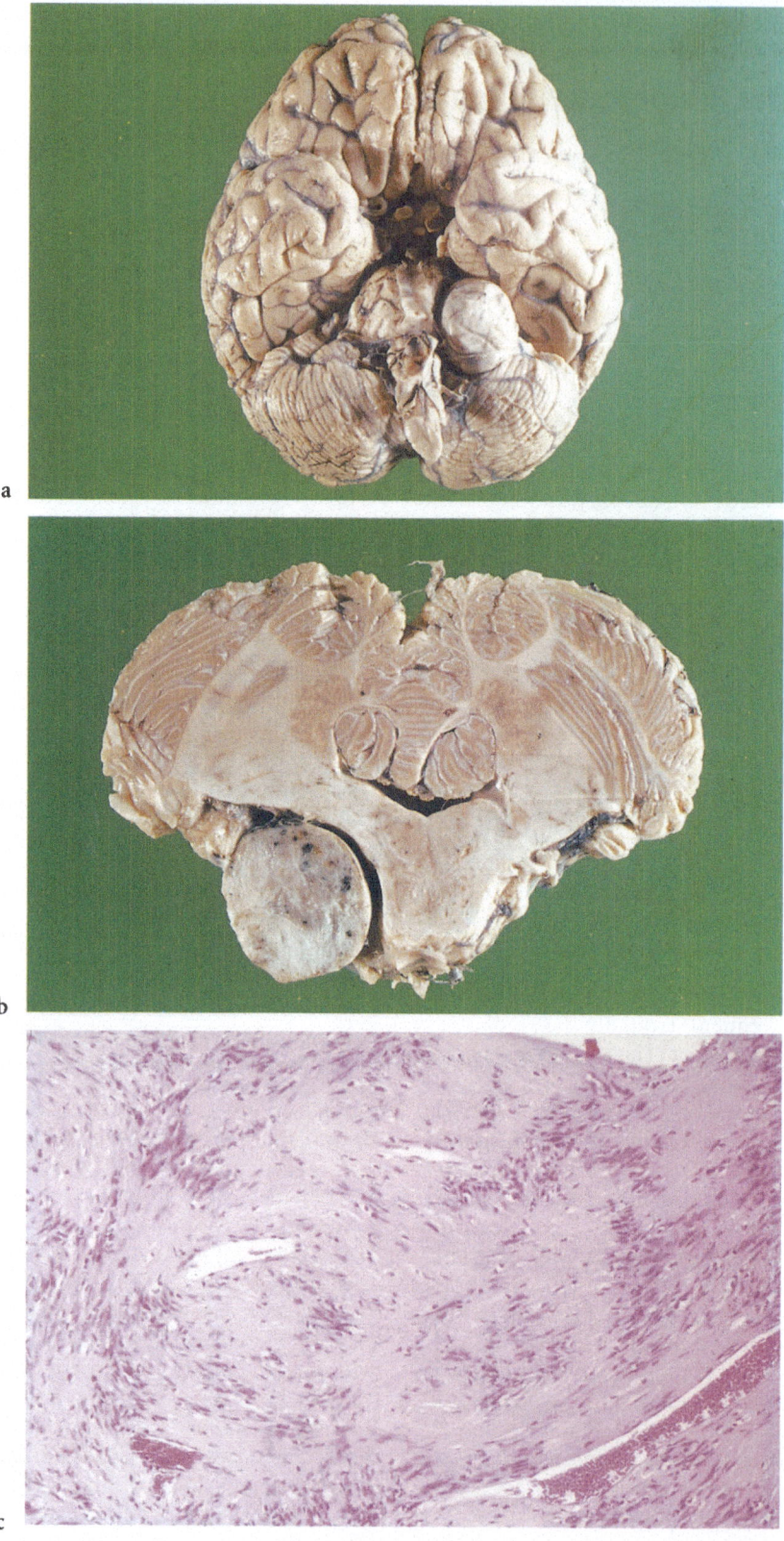

Fig. 265. a, b Typical, clinically asymptomatic acoustic neurinoma which had not been detected before autopsy. **c** Rhythmic, palisaded arrangement of the cell nuclei (Verocay bodies) in mainly spindle-shaped cells. Paraffin: H & E

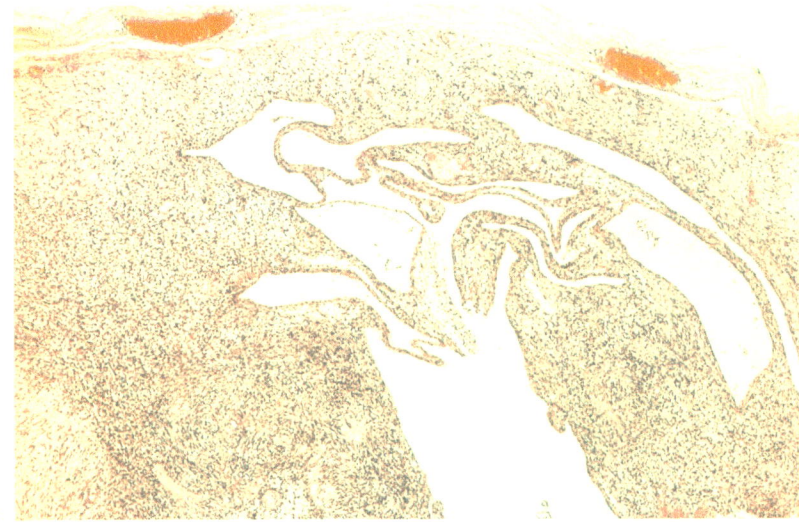

Fig. 266 a–d. Cellular Schwannoma (neurinoma) at the level of Th 9/10 on the *left* with a history of preceding surgery of a neurinoma at the level of L 1 in a 39-year-old male. **a** The tumor is surrounded at its surface by a thick capsule. Several cystic spaces are bordered by thin tissue components without formation of a limiting membrane. **b–d** s. p. 310

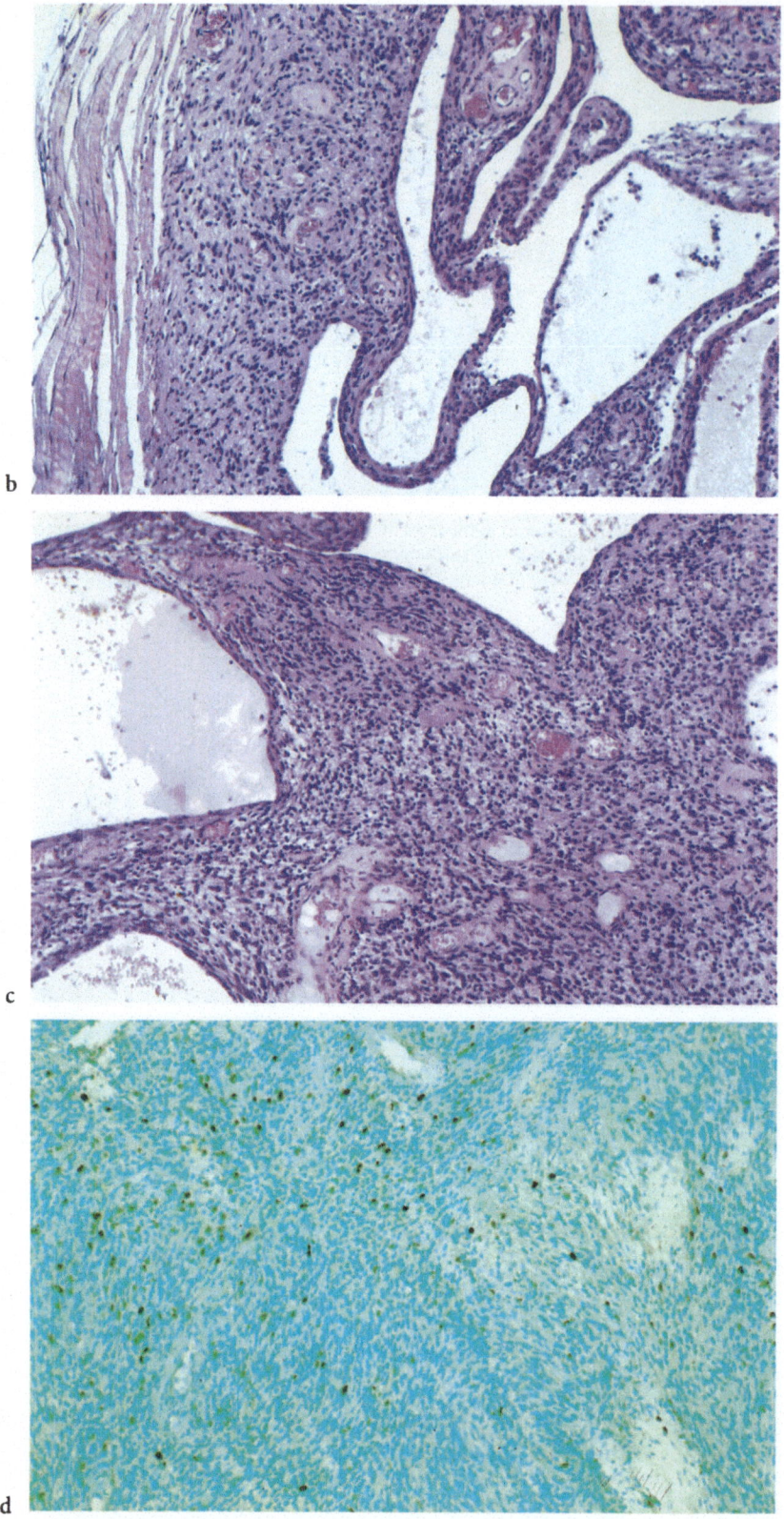

Fig. 266 *(continued)*. **b, c** The pseudocystic cavities are covered by flat cells. The tumor cells correspond neither to the reticular Antoni-type B nor to the fibrillar Antoni-type A. **d** The immunohistochemical reaction with the antibody MIB I against the proliferation associated antigen Ki67 reveals a labeling of a considerable portion of the tumor cell nuclei. But this component varies depending on the cell density

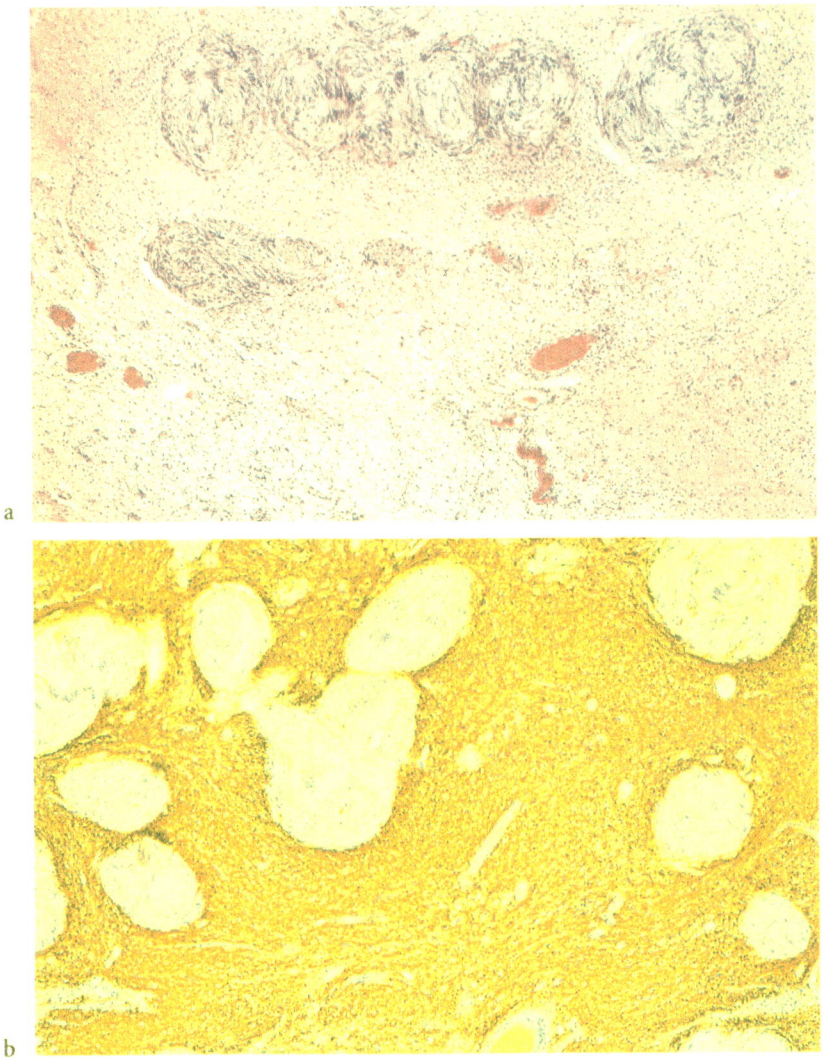

Fig. 267a–d. Intramedullary neurinoma in a 40-year-old man. **a** The neurinoma has grown into the spinal cord. The surrounding cord shows prominent gliosis. Paraffin: H & E. **b** The immunohistochemical reaction with antibodies against the glial fibrillary protein (GFAP) reveals an intense reaction of the spinal cord tissue (gliosis) whereas the tumor cells are not immunoreactive. **c, d** s. p. 312

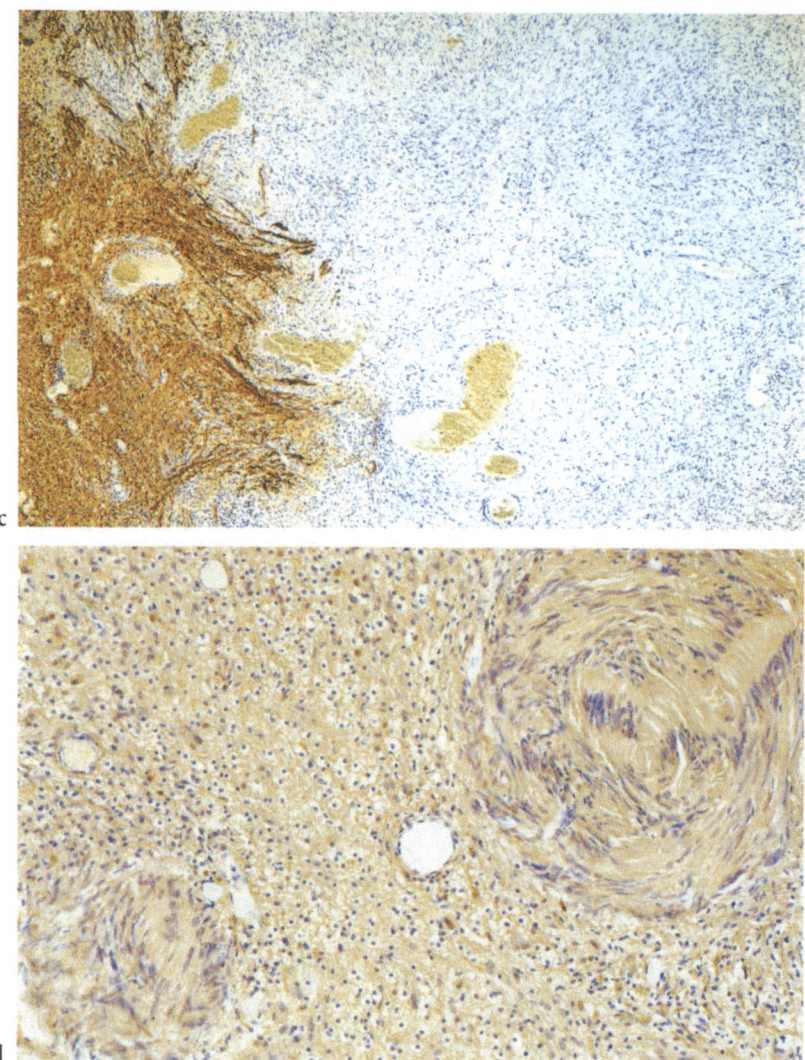

Fig. 267 *(continued)*. **c** Focally the intraspinal neurinoma grows diffusely or in stripes into the adjacent spinal cord tissue. GFAP-reaction. **d** Immunohistochemical reaction against protein S100. The neurinoma cells show only weak immunoreactivity, as does the surrounding spinal cord tissue. At several sites, the typical palisaded pattern of arrangement of the tumor cell nuclei is detectable, so that there is no doubt about the diagnosis of a neurinoma

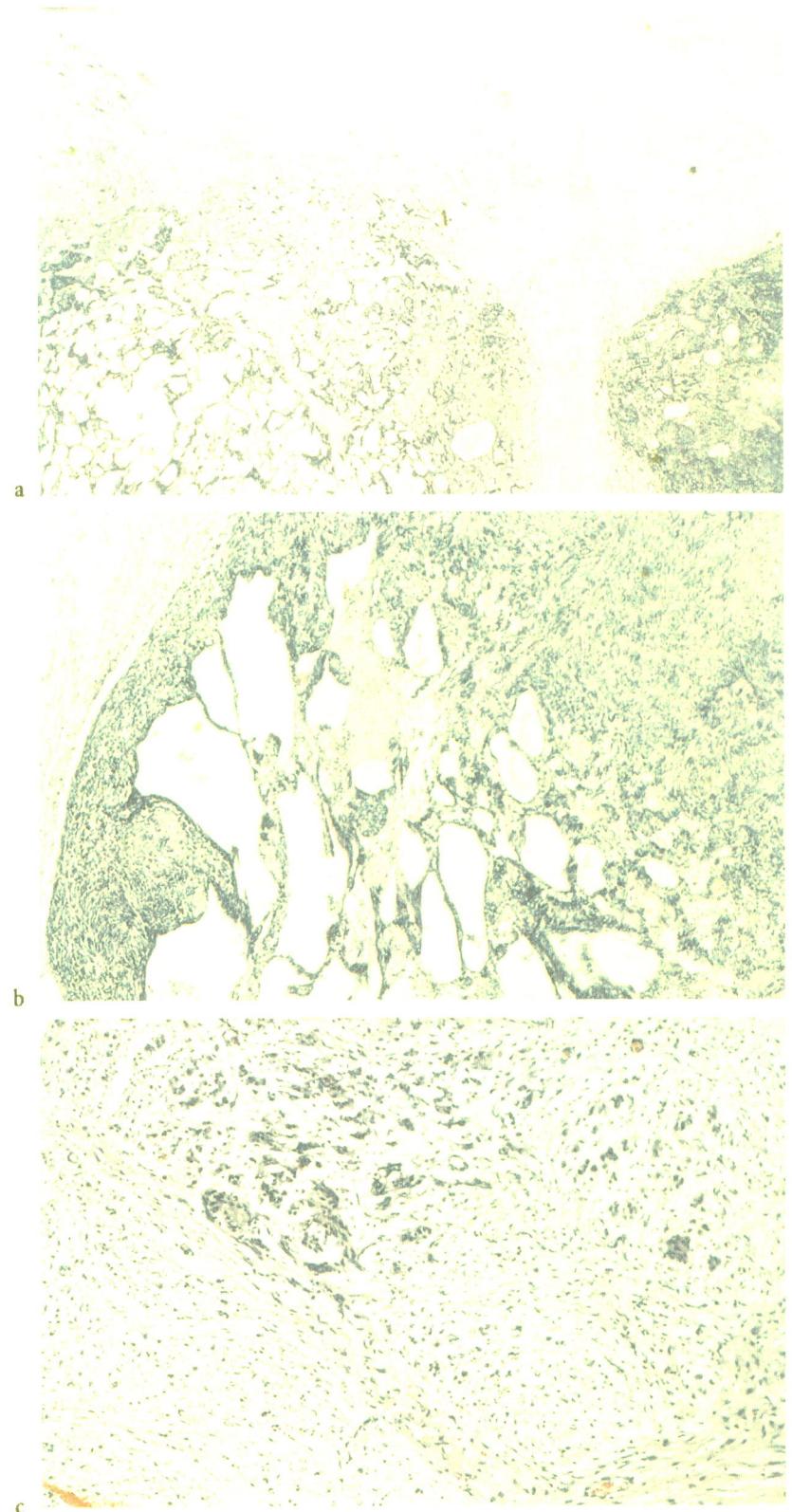

Fig. 268a – f. Plexiform neurofibroma of the ulnar nerve in a 58-year-old female. Focally there are partly compact, partly pseudocystic neurinoma-like components, which are isolated, but transitions into less cellular, loose areas rich in collagen do occur. The old fascicular borders in **d** are still well defined, but not so clearly preserved in **f**, characterizing the plexiform neurofibroma **d – f** s. p. 314

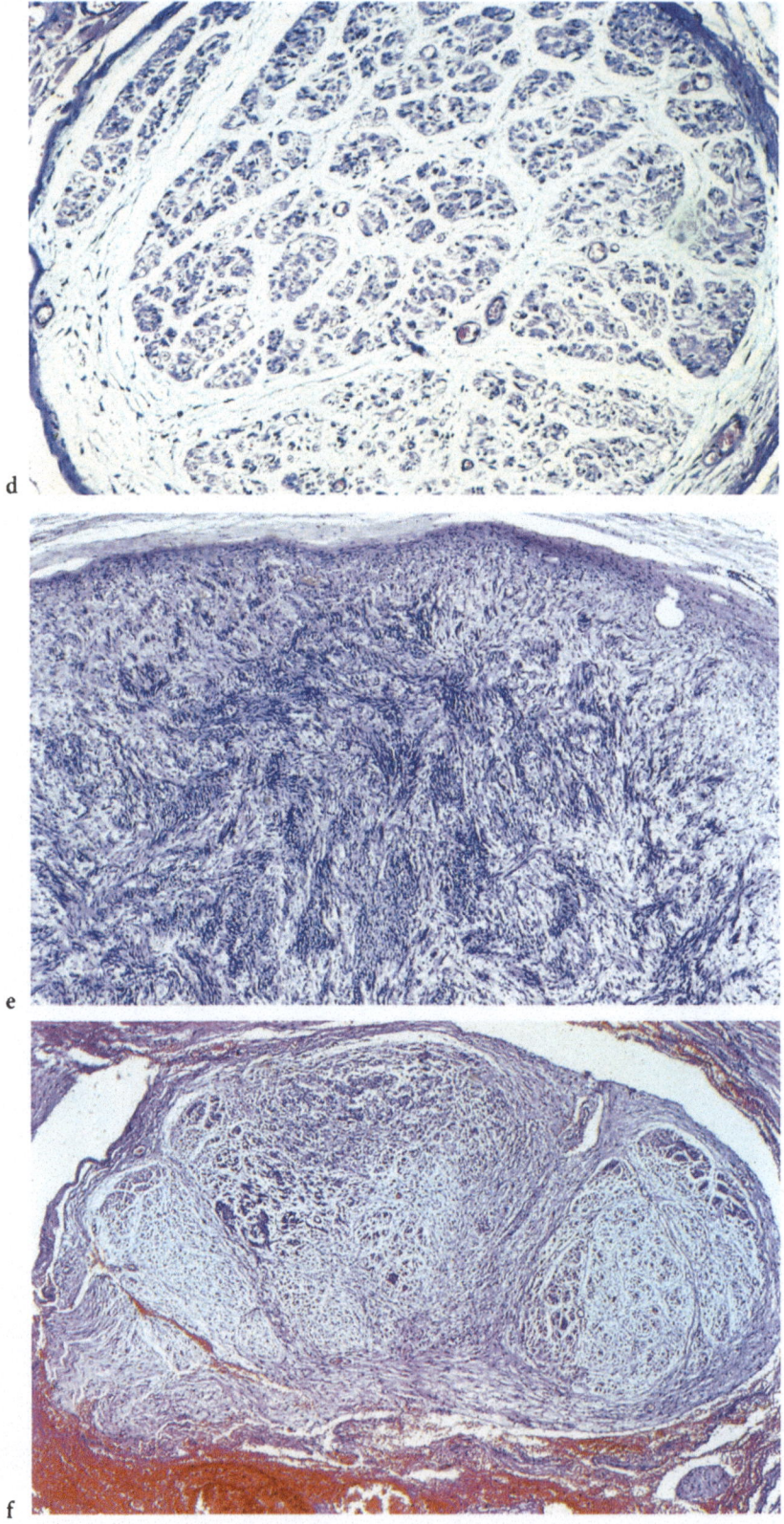

Fig. 268 d–f *(continued)*. Legend s. p. 313

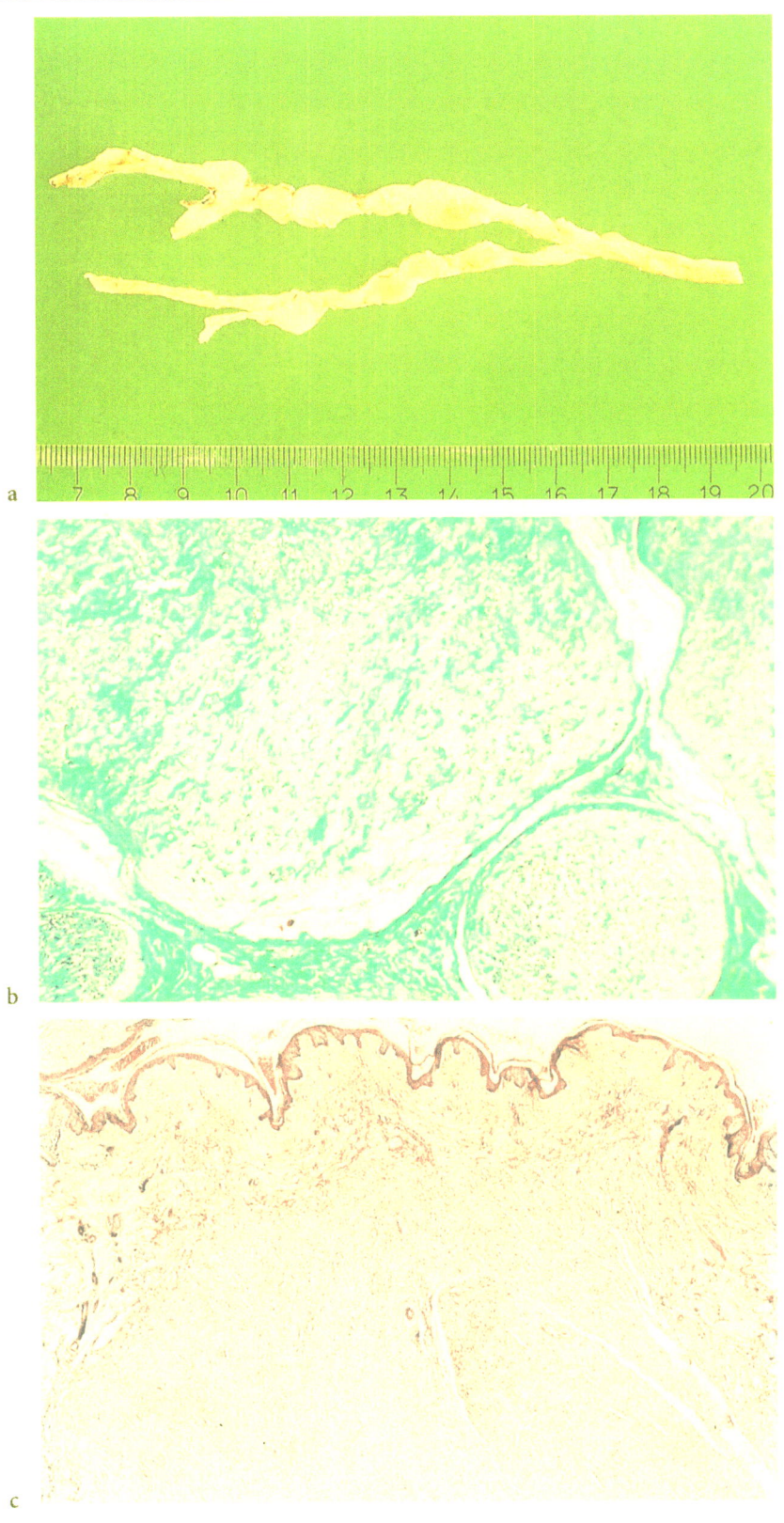

Fig. 269a–f. Neurofibromatosis type 1. **a** Plexiform neurofibromas with multiple, circumscribed enlargements of nerve fascicles. **b** Normal nerve fascicles adjacent to two severely enlarged ones with neurofibromatous changes. **c, d** Neurofibromas in the skin of a patient with neurofibromatosis type 1. **c:** H & E, **d:** EvG. **e** Benign adenoma of the adrenal gland. H & E. **f** Ganglioneuroma in the adrenal medulla. H & E **d–f** s. p. 316

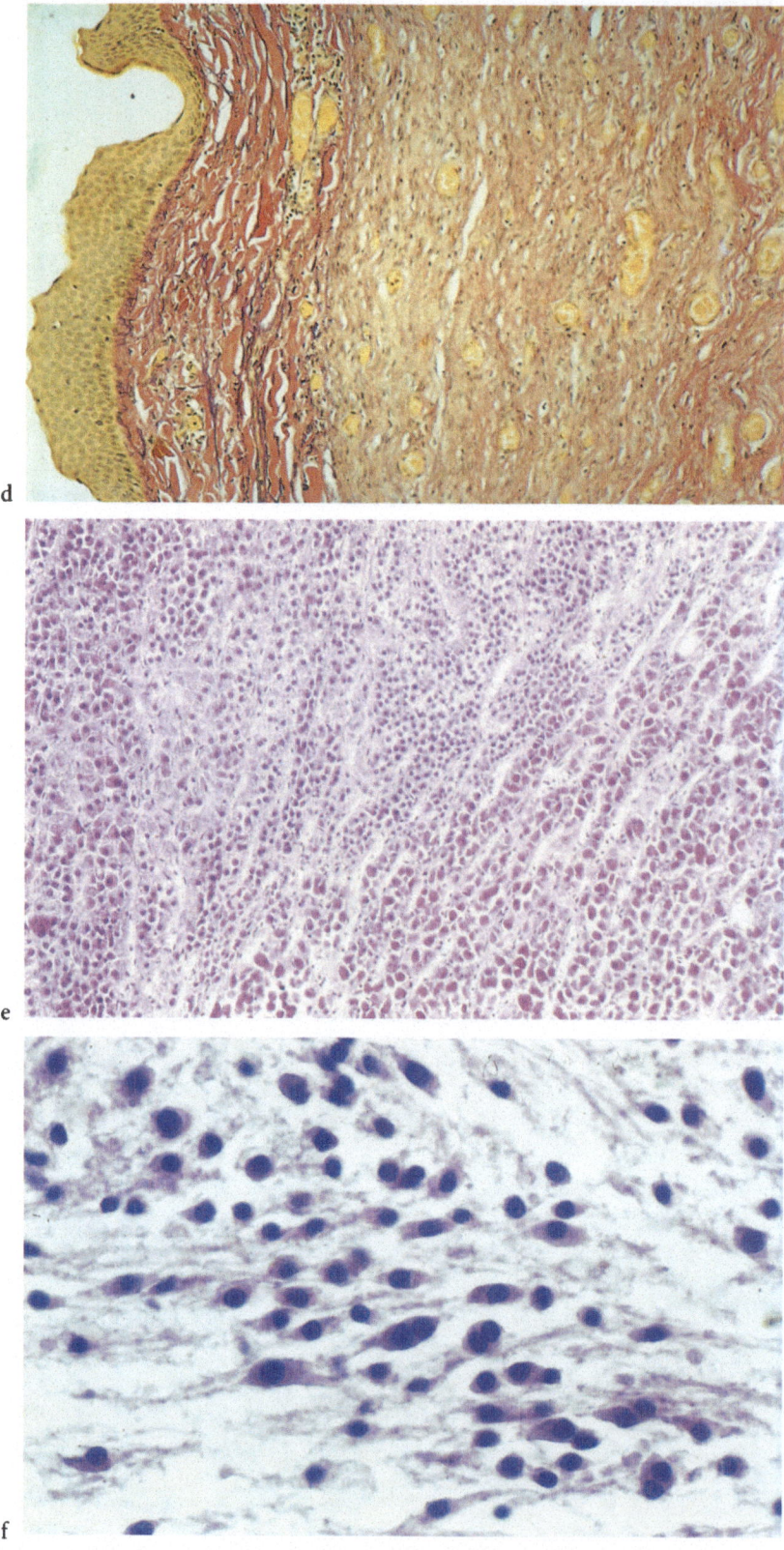

Fig. 269 d–f (continued). Legend s. p. 315

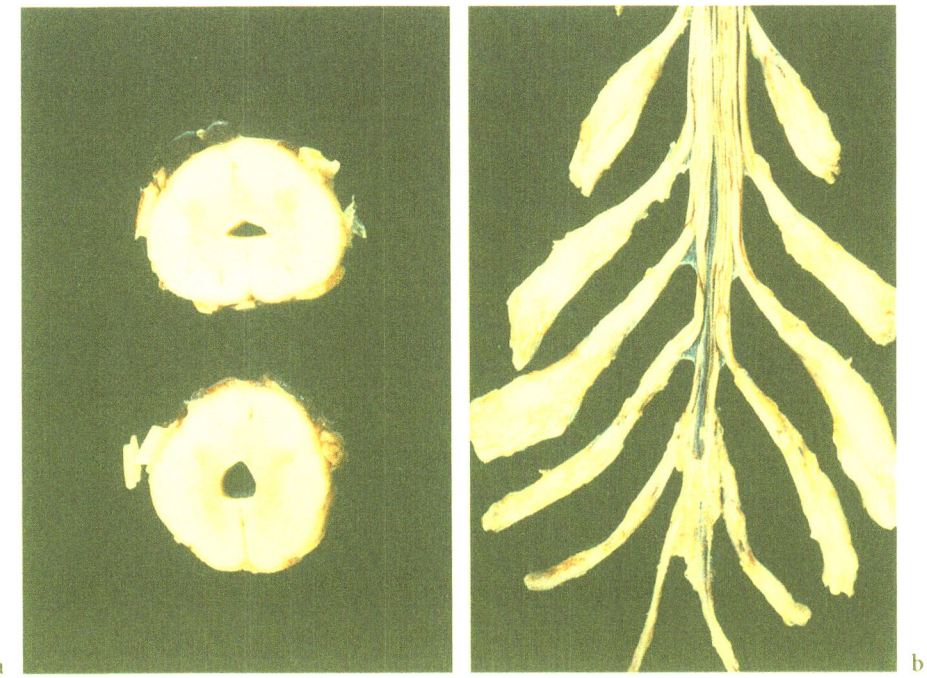

Fig. 270 a, b. Neurofibromatosis in a 32-year-old patient. **a** Hydromyelia of intermediate severity at the thoracic medulla. **b** Prominent enlargement of several nerve roots in the cauda equina

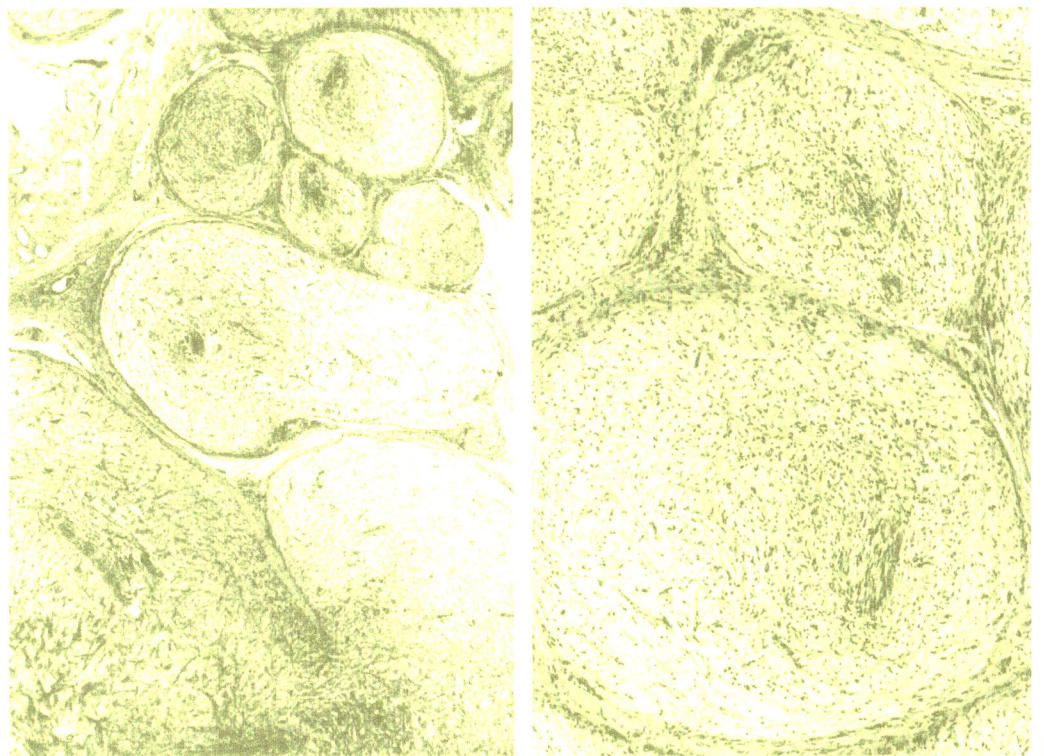

Fig. 271 a, b. Neurofibromatosis in a 4-year-old boy. Plexiform neurofibromas in several nerve fascicles. Some nerve fascicles are severely enlarged whereas others are hardly affected. The number of fibroblast-like cells in the endoneurium and the endoneurial connective tissue is severely increased. The cells are surrounded by mucoid substances. The perineurium appears to be largely preserved. **a** × 50; **b** × 160

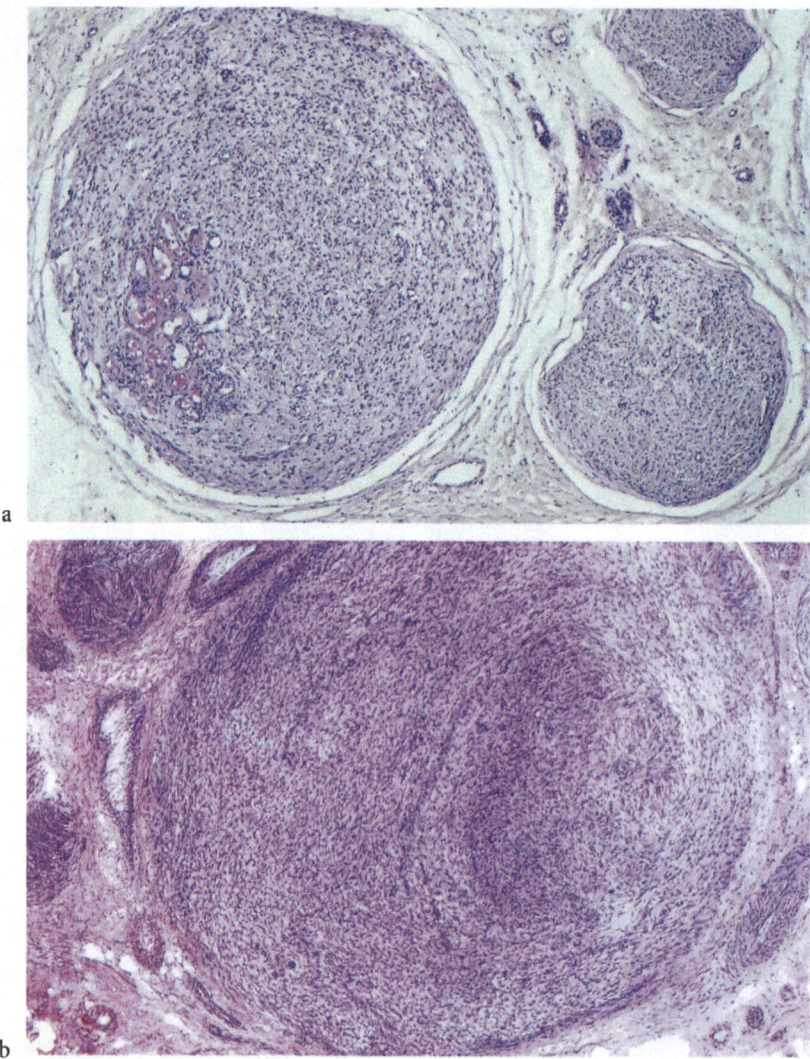

Fig. 272 a, b. Early stage of a nerve involvement in neurofibromatosis of a 72-year-old female. At circumscribed sites, tumor cells have grown in larger numbers whereas the remainder of the nerve fascicles appear less severely, but more evenly affected

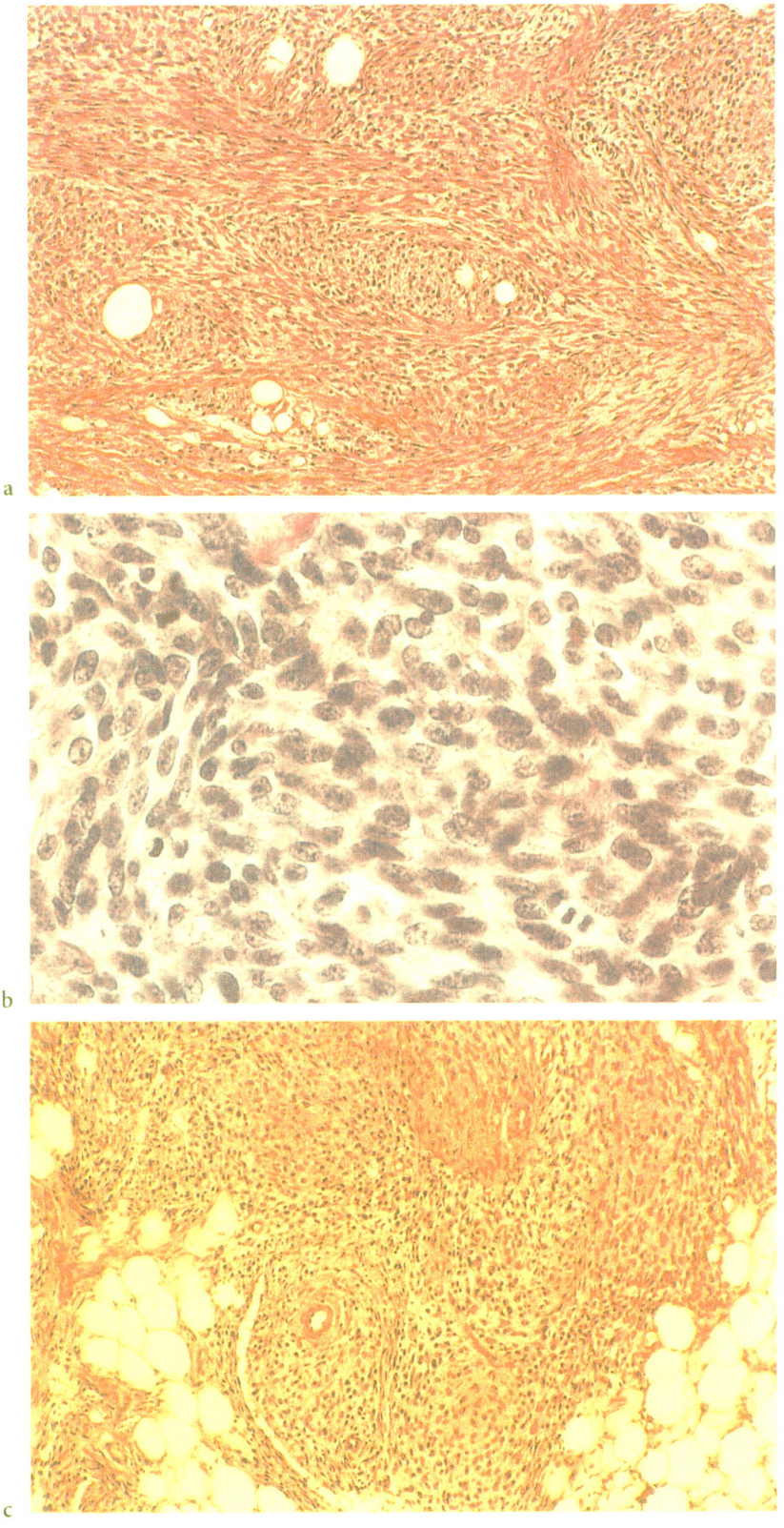

Fig. 273a–f. Malignant peripheral nerve sheath tumor (MPNST). a The tumor cells are mainly arranged in strands which are oriented longitudinally, obliquely, or transversely. **b** The nucleocytoplasmic ratio is altered in favor of the nuclei. Mitoses can be repeatedly seen. **c** The adjacent fat tissue is infiltrated, **d** as is the muscle tissue. **e** Because of dedifferentiation few tumor cells only are weakly immunoreactive for protein S100. **f** The antibody reaction with MIB1 against the proliferation associated antigen Ki67 reveals a positive reaction in roughly 8% of the tumor cell nuclei **d–f** s. p. 320

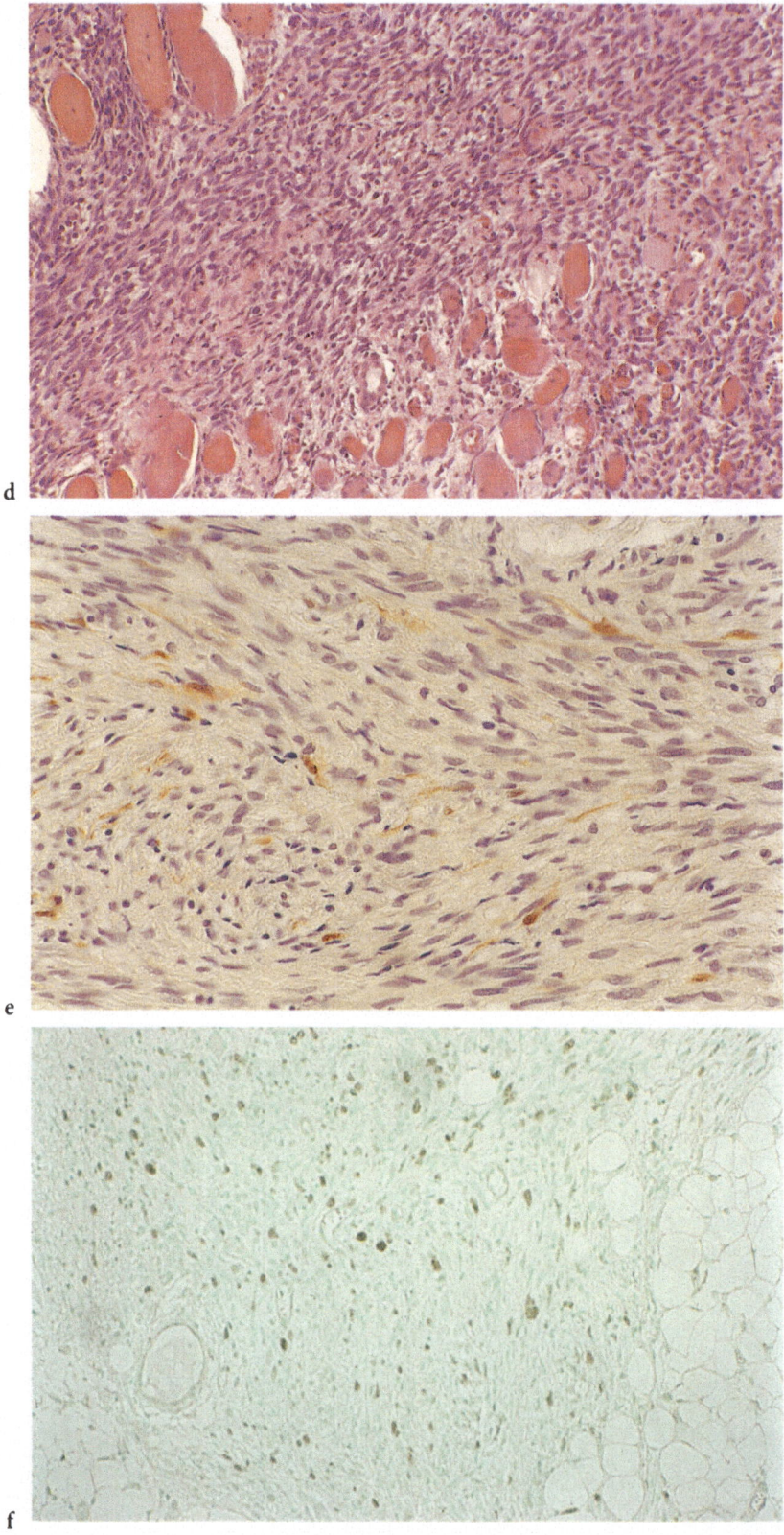

Fig. 273 d – f *(continued).* Legend s. p. 319

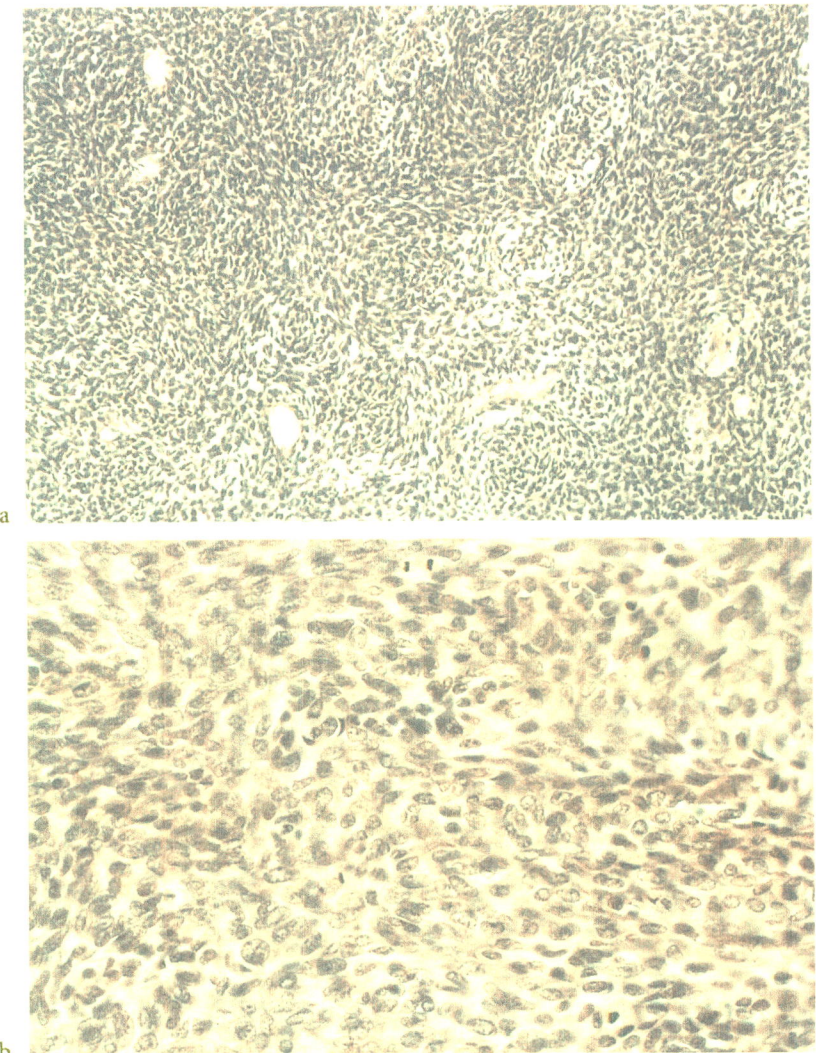

Fig. 274a, b. Malignant central (intracerebral) Schwannoma in a 24-year-old male. **a** The tumor shows high cellularity. The tumor cells are focally still aligned in parallel formations. **b** The ratio between the nucleocytoplasm ratio is clearly altered in favor of the nuclei. Mitoses can be repeatedly seen

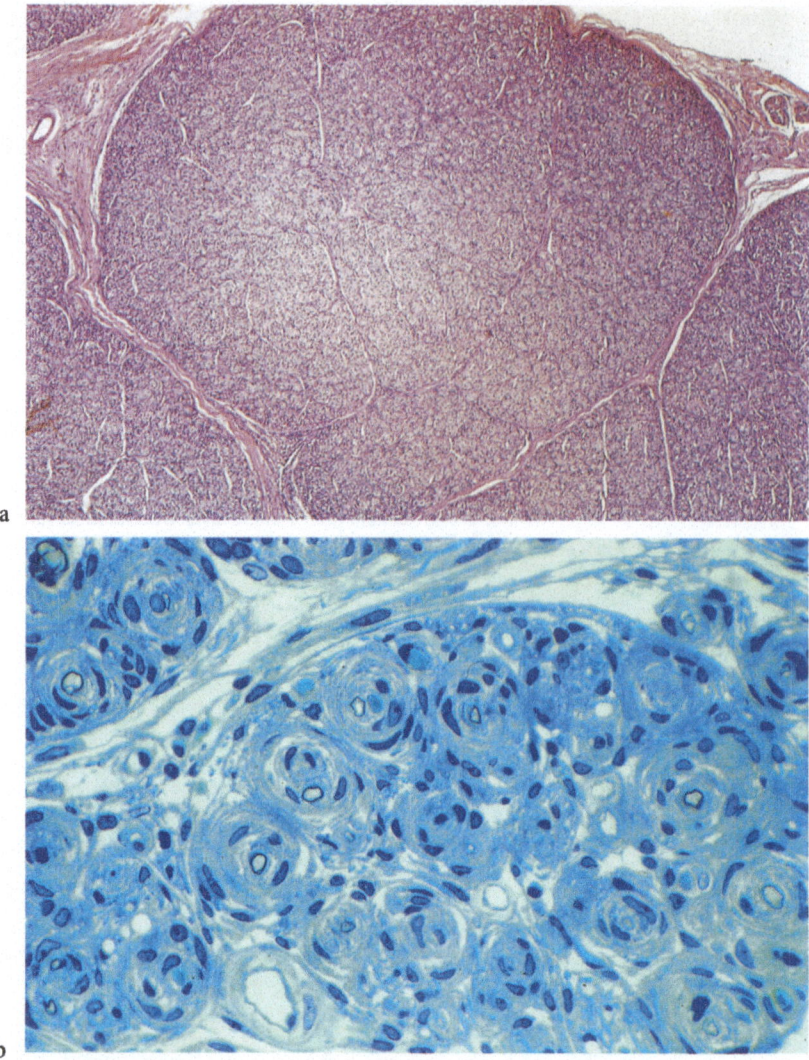

Fig. 275 a, b. Perineurioma in the radial nerve between the branches to the triceps brachii and the brachioradialis muscles in a 5-year-old boy with spontaneous paresis of the radial nerve for 2 years. **a** The nerve fascicles are equally affected and enlarged as can be seen in hypertrophic neuropathy. Paraffin: H & E. **b** Many myelinated or unmyelinated nerve fibers are individually surrounded by circumferentially arranged perineurial cells. The cell adjacent to the capillary in the *lower left* appears to be less dense than the cells surrounding the nerve fibers. Semithin section: toluidine blue

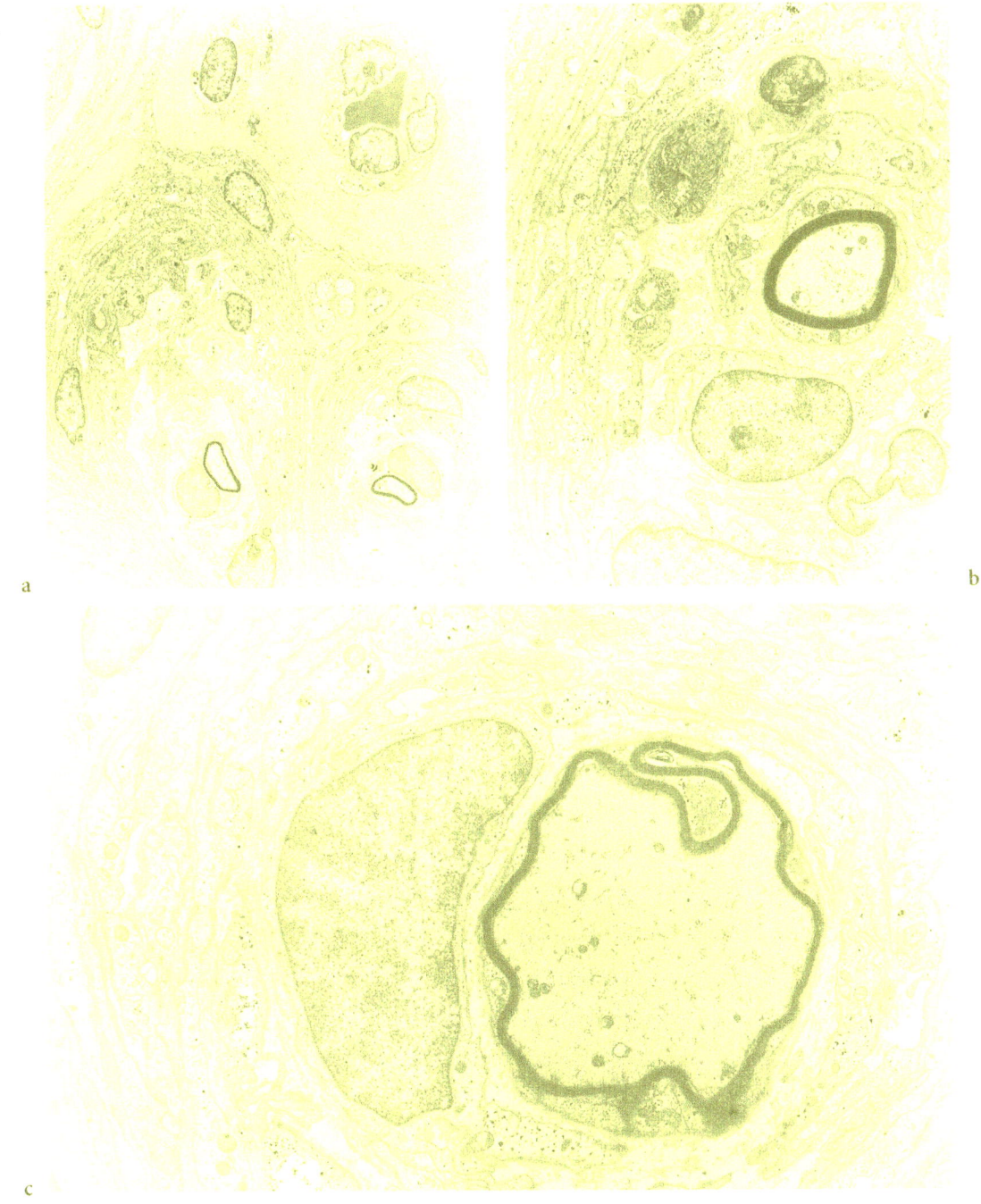

Fig. 276a–c. Perineurioma in the spinal root of L5 in a 13-year-old patient with multiple perineuriomas according to clinical data. **a** Two thinly myelinated nerve fibers are surrounded by numerous unevenly arranged or flat cell processes resembling perineurial cells. The unmyelinated axons lying above and between both minifascicles and the capillary in the upper right corner are not similarly ensheathed. × 2,300. **b** Higher magnification of a minifascicle; several cells situated within the minifascicle are not covered by a basal lamina. The ensheathing flat cells and their processes, however, are at least partially covered by a basal lamina. × 6,500. **c** A remyelinated or regenerated axon with a disproportionately thin myelin sheath shows an increased density of neurofilaments and is concentrically surrounded more or less completely by numerous cells and their processes which are usually only incompletely covered by a basal lamina. Interspersed are remarkably few collagen fibrils. × 9,400

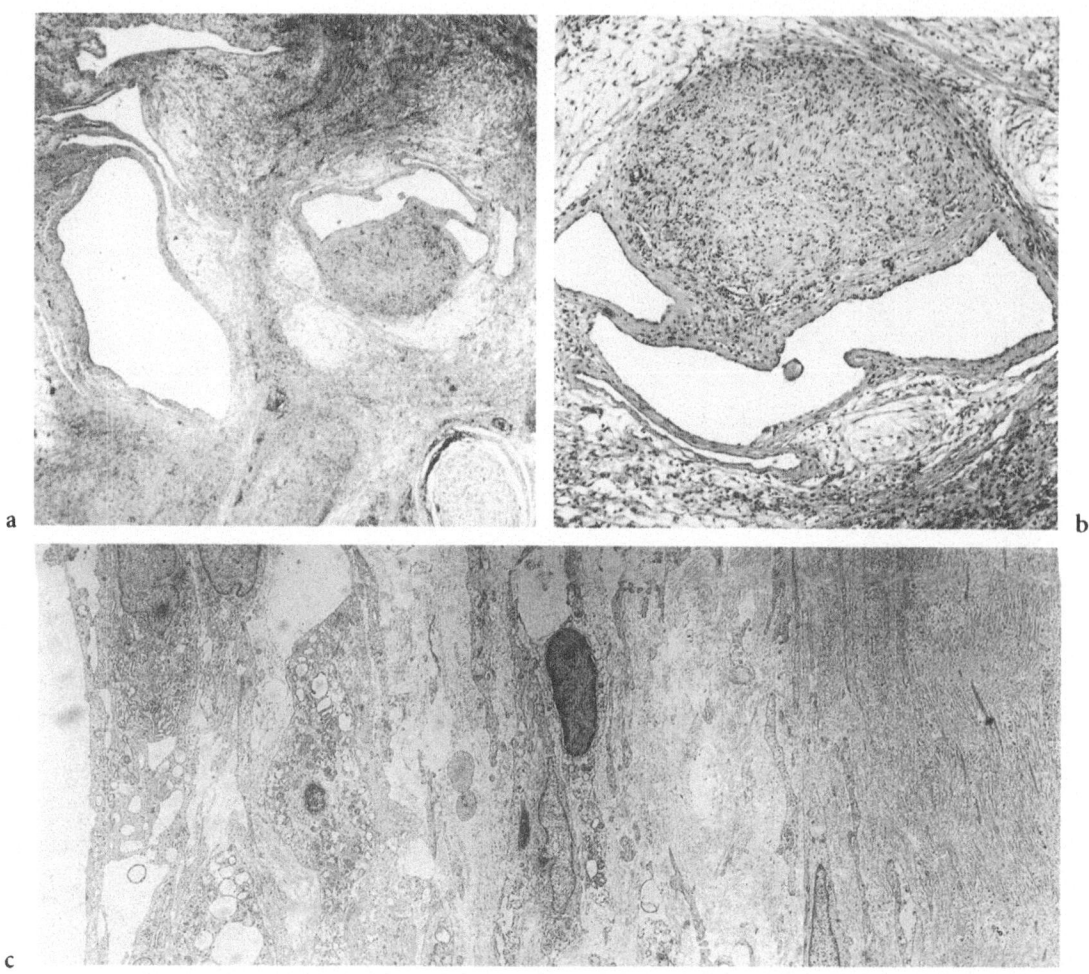

Fig. 277. a, b Neuropathia pseudocystica of the common peroneal nerve (at the capitulum fibulae) in a 57-year-old female. The cysts are of uneven size and are covered by flat cells resembling synovial cells (**a, b**). **c** The covering cells of the cystic cavities are not covered by a basal lamina at their outer surface. But they repeatedly show special contacts with adjacent cells. These cells may contain several vacuoles. Numerous collagen fibrils are seen at the abluminal side. **a, b** paraffin: H & E; **a** × 76; **b** × 90; **c** × 2,400

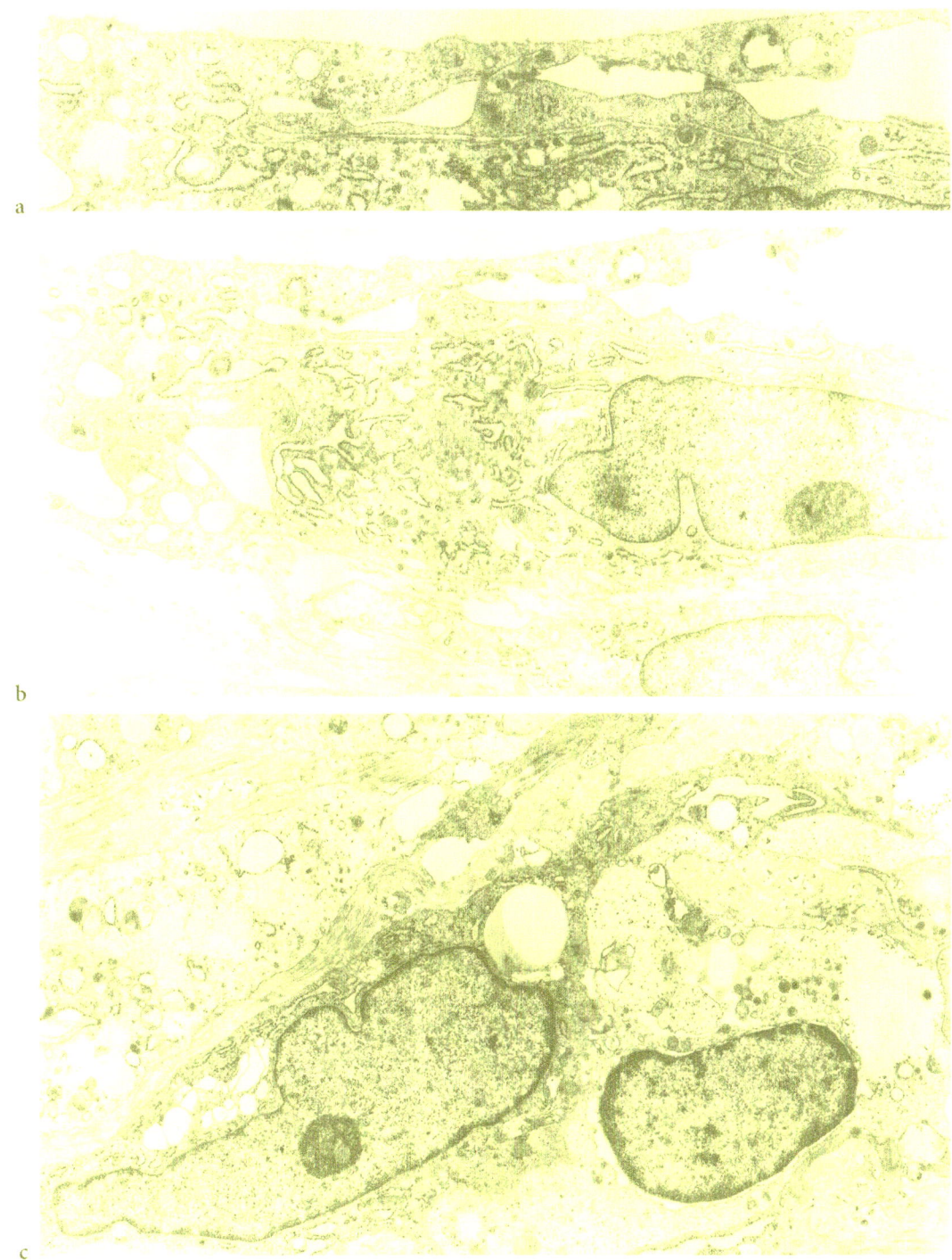

Fig. 278 a – c. Same case as in Fig. 277. **a, b** The cells bordering the cystic spaces are connected by flat processes with the cells located underneath. An indistinct basal lamina is focally seen between the processes. **c** The cytoplasm of the cells in the pseudocystic membrane is of uneven electron density. Lipid droplets and electron dense granules may occur focally. Some cells are rich in organelles comprising a well developed ergastoplasma whereas others show vacuoles and other regressive changes. **a** × 10,000; **b, c** × 7,700

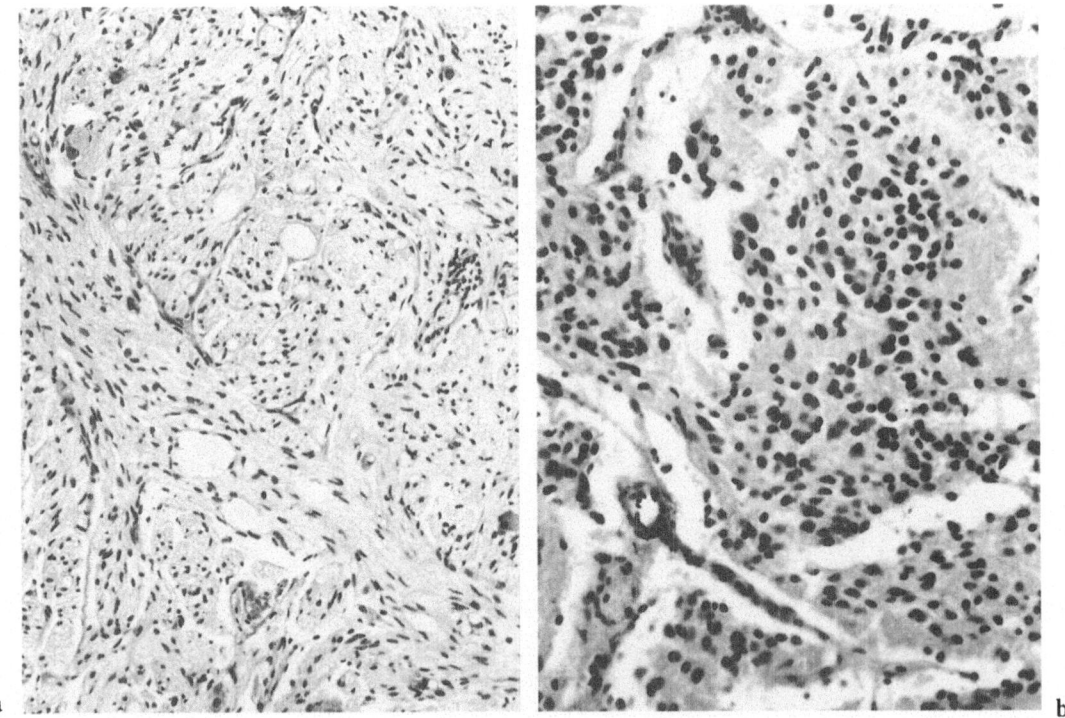

Fig. 279 a, b. Metastasis of a ganglioneuroblastoma in the truncus coeliacus of a 5-year-old boy (stage IV; grade I according to Hughes). The cells are focally aligned in strands or bundles or they show an alveolar pattern of growth. **a** × 160; **b** × 210

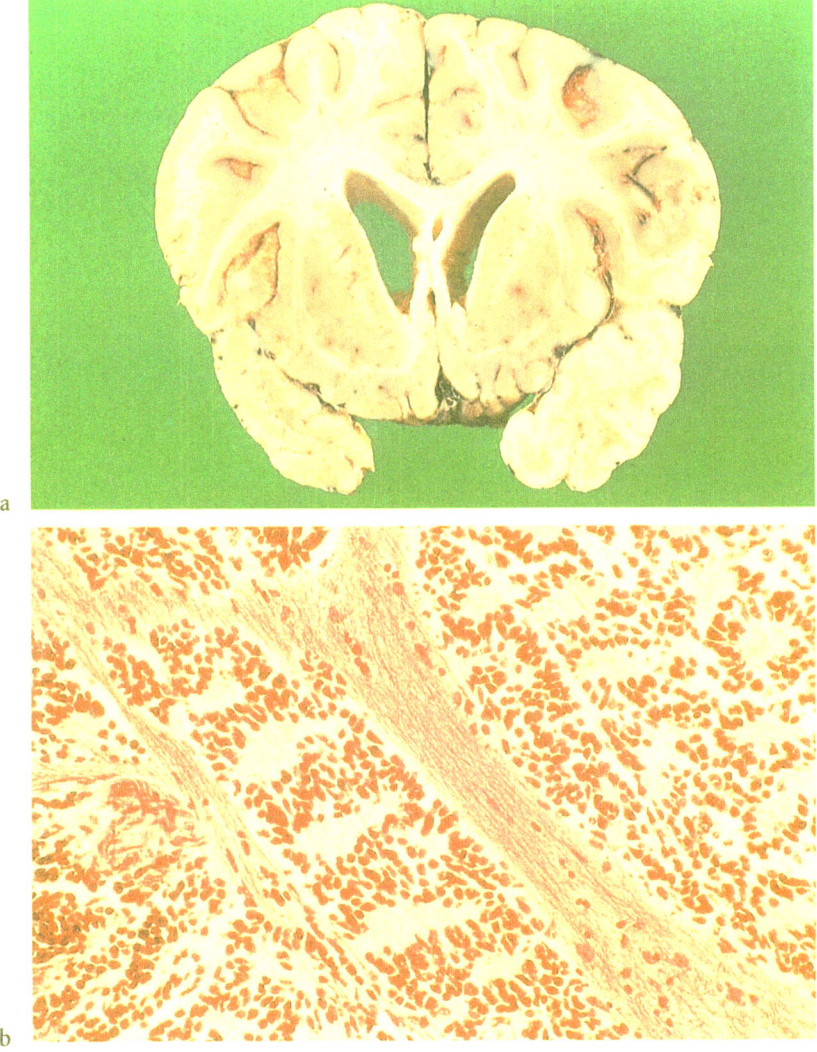

Fig. 280 a, b. Central metastases of a peripheral neuroblastoma. **a** There are multiple nodules in the leptomeninges in addition to a diffuse pattern of infiltration. **b** The tumor consists of undifferentiated small cells which are frequently arranged in pseudorosettes. Occasionally fine, silver impregnated nerve cell processes (neurites) may be seen in the center of the rosettes. Cerebellar metastasis: silver impregnation according to Bodian

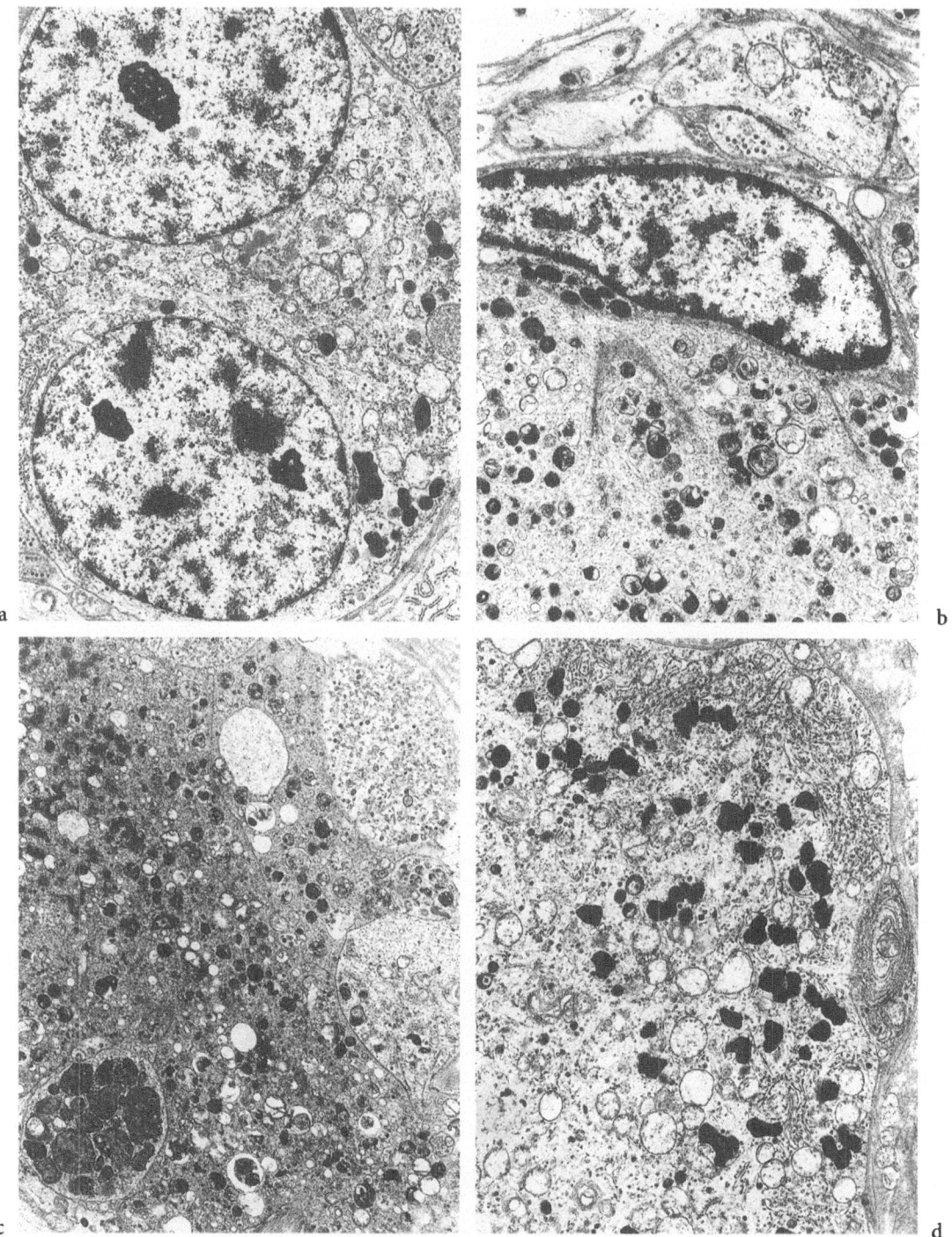

Fig. 281a–d. Ganglioneuroblastoma in a 4-year-old girl. The cells contain electron-dense bodies of uneven size as well as lamellated figures. Adjacent, neuronal processes containing neurosecretory granules can also be seen. In **a,** a cell is shown with two nuclei, in **c** a process is illustrated with multiple pleomorphic electron dense lysosome-like bodies. **a** × 6,200; **b** × 9,000; **c** × 6,100; **d** × 7,600

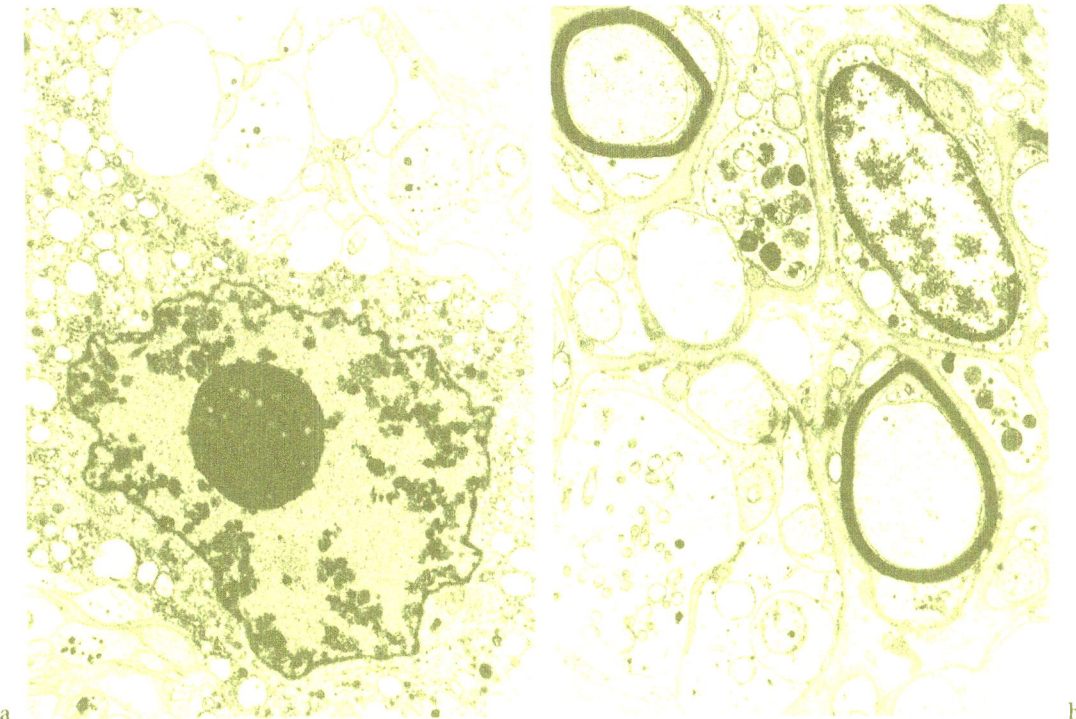

a   b

Fig. 282 a, b. Same case as in Fig. 281. **a** Numerous unmyelinated axons contain neurosecretory granules and vesicles of different sizes. The nucleus of the cell in the center includes an extraordinarily large nucleolus and unevenly distributed small heterochromatin particles in an otherwise relatively light caryoplasm. The nuclear membrane appears especially electron dense. (Many mitochondria are artificially swollen.) × 6,100. **b** This group of nerve fibers in the ganglioneuroblastoma appears relatively well preserved. Myelinated fibers are seen adjacent to unmyelinated ones. Some axons or Schwann cell processes contain lysosome-like electron-dense bodies. × 7,300

References

1. Abel A, Bone LJ, Messing A, Scherer SS, Fischbeck KH (1999) Studies in transgenic mice indicate a loss of connexin32 function in X-linked Charcot-Marie-Tooth disease. J Neuropathol Exp Neurol 58:702–710

2. Adlkofer K, Martini R, Aguzzi A, Zielasek J, Toyka KV, Suter U (1995) Hypermyelination and demyelinating peripheral neuropathy in Pmp22-deficient mice. Nat Genet 11:274–280

3. Aguayo AJ, Dickson R, Trecarten J, Attiwell M, Bray GM, Richardson P (1978) Ensheathment and myelination of regenerating PNS fibres by transplanted optic nerve glia. Neurosci Lett 9:97–104

4. Aicardi J, Castelein P (1979) Infantile neuroaxonal dystrophy. Brain 102:727–748

5. Albin R, Albers J, Greenberg H, Townsend J, Lynn R, Burke J, Allessi A (1987) Acute sensory neuropathy-neuronopathy from pyridoxine overdose. Neurology 37:1729–1732

6. al-Chalabi A, Powell JF, Leigh PN (1995) Neurofilaments, free radicals, excitotoxins, and amyotrophic lateral sclerosis. Muscle Nerve 18:540–545

7. Alderson K, Holds JB, Anderson RL (1991) Botulinum-induced alteration of nerve-muscle interactions in the human orbicularis oculi following treatment for blepharospasm. Neurology 41:1800–1805

8. Alexianu M, Christodorescu D, Vasilescu C, Dan A, Petrovici A, Magureanu S, Savu C (1983) Sensorimotor neuropathy in a patient with Marinesco-Sjögren syndrome. Eur Neurol 22:222–226

9. al-Hakim M, Cohen M, Daroff RB (1993) Postmortem examination of relapsing acute Guillain-Barré syndrome. Muscle Nerve 16:173–176

10. Allcutt DA, Hoffman HJ, Isla A, Becker LE, Humphreys RP (1991) Acoustic Schwannomas in children. Neurosurgery 29:14–18

11. Almsaddi M, Bertorini TE, Seltzer WK (1998) Demyelinating neuropathy in a patient with multiple sclerosis and genotypical HMSN I. Neuromusc Disord 8:87–89

12. ALS-CNTF Treatment Study Group (1996) A double-blind placebo-controlled clinical trial of subcutaneous recombinant human ciliary neurotrophic factor (rHCNTF) in amyotrophic lateral sclerosis. ALS CNTF Treatment Study Group. Neurology 46:1244–1249

13. Alter M (1990) The epidemiology of Guillain-Barré syndrome. Ann Neurol 27 Suppl:S7–S12

14. An SF, Ciardi A, Scaravilli F (1994) PCR detection of HIV proviral DNA (gag) in the brains of patients with AIDS: comparison between results using fresh frozen and paraffin wax embedded specimens. J Clin Pathol 47:990–994

15. Anan I, El-Salhy M, Ando Y, Forsgren S, Nyhlin N, Terazaki H, Sakashita N, Suhr OB (1999) Colonic enteric nervous system in patients with familial amyloidotic neuropathy. Acta Neuropathol (Berl) 98:48–54

16. Anderson B, Robertson DM (1979) Melanin containing neurofibroma: case report with evidence of Schwann cell origin of melanin. Can J Neurol Sci 6:139–143

17. Anderson NE, Rosenblum MK, Graus F, Wiley RG, Posner JB (1988) Autoantibodies in paraneoplastic syndromes associated with small-cell lung cancer. Neurology 38:1391–1398

18. Anderson PN, Woodham P, Turmaine M (1989) Peripheral nerve regeneration through optic nerve grafts. Acta Neuropathol (Berl) 77:525–534

19. Ansselin AD, Fink T, Davey DF (1997) Peripheral nerve regeneration through nerve guides seeded with adult Schwann cells. Neuropathol Appl Neurobiol 23:387–398

20. Antel JP, Moumdjian R (1989) Paraneoplastic syndromes: a role for the immune system. J Neurol 236:1–3

21. Arakawa Y, Sendtner M, Thoenen H (1990) Survival effect of ciliary neurotrophic factor (CNTF) on chick embryonic motoneurons in culture: comparison with other neurotrophic factors and cytokines. J Neurosci 10:3507–3515

22. Arasaki K, Kusunoki S, Kudo N, Kanazawa I (1993) Acute conduction block in vitro following exposure to antiganglioside sera. Muscle Nerve 16:587–593

23. Archelos JJ, Maurer M, Jung S, Toyka KV, Hartung HP (1993) Suppression of experimental allergic neuritis by an antibody to the intracellular adhesion molecule ICAM-1. Brain 116:1043–1058

24. Argov Z, Soffer D, Eisenberg S, Zimmerman Y (1986) Chronic demyelinating peripheral neuropathy in cerebrotendinous xanthomatosis. Ann Neurol 20:89–91

25. Arvidson B (1992) Inorganic mercury is transported from muscular nerve terminals to spinal and brainstem motoneurons. Muscle Nerve 15:1089–1094

26. Asbury AK, Gale MK, Cox SC, Baringer JR, Berg BO (1972) Giant axonal neuropathy – a unique case with segmental neurofilamentous masses. Acta Neuropathol (Berl) 20:237–247

27. Asbury AK, Johnson PC (1978) Pathology of peripheral nerve. Major Probl Pathol 9:1–311

28. Asbury AK, Porte DJ (1992) Proceedings of a consensus development conference on standardized measures in diabetic neuropathy. Neurology 42:1823–1839

29. Asbury AK, Victor M, Adams RD (1963) Uremic polyneuropathy. Arch Neurol 8:413–428

30. Ashby J, Tinwell H (1995) Is thalidomide mutagenic? [letter]. Nature 375:453

31. Askin FB, Rosai J, Sibley RK, Dehner LP, McAlister WH (1979) Malignant small cell tumor of the thoracopulmonary region in childhood: a distinctive clinicopathologic entity of uncertain histogenesis. Cancer 43:2438–2451

32. Atsumi T (1981) The ultrastructure of intramuscular nerves in amyotrophic lateral sclerosis. Acta Neuropathol (Berl) 55:193–198

33. Atsumi T, Miyatake T (1987) Morphometry of the degenerative process in the hypoglossal nerves in amyotrophic lateral sclerosis. Acta Neuropathol (Berl) 73:25–31

34. Auer RN, Budny J, Drake CG, Ball MJ (1982) Frontal lobe perivascular Schwannoma. Case report. J Neurosurg 56:154–157

35. Auer-Grumbach M, Wagner K, Fazekas F, Löscher WN, Strasser-Fuchs S, Hartung HP (1999) Hereditary motorsensory neuropathies (Charcot-Marie-Tooth syndrome) and related neuropathies. Current classification and genotype-phenotype correlation. Nervenarzt 70:1052–1061

36. Awasthi D, Kline DG, Beckman EN (1991) Neuromuscular hamartoma (benign "triton" tumor) of the brachial plexus. Case report. J Neurosurg 75:795–797

37. Baechner D, Liehr T, Hameister H, Altenberger H, Grehl H, Suter U, Rautenstrauss B (1995) Widespread expression of the peripheral myelin protein-22 gene (PMP22) in neural and non-neural tissues during murine development. J Neurosci Res 42:733–741

38. Baethmann M, Göhlich-Ratmann G, Schröder JM, Kalaydjieva L, Voit T (1998) HMSNL in a 13-year-old Bulgarian girl. Neuromusc Disord 8:90–94

39. Bailey RO, Baltch AL, Venkatesh R, Singh JK, Bishop MB (1988) Sensory motor neuropathy associated with AIDS. Neurology 38:886–891

40. Bain PG, Britton TC, Jenkins IH, Thompson PD, Rothwell JC, Thomas PK, Brooks DJ, Marsden CD (1996) Tremor associated with benign IgM paraproteinaemic neuropathy. Brain 119:789–799

41. Bakshi R, Graves MC (1997) Guillain-Barré syndrome after combined tetanus-diphtheria toxoid vaccination. J Neurol Sci 147:201–202

42. Baldeweg T, Riccio M, Gruzelier J, Hawkins D, Burgess A, Irving G, Stygall J, Catt S, Catalan J (1995) Neurophysiological evaluation of zidovudine in asymptomatic HIV-1 infection: a longitudinal placebo-controlled study. J Neurol Sci 132:162–169

43. Barakat I, Deruaz JP, de Tribolet N (1995) Differential expression of triiodothyronine receptors of Schwannoma and neurofibroma: role of Schwann cell-axon interaction. Acta Neuropathol 90:142–149

44. Barbin G, Manthorpe M, Varon S (1984) Purification of the chick eye ciliary neuronotrophic factor. J Neurochem 43:1468–1478

45. Bardosi A, Creutzfeldt W, DiMauro S, Felgenhauer K, Friede RL, Goebel HH, Kohlschütter A, Mayer G, Rahlf G, Servidei S et al. (1987) Myo-, neuro-, gastrointestinal encephalopathy (MNGIE syndrome) due to partial deficiency of cytochrome-c-oxidase. A new mitochondrial multisystem disorder. Acta Neuropathol (Berl) 74:248–258

46. Baumann N, Masson M, Carreau V, Lefevre M, Herschkowitz N, Turpin JC (1991) Adult forms of metachromatic leukodystrophy: clinical and biochemical approach. Dev Neurosci 13:211–215

47. Baumgartner MR, Jansen GA, Verhoeven NM, Mooyer PA, Jakobs C, Roels F, Espeel M, Fourmaintraux A, Bellet H, Wanders RJ, Saudubray JM (2000) Atypical Refsum disease with pipecolic acidemia and abnormal catalase distribution. Ann Neurol 47:109–113

48. Beckmann A, Hartmann C, Schröder JM (1999) DDD-PCR for the gene dosage determination of PMP22 in DNA from long-term stored, paraffin embedded tissue (abstract). J Periph Nerv Sys 4:285–286

49. Beckmann A, Schröder JM (2000) Screening for Charcot-Marie-Tooth type 1A and hereditary neuropathy with liability to pressure palsy in archival nerve biopsy samples by direct-double-differential PCR. Acta Neuropathol 100:459–463

50. Beggs J, Johnson PC, Olafsen A, Watkins CJ (1992) Innervation of the vasa nervorum: changes in human diabetics. J Neuropathol Exp Neurol 51:612–629

51. Beggs J, Johnson PC, Olafsen A, Watkins CJ, Cleary C (1991) Transperineurial arterioles in human sural nerve. J Neuropathol Exp Neurol 50:704–718

52. Beggs JL, Johnson PC, Olafsen AG, Watkins CJ, Targovnik JH, Koep LJ (1989) Regression of perineurial cell basement membrane in a human diabetic following isogenic pancreas transplant. Acta Neuropathol (Berl) 79:108–112

53. Behar R, Wiley C, McCutchan JA (1987) Cytomegalovirus polyradiculoneuropathy in acquired immune deficiency syndrome. Neurology 37:557–561

54. Behse F, Buchthal F, Carlsen F (1977) Nerve biopsy and conduction studies in diabetic neuropathy. J Neurol Neurosurg Psychiatry 40:1072–1082

55. Ben Hamida M, Hentati F, Ben Hamida C (1990) Hereditary motor system diseases (chronic juvenile amyotrophic lateral sclerosis). Conditions combining a bilateral pyramidal syndrome with limb and bulbar amyotrophy. Brain 113:347–363

56. Ben Hamida M, Letaief F, Hentati F, Ben Hamida C (1987) Morphometric study of the sensory nerve in classical (or Charcot disease) and juvenile amyotrophic lateral sclerosis. J Neurol Sci 78:313–329

57. Bendixen BH, Younger DS, Hair LS, Gutierrez C, Meyers ML, Homma S, Jaffe IA (1992) Cholesterol emboli neuropathy. Neurology 42:428–430

58. Benhaiem-Sigaux N, Ricolfi F, Keravel Y, Poirier J (1996) Epithelioid Schwannoma of the acoustic nerve. Clin Neuropathol 15:231–233

59. Benke PJ, Reyes PF, Parker JC Jr (1981) New form of adrenoleukodystrophy. Hum Genet 58:204–208

60. Bennett GJ (1994) Hypotheses on the pathogenesis of herpes zoster-associated pain. Ann Neurol 35 Suppl: S38–S41

61. Bennett JL, Mahalingam R, Wellish MC, Gilden DH (1996) Epstein-Barr virus-associated acute autonomic neuropathy. Ann Neurol 40:453–455

62. Benstead TJ, Dyck PJ, Low P (1988) Chronic hypoxia induces selective maldevelopment of peripheral myelin in rat. J Neuropathol Exp Neurol 47:599–608

63. Berciano J, Figols J, Combarros O, Calleja J, Pascual J, Oterino A (1996) Plexiform neurofibroma of the cauda equina presenting as peroneal muscular atrophy. Muscle Nerve 19:250–253

64. Berciano J, Figols J, Garcia A, Calle E, Illa I, Lafarga M, Berciano MT (1997) Fulminant Guillain-Barré syndrome with universal inexcitability of peripheral

nerves: a clinicopathological study. Muscle Nerve 20: 846–857

65. Berciano MT, Calle E, Andres MA, Berciano J, Lafarga M (1996) Schwann cell nuclear remodelling and formation of nuclear and coiled bodies in Guillain-Barré syndrome. Acta Neuropathol (Berl) 92:386–394

66. Berg BO, Rosenberg SH, Asbury AK (1972) Giant axonal neuropathy. Pediatrics 49:894–899

67. Berger AR, Schaumburg HH, Schroeder C, Apfel S, Reynolds R (1992) Dose response, coasting, and differential fiber vulnerability in human toxic neuropathy: a prospective study of pyridoxine neurotoxicity. Neurology 42:1367–1370

68. Bergmann C, Senderek J, Hermanns B, Jauch A, Janssen B, Schröder JM, Karch D (1999) A unique combination of X-chromosomal neuromuscular disorders: Becker muscular dystrophy in a male with X-linked Charcot-Marie-Tooth disease. Muscle Nerve 23:818–823

69. Bergmann KC (1988) Erkrankungen der Lunge (11). Wesen und Bedeutung der Bronchialschleimhautentzündung bei chronisch-obstruktiven Atemwegserkrankungen. Deutsches Ärzteblatt 85:B-2477–2482

70. Bergoffen J, Scherer SS, Wang S, Scott MO, Bone LJ, Paul DL, Chen K, Lensch MW, Chance PF, Fischbeck KH (1993) Connexin mutations in X-linked Charcot-Marie-Tooth disease. Science 262:2039–2042

71. Berlit P (1992) Clinical and laboratory findings with giant cell arteritis. J Neurol Sci 111:1–12

72. Berrettini S, Ravecca F, Sellari-Franceschini S, Bruschini P, Casani A, Padolecchia R (1996) Acoustic neuroma: correlations between morphology and otoneurological manifestations. J Neurol Sci 144:24–33

73. Berthold CH (1978) Morphology of normal peripheral axons. In: Waxman SG (ed) Physiology and pathology of axons. Raven Press, New York, pp 3–63

74. Berthold CH, Skoglund S (1967) Histochemical and ultrastructural demonstration of mitochondria in the paranodal region of developing feline spinal roots and nerves. Acta Soc Med Ups 72:37–70

75. Bertram M, Schröder JM (1993) Developmental changes at the node and paranode in human sural nerves: morphometric and fine-structural evaluation. Cell Tissue Res 273:499–509

76. Bertrand C, Molina-Negro P, Bouvier G, Gorczyca W (1987) Observations and analysis of results in 131 cases of spasmodic torticollis after selective denervation. Appl Neurophysiol 50:319–323

77. Best PV (1987) Malignant triton tumour in the cerebellopontine angle. Report of a case. Acta Neuropathol (Berl) 74:92–96

78. Bharucha VA, Peden KW, Tennekoon GI (1994) SV40 large T antigen with c-Jun down-regulates myelin Po gene expression: a mechanism for papovaviral T antigen-mediated demyelination. Neuron 12:627–637

79. Bhigjee AI, Bill PL, Wiley CA, Windsor IM, Matthias DA, Amenomori T, Wachsman W, Moorhouse D (1993) Peripheral nerve lesions in HTLV-I associated myelopathy (HAM/TSP). Muscle Nerve 16:21–26

80. Bigner DD, McLendon RE, Brunner JM (1998) Russell and Rubinstein's Pathology of Tumors of the Nervous System (vol 1). Arnold, London, Sydney, Auckland

81. Bijlsma EK, Brouwer-Mladin R, Bosch DA, Westerveld A, Hulsebos TJ (1992) Molecular characterization of chromosome 22 deletions in Schwannomas. Genes Chromosomes Cancer 5:201–205

82. Bilbao JM, Khoury NJ, Hudson AR, Briggs SJ (1984) Perineurioma (localized hypertrophic neuropathy). Arch Pathol Lab Med 108:557–560

83. Birouk N, LeGuern E, Maisonobe T, Rouger H, Gouider R, Tardieu S, Gugenheim M, Routon MC, Leger JM, Agid Y, Brice A, Bouche P (1998) X-linked Charcot-Marie-Tooth disease with connexin 32 mutations: clinical and electrophysiologic study. Neurology 50:1074–1082

84. Bischoff A, Fierz U, Regli F, Ulrich J (1968) Peripher-neurologische Störungen bei der Fabryschen Krankheit (Angiokeratoma corporis diffusum universale). Klin Wschr 46:666–671

85. De Blaquière G, Santamaria L, Curtis J, Terenghi G, Polak J, Turk J (1994) A morphological and functional assessment of myobacterium leprae-induced nerve damage in a guinea-pig model of leprous neuritis. Neuropathol Appl Neurobiol 20:261–271

86. Blasi J, Chapman ER, Link E, Binz T, Yamasaki S, De Camilli P, Sudhof TC, Niemann H, Jahn R (1993) Botulinum neurotoxin A selectively cleaves the synaptic protein SNAP-25 (see comments). Nature 365:160–163

87. Blexrud MD, Lee DA, Windebank AJ, Brunden KR (1990) Kinetics of production of a novel growth factor after peripheral nerve injury. J Neurol Sci 98:287–299

88. Blinzinger K, Kreutzberg G (1968) Displacement of synaptic terminals from regenerating motoneurons by microglial cells. Z Zellforsch Mikrosk Anat 85:145–157

89. Blum AS, Dal Pan GJ, Feinberg J, Raines C, Mayjo K, Cornblath DR, McArthur JC (1996) Low-dose zalcitabine-related toxic neuropathy: frequency, natural history, and risk factors. Neurology 46:999–1003

90. Bodzioch M, Orso E, Klucken J, Langmann T, Bottcher A, Diederich W, Drobnik W, Barlage S, Buchler C, Porsch-Ozcurumez M, Kaminski WE, Hahmann HW, Oette K, Rothe G, Aslanidis C, Lackner KJ, Schmitz G (1999) The gene encoding ATP-binding cassette transporter 1 is mutated in Tangier disease (see comments). Nat Genet 22:347–351

91. Bolino A, Muglia M, Conforti FL, LeGuern E, Salih MA, Georgiou DM, Christodoulou K, Hausmanowa-Petrusewicz I, Mandich P, Schenone A, Gambardella A, Bono F, Quattrone A, Devoto M, Monaco AP (2000) Charcot-Marie-Tooth type 4B is caused by mutations in the gene encoding myotubularin-related protein-2. Nat Genet 25:17–19

92. Bollensen E, Steck AJ, Schachner M (1988) Reactivity with the peripheral myelin glycoprotein Po in serum from patients with monoclonal IgM gammopathy and polyneuropathy. Neurology 38:1266–1270

93. Bolton CF, Gilbert JJ, Hahn AF, Sibbald WJ (1984) Polyneuropathy in critically ill patients. J Neurol Neurosurg Psychiatry 47:1223–1231

94. Bolton CF, Young GB, Zochodne DW (1993) The neurological complications of sepsis. Ann Neurol 33:94–100

95. Boltshauser E, Bischoff A, Isler W (1977) Giant axonal neuropathy. Report of a case with normal hair. J Neurol Sci 31:269–278

96. Bone LJ, Dahl N, Lensch MW, Chance PF, Kelly T, Le Guern E, Magi S, Parry G, Shapiro H, Wang S et al. (1995) New connexin32 mutations associated with X-linked Charcot-Marie-Tooth disease. Neurology 45:1863–1866

97. Borchard F (1978) The adrenergic nerves of the normal and the hypertrophied heart. Norm Pathol Anat (Stuttg) 33:1–68

98. Borg K, Ahlberg G, Anvret M, Edström L (1998) Welander distal myopathy-an overview. Neuromusc Disord 8:115–118

99. Borg K, Borg J, Lindbloom U (1987) Sensory involvement in distal myopathy (Welander). J Neurol Sci 80: 323–332

100. Borg K, Solders G, Borg J, Edström L, Kristensson K (1989) Neurogenic involvement in distal myopathy (Welander). Histochemical and morphological observations on muscle and nerve biopsies. J Neurol Sci 91:53–70

101. Bort S, Nelis E, Timmerman V, Sevilla T, Cruz-Martinez A, Martinez F, Millan JM, Arpa J, Vilchez JJ, Prieto F, Van Broeckhoven C, Palau F (1997) Mutational analysis of the MPZ, PMP22 and Cx32 genes in patients of Spanish ancestry with Charcot-Marie-Tooth disease and hereditary neuropathy with liability to pressure palsies. Hum Genet 99:746–754

102. Bort S, Sevilla T, Garcia-Planells J (1996) Déjérine-Sottas Neuropathy associated with de novo S79P mutation of the peripheral myelin protein 22 (PMP22) gene. Hum Mut 1:S95-S98

103. Bosboom WM, Van den Berg LH, De Boer L, Van Son MJ, Veldman H, Franssen H, Logtenberg T, Wokke JH (1999) The diagnostic value of sural nerve T cells in chronic inflammatory demyelinating polyneuropathy. Neurology 53:837–845

104. Bostock H, Sharief MK, Reid G, Murray NM (1995) Axonal ion channel dysfunction in amyotrophic lateral sclerosis. Brain 118:217–225

105. Bouche P, Leger JM, Travers MA, Cathala HP, Castaigne P (1986) Peripheral neuropathy in systemic vasculitis: clinical and electrophysiologic study of 22 patients. Neurology 36:1598–1602

106. Bowe CM, Hildebrand C, Kocsis JD, Waxman SG (1989) Morphological and physiological properties of neurons after long-term axonal regeneration: observations on chronic and delayed sequelae of peripheral nerve injury. J Neurol Sci 91:259–292

107. Boysen G, Galassi G, Kamieniecka Z, Schlaeger J, Trojaborg W (1979) Familial amyloidosis with cranial neuropathy and corneal lattice dystrophy. J Neurol Neurosurg Psychiatry 42:1020–1030

108. Bradley JL, Thomas PK, King RH, Muddle JR, Ward JD, Tesfaye S, Boulton AJ, Tsigos C, Young RJ (1995) Myelinated nerve fibre regeneration in diabetic sensory polyneuropathy: correlation with type of diabetes. Acta Neuropathol (Berl) 90:403–410

109. Bradley JL, Thomas PK, King RH, Watkins PJ (1994) A comparison of perineurial and vascular basal laminal changes in diabetic neuropathy. Acta Neuropathol (Berl) 88:426–432

110. Bradley WG, Badger GJ, Tandan R, Fillyaw MJ, Young J, Fries TJ, Krusinski PB, Witarsa M, Boerman J, Blair CJ (1988) Double-blind controlled trials of Cronassial in chronic neuromuscular diseases and ataxia. Neurology 38:1731–1739

111. Brady RO (1993) Fabry disease. In: Dyck PJ, Thomas PK (eds) Peripheral Neuropathy. Saunders, Philadelphia London Toronto, pp 1169–1178

112. Brashear A, Unverzagt FW, Farber MO, Bonnin JM, Garcia JG, Grober E (1996) Ethylene oxide neurotoxicity: a cluster of 12 nurses with peripheral and central nervous system toxicity. Neurology 46:992–998

113. Braun PE, Frail DE, Latov N (1982) Myelin-associated glycoprotein is the antigen for a monoclonal IgM in polyneuropathy. J Neurochem 39:1261–1265

114. Braun V, Richter HP (1996) Erstmaliger Nachweis der Möglichkeit einer spontanen funktionellen Regeneration motorischer Nerven beim Menschen. In: Schmelzle R, Bschorer R (eds) Plastische und Wiederherstellungschirurgie – Ein Jahrbuch. Uni-MED Verlag, Lorch, pp 48–51

115. Braun V, Richter HP, Schröder JM (1995) Selective peripheral denervation for spasmodic torticollis: is the outcome predictable? J Neurol 242:504–507

116. Brett M, Persey MR, Reilly MM, Revesz T, Booth DR, Booth SE, Hawkins PN, Pepys MB, Morgan-Hughes JA (1999) Transthyretin Leu12Pro is associated with systemic, neuropathic and leptomeningeal amyloidosis. Brain 122:183–190

117. Briggs L, Garcia JH, Conger KA, Pinto de Moraes H, Geer JC, Hollander W (1985) Innervation of brain intraparenchymal vessels in subhuman primates: ultrastructural observations. Stroke 16:297–301

118. Bristol DC, Fraher JP (1989) Experimental traction injuries of ventral spinal nerve roots. A scanning electron microscopic study. Neuropathol Appl Neurobiol 15: 549–561

119. Brodeur GM, Shimada, H (1998) Pheochromocytomas and paragangliomas. In: Bigner DD, McLendon RE, Bruner JM (eds) Russell and Rubinstein's Pathology of Tumors of the Nervous System (vol 2). Arnold, London Sydney Auckland, pp 535–560

120. Bronson RT, Lake BD, Cook S, Taylor S, Davisson MT (1993) Motor neuron degeneration of mice is a model of neuronal ceroid lipofuscinosis (Batten's disease). Ann Neurol 33:381–385

121. Brook G, Duchen L (1990) End-plates, transmissions and contractile characteristics of muscles without spindles in the hereditary sensory neuropathy of the sprawling mouse. Brain 113:867–891

122. Brooks JS, Freeman M, Enterline HT (1985) Malignant "Triton" tumors. Natural history and immunohistochemistry of nine new cases with literature review. Cancer 55:2543–2549

123. Brooks-Wilson A, Marcil M, Clee SM, Zhang LH, Roomp K, van Dam M, Yu L, Brewer C, Collins JA, Molhuizen HO, Loubser O, Ouelette BF, Fichter K, Ashbourne-Excoffon KJ, Sensen CW, Scherer S, Mott S, Denis M, Martindale D, Frohlich J, Morgan K, Koop B, Pimstone S, Kastelein JJ, Hayden MR et al. (1999) Mutations in ABC1 in Tangier disease and familial high-density lipoprotein deficiency (see comments). Nat Genet 22: 336–345

124. Brosnan JV, King RH, Thomas PK, Craggs RI (1988) Disease patterns in experimental allergic neuritis (EAN) in the Lewis rat. Is EAN a good model for the Guillain-Barré syndrome? J Neurol Sci 88:261–276

125. Brown H, Flynn JE (1973) Abdominal pedicle flap for hand neuromas and entrapped nerves. J Bone Joint Surg Am 55:575–579

126. Brown MC, Perry VH, Lunn ER, Gordon S, Heumann R (1991) Macrophage dependence of peripheral sensory nerve regeneration: possible involvement of nerve growth factor. Neuron 6:359–370

127. Brown MJ, Martin JR, Asbury AK (1976) Painful diabetic neuropathy. A morphometric study. Arch Neurol 33: 164–171

128. Bruyn GW, Bots GT, Went LN, Klinkhamer PJ (1992) Hereditary spastic dystonia with Leber's hereditary optic neuropathy: neuropathological findings. J Neurol Sci 113:55–61

129. Bruzzone R, White TW, Scherer SS, Fischbeck KH, Paul DL (1994) Null mutations of connexin32 in patients with X-linked Charcot-Marie-Tooth disease. Neuron 13:1253–1260

130. Busard H, Gabreels-Festen A, Van 't Hof M, Renier W, Gabreels F (1990) Polyglucosan bodies in sural nerve biopsies. Acta neuropathol (Berl) 80:554–557

131. Butinar D, Zidar J, Leonardis L, Popovic M, Kalaydjieva L, Angelicheva D, Sininger Y, Keats B, Starr A (1999) Hereditary auditory, vestibular, motor, and sensory neuropathy in a Slovenian Roma (Gypsy) kindred. Ann Neurol 46:36–44

132. Buxton PH, Hayward M (1967) Polyneuritis cranialis associated with industrial trichloroethylene poisoning. J Neurol Neurosurg Psychiatry 30:511–518

133. Byrnes ML, Thickbroom GW, Wilson SA, Sacco P, Shipman JM, Stell R, Mastaglia FL (1998) The corticomotor representation of upper limb muscles in writer's cramp and changes following botulinum toxin injection. Brain 121:977–988

134. Calabresi PA, Silvestri G, DiMauro S, Griggs RC (1994) Ekbom's syndrome: lipomas, ataxia, and neuropathy with MERRF (see comments). Muscle Nerve 17:943–945

135. Calcutt NA, Carrington AL, Ettlinger CB, Tomlinson DR (1992) The effect of mixed bovine brain gangliosides on hypoxic conduction block in control and streptozotocin-diabetic rats. J Neurol Sci 109:96–101

136. Campuzano V, Montermini L, Molto MDea (1996) Friedreich's ataxia: autosomal recessive disease caused by an intronic GAA triplet repeat expansion. Science 271:1423–1427

137. Carney JA (1990) Psammomatous melanotic Schwannoma. A distinctive, heritable tumor with special associations, including cardiac myxoma and the Cushing syndrome. Am J Surg Pathol 14:206–222

138. Carpo M, Pedotti R, Lolli F, Pitrola A, Allaria S, Scarlato G, Nobile-Orazio E (1998) Clinical correlate and fine specificity of anti-GQ1b antibodies in peripheral neuropathy. J Neurol Sci 155:186–191

139. Caruso G, Santoro L, Perretti A, Massini R, Pelosi L, Crisci C, Ragno M, Campanella G, Filla A (1987) Friedreich's ataxia: electrophysiologic and histologic findings in patients and relatives. Muscle Nerve 10:503–515

140. Casadei GP, Scheithauer BW, Hirose T, Manfrini M, Van Houton C, Wood MB (1995) Cellular Schwannoma. A clinicopathologic, DNA flow cytometric, and proliferation marker study of 70 patients. Cancer 75:1109–1119

141. Caselli RJ, Daube JR, Hunder GG, Whisnant JP (1988) Peripheral neuropathic syndromes in giant cell (temporal) arteritis. Neurology 38:685–689

142. Cavanagh JB (1999) Corpora-amylacea and the family of polyglucosan diseases. Brain Res Brain Res Rev 29:265–295

143. Cavanagh JB, Buxton PH (1989) Trichloroethylene cranial neuropathy: is it really a toxic neuropathy or does it activate latent herpes virus? J Neurol Neurosurg Psychiatry 52:297–303

144. Cavanagh JB, Tomiwa K, Munro PM (1987) Nuclear and nucleolar damage in adriamycin-induced toxicity to rat sensory ganglion cells. Neuropathol Appl Neurobiol 13:23–38

145. Caviglia AG, Monti G, Navassa G, Colzani M, Gomitoni A, Villa P, Zerbi D (1986) Chronic-relapsing polyneuropathy in the course of cryoglobulinemia. Clinical aspects and plasmapheretic treatment. Ric Clin Lab 16:385–387

146. Ceballos-Baumann AO, Sheean G, Passingham RE, Marsden CD, Brooks DJ (1997) Botulinum toxin does not reverse the cortical dysfunction associated with writer's cramp. A PET study. Brain 120:571–582

147. Ceuterick C, Martin JJ (1992) Electron microscopic features of skin in neurometabolic disorders. J Neurol Sci 112:15–29

148. Ceuterick C, Martin JJ (1994) Nerve biopsy findings in Niemann-Pick type II (NPC) (letter; comment). Acta Neuropathol (Berl) 88:602–603

149. Ceuterick de Groote C, Martin JJ (1998) Extracerebral biopsy in lysosomal and peroxisomal disorders. Ultrastructural findings. Brain Pathol 8:121–132

150. Chad DA, Lacomis D (1994) Critically ill patients with newly acquired weakness: the clinicopathological spectrum (editorial; comment). Ann Neurol 35:257–259

151. Chalk CH, Homburger HA, Dyck PJ (1993) Anti-neutrophil cytoplasmic antibodies in vasculitis peripheral neuropathy. Neurology 43:1826–1827

152. Chalk CH, Lennon VA, Stevens JC, Windebank AJ (1993) Seronegativity for type 1 antineuronal nuclear antibodies ('anti-Hu') in subacute sensory neuronopathy patients without cancer (see comments). Neurology 43:2209–2211

153. Challa VR, Jona JZ, Markesbery WR (1977) Ultrastructural observations of the myenteric plexus in infantile hypertrophic pyloric stenosis. Am J Pathol 88:309–322

154. Chalmers RM, Harding AE (1996) A case-control study of Leber's hereditary optic neuropathy. Brain 119:1481–1486

155. Chance PF, Abbas N, Lensch MW, Pentao L, Roa BB, Patel PI, Lupski JR (1994) Two autosomal dominant neuropathies result from reciprocal DNA duplication/deletion of a region on chromosome 17. Hum Mol Genet 3:223–228

156. Chance PF, Bird TD, Matsunami N, Lensch MW, Brothman AR, Feldman GM (1992) Trisomy 17p associated with Charcot-Marie-Tooth neuropathy type 1A phenotype: evidence for gene dosage as a mechanism in CMT1A. Neurology 42:2295–2299

157. Chance PF, Bird TD, O'Connell P, Lipe H, Lalouel JM, Leppert M (1990) Genetic linkage and heterogeneity in type I Charcot-Marie-Tooth disease (hereditary motor and sensory neuropathy type I). Am J Hum Genet 47:915–925

158. Chance PF, Matsunami N, Lensch W, Smith B, Bird TD (1992) Analysis of the DNA duplication 17p11.2 in Charcot-Marie-Tooth neuropathy type 1 pedigrees: additional evidence for a third autosomal CMT1 locus. Neurology 42:2037–2041

159. Charnas L, Trapp B, Griffin J (1988) Congenital absence of peripheral myelin: abnormal Schwann cell development causes lethal arthrogryposis multiplex congenita. Neurology 38:966–974

160. Chaudhry V, Cornblath DR (1992) Wallerian degeneration in human nerves: serial electrophysiological studies. Muscle Nerve 15:687–693

161. Chen CM, Chang HS, Lyu RK, Tang LM, Chen ST (1997) Myasthenia gravis and Charcot-Marie-Tooth disease type 1A: an unusual combination of diseases. Muscle Nerve 20:1457–1459

162. Cheong DM, Vaccaro CA, Salanga VD, Wexner SD, Phillips RC, Hanson MR, Waxner SD (1995) Electrodiagnostic evaluation of fecal incontinence (published erratum appears in Muscle Nerve 1995 Nov;18(11):1368). Muscle Nerve 18:612–619

163. Chiba A, Kusunoki S, Obata H, Machinami R, Kanazawa I (1993) Serum anti-GQ1b IgG antibody is associated with ophthalmoplegia in Miller Fisher syndrome and Guillain-Barré syndrome: clinical and immunohistochemical studies. Neurology 43:1911–1917

164. Chiba A, Kusunoki S, Obata H, Machinami R, Kanazawa I (1993) Serum anti-GQ1b IgG antibody is associated with ophthalmoplegia in Miller Fisher syndrome and Guillain-Barré syndrome: clinical and immunohistochemical studies. Neurology 43:1911–1917

165. Chitre MB, Rajshekhar V, Chandi SM, Chandy MJ (1992) Cystic cerebellar Schwannoma. Br J Neurosurg 6: 477–479

166. Chou SM (1992) Immunohistochemical and ultrastructural classification of peripheral neuropathies with onion-bulbs. Clin Neuropathol 11:109–114

167. Chou SM, Gilbert EF, Chun RW, Laxova R, Tuffli GA, Sufit RL, Krassikot N (1990) Infantile olivopontocerebellar atrophy with spinal muscular atrophy (infantile OPCA + SMA). Clin Neuropathol 9:21–32

168. Christodoulou K, Kyriakides T, Hristova AH, Georgiou DM, Kalaydjieva L, Yshpekova B, Ivanova T, Weber JL, Middleton LT (1995) Mapping of a distal form of spinal muscular atrophy with upper limb predominance to chromosome 7p. Hum Mol Genet 4:1629–1632

169. Churg J, Strauss L (1951) Allergic granulomatosis, allergic angiitis and periarteritis nodosa. Amer J Path 27:277

170. Cinar Y, Hekimoglu F, Ince B, Ince U, Onganer E (1998) A case of a hereditary, late progressing sensory autonomic neuropathy. Clin Neuropathol 17:12–14

171. Clark AW, Tran PM, Parhad IM, Krekoski CA, Julien JP (1990) Neuronal gene expression in amyotrophic lateral sclerosis. Brain Res Mol Brain Res 7:75–83

172. Classen CF (1990) Hereditäre sensorisch-autonome Neuropathie Typ II: 2 Beobachtungen. Pädiat Prax 40: 399–406

173. Cock HR, Cooper JM, Schapira AHV (1999) Functional consequences of the 3460-bp mitochondrial DNA mutation associated with Leber's hereditary optic neuropathy. J Neurol Sci 165:10–17

174. Cock HR, Tabrizi SJ, Cooper JM, Schapira AH (1998) The influence of nuclear background on the biochemical expression of 3460 Leber's hereditary optic neuropathy. Ann Neurol 44:187–193

175. Cohen BA, McArthur JC, Grohman S, Patterson B, Glass JD (1993) Neurologic prognosis of cytomegalovirus polyradiculomyelopathy in AIDS (see comments). Neurology 43:493–499

176. Cohen J, Low P, Fealey R, Sheps S, Jiang NS (1987) Somatic and autonomic function in progressive autonomic failure and multiple system atrophy. Ann Neurol 22: 692–699

177. Cohen-Cory S, Fraser SE (1995) Effects of brain-derived neurotrophic factor on optic axon branching and remodelling in vivo. Nature 378:192–196

178. Combarros O, Pascual J, de Pablos C, Ortega F, Berciano J (1996) Taste loss as an initial symptom of Guillain-Barré syndrome. Neurology 47:1604–1605

179. Comella CL, Buchman AS, Tanner CM, Brown-Toms NC, Goetz CG (1992) Botulinum toxin injection for spasmodic torticollis: increased magnitude of benefit with electromyographic assistance. Neurology 42:878–882

180. Comola M, Nemni R, Sher E, Quattrini A, Faravelli A, Comi G, Corbo M, Clementi F, Canal N (1993) Lambert-Eaton myasthenic syndrome and polyneuropathy in a patient with epidermoid carcinoma of the lung. Eur J Neurol 33:121–125

181. Connolly AM, Pestronk A, Mehta S, Yee WC, Green BJ, Fellin C, Olney RK, Miller RG, Devor WN (1997) Serum IgM monoclonal autoantibody binding to the 301 to 314 amino acid epitope of beta-tubulin: clinical association with slowly progressive demyelinating polyneuropathy. Neurology 48:243–248

182. Connolly AM, Pestronk A, Trotter JL, Feldman EL, Cornblath DR, Olney RK (1993) High-titer selective serum anti-beta-tubulin antibodies in chronic inflammatory demyelinating polyneuropathy. Neurology 43:557–562

183. Constantin G, Piccio L, Bussini S, Pizzuti A, Scarpini E, Baron P, Conti G, Pizzul S, Scarlato G (1999) Induction of adhesion molecules on human Schwann cells by proinflammatory cytokines, an immunofluorescence study. J Neurol Sci 170:124–130

184. Conti AM, Fischer SJ, Windebank AJ (1997) Inhibition of axonal growth from sensory neurons by excess nerve growth factor. Ann Neurol 42:838–846

185. Corbo M, Abouzahr MK, Latov N, Iannaccone S, Quattrini A, Nemni R, Canal N, Hays AP (1997) Motor nerve biopsy studies in motor neuropathy and motor neuron disease. Muscle Nerve 20:15–21

186. Cornblath D (1991) Research criteria for diagnosis of chronic inflammatory demyelinating polyneuropathy (CIDP). Neurology 41:617–618

187. Cornblath DR, McArthur JC (1988) Predominantly sensory neuropathy in patients with AIDS and AIDS-related complex. Neurology 38:794–796

188. Cornell J, Sellars S, Beighton P (1984) Autosomal recessive inheritance of Charcot-Marie-Tooth disease associated with sensorineural deafness. Clin Genet 25: 163–165

189. Corse AM, Chaudhry V, Crawford TO, Cornblath DR, Kuncl RW, Griffin JW (1996) Sensory nerve pathology in multifocal motor neuropathy (see comments). Ann Neurol 39:319–325

190. Costeff H, Gadoth N, Apter N, Prialnic M, Savir H (1989) A familial syndrome of infantile optic atrophy, movement disorder, and spastic paraplegia. Neurology 39: 595–597

191. Cowchock FS, Duckett SW, Streletz LJ, Graziani LJ, Jackson LG (1985) X-linked motor-sensory neuropathy type-II with deafness and mental retardation: a new disorder. Am J Med Genet 20:307–315

192. Craddock C, Pasvol G, Bull R, Protheroe A, Hopkin J (1987) Cardiorespiratory arrest and autonomic neuropathy in AIDS. Lancet 2:16–18

193. Cras P, Ceuterick de Groote C, Van Vyve M, Vercruyssen A, Martin JJ (1990) Malignant pigmented spinal nerve

root Schwannoma metastasizing in the brain and viscera. Clin Neuropathol 9:290–294

194. Créange A, Zeller J, Rostaing-Rigattieri S, Brugières P, Degos J-D, Revuz J, Wolkenstein P (1999) Neurological complications of neurofibromatosis type 1. Brain 122: 473–481

195. Croen KD, Ostrove JM, Dragovic LJ, Straus SE (1988) Patterns of gene expression and sites of latency in human nerve ganglia are different for varicella-zoster and herpes simplex viruses. Proc Natl Acad Sci USA 85:9773–9777

196. Cros D, Harnden P, Pouget J, Pellissier JF, Gastaut JL, Serratrice G (1988) Peripheral neuropathy in myotonic dystrophy: a nerve biopsy study. Ann Neurol 23:470–476

197. Cros D, Triggs WJ (1994) There are no neurophysiologic features characteristic of "axonal" Guillain-Barré syndrome. Muscle Nerve 17:675–677

198. Cruz-Martinez A, Anciones B, Palau F (1997) GAA trinucleotide repeat expansion in variant Friedreich's ataxia families. Muscle Nerve 20:1121–1126

199. Crystal HA, Schaumburg HH, Grober E, Fuld PA, Lipton RB (1988) Cognitive impairment and sensory loss associated with chronic low-level ethylene oxide exposure. Neurology 38:567–569

200. Cummings JF, George C, de Lahunta A, Valentine BA, Bookbinder PF (1989) Focal spinal muscular atrophy in two German shepherd pups. Acta Neuropathol (Berl) 79:113–116

201. Cuppini R, Cecchini T, Ciaroni S, Ambrogini P, Del Grande P (1993) Nodal and terminal sprouting by regenerating nerve in vitamin E-deficient rats. J Neurol Sci 117: 61–67

202. Cusimano MD, Bilbao JM, Cohen SM (1988) Hypertrophic brachial plexus neuritis: a pathological study of two cases. Ann Neurol 24:615–622

203. da Luz NW, Vieira G, Rinaldi B (1981) Phlebectasia within the sural nerve. J Cardiovasc Surg (Torino) 22: 213–216

204. da Silveira CM, Salisbury DM, de Quadros CA (1997) Measles vaccination and Guillain-Barré syndrome (see comments). Lancet 349:14–16

205. Dalakas MC (1986) Chronic idiopathic ataxic neuropathy. Ann Neurol 19:545–554

206. Dalakas MC (1988) Morphologic changes in the muscles of patients with postpoliomyelitis neuromuscular symptoms. Neurology 38:99–104

207. Dalakas MC, Leon-Monzon ME, Bernardini I, Gahl WA, Jay CA (1994) Zidovudine-induced mitochondrial myopathy is associated with muscle carnitine deficiency and lipid storage (see comments). Ann Neurol 35: 482–487

208. Darnell RB (1993) The polymerase chain reaction: application to nervous system disease. Ann Neurol 34: 513–523

209. Davies AM, Bandtlow C, Heumann R, Korsching S, Rohrer H, Thoenen H (1987) Timing and site of nerve growth factor synthesis in developing skin in relation to innervation and expression of the receptor. Nature 326:353–358

210. Davies L, Spies JM, Pollard JD, McLeod JG (1996) Vasculitis confined to peripheral nerves. Brain 119:1441–1448

211. Davis DG, Markesbery WR (1992) Perivascular siderophages in skeletal muscle from a patient with diabetic neuropathy. Acta Neuropathol (Berl) 84:216–220

212. De Blaquière G, Santamaria L, Curtis J, Terenghi G, Polak J, Turk J (1994) A morphological and functional assessment of myobacterium leprae-induced nerve damage in a guinea-pig model of leprous neuritis. Neuropathol Appl Neurobiol 20:261–271

213. de Iongh RU (1990) A quantitative ultrastructural study of motor and sensory lumbosacral nerve roots in the thalidomide-treated rabbit fetus. J Neuropathol Exp Neurol 49:564–581

214. DeAngelis LM, Kelleher MB, Post KD, Fetell MR (1987) Multiple paragangliomas in neurofibromatosis: a new neuroendocrine neoplasia. Neurology 37:129–133

215. Delhaas T, Kamphuis DJ, Witkamp TD (1998) Transitory spinal cord swelling in a 6-year-old boy with Guillain-Barré syndrome. Pediatr Radiol 28:544–546

216. Denny-Brown D (1951) Hereditary sensory radicular neuropathy. J Neurol Neurosurg Psychiatr 14:237–252

217. DePaul R, Abbs JH, Caligiuri M, Gracco VL, Brooks BR (1988) Hypoglossal, trigeminal, and facial motoneuron involvement in amyotrophic lateral sclerosis. Neurology 38:281–283

218. Deruaz JP, Janzer RC, Costa J (1993) Cellular Schwannomas of the intracranial and intraspinal compartment: morphological and immunological characteristics compared with classical benign Schwannomas. J Neuropathol Exp Neurol 52:114–118

219. Desai HB, Donat J, Shokeir MH, Munoz DG (1990) Amyotrophic lateral sclerosis in a patient with fragile X syndrome. Neurology 40:378–80

220. Dettmers C, Fatepour D, Faust H, Jerusalem F (1993) Sympathetic skin response abnormalities in amyotrophic lateral sclerosis (see comments). Muscle Nerve 16: 930–934

221. Deuschl G, Seifert C, Heinen F, Illert M, Lucking CH (1992) Reciprocal inhibition of forearm flexor muscles in spasmodic torticollis. J Neurol Sci 113:85–90

222. Di Trapani G, Carnevale A, Cioffi RP, Massaro AR, Profice P (1996) Multiple sclerosis associated with peripheral demyelinating neuropathy. Clin Neuropathol 15:135–138

223. Di Troia A, Carpo M, Meucci N, Pellegrino C, Allaria S, Gemignani F, Marbini A, Mantegazza R, Sciolla R, Manfredini E, Scarlato G, Nobile-Orazio E (1999) Clinical features and anti-neural reactivity in neuropathy associated with IgG monoclonal gammopathy of undetermined significance. J Neurol Sci 164:64–71

224. Dias-Tosta E, Kuckelhaus CS, Amaral K (1999) Myasthenia gravis and peripheral neuropathy in an Amazon indigenous female. Neuromuscul Disord 9:262–263

225. Dichgans M, Gasser T (1999) Klinische Befunde und diagnostisches Vorgehen bei CADASIL. Akt Neurologie 26:260–269

226. Dieler R, Schröder JM (1989) Myenteric plexus neuropathy in infantile hypertrophic pyloric stenosis. Acta Neuropathol (Berl) 78:649–661

227. Dieler R, Schröder JM (1990) Abnormal sensory and motor reinnervation of rat muscle spindles following nerve transection and suture. Acta Neuropathol (Berl) 80:163–171

228. Dieler R, Schröder JM (1990) Lacunar dilatations of intrafusal and extrafusal terminal cisternae, annulate lamellae, confronting cisternae and tubulofilamentous inclusions within the spectrum of muscle and nerve fiber changes in myotonic dystrophy. Pathol Res Pract 186:371–382

229. Dieler R, Schröder JM, Reddemann K (1990) Electron-dense lipidic capillary deposits in Rett Syndrome. Acta Neuropathol 79:573-578

230. Dieler R, Schröder JM, Skopnik H, Steinau G (1990) Infantile hypertrophic pyloric stenosis: myopathic type. Acta Neuropathol (Berl) 80:295-306

231. Dieler R, Völker A, Schröder JM (1992) Scanning electron microscopic study of denervated and reinnervated intrafusal muscle fibers in rats. Muscle Nerve 15:433-441

232. Dittrich F, Thoenen H, Sendtner M (1994) Ciliary neurotrophic factor: pharmacokinetics and acute-phase response in rat (see comments). Ann Neurol 35:151-163

233. Dole MG, Jasty R, Cooper MJ, Thompson CB, Nunez G, Castle VP (1995) Bcl-xL is expressed in neuroblastoma cells and modulates chemotherapy-induced apoptosis. Cancer Res 55:2576-2582

234. Dolly JO, Black J, Williams RS, Melling J (1984) Acceptors for botulinum neurotoxin reside on motor nerve terminals and mediate its internalization. Nature 307:457-460

235. Donaghy M, Hakin RN, Bamford JM, Garner A, Kirkby GR, Noble BA, Tazir-Melboucy M, King RH, Thomas PK (1987) Hereditary sensory neuropathy with neurotrophic keratitis. Description of an autosomal recessive disorder with a selective reduction of small myelinated nerve fibres and a discussion of the classification of the hereditary sensory neuropathies. Brain 110:563-583

236. Donaghy M, King RH, McKeran RO, Schwartz MS, Thomas PK (1990) Cerebrotendinous xanthomatosis: clinical, electrophysiological and nerve biopsy findings, and response to treatment with chenodeoxycholic acid. J Neurol 237:216-219

237. Donofrio PD, Kelly JJ Jr (1989) AAEE case report 17: Peripheral neuropathy in monoclonal gammopathy of undetermined significance. Muscle Nerve 12:1-8

238. Donofrio PD, Stanton C, Miller VS, Oestreich L, Lefkowitz DS, Walker FO, Ely EW (1992) Demyelinating polyneuropathy in eosinophilia-myalgia syndrome. Muscle Nerve 15:796-805

239. Dotson R, Ochoa J, Marchettini P, Cline M (1990) Sympathetic neural outflow directly recorded in patients with primary autonomic failure: clinical observations, microneurography, and histopathology. Neurology 40:1079-1085

240. Drachman DB, Kuncl RW (1989) Amyotrophic lateral sclerosis: an unconventional autoimmune disease? Ann Neurol 26:269-274

241. Drlicek M, Bodenteich A, Setinek U, Tucek G, Urbanits S, Grisold W (2000) T cell-mediated paraneoplastic ganglionitis - an autopsy case. Acta Neuropathol (Berl) 99:599-602

242. Dropcho EJ, Stanton C, Oh SJ (1989) Neuronal antinuclear antibodies in a patient with Lambert-Eaton myasthenic syndrome and small-cell lung carcinoma. Neurology 39:249-251

243. Dubas F, Saint-Andre JP, Pouplard-Barthelaix A, Delestre F, Emile J (1990) Intravascular malignant lymphomatosis (so-called malignant angioendotheliomatosis): a case confined to the lumbosacral spinal cord and nerve roots. Clin Neuropathol 9:115-120

244. Duchen LW (1971) Changes in the electron microscopic structure of slow and fast skeletal muscle fibres of the mouse after the local injection of botulinum toxin. J Neurol Sci 14:61-74

245. Duchen LW (1971) An electron microscopic study of the changes induced by botulinum toxin in the motor end-plates of slow and fast skeletal muscle fibres of the mouse. J Neurol Sci 14:47-60

246. Duckers HJ, Verhaagen J, de Bruijn E, Gispen WH (1994) Effective use of a neurotrophic ACTH4-9 analogue in the treatment of a peripheral demyelinating syndrome (experimental allergic neuritis). An intervention study. Brain 117:365-374

247. Dulaney JT, Moser HW (1978) Sulfatide lipidosis: metachromatic leukodystrophy. In: Stanbury JB, Wyngaarden JB, Fredrickson DS (eds) The metabolic basis of inherited disease (vol 4) McGraw-Hill, New York

248. Dunn HG (1973) Nerve conduction studies in children with Friedreich's ataxia and ataxia-telangiectasia. Dev Med Child Neurol 15:324-337

249. Duyckaerts C, Durr A, Cancel G, Brice A (1999) Nuclear inclusions in spinocerebellar ataxia type 1. Acta Neuropathol (Berl) 97:201-207

250. Dyck PJ (1989) Hypoxic neuropathy: does hypoxia play a role in diabetic neuropathy? The 1988 Robert Wartenberg lecture. Neurology 39:111-118

251. Dyck PJ, Chance P, Lebo R, Carney JA (1993) Hereditary motor and sensory neuropathies. In: Dyck PJ, Thomas PK, Griffin JW, Low PA, Poduslo JF (eds) Peripheral Neuropathy, (vol 3) W.B. Saunders Company, Philadelphia, pp 1094-1136

252. Dyck PJ, Conn DL, Okazaki H (1972) Necrotizing angiopathic neuropathy. Three-dimensional morphology of fiber degeneration related to sites of occluded vessels. Mayo Clin Proc 47:461-475

253. Dyck PJ, Giannini C (1996) Pathologic alterations in the diabetic neuropathies of humans: a review (see comments). J Neuropathol Exp Neurol 55:1181-1193

254. Dyck PJ, Johnson WJ, Lambert EH, O'Brien PC (1971) Segmental demyelination secondary to axonal degeneration in uremic neuropathy. Mayo Clin Proc 46:400-431

255. Dyck PJ, Lais AC (1971) Evidence for segmental demyelination secondary to axonal degeneration in Friedreich's ataxia. ICS No. 295: Clinical Studies in Myology, Part 2 of the Proc. of the Second Intern. Congr. on Muscle Diseases, Perth, Australia, pp 22-26

256. Dyck PJ, Lambert EH (1970) Polyneuropathy associated with hypothyroidism. J Neuropathol Exp Neurol 29:631-658

257. Dyck PJ, Lofgren EP (1966) Method of fascicular biopsy of human peripheral nerve for electrophysiologic and histologic study. Mayo Clin Proc 41:778-784

258. Dyck PJ, Low PA, Stevens JC (1983) "Burning feet" as the only manifestation of dominantly inherited sensory neuropathy. Mayo Clin Proc 58:426-429

259. Dyck PJ, Ott J, Moore SB, Swanson CJ, Lambert EH (1983) Linkage evidence for genetic heterogeneity among kinships with hereditary motor and sensory neuropathy, type I. Mayo Clin Proc 58:430-435

260. Dyck PJ, Thomas PK (1993) Peripheral neuropathy, 3rd ed. Saunders, Philadelphia London Toronto

261. Dyck PJ, Thomas PK (1999) Diabetic neuropathy - book review. Muscle Nerve 22:972-973

262. Dyck PJ, Thomas PK, Asbury AK, Winegrad AI, Porte D (1987) Diabetic Neuropathy. Saunders Company, Philadelphia

263. Edery P, Pelet A, Mulligan LM, Abel L, Attie T, Dow E, Bonneau D, David A, Flintoff W, Jan D et al. (1994) Long

segment and short segment familial Hirschsprung's disease: variable clinical expression at the RET locus. J Med Genet 31:602–606

264. Edvinsson L, Ekman R, Jansen I, Ottosson A, Uddman R (1987) Peptide-containing nerve fibers in human cerebral arteries: immunocytochemistry, radioimmunoassay, and in vitro pharmacology. Ann Neurol 21: 431–437

265. Edvinsson L, Hara H, Uddman R (1989) Retrograde tracing of nerve fibers to the rat middle cerebral artery with true blue: colocalization with different peptides. J Cereb Blood Flow Metab 9:212–218

266. Eggers C, Hagel C, Pfeiffer G (1998) Anti-Hu-associated paraneoplastic sensory neuropathy with peripheral nerve demyelination and microvasculitis. J Neurol Sci 155:178–181

267. Elbadawi A, Yalla SV, Resnick NM (1993) Structural basis of geriatric voiding dysfunction. IV. Bladder outlet obstruction. J Urol 150:1681–1695

268. Enders U, Karch H, Toyka KV, Michels M, Zielasek J, Pette M, Heesemann J, Hartung HP (1993) The spectrum of immune responses to Campylobacter jejuni and glycoconjugates in Guillain-Barré syndrome and in other neuroimmunological disorders (see comments). Ann Neurol 34:136–144

269. Engelhardt JI, Tajti J, Appel SH (1993) Lymphocytic infiltrates in the spinal cord in amyotrophic lateral sclerosis. Arch Neurol 50:30–36

270. England JD, Asbury AK, Rhee EK, Sumner AJ (1988) Lethal retrograde axoplasmic transport of doxorubicin (adriamycin) to motor neurons. A toxic motor neuronopathy. Brain 111:915–926

271. England JD, Rhee EK, Said G, Sumner AJ (1988) Schwann cell degeneration induced by doxorubicin (adriamycin). Brain 111:901–913

272. Engstrom JW, Layzer RB, Olney RK, Edwards MB (1993) Idiopathic, progressive mononeuropathy in young people. Arch Neurol 50:20–23

273. Enzinger FM, Weiss SW (1995) Soft tissue tumors, 3rd ed. Mosby-Year Book, St. Louis

274. Eriksen CA, Anders CJ (1991) Audit of results of operations for infantile pyloric stenosis in a district general hospital (see comments). Arch Dis Child 66: 130–133

275. Ernfors P, Lee KF, Kucera J, Jaenisch R (1994) Lack of neurotrophin-3 leads to deficiencies in the peripheral nervous system and loss of limb proprioceptive afferents. Cell 77:503–512

276. Esiri MM, Tomlinson AH (1972) Herpes Zoster. Demonstration of virus in trigeminal nerve and ganglion by immunofluorescence and electron microscopy. J Neurol Sci 15:35–48

277. Estrada R, Galarraga J, Orozco G, Nodarse A, Auburger G (1999) Spinocerebellar ataxia 2 (SCA2): morphometric analyses in 11 autopsies. Acta Neuropathol (Berl) 97:306–910

278. Evangelista T, Carvalho M, Conceicao I, Pinto A, de Lurdes M, Luis ML (1996) Motor neuropathies mimicking amyotrophic lateral sclerosis/motor neuron disease. J Neurol Sci 139 Suppl:95–98

279. Evans PJ, Mackinnon SE, Best TJ, Wade JA, Awerbuck DC, Makino AP, Hunter DA, Midha R (1995) Regeneration across preserved peripheral nerve grafts. Muscle Nerve 18:1128–1138

280. Fabian VA, Wood B, Crowley P, Kakulas BA (1997) Herpes zoster brachial plexus neuritis. Clin Neuropathol 16:61–64

281. Fadic R, Russell JA, Vedanarayanan VV, Lehar M, Kuncl RW, Johns DR (1997) Sensory ataxic neuropathy as the presenting feature of a novel mitochondrial disease. Neurology 49:239–245

282. Farrell DF, Hamilton SR, Knauss TA, Sanocki E, Deeb SS (1993) X-linked adrenoleukodystrophy: adult cerebral variant. Neurology 43:1518–1522

283. Farrell DF, Starr A (1968) Delayed neurological sequelae of electrical injuries. Neurology 18:601–606

284. Feasby TE (1996) Axonal CIDP: a premature concept? Muscle Nerve 19:372–374

285. Feibel JH, Campa JF (1976) Thyrotoxic neuropathy (Basedow's paraplegia). J Neurol Neurosurg Psychiatry 39:491–497

286. Feldman D, Anderson TD (1994) Schwann cell mitochondrial alterations in peripheral nerves of rabbits treated with 2′,3′-dideoxycytidine. Acta Neuropathol (Berl) 87:71–80

287. Fetter M, Dichgans J (1996) Vestibular neuritis spares the inferior division of the vestibular nerve. Brain 110:755–763

288. Fialkow PJ, Sagebiel RW, Gartler SM, Rimoin DL (1971) Multiple cell origin of hereditary neurofibromas. N Engl J Med 284:298–300

289. Fidzianska A, Toniolo D, Hausmanowa-Petrusewicz I (1998) Ultrastructural abnormality of sarcolemmal nuclei in Emery-Dreifuss muscular dystrophy (EDMD). J Neurol Sci 159:88–93

290. Filla A, De Michele G, Banfi S, Santoro L, Perretti A, Cavalcanti F, Pianese L, Castaldo I, Barbieri F, Campanella G et al. (1995) Has spinocerebellar ataxia type 2 a distinct phenotype? Genetic and clinical study of an Italian family. Neurology 45:793–796

291. Filla A, De Michele G, Campanella G, Perretti A, Santoro L, Serlenga L, Ragno M, Calabrese O, Castaldo I, De Joanna G, Cocozza S (1996) Autosomal dominant cerebellar ataxia type I. Clinical and molecular study in 36 Italian families including a comparison between SCA1 and SCA2 phenotypes. J Neurol Sci 142:140–147

292. Fine EJ, Soria E, Paroski MW, Petryk D, Thomasula L (1990) The neurophysiological profile of vitamin B12 deficiency. Muscle Nerve 13:158–164

293. Fischbeck KH, Abel A, Lin GS, Scherer SS (1999) X-linked Charcot-Marie-Tooth disease and connexin32. Ann N Y Acad Sci 883:36–41

294. Fischbeck KH, ar-Rushdi N, Pericak-Vance M, Rozear M, Roses AD, Fryns JP (1986) X-linked neuropathy: gene localization with DNA probes. Ann Neurol 20: 527–532

295. Fisher GT, Boswick JA Jr (1983) Neuroma formation following digital amputations. J Trauma 23:136–142

296. Fishman PS, Carrigan DR (1988) Motoneuron uptake from the circulation of the binding fragment of tetanus toxin. Arch Neurol 45:558–561

297. Flanigan KM, Crawford TO, Griffin JW, Goebel HH, Kohlschutter A, Ranells J, Camfield PR, Ptacek LJ (1998) Localization of the giant axonal neuropathy gene to chromosome 16q24. Ann Neurol 43:143–148

298. Flanigan KM, Johns DR (1993) Association of the 11778 mitochondrial DNA mutation and demyelinating disease. Neurology 43:2720–2722

299. Fletcher NA, Harding AE, Marsden CD (1991) The relationship between trauma and idiopathic torsion dystonia. Neurol Neurosurg Psychiat 54:713–717

300. Florence G, Seylaz J (1992) Rapid autoregulation of cerebral blood flow: a laser-Doppler flowmetry study. J Cereb Blood Flow Metab 12:674–680

301. Fois A, Balestri P, Farnetani MA, Berardi R, Mattei R, Laurenzi E, Alessandrini C, Gerli R, Ribuffo A, Calvieri S (1985) Giant axonal neuropathy. Endocrinological and histological studies. Eur J Pediatr 144:274–280

302. Folkerth RD, Alroy J, Lomakina I, Skutelsky E, Raghavan SS, Kolodny EH (1995) Mucolipidosis IV: morphology and histochemistry of an autopsy case. J Neuropathol Exp Neurol 54:154–164

303. Folkerth RD, Guttentag SH, Kupsky WJ, Kinney HC (1993) Arthrogryposis multiplex congenita with posterior column degeneration and peripheral neuropathy: a case report. Clin Neuropathol 12:25–33

304. Fontaine B, Hanson MP, VonSattel JP, Martuza RL, Gusella JF (1991) Loss of chromosome 22 alleles in human sporadic spinal Schwannomas. Ann Neurol 29: 183–186

305. Fressinaud C, Vallat JM, Durand J, Archambeaud-Mouveroux F, Rigaud M (1987) Changes in composition of endoneurial and perineurial fatty acids during glycerol-induced Wallerian degeneration and regeneration in the sciatic nerve of the adult rat. J Neurochem 49: 797–801

306. Fressinaud C, Vallat JM, Masson M, Jauberteau MO, Baumann N, Hugon J (1992) Adult-onset metachromatic leukodystrophy presenting as isolated peripheral neuropathy. Neurology 42:1396–1398

307. Friedman JM, Fialkow PJ, Greene CL, Weinberg MN (1982) Probable clonal origin of neurofibrosarcoma in a patient with hereditary neurofibromatosis. J Natl Cancer Inst 69:1289–1292

308. Fross RD, Daube JR (1987) Neuropathy in the Miller Fisher syndrome: clinical and electrophysiologic findings. Neurology 37:1493–1498

309. Fujita T, Kanno T, Kobayashi S (1988) The paraneuron. Springer, Berlin Heidelberg New York

310. Fuller GN, Jacobs JM (1989) Cytomembranous inclusions in the peripheral nerves in AIDS. Acta Neuropathol (Berl) 79:336–339

311. Fuller GN, Jacobs JM, Lewis PD, Lane RJ (1992) Pseudo-axonal Guillain-Barré syndrome: severe demyelination mimicking axonopathy. A case with pupillary involvement. J Neurol Neurosurg Psychiatry 55:1079–1083

312. Furneaux HF, Reich L, Posner JB (1990) Autoantibody synthesis in the central nervous system of patients with paraneoplastic syndromes. Neurology 40:1085–1091

313. Gabreels-Festen AA, Bolhuis PA, Hoogendijk JE, Valentijn LJ, Eshuis EJ, Gabreels FJ (1995) Charcot-Marie-Tooth disease type 1A: morphological phenotype of the 17p duplication versus PMP22 point mutations. Acta Neuropathol (Berl) 90:645–649

314. Gabreels-Festen AA, Gabreels FJ, Jennekens FG, Joosten EM, Janssen-van Kempen TW (1992) Autosomal recessive form of hereditary motor and sensory neuropathy type I. Neurology 42:1755–1761

315. Gabreels-Festen AA, Hoogendijk JE, Meijerink PH, Gabreels FJ, Bolhuis PA, van Beersum S, Kulkens T, Nelis E, Jennekens FG, de Visser M, van Engelen BG, Van Broeckhoven C, Mariman EC (1996) Two divergent

316. types of nerve pathology in patients with different P0 mutations in Charcot-Marie-Tooth disease. Neurology 47:761–765

316. Gal A, Mucke J, Theile H, Wieacker PF, Ropers HH, Wienker TF (1985) X-linked dominant Charcot-Marie-Tooth disease: suggestion of linkage with a cloned DNA sequence from the proximal Xq. Hum Genet 70:38–42

317. Gallant PE (1992) The direct effects of graded axonal compression on axoplasm and fast axoplasmic transport. J Neuropathol Exp Neurol 51:220–230

318. Galloway G, Giuliani MJ, Burns DK, Lacomis D (1998) Neuropathy associated with hyperoxaluria: improvement after combined renal and liver transplantations. Brain Pathol 8:247–251

319. Garcia-Merino A, Cabello A, Mora JS, Liano H (1991) Continuous muscle fiber activity, peripheral neuropathy, and thymoma (see comments). Ann Neurol 29: 215–218

320. Garnaas KR, Windebank AJ, Blexrud MD, Kurtz SB (1991) Ultrastructural changes produced in dorsal root ganglia in vitro by exposure to ethylene oxide from hemodialyzers. J Neuropathol Exp Neurol 50:256–262

321. Garofalo O, Kennedy PG, Swash M, Martin JE, Luthert P, Anderton BH, Leigh PN (1991) Ubiquitin and heat shock protein expression in amyotrophic lateral sclerosis. Neuropathol Appl Neurobiol 17:39–45

322. Gelot A, Vallat JM, Tabaraud F, Rocchiccioli F (1995) Axonal neuropathy and late detection of Refsum's disease. Muscle Nerve 18:667–670

323. Gervaix A, Caflisch M, Suter S, Haenggeli CA (1993) Guillain-Barré syndrome following immunisation with Haemophilus influenzae type b conjugate vaccine. Eur J Pediatr 152:613–614

324. Gherardi R, Gaulard P, Prost C, Rocha D, Imbert M, Andre C, Rochant H, Farcet JP (1986) T-cell lymphoma revealed by a peripheral neuropathy. A report of two cases with an immunohistologic study on lymph node and nerve biopsies. Cancer 58:2710–2716

325. Gherardi R, Lebargy F, Gaulard P, Mhiri C, Bernaudin JF, Gray F (1989) Necrotizing vasculitis and HIV replication in peripheral nerves (letter). N Engl J Med 321: 685–686

326. Gherardi RK, Chariot P, Vanderstigel M, Malapert D, Verroust J, Astier A, Brun-Buisson C, Schaeffer A (1990) Organic arsenic-induced Guillain-Barré-like syndrome due to melarsoprol: a clinical, electrophysiological, pathological study. Muscle Nerve 13:637–645

327. Giannini C, Dyck PJ (1994) Ultrastructural morphometric abnormalities of sural nerve endoneurial microvessels in diabetes mellitus. Ann Neurol 36:408–415

328. Giannini C, Monaco S, Kirschfink M, Rother KO, Lorbacher de Ruiz H, Nardelli E, Bonetti B, Salviati A, Zanette GP, Rizzuto N (1992) Inherited neuroaxonal dystrophy in C6 deficient rabbits. J Neuropathol Exp Neurol 51: 514–522

329. Gibbels E, Behse F, Kentenich M, Haupt WF (1993) Chronic multifocal neuropathy with persistent conduction block (Lewis-Sumner syndrome). A clinico-morphologic study of two further cases with review of the literature. Clin Neuropathol 12:343–352

330. Gibbels E, Behse F, Klingmuller G, Henke-Lubke U, Haupt WF, Gollmer E (1988) Sural nerve biopsy findings in leprosy: a qualitative and quantitative light and electron microscope study in 4 treated cases of the lepromatous spectrum. Clin Neuropathol 7:120–130

331. Gibbels E, Schaefer HE, Runne U, Schröder JM, Haupt WF, Assmann G (1985) Severe polyneuropathy in Tangier disease mimicking syringomyelia or leprosy. Clinical, biochemical, electrophysiological, and morphological evaluation, including electron microscopy of nerve, muscle, and skin biopsies. J Neurol 232:283–294

332. Giese KP, Martini R, Lemke G, Soriano P, Schachner M (1992) Mouse Po gene disruption leads to hypomyelination, abnormal expression of recognition molecules, and degeneration of myelin and axons. Cell 71:565–576

333. Giess R, Goetz R, Schrank B, Ochs G, Sendtner M, Toyka K (1998) Potential implications of a ciliary neurotrophic factor gene mutation in a German population of patients with motor neuron disease. Muscle Nerve 21: 236–238

334. Giftochristos N, David S (1988) Immature optic nerve glia of rat do not promote axonal regeneration when transplanted into a peripheral nerve. Brain Res 467: 149–153

335. Giladi N (1997) The mechanism of action of botulinum toxin type A in focal dystonia is most probably through its dual effect on efferent (motor) and afferent pathways at the injected site. J Neurol Sci 152:132–135

336. Gilden DH, Rozenman Y, Murray R, Devlin M, Vafai A (1987) Detection of varicella-zoster virus nucleic acid in neurons of normal human thoracic ganglia. Ann Neurol 22:377–380

337. Ginsberg AH, Gale MJ Jr, Rose LM, Clark EA (1989) T-cell alterations in late postpoliomyelitis. Arch Neurol 46:497–501

338. Giovannoni G, Hartung HP (1996) The immunopathogenesis of multiple sclerosis and Guillain-Barré syndrome. Curr Opin Neurol 9:165–177

339. Glanzman RL, Gelb DJ, Drury I, Bromberg MB, Truong DD (1990) Brachial plexopathy after botulinum toxin injections. Neurology 40:1143

340. Glazner GW, Ishii DN (1995) Insulinlike growth factor gene expression in rat muscle during reinnervation. Muscle Nerve 18:1433–1442

341. Goadsby PJ, Edvinsson L (1993) The trigeminovascular system and migraine: studies characterizing cerebrovascular and neuropeptide changes seen in humans and cats. Ann Neurol 33:48–56

342. Goebel HH, Besser R (1988) Traumatic fascicular neuroma. Acta Neuropathol (Berl) 75:321–324

343. Goebel HH, Kohlschutter A, Schulte FJ (1980) Rectal biopsy findings in infantile neuroaxonal dystrophy. Neuropediatrics 11:388–392

344. Goebel HH, Meyermann R, Rosin R, Schlote W (1997) Characteristic morphologic manifestation of CADASIL, cerebral autosomal-dominant arteriopathy with subcortical infarcts and leukoencephalopathy, in skeletal muscle and skin. Muscle Nerve 20:625–627

345. Goebel HH, Veit S, Dyck PJ (1980) Confirmation of virtual unmyelinated fiber absence in hereditary sensory neuropathy type IV. J Neuropathol Exp Neurol 39: 670–675

346. Goihman-Yahr M, Requena MA, Vallecalle-Suegart E, Convit J (1972) Autoimmune diseases and thalidomide. I. Experimental allergic encephalomyelitis and experimental allergic neuritis of the guinea pig. Int J Lepr Other Mycobact Dis 40:133–141

347. Goihman-Yahr M, Requena MA, Vallecalle-Suegart E, Convit J (1974) Autoimmune diseases and thalidomide. II. Adjuvant disease, experimental allergic encephalomyelitis and experimental allergic neuritis of the rat. Int J Lepr Other Mycobact Dis 42:266–275

348. Gold BG, Mobley WC, Matheson SF (1991) Regulation of axonal caliber, neurofilament content, and nuclear localization in mature sensory neurons by nerve growth factor. J Neurosci 11:943–955

349. Gombault A (1980) Contribution à l'etude anatomique de la névrite parenchymateuse subaigue ou chronique. Névrite segmentaire péri-axile (suite). Arch Neurol (Paris) I:177–190

350. Gonzales-Darder J, Barbera J, Abellan MJ, Mora A (1987) Centrocentral anastomosis in the prevention and treatment of painful terminal neuroma. An experimental study in the rat. J Neurosurg 63:754–758

351. Gorson KC, Ropper AH, Muriello MA, Blair R (1996) Prospective evaluation of MRI lumbosacral nerve root enhancement in acute Guillain-Barré syndrome (see comments). Neurology 47:813–817

352. Govoni V, Granieri E, Tola MR, Paolino E, Casetta I, Fainardi E, Monetti VC (1997) Exogenous gangliosides and Guillain-Barré syndrome. An observational study in the local health district of Ferrara, Italy. Brain 120:1123–1130

353. Grabow JD, Chou SM (1968) Thyrotropin hormone deficiency with a peripheral neuropathy. Arch Neurol 19: 284–291

354. Graeber MB, Streit WJ, Kreutzberg GW (1989) Formation of microglia-derived brain macrophages is blocked by adriamycin. Acta Neuropathol (Berl) 78:348–358

355. Grafe MR, Wiley CA (1989) Spinal cord and peripheral nerve pathology in AIDS: the roles of cytomegalovirus and human immunodeficiency virus. Ann Neurol 25: 561–566

356. Greenberg SJ, Kandt RS, D'Sonza BJ (1987) Birth injuryinduced glossolaryngeal paresis. Neurology 37: 533–535

357. Greene DA, Arezzo JC, Brown MB (1999) Effect of aldose reductase inhibition on nerve conduction and morphometry in diabetic neuropathy. Zenarestat Study Group. Neurology 53:580–591

358. Greene P, Kang U, Fahn S, Brin M, Moskowitz C, Flaster E (1990) Double-blind, placebo-controlled trial of botulinum toxin injections for the treatment of spasmodic torticollis. Neurology 40:1213–1218

359. Gregory R, Thomas PK, King RH, Hallam PL, Malcolm S, Hughes RA, Harding AE (1993) Coexistence of hereditary motor and sensory neuropathy type Ia and IgM paraproteinemic neuropathy. Ann Neurol 33:649–652

360. Grehl H, Schröder JM (1991) Significance of degenerating endoneurial cells in peripheral neuropathy. Acta Neuropathol (Berl) 81:680–685

361. Griffin JW, Cornblath DR, Alexander E, Campbell J, Low PA, Bird S, Feldman EL (1990) Ataxic sensory neuropathy and dorsal root ganglionitis associated with Sjögren's syndrome. Ann Neurol 27:304–315

362. Griffin JW, Goren E, Schaumburg H, Engel WK, Loriaux L (1977) Adrenomyeloneuropathy: a probable variant of adrenoleukodystrophy. I. Clinical and endocrinologic aspects. Neurology 27:1107–1113

363. Griffin JW, Ho TW (1993) The Guillain-Barré syndrome at 75: the Campylobacter connection (editorial; comment). Ann Neurol 34:125–127

364. Griffin JW, Li CY, Ho TW, Tian M, Gao CY, Xue P, Mishu B, Cornblath DR, Macko C, McKhann GM, Asbury AK

(1996) Pathology of the motor-sensory axonal Guillain-Barré syndrome (see comments). Ann Neurol 39:17–28

365. Griffin JW, Li CY, Ho TW, Xue P, Macko C, Gao CY, Yang C, Tian M, Mishu B, Cornblath DR (1995) Guillain-Barré syndrome in northern China. The spectrum of neuropathological changes in clinically defined cases (see comments). Brain 118:577–595

366. Grisold W, Drlicek M, Liszka U, Popp W (1989) Anti-Purkinje cell antibodies are specific for small-cell lung cancer but not for paraneoplastic neurological disorders (letter). J Neurol 236:64

367. Grisold W, Drlicek M, Popp W, Jellinger K (1987) Antineuronal antibodies in small cell lung carcinoma – a significance for paraneoplastic syndromes? Acta Neuropathol (Berl) 75:199–202

368. Grisold W, Udo Z, Markus D (1997) Should every unclear neuromuscular symptom be termed "paraneoplastic"? (letter; comment). Muscle Nerve 20:1204–1205

369. Groen RJ, Sie OG, van Weerden TW (1993) Dominant inherited distal spinal muscular atrophy with atrophic and hypertrophic calves. J Neurol Sci 114:81–84

370. Grosfeld JL, Skinner MA, Rescorla FJ, West KW, Scherer LR, 3rd (1994) Mediastinal tumors in children: experience with 196 cases. Ann Surg Oncol 1:121–127

371. Grünewald RA, Yoneda Y, Shipman JM, Sagar HJ (1997) Idiopathic focal dystonia: a disorder of muscle spindle afferent processing? Brain 120:2179–2185

372. Guidetti D, Vescovini E, Motti L, Ghidoni E, Gemignani F, Marbini A, Patrosso MC, Ferlini A, Solime F (1996) X-linked bulbar and spinal muscular atrophy, or Kennedy disease: clinical, neurophysiological, neuropathological, neuropsychological and molecular study of a large family. J Neurol Sci 135:140–148

373. Gunzler V (1992) Thalidomide in human immunodeficiency virus (HIV) patients. A review of safety considerations. Drug Saf 7:116–134

374. Gutmann DH, Collins FS (1992) Recent progress toward understanding the molecular biology of von Recklinghausen neurofibromatosis. Ann Neurol 31:555–561

375. Gutmann L, Medawar PB (1942) The chemical inhibition of fibre regeneration and neuroma formation in peripheral nerves. J Neurol Psychiat 5:130–141

376. Haanpaa M, Hakkinen V, Nurmikko T (1997) Motor involvement in acute herpes zoster. Muscle Nerve 20: 1433–1438

377. Haas JE, Johnson ES, Farrell DL (1982) Neonatal-onset adrenoleukodystrophy in a girl. Ann Neurol 12:449–457

378. Haberhausen G, Damian MS, Leweke F, Muller U (1995) Spinocerebellar ataxia, type 3 (SCA3) is genetically identical to Machado-Joseph disease (MJD). J Neurol Sci 132:71–75

379. Hahn AF, Brown WF, Koopman WJ, Feasby TE (1990) X-linked dominant hereditary motor and sensory neuropathy. Brain 113:1511–1525

380. Hahn AF, Feasby TE, Lovgren D, Wilkie L (1993) Adoptive transfer of experimental allergic neuritis in the immune suppressed host. Acta Neuropathol (Berl) 86: 596–601

381. Hahn AF, Feasby TE, Wilkie L, Lovgren D (1993) Antigalactocerebroside antibody increases demyelination in adoptive transfer experimental allergic neuritis. Muscle Nerve 16:1174–1180

382. Hahn AF, Gilbert JJ, Kwarciak C, Gillett J, Bolton CF, Rupar CA, Callahan JW (1994) Nerve biopsy findings in

383. Hahn AF, Gordon BA, Gilbert JJ, Hinton GG (1981) The AB-variant of metachromatic leukodystrophy (postulated activator protein deficiency). Light and electron microscopic findings in a sural nerve biopsy. Acta Neuropathol (Berl) 55:281–287

384. Hall SM, Hughes RA, Atkinson PF, McColl I, Gale A (1992) Motor nerve biopsy in severe Guillain-Barré syndrome. Ann Neurol 31:441–444

385. Halperin J, Luft BJ, Volkman DJ, Dattwyler RJ (1990) Lyme neuroborreliosis. Peripheral nervous system manifestations. Brain 113:1207–1221

386. Han DH, Kim DG, Chi JG, Park SH, Jung HW, Kim YG (1992) Malignant triton tumor of the acoustic nerve. Case report. J Neurosurg 76:874–877

387. Hara H, Jansen I, Ekman R, Hamel E, MacKenzie ET, Uddman R, Edvinsson L (1989) Acetylcholine and vasoactive intestinal peptide in cerebral blood vessels: effect of extirpation of the sphenopalatine ganglion. J Cereb Blood Flow Metab 9:204–211

388. Hardie RJ, Pullon HW, Harding AE, Owen JS, Pires M, Daniels GL, Imai Y, Misra VP, King RH, Jacobs JM et al. (1991) Neuroacanthocytosis. A clinical, haematological and pathological study of 19 cases. Brain 114:13–49

389. Hardiman O, Halperin JJ, Farrell MA, Shapiro BE, Wray SH, Brown RH Jr (1993) Neuropathic findings in oculopharyngeal muscular dystrophy. A report of seven cases and a review of the literature. Arch Neurol 50: 481–488

390. Harding AE (1981) Friedreich's ataxia: a clinical and genetic study of 90 families with an analysis of early diagnostic criteria and intrafamilial clustering of clinical features. Brain 104:589–620

391. Harding AE, Sweeney MG, Miller DH, Mumford CJ, Kellar-Wood H, Menard D, McDonald WI, Compston DA (1992) Occurrence of a multiple sclerosis-like illness in women who have a Leber's hereditary optic neuropathy mitochondrial DNA mutation. Brain 115: 979–989

392. Harding AE, Thomas PK (1980) Distal and scapuloperoneal distributions of muscle involvement occurring within a family with type I hereditary motor and sensory neuropathy. J Neurol 224:17–23

393. Harding AE, Thomas PK (1980) Hereditary distal spinal muscular atrophy. A report on 34 cases and a review of the literature. J Neurol Sci 45:337–348

394. Harkin J, Reed RJ (1983) Tumors of the peripheral nervous system. Supplementum. AFIP, Washington DC

395. Harris CP, Alderson K, Nebeker J, Holds JB, Anderson RL (1991) Histologic features of human orbicularis oculi treated with botulinum A toxin. Arch Ophthalmol 109:393–395

396. Hart IK, Waters C, Vincent A, Newland C, Beeson D, Pongs O, Morris C, Newsom-Davis J (1997) Autoantibodies detected to expressed K+ channels are implicated in neuromyotonia. Ann Neurol 41:238–246

397. Hartmann HA, McMahon S, Sun DY, Abbs JH, Uemura E (1989) Neuronal RNA in nucleus ambiguus and nucleus hypoglossus of patients with amyotrophic lateral sclerosis. J Neuropathol Exp Neurol 48:669–673

398. Hartung HP, Heininger K, Toyka KV (1988) Neuromuskuläre Manifestationen der HIV-1 und HTLV-I Infektionen. Dtsch Med Wochenschr 113:1975–1981

399. Hartung HP, Pollard JD, Harvey GK, Toyka KV (1995) Immunopathogenesis and treatment of the Guillain-Barré syndrome – part II. Muscle Nerve 18:154–164

400. Hassan SM, Jennekens FG, Veldman H (1995) Botulinum toxin-induced myopathy in the rat (see comments). Brain 118:533–545

401. Hassan SM, Kerkhoff H, Troost D, Veldman H, Jennekens FG (1994) Basic fibroblast growth factor immunoreactivity in the peripheral motor system of the rat. Acta Neuropathol (Berl) 87:405–410

402. Hayasaka K, Himoro M, Sato W, Takada G, Uyemura K, Shimizu N, Bird TD, Conneally PM, Chance PF (1993) Charcot-Marie-Tooth neuropathy type 1B is associated with mutations of the myelin P0 gene (see comments). Nat Genet 5:31–34

403. Hayasaka K, Himoro M, Sawaishi Y, Nanao K, Takahashi T, Takada G, Nicholson GA, Ouvrier RA, Tachi N (1993) De novo mutation of the myelin P0 gene in Dejerine-Sottas disease (hereditary motor and sensory neuropathy type III). Nat Genet 5:266–268

404. Hays AP, Latov N, Takatsu M, Sherman WH (1987) Experimental demyelination of nerve induced by serum of patients with neuropathy and an anti-MAG IgM M-protein. Neurology 37:242–256

405. Heads T, Pollock M, Robertson A, Sutherland WH, Allpress S (1991) Sensory nerve pathology in amyotrophic lateral sclerosis. Acta Neuropathol (Berl) 82:316–320

406. Heath JP, Ewing DJ, Cull RE (1988) Abnormalities of autonomic function in the Lambert Eaton myasthenic syndrome. J Neurol Neurosurg Psychiatry 51:436–439

407. Helliwell TR, Gunhan O, Edwards RH (1990) Mast cells in neuromuscular diseases. J Neurol Sci 98:267–276

408. Hemachudha T, Griffin DE, Chen WW, Johnson RT (1988) Immunologic studies of rabies vaccination-induced Guillain-Barré syndrome. Neurology 38:375–378

409. Hermosilla E, Lagueny A, Vital C, Vital A, Ferrer X, Steck A, Julien J (1996) Peripheral neuropathy associated with monoclonal IgG of undetermined significance (Clinical, electrophysiologic, pathologic and therapeutic study of 14 cases). J Periph Nerv Sys 2:139–148

410. Herrera GA, de Moraes HP (1984) Neurogenic sarcomas in patients with neurofibromatosis (von Recklinghausen's disease). Light, electron microscopy and immunohistochemistry study. Virchows Arch A Pathol Anat Histopathol 403:361–376

411. Higami Y, Shimokawa I, Kishikawa M, Okimoto T, Ohtani H, Tomita M, Tsujino A, Ikeda T (1998) Malignant peripheral nerve sheath tumors developing multifocally in the central nervous system in a patient with neurofibromatosis type 2. Clin Neuropathol 17:115–120

412. Higashi Y, Murayama S, Pentchev PG, Suzuki K (1995) Peripheral nerve pathology in Niemann-Pick type C mouse. Acta Neuropathol (Berl) 90:158–163

413. Himmelmann F, Schröder JM (1992) Colchicine myopathy in a case of familial Mediterranean fever: immunohistochemical and ultrastructural study of accumulated tubulin-immunoreactive material. Acta Neuropathol (Berl) 83:440–444

414. Hinchey JA, Preston DC, Logigian EL (1996) Idiopathic lumbosacral neuropathy: a cause of persistent leg pain. Muscle Nerve 19:1484–1486

415. Hirano M, Cleary JM, Stewart AM, Lincoff NS, Odel JG, Santiesteban R, Santiago Luis R (1994) Mitochondrial DNA mutations in an outbreak of optic neuropathy in Cuba (see comments). Neurology 44:843–845

416. Hirata H, Hibasami H, Hineno T, Shi D, Morita A, Inada H, Fujisawa K, Nakashima K, Ogihara Y (1995) Role of ornithine decarboxylase in proliferation of Schwann cells during Wallerian degeneration and its enhancement by nerve expansion. Muscle Nerve 18:1341–1343

417. Hirose T, Sano T, Hizawa K (1988) Heterogeneity of malignant Schwannomas. Ultrastruct Pathol 12:107–116

418. Hoffer A (1993) Isoniazid and pyridoxine (letter; comment). Cmaj 149:1232

419. Hoffmann CFE, Marani E, Oestreicher AB, Thomeer RTWM (1993) Ventral root avulsion versus transection at the cervical 7 level of the cat spinal cord. Resto Neurol Neurosci 5:291–302

420. Hofstra RM, Landsvater RM, Ceccherini I, Stulp RP, Stelwagen T, Luo Y, Pasini B, Hoppener JW, van Amstel HK, Romeo G et al. (1994) A mutation in the RET proto-oncogene associated with multiple endocrine neoplasia type 2B and sporadic medullary thyroid carcinoma (see comments). Nature 367:375–376

421. Holds JB, Alderson K, Fogg SG, Anderson RL (1990) Motor nerve sprouting in human orbicularis muscle after botulinum A injection. Invest Ophthalmol Vis Sci 31:964–967

422. Holds JB, Fogg SG, Anderson RL (1990) Botulinum A toxin injection. Failures in clinical practice and a biomechanical system for the study of toxin-induced paralysis. Ophthal Plast Reconstr Surg 6:252–259

423. Holland NR, Crawford TO, Hauer P, Cornblath DR, Griffin JW, McArthur JC (1998) Small-fiber sensory neuropathies: clinical course and neuropathology of idiopathic cases. Ann Neurol 44:47–59

424. Holmberg M, Duyckaerts C, Durr A, Cancel G, Gourfinkel-An I, Damier P, Faucheux B, Trottier Y, Hirsch EC, Agid Y, Brice A (1998) Spinocerebellar ataxia type 7 (SCA7): a neurodegenerative disorder with neuronal intranuclear inclusions. Hum Mol Genet 7:913–918

425. Holtzman RNN, Zablozki V, Yang WC, Leeds E (1987) Lateral pontine segmental hemorrhage presenting as isolated trigeminal sensory neuropathy. Neurology 37:704–706

426. Honavar M, Tharakan JK, Hughes RA, Leibowitz S, Winer JB (1991) A clinicopathological study of the Guillain-Barré syndrome. Nine cases and literature review. Brain 114:1245–1269

427. Honavar M, Tharakan JK, Hughes RA, Leibowitz S, Winer JB (1991) A clinicopathological study of the Guillain-Barré syndrome. Nine cases and literature review. Brain 114:1245–1269

428. Hopkins SJ, Rothwell NJ (1995) Cytokines and the nervous system. I: Expression and recognition (see comments). Trends Neurosci 18:83–88

429. Horoupian DS (1989) Hereditary sensory neuropathy with deafness: a familial multisystem atrophy. Neurology 39:244–248

430. Houi H, Mochio S, Kobayashi T (1993) Gangliosides attenuate vincristine neurotoxicity on dorsal root ganglion cells. Muscle Nerve 16:11–14

431. Hozumi I, Nishizawa M, Ariga T, Inoue Y, Ohnishi Y, Yokoyama A, Shibata A, Miyatake T (1989) Accumulation of glycosphingolipids in spinal and sympathetic ganglia of a symptomatic heterozygote of Fabry's disease. J Neurol Sci 90:273–280

432. Hughes R, Atkinson P, Coates P, Hall S, Leibowitz S (1992) Sural nerve biopsies in Guillain-Barré syndrome: axonal degeneration and macrophage-associated demyelination and absence of cytomegalovirus genome (see comments). Muscle Nerve 15:568–575

433. Hughes RAC (1990) Guillain-Barré syndrome. Springer, Berlin Heidelberg New York

434. Hund E, Grau A, Fogel W, Forsting M, Cantz M, Kustermann-Kuhn B, Harzer K, Navon R, Goebel HH, Meinck HM (1997) Progressive cerebellar ataxia, proximal neurogenic weakness and ocular motor disturbances: hexosaminidase A deficiency with late clinical onset in four siblings. J Neurol Sci 145:25–31

435. Hurwitz ES, Holman RC, Nelson DB, Schonberger LB (1983) National surveillance for Guillain-Barré syndrome: January 1978–March 1979. Neurology 33:150–157

436. Hutchinson M, O'Riordan J, Javed M, Quin E, Macerlaine D, Wilcox T, Parfrey N, Nagy TG, Tournier-Lasserve E (1995) Familial hemiplegic migraine and autosomal dominant arteriopathy with leukoencephalopathy (CADASIL). Ann Neurol 38:817–824

437. Iannaccone S, Ferini-Strambi L, Nemni R, Marchettini P, Corbo M, Pinto P, Smirne S (1992) Peripheral motor-sensory neuropathy in membranous lipodystrophy (Nasu's disease): a case report. Clin Neuropathol 11: 49–53

438. Ichimura M, Yamamoto M, Kobayashi Y, Kawakami O, Niimi Y, Hattori N, Nagamatsu M, Hashizume Y, Sobue G (1998) Tissue distribution of pathological lesions and hu antigen expression in paraneoplastic sensory neuronopathy. Acta Neuropathol 95:641–648

439. IGPSG (1995) Chronic symmetric symptomatic polyneuropathy in the elderly: a field screening investigation in two Italian regions. I. Prevalence and general characteristics of the sample. Italian General Practitioner Study Group (IGPSG). Neurology 45:1832–1836

440. Ikeda K, Iwasaki Y, Shiojima T, Kinoshita M (1996) Neuroprotective effect of various cytokines on developing spinal motoneurons following axotomy. J Neurol Sci 135: 109–113

441. Illa I, Ortiz N, Gallard E, Juarez C, Grau JM, Dalakas MC (1995) Acute axonal Guillain-Barré syndrome with IgG antibodies against motor axons following parenteral gangliosides. Ann Neurol 38:218–224

442. Ilyas AA, Mithen FA, Dalakas MC, Chen ZW, Cook SD (1992) Antibodies to acidic glycolipids in Guillain-Barré syndrome and chronic inflammatory demyelinating polyneuropathy. J Neurol Sci 107:111–121

443. Ince PG, Shaw PJ, Fawcett PR, Bates D (1987) Demyelinating neuropathy due to primary IgM kappa B cell lymphoma of peripheral nerve. Neurology 37:1231–1235

444. Inoue A, Koh C, Iwahashi T (1999) Detection of serum anticerebellar antibodies in patients with Miller Fisher syndrome. Eur Neurol 42:230–234

445. Ionasescu V, Searby C, Ionasescu R, Meschino W (1995) New point mutations and deletions of the connexin 32 gene in X-linked Charcot-Marie-Tooth neuropathy. Neuromuscul Disord 5:297–299

446. Ionasescu VV, Ionasescu R, Searby C, Neahring R (1995) Dejerine-Sottas disease with de novo dominant point mutation of the PMP22 gene. Neurology 45:1766–1767

447. Ionasescu VV, Searby C, Greenberg SA (1996) Dejerine-Sottas disease with sensorineural hearing loss, nystagmus, and peripheral facial nerve weakness: de novo dominant point mutation of the PMP22 gene. J Med Genet 33:1048–1049

448. Ionasescu VV, Searby C, Ionasescu R, Neuhaus IM, Werner R (1996) Mutations of the noncoding region of the connexin32 gene in X-linked dominant Charcot-Marie-Tooth neuropathy. Neurology 47:541–544

449. Ionasescu VV, Searby CC, Ionasescu R, Chatkupt S, Patel N, Koenigsberger R (1997) Dejerine-Sottas neuropathy in mother and son with same point mutation of PMP22 gene. Muscle Nerve 20:97–99

450. Ionasescu VV, Trofatter J, Haines JL, Ionasescu R, Searby C (1992) Mapping of the gene for X-linked dominant Charcot-Marie-Tooth neuropathy. Neurology 42:903–908

451. Ionasescu VV, Trofatter J, Haines JL, Summers AM, Ionasescu R, Searby C (1992) X-linked recessive Charcot-Marie-Tooth neuropathy: clinical and genetic study. Muscle Nerve 15:368–373

452. Itoh T, Sobue G, Ken E, Mitsuma T, Takahashi A, Trojanowski JQ (1992) Phosphorylated high molecular weight neurofilament protein in the peripheral motor, sensory and sympathetic neuronal perikarya: system-dependent normal variations and changes in amyotrophic lateral sclerosis and multiple system atrophy. Acta Neuropathol (Berl) 83:240–245

453. Iwashita H, Inoue N, Araki S, Kuroiwa Y (1970) Optic atrophy, neural deafness, and distal neurogenic amyotrophy; report of a family with two affected siblings. Arch Neurol 22:357–364

454. Jablecki CK, Berry C, Leach J (1989) Survival prediction in amyotrophic lateral sclerosis (see comments). Muscle Nerve 12:833–841

455. Jackson M, Al-Chalabi A, Enayat ZE, Chioza B, Leigh PN, Morrison KE (1997) Copper/zinc superoxide dismutase 1 and sporadic amyotrophic lateral sclerosis: analysis of 155 cases and identification of a novel insertion mutation. Ann Neurol 42:803–807

456. Jacobs BC, Rothbarth PH, van der Meche FG, Herbrink P, Schmitz PI, de Klerk MA, van Doorn PA (1998) The spectrum of antecedent infections in Guillain-Barré syndrome: a case-control study. Neurology 51:1110–1115

457. Jacobs JM (1996) Morphological changes at paranodes in IgM paraproteinaemic neuropathy. Microsc Res Tech 34:544–553

458. Jacobs JM, Laing JH, Harrison DH (1996) Regeneration through a long nerve graft used in the correction of facial palsy. A qualitative and quantitative study. Brain 119:271–279

459. Jacobs JM, Love S (1985) Qualitative and quantitative morphology of human sural nerve at different ages. Brain 108:897–924

460. Jacobs JM, Scadding JW (1990) Morphological changes in IgM paraproteinaemic neuropathy. Acta Neuropathol (Berl) 80:77–84

461. Jacobs JM, Shetty VP, Antia NH (1987) Myelin changes in leprous neuropathy. Acta Neuropathol (Berl) 74:75–80

462. Jacobs JM, Shetty VP, Antia NH (1987) Teased fibre studies in leprous neuropathy. J Neurol Sci 79:301–313

463. Jacobs JM, Shetty VP, Antia NH (1993) A morphological study of nerve biopsies from cases of multibacillary leprosy given multidrug therapy. Acta Neuropathol (Berl) 85:533–541

464. Jacobs JM, Wilson J (1992) An unusual demyelinating neuropathy in a patient with Waardenburg's syndrome. Acta Neuropathol (Berl) 83:670–674

465. Jamal GA, Hansen S, Weir AI, Ballantyne JP (1987) The neurophysiologic investigation of small fiber neuropathies. Muscle Nerve 10:537-545

466. Jaradeh S, Dyck PJ (1992) Hereditary motor and sensory neuropathy with treatable extrapyramidal features. Arch Neurol 49:175-178

467. Jay V, Vajsar J, Haslam R (1996) Axonal neuropathy with perineurial hyperplasia: report of a case with multifocal involvement (published erratum appears in J Child Neurol 1996 Nov;11(6):489). J Child Neurol 11: 400-403

468. Jellinger K, Grisold W, Armstrong D, Rett A (1990) Peripheral nerve involvement in the Rett syndrome. Brain Dev 12:109-114

469. Jellinger K, Paulus W, Grisold W, Paschke E (1990) New phenotype of adult alpha-L-iduronidase deficiency (mucopolysaccharidosis I) masquerading as Friedreich's ataxia with cardiopathy. Clin Neuropathol 9:163-169

470. Jestico JV, Urry PA, Efphimiou J (1985) An hereditary sensory and autonomic neuropathy transmitted as an X-linked recessive trait. J Neurol Neurosurg Psychiatry 48:1259-1264

471. Jia J, Pollock M (1997) The pathogenesis of non-freezing cold nerve injury. Observations in the rat. Brain 120: 631-646

472. Jitpimolmard S, Small J, King RH, Geddes J, Misra P, McLaughlin J, Muddle JR, Cole M, Harding AE, Thomas PK (1993) The sensory neuropathy of Friedreich's ataxia: an autopsy study of a case with prolonged survival. Acta Neuropathol (Berl) 86:29-35

473. Johnson PC, Beggs JL (1993) Pathology of the autonomic nerve innervating the vasa nervorum in diabetic neuropathy. Diabet Med 10 Suppl 2:56S-61S

474. Jona JZ (1978) Electron microscopic observations in infantile hypertrophic pyloric stenosis (IHPS). J Pediatr Surg 13:17-20

475. Joutel A, Corpechot C, Ducros A, Vahedi K, Chabriat H, Mouton P, Alamowitch S, Domenga V, Cecillion M, Marechal E, Maciazek J, Vayssiere C, Cruaud C, Cabanis EA, Ruchoux MM, Weissenbach J, Bach JF, Bousser MG, Tournier-Lasserve E (1996) Notch3 mutations in CADASIL, a hereditary adult-onset condition causing stroke and dementia (see comments). Nature 383:707-710

476. Jurgens H, Bier V, Harms D, Beck J, Brandeis W, Etspuler G, Gadner H, Schmidt D, Treuner J, Winkler K et al. (1988) Malignant peripheral neuroectodermal tumors. A retrospective analysis of 42 patients. Cancer 61: 349-357

477. Kafka SP, Condemi JJ, Marsh DO, Leddy JP (1994) Mononeuritis multiplex and vasculitis. Association with antineutrophil cytoplasmic autoantibody (see comments). Arch Neurol 51:565-568

478. Kahn R (1992) Proceedings of a consensus development conference on standardized measures in diabetic neuropathy. Muscle Nerve 15:1143-1146

479. Kaji R, Kohara N, Katayama M, Kubori T, Mezaki T, Shibasaki H, Kimura J (1995) Muscle afferent block by intramuscular injection of lidocaine for the treatment of writer's cramp. Muscle Nerve 18:234-235

480. Kaji R, Oka N, Tsuji T, Mezaki T, Nishio T, Akiguchi I, Kimura J (1993) Pathological findings at the site of conduction block in multifocal motor neuropathy (see comments). Ann Neurol 33:152-158

481. Kalaydjieva L, Gresham D, Gooding R, Heather L, Baas F, de Jonge R, Blechschmidt K, Angelicheva D, Chandler D, Worsley P, Rosenthal A, King RH, Thomas PK (2000) N-myc downstream-regulated gene 1 is mutated in hereditary motor and sensory neuropathy-Lom. Am J Hum Genet 67:47-58

482. Kalaydjieva L, Nikolova A, Turnev I, Petrova J, Hristova A, Ishpekova B, Petkova I, Shmarov A, Stancheva S, Middleton L, Merlini L, Trogu A, Muddle JR, King RH, Thomas PK (1998) Hereditary motor and sensory neuropathy – Lom, a novel demyelinating neuropathy associated with deafness in gypsies. Clinical, electrophysiological and nerve biopsy findings. Brain 121:399-408

483. Kalichman MW, Chalk CH, Mizisin AP (1999) Classification of teased nerve fibers for multicenter clinical trials. J Peripher Nerv Syst 4:233-244

484. Kalichman MW, Powell HC, Mizisin AP (1998) Reactive, degenerative, and proliferative Schwann cell responses in experimental galactose and human diabetic neuropathy. Acta Neuropathol (Berl) 95:47-56

485. Kanda T, Hayashi H, Tanabe H, Tsubaki T, Oda M (1989) A fulminant case of Guillain-Barré syndrome: topographic and fibre size related analysis of demyelinating changes. J Neurol Neurosurg Psychiatry 52:857-864

486. Kanda T, Isozaki E, Kato S, Tanabe H, Oda M (1989) Type III Machado-Joseph disease in a Japanese family: a clinicopathological study with special reference to the peripheral nervous system. Clin Neuropathol 8:134-141

487. Kanda T, Oda M, Yonezawa M, Tamagawa K, Isa F, Hanakago R, Tsukagoshi H (1990) Peripheral neuropathy in xeroderma pigmentosum. Brain 113:1025-1044

488. Kanda T, Tsukagoshi H, Oda M, Miyamoto K, Tanabe H (1996) Changes of unmyelinated nerve fibers in sural nerve in amyotrophic lateral sclerosis, Parkinson's disease and multiple system atrophy. Acta Neuropathol (Berl) 91:145-154

489. Kanda T, Usui S, Beppu H, Miyamoto K, Yamawaki M, Oda M (1998) Blood-nerve barrier in IgM paraproteinemic neuropathy: a clinicopathologic assessment. Acta Neuropathol (Berl) 95:184-192

490. Kaplan JE, Schonberger LB, Hurwitz ES, Katona P (1983) Guillain-Barré syndrome in the United States, 1978–1981: additional observations from the national surveillance system. Neurology 33:633-637

491. Kaslow RA, Sullivan-Bolyai JZ, Holman RC, Hafkin B, Dicker RC, Schonberger LB (1987) Risk factors for Guillain-Barré syndrome. Neurology 37:685-688

492. Kato S, Horiuchi S, Nakashima K, Hirano A, Shibata N, Nakano I, Saito M, Kato M, Asayama K, Ohama E (1999) Astrocytic hyaline inclusions contain advanced glycation endproducts in familial amyotrophic lateral sclerosis with superoxide dismutase 1 gene mutation: immunohistochemical and immunoelectron microscopical analyses. Acta Neuropathol (Berl) 97:260-266

493. Katsetos CD, Karkavelas G, Frankfurter A, Vlachos IN, Vogeley K, Schober R, Wechsler W, Urich H (1994) The stromal Schwann cell during maturation of peripheral neuroblastomas. Immunohistochemical observations with antibodies to the neuronal class III beta-tubulin isotype (beta III) and S-100 protein. Clin Neuropathol 13:171-180

494. Katz DA, Scheinberg L, Horoupian DS, Salen G (1985) Peripheral neuropathy in cerebrotendinous xanthomatosis. Arch Neurol 42:1008-1010

495. Kawana T, Nada O, Ikeda K (1988) An immunohistochemical study of glial fibrillary acidic (GFA) protein and S-100 protein in the colon affected by Hirschsprung's disease. Acta Neuropathol (Berl) 76:159–165

496. Kawata A, Kato S, Hayashi H, Hirai S (1997) Prominent sensory and autonomic disturbances in familial amyotrophic lateral sclerosis with a Gly93Ser mutation in the SOD1 gene. J Neurol Sci 153:82–85

497. Keller MP, Chance PF (1999) Inherited neuropathies: from gene to disease. Brain Pathol 9:327–341

498. Kelly JJ, Adelman LS, Berkman E, Bhan I (1988) Polyneuropathies associated with IgM monoclonal gammopathies. Arch Neurol 45:1355–1359

499. Kelsell DP, Dunlop J, Stevens HP, Lench NJ, Liang JN, Parry G, Mueller RF, Leigh IM (1997) Connexin 26 mutations in hereditary non-syndromic sensorineural deafness. Nature 387:80–83

500. Kennedy PGE (1987) Neurological complications of varicella-zoster virus. In: Kennedy PGE, Johnson RT (eds) Infections of the nervous system. Butterworths, London, pp 177–208

501. Kennedy WR, Wendelschafer-Crabb G, Johnson T (1996) Quantitation of epidermal nerves in diabetic neuropathy. Neurology 47:1042–1048

502. Kennett RP, Gilliatt RW (1991) Nerve conduction studies in experimental non-freezing cold injury: I. Local nerve cooling. Muscle Nerve 14:553–562

503. Kerkhoff H, Hassan SM, Troost D, Van Etten RW, Veldman H, Jennekens FG (1994) Insulin-like and fibroblast growth factors in spinal cords, nerve roots and skeletal muscle of human controls and patients with amyotrophic lateral sclerosis. Acta Neuropathol (Berl) 87: 411–421

504. Khalili-Shirazi A, Hughes RA, Brostoff SW, Linington C, Gregson N (1992) T cell responses to myelin proteins in Guillain-Barré syndrome. J Neurol Sci 111:200–203

505. Khella SL, Frost S, Hermann GA, Leventhal L, Whyatt S, Sajid MA, Scherer SS (1995) Hepatitis C infection, cryoglobulinemia, and vasculitic neuropathy. Treatment with interferon alfa: case report and literature review. Neurology 45:407–411

506. Kida E, Barcikowska M, Joachimowicz-Jaskowiak E, Michalska T, Siekierzynska A, Walasik A, Roszkowski K, Figura-Chojak E (1994) Subacute sensory neuronopathy in small cell cancer of the lung. Immunocytochemical study of 2 cases. Clin Neuropathol 13:64–70

507. Kimura S, Sasaki Y, Warlo I, Goebel HH (1987) Axonal pathology of the skin in infantile neuroaxonal dystrophy. Acta Neuropathol (Berl) 75:212–215

508. King RH, Llewelyn JG, Thomas PK, Gilbey SG, Watkins PJ (1989) Diabetic neuropathy: abnormalities of Schwann cell and perineurial basal laminae. Implications for diabetic vasculopathy. Neuropathol Appl Neurobiol 15:339–355

509. King RH, Sarsilmaz M, Thomas PK, Jacobs JM, Muddle JR, Duncan ID (1993) Axonal neurofilamentous accumulations: a comparison between human and canine giant axonal neuropathy and 2,5-HD neuropathy. Neuropathol Appl Neurobiol 19:224–232

510. King RHM, Pollard JD, Thomas PK (1975) Aberrant remyelination in chronic relapsing experimental allergic neuritis. Neuropathol appl Neurobiol 1:367–378

511. King RHM, Tournev I, Colomer J, Merlini L, Kalaydjieva L, Thomas PK (1999) Ultrastructural changes in peripheral nerve in hereditary motor and sensory neuropathy-Lom. Neuropathol Appl Neurobiol 25:306–312

512. Kinnunen E, Junttila O, Haukka J, Hovi T (1998) Nationwide oral poliovirus vaccination campaign and the incidence of Guillain-Barré Syndrome. Am J Epidemiol 147:69–73

513. Kinoshita A, Hayashi M, Oda M, Tanabe H (1995) Clinicopathological study of the peripheral nervous system in Machado-Joseph disease. J Neurol Sci 130:48–58

514. Kissel JT, Mendel JR (1995) Neuropathies associated with monoclonal gammopathies (Review Article). Neuromus Disord 6:3–18

515. Kissel JT, Riethman JL, Omerza J, Rammohan KW, Mendell JR (1989) Peripheral nerve vasculitis: immune characterization of the vascular lesions (see comments). Ann Neurol 25:291–297

516. Kitajima I, Kuriyama M, Usuki F, Izumo S, Osame M, Suganuma T, Murata F, Nagamatsu K (1989) Nasu-Hakola disease (membranous lipodystrophy). Clinical, histopathological and biochemical studies of three cases. J Neurol Sci 91:35–52

517. Kitamura J, Kubuki Y, Tsuruta K, Kurihara T, Matsukura S (1989) A new family with Joseph disease in Japan. Homovanillic acid, magnetic resonance, and sleep apnea studies. Arch Neurol 46:425–428

518. Kjellstrom C, Conradi NG (1993) Decreased axonal calibres without axonal loss in optic nerve following chronic alcohol feeding in adult rats: a morphometric study. Acta Neuropathol (Berl) 85:117–121

519. Kleihues P, Burger PC, Scheithauer BW (1993) Histological typing of tumours of the central nervous system. 2nd ed. Spinger, Berlin Heidelberg New York

520. Kleihues P, Cavanee WK (2000) Pathology and genetics: tumours of the nervous system. IARC, Lyon

521. Klemm H (1970) Das Perineurium als Diffusionsbarriere gegenüber Peroxydase bei epi- und endoneuraler Applikation. Z Zellforsch Mikrosk Anat 108:431–445

522. Klopstock T, Jaksch M, Gasser T (1999) Age and cause of death in mitochondrial diseases. Neurology 53: 855–857

523. Knorr-Held S, Meier C (1990) Mast cells in human polyneuropathies: their density and regional distribution. Clin Neuropathol 9:121–124

524. Kocen RS, King RH, Thomas PK, Haas LF (1973) Nerve biopsy findings in two cases of Tangier disease. Acta Neuropathol (Berl) 26:317–327

525. Kocen RS, Thomas PK (1970) Peripheral nerve involvement in Fabry's disease. Arch Neurol 22:81–88

526. Koch T, Schultz P, Williams R, Lampert P (1977) Giant axonal neuropathy: a childhood disorder of microfilaments. Ann Neurol 1:438–451

527. Koeppen AH, Dickson AC, Lamarche JB, Robitaille Y (1999) Synapses in the hereditary ataxias. J Neuropathol Exp Neurol 58:748–764

528. Konishi T, Saida K, Ohnishi A, Nishitani H (1982) Perineuritis in mononeuritis multiplex with cryoglobulinemia. Muscle Nerve 5:173–177

529. Korinthenberg R, Sauer M, Ketelsen UP, Hanemann CO, Stoll G, Graf M, Baborie A, Volk B, Wirth B, Rudnik-Schoneborn S, Zerres K (1997) Congenital axonal neuropathy caused by deletions in the spinal muscular atrophy region. Ann Neurol 42:364–368

530. Kornberg AJ, Pestronk A, Bieser K, Ho TW, McKhann GM, Wu HS, Jiang Z (1994) The clinical correlates of

high-titer IgG anti-GM1 antibodies (see comments). Ann Neurol 35:234–237

531. Koskinen T, Sainio K, Rapola J, Pihko H, Paetau A (1994) Sensory neuropathy in infantile onset spinocerebellar ataxia (IOSCA). Muscle Nerve 17:509–515

532. Krajewski S, Chatten J, Hanada M, Reed JC (1995) Immunohistochemical analysis of the Bcl-2 oncoprotein in human. Lab Invest 72:42–54

533. Krämer E (1992) Experimentelle Untersuchungen zur lokaltoxischen Wirkung von Ethanol am peripheren Nerven. Universitätsklinikum, Institut für Neuropathologie. Rheinisch-Westfälische Technische Hochschule, Aachen

534. Kramer W (1970) Tumours of nerves. In: Vinken PJ, Bruyn GW (eds) Handbook of clinical neurology. (Diseases of nerves II, vol 8) pp 412–512

535. Krarup C, Loeb GE, Pezeshkpour GH (1989) Conduction studies in peripheral cat nerve using implanted electrodes: III. The effects of prolonged constriction on the distal nerve segment. Muscle Nerve 12:915–928

536. Krendel DA, Stahl RL, Chan WC (1991) Lymphomatous polyneuropathy. Biopsy of clinically involved nerve and successful treatment. Arch Neurol 48:330–332

537. Kretzschmar HA, Berg BO, Davis RL (1987) Giant axonal neuropathy. A neuropathological study. Acta Neuropathol 73:138–144

538. Krinke G, Naylor DC, Skorpil V (1985) Pyridoxine megavitaminosis: an analysis of the early changes induced with massive doses of vitamin B6 in rat primary sensory neurons. J Neuropathol Exp Neurol 44: 117–129

539. Kristoferitsch W, Sluga E, Graf M, Partsch H, Neumann R, Stanek G, Budka H (1988) Neuropathy associated with acrodermatitis chronica atrophicans. Clinical and morphological features. Ann N Y Acad Sci 539:35–45

540. Krücke W (1942) Zur Histopathologie der neuralen Muskelatrophie, der hypertrophischen Neuritis und Neurofibromatose. Arch Psychiat 115:180–236

541. Krücke W (1974) Pathologie der peripheren Nerven. In: Olivecrona H, Tönnis W, Krenkel W (eds) Handbuch der Neurochirurgie, Bd VII/3. Springer, Berlin Heidelberg New York, pp 1–267

542. Krücke W, Hartrott HHv, Schröder JM, Thomas E, Gibbels E, Scheid W (1971) Licht- und elektronenmikroskopische Untersuchungen zum Spätstadium der Thalidomidneuropathie. Fortschr Neurol Psychiatr Grenzgeb 39:15–50

543. Krüttgen A, Grotzinger J, Kurapkat G, Weis J, Simon R, Thier M, Schröder M, Heinrich P, Wollmer A, Comeau M, et al. (1995) Human ciliary neurotrophic factor: a structure-function analysis. Biochem J 309:215–220

544. Kubis N, Durr A, Gugenheim M, Chneiweiss H, Mazzetti P, Brice A, Bouche P (1999) Polyneuropathy in autosomal dominant cerebellar ataxias: phenotype-genotype correlation. Muscle Nerve 22:712–717

545. Kuhn G, Lie A, Wilms S, Muller HW (1993) Coexpression of PMP22 gene with MBP and Po during de novo myelination and nerve repair. Glia 8:256–264

546. Kulkens T, Bolhuis PA, Wolterman RA, Kemp S, te Nijenhuis S, Valentijn LJ, Hensels GW, Jennekens FG, de Visser M, Hoogendijk JE, et al. (1993) Deletion of the serine 34 codon from the major peripheral myelin protein Po gene in Charcot-Marie-Tooth disease type 1B. Nat Genet 5:35–39

547. Kuncl RW, Duncan G, Watson D, Alderson K, Rogawski MA, Peper M (1987) Colchicine myopathy and neuropathy. N Engl J Med 316:1562–1568

548. Kuritzky A, Berginer VM, Korczyn AD (1979) Peripheral neuropathy in cerebrotendinous xanthomatosis. Neurology 29:880–881

549. Kuroda Y, Nakata H, Kakigi R, Oda K, Shibasaki H, Nakashiro H (1989) Human neurolymphomatosis by adult T-cell leukemia (see comments). Neurology 39: 144–146

550. Kuroiwa Y, Wada T, Tohgi H (1987) Measurement of blood pressure and heart-rate variation while resting supine and standing for the evaluation of autonomic dysfunction. J Neurol 235:65–68

551. Kurtzke JF (1982) The current neurologic burden of illness and injury in the United States. Neurology 32:1207–1214

552. Kusaka H, Imai T (1993) Pathology of motor neurons in amyotrophic lateral sclerosis with dementia. Clin Neuropathol 12:164–168

553. Kusunoki S, Iwamori M, Chiba A, Hitoshi S, Arita M, Kanazawa I (1996) GM1b is a new member of antigen for serum antibody in Guillain-Barré syndrome. Neurology 47:237–242

554. Kusunoki S, Kohriyama T, Pachner AR, Latov N, Yu RK (1987) Neuropathy and IgM paraproteinemia: differential binding of IgM M-proteins to peripheral nerve glycolipids. Neurology 37:1795–1797

555. Kuwabara S, Yuki N, Koga M, Hattori T, Matsuura D, Miyake M, Noda M (1998) IgG anti-GM1 antibody is associated with reversible conduction failure and axonal degeneration in Guillain-Barré syndrome. Ann Neurol 44:202–208

556. Kuzuhara S, Kanazawa I, Nakanishi T, Egashira T (1983) Ethylene oxide polyneuropathy. Neurology 33:377–380

557. Lach B, Rippstein P, Atack D, Afar DE, Gregor A (1993) Immunoelectron microscopic localization of monoclonal IgM antibodies in gammopathy associated with peripheral demyelinative neuropathy. Acta Neuropathol (Berl) 85:298–307

558. Laeng RH, Altermatt HJ, Scheithauer BW, Zimmermann DR (1998) Amyloidomas of the nervous system: a monoclonal B-cell disorder with monotypic amyloid light chain lambda amyloid production. Cancer 82:362–374

559. Lam A, Fuller F, Miller J, Kloss J, Manthorpe M, Varon S, Cordell B (1991) Sequence and structural organization of the human gene encoding ciliary neurotrophic factor. Gene 102:271–276

560. Lamarche JB, Lemieux B, Lieu HB (1984) The neuropathology of "typical" Friedreich's ataxia in Quebec. Can J Neurol Sci 11:592–600

561. Lamb NL, Patten BM (1991) Clinical correlations of anti-GM1 antibodies in amyotrophic lateral sclerosis and neuropathies. Muscle Nerve 14:1021–1027

562. Lambert P, Blumberg JM, Pentschew A (1964) An electron microscopic study of dystrophic axons in the gracile and cuneate nuclei of vitamin E-deficient rats: axonal dystrophy in vitamin E deficiency. J Neuropathol Exp Neurol 23:60–77

563. Lammie GA, Rakshi J, Rossor MN, Harding AE, Scaravilli F (1995) Cerebral autosomal dominant arteriopathy with subcortical infarcts and leukoencephalopathy (CADASIL) – confirmation by cerebral biopsy in 2 cases. Clin Neuropathol 14:201–206

564. Lamont PJ, Davis MB, Wood NW (1997) Identification and sizing of the GAA trinucleotide repeat expansion of Friedreich's ataxia in 56 patients. Clinical and genetic correlates. Brain 120:673–680

565. Lampert PW (1969) Mechanism of demyelination in experimental allergic neuritis. Electron microscopic studies. Lab Invest 20:127–138

566. Lampert PW, Schochet SS Jr (1968) Demyelination and remyelination in lead neuropathy. Electron microscopic studies. J Neuropathol Exp Neurol 27:527–545

567. Landi G, D'Alessandro R, Dossi BC, Ricci S, Simone IL, Ciccone A (1993) Guillain-Barré syndrome after exogenous gangliosides in Italy (see comments). BMJ 307:1463–1464

568. Landrieu P, Said G (1984) Peripheral neuropathy in type A Niemann-Pick disease. A morphological study. Acta Neuropathol (Berl) 63:66–71

569. Landrieu P, Said G, Allaire C (1990) Dominantly transmitted congenital indifference to pain. Ann Neurol 27:574–578

570. Lane RJ, McLean KA, Moss J, Woodrow DF (1993) Myopathy in HIV infection: the role of zidovudine and the significance of tubuloreticular inclusions. Neuropathol Appl Neurobiol 19:406–413

571. Lange DJ, Trojaborg W, Latov N, Hays AP, Younger DS, Uncini A, Blake DM, Hirano M, Burns SM, Lovelace RE et al. (1992) Multifocal motor neuropathy with conduction block: is it a distinct clinical entity? (see comments). Neurology 42:497–505

572. Lanska MJ, Lanska DJ, Schmidley JW (1988) Syphilitic polyradiculopathy in an HIV-positive man. Neurology 38:1297–1301

573. Lantos PL, Vandenberg SR, Kleihues P (1997) Tumours of the nervous system. In: Graham DI, Lantos PL (eds) Greenfield's neuropathology, vol 2. Arnold, London Sydney Auckland, pp 583–879

574. Larson WL, Beydoun A, Albers JW, Wald JJ (1997) Collet-Sicard syndrome mimicking neuralgic amyotrophy. Muscle Nerve 20:1173–1177

575. Laskin WB, Weiss SW, Bratthauer GL (1991) Epithelioid variant of malignant peripheral nerve sheath tumor (malignant epithelioid Schwannoma). Am J Surg Pathol 15:1136–1345

576. Lassmann H, Fierz W, Neuchrist C, Meyermann R (1991) Chronic relapsing experimental allergic neuritis induced by repeated transfer of P2-protein reactive T cell lines. Brain 114:429–442

577. Latour P, Lévy N, Paret M, Chapon F, Chazot G, Clavelou P, Couratier P, Dumas R, Ollagnon E, Pouget J, Setiey A, Vallat JM, Boucherat M, Fontes M, Vandenberghe A (1997) Mutations in the X-linked form of Charcot-Marie-Tooth disease in the French population. Neurogenetics 1:117–123

578. Latov N, Hays AP, Donofrio PD, Liao J, Ito H, McGinnis S, Konstadoulakis M, Freddo L, Shy ME, Manoussos K et al. (1988) Monoclonal IgM with unique specificity to gangliosides GM1 and GD1b and to lacto-N-tetraose associated with human motor neuron disease (published erratum appears in Neurology 1988 Sep; 38(9):1506). Neurology 38:763–768

579. Latov N, Wokke JHJ, Kelly JJ Jr (1998) Immunological and infectious diseases of the peripheral nerves. University Press, Cambridge

580. Lauria G, Pareyson D, Grisoli M, Sghirlanzoni A (2000) Clinical and magnetic resonance imaging findings in chronic sensory ganglionopathies. Ann Neurol 47:104–109

581. Lazarus SS, Trombetta LD (1978) Ultrastructural identification of a benign perineurial cell tumor. Cancer 41:1823–1829

582. Le Guern E, Ravise N, Gugenheim M, Vignal A, Penet C, Bouche P, Weissenbach J, Agid Y, Brice A (1994) Linkage analyses between dominant X-linked Charcot-Marie-Tooth disease, 15 Xq11-Xq21 microsatellites in a new large family: three new markers are closely linked to the gene. Neuromuscul Disord 4:463–469

583. Leandri M, Eldridge P, Miles J (1998) Recovery of nerve conduction following microvascular decompression for trigeminal neuralgia. Neurology 51:1641–1646

584. Lee DA, Zurawel RH, Windebank AJ (1995) Ciliary neurotrophic factor expression in Schwann cells is induced by axonal contact. J Neurochem 65:564–568

585. Lee HC, Coulter CL, Adickes ED, Porterfield J, Robertson D, Bravo E, Pettinger WA (1996) Autonomic ganglionitis with severe hypertension, migraine, and episodic but fatal hypotension (see comments). Neurology 47:817–821

586. Lefaucheur JP, Authier FJ, Verroust J, Gherardi RK (1997) Zidovudine and human immunodeficiency virus-associated peripheral neuropathies: low intake in patients with mononeuropathy multiplex and no evidence for neurotoxicity. Muscle Nerve 20:106–109

587. Leone M, Rocca WA, Rosso MG, Mantel N, Schoenberg BS, Schiffer D (1988) Friedreich's disease: survival analysis in an Italian population. Neurology 38:1433–1438

588. Lesourd A, Mikol J, Bishopric G, Dubost C, Brocheriou C (1988) Multiple endocrine neoplasia (MEN) type II b: report of a case observed at autopsy with immunohistochemical study of mucosal neuromas. Clin Neuropathol 7:238–243

589. Levade T, Graber D, Flurin V, Delisle MB, Pieraggi MT, Testut MF, Carrière JP, Salvayre R (1994) Human beta-mannosidase deficiency associated with peripheral neuropathy. Ann Neurol 35:116–119

590. Levi-Montalcini R (1987) The nerve growth factor 35 years later. Science 237:1154–1162

591. Levin KH, Lutz G (1996) Angiotropic large-cell lymphoma with peripheral nerve and skeletal muscle involvement: early diagnosis and treatment. Neurology 47:1009–1011

592. Liehr T, Grehl H, Rautenstrauss B (1997) Accumulation of peripheral myelin protein 22 (PMP22) in onion bulbs of nerves biopsied from patients with different subtypes of Charcot-Marie-Tooth disease type 1 (letter; comment). Acta Neuropathol (Berl) 94:514–516

593. Liehr T, Grehl H, Rautenstrauss B (1997) Molecular diagnosis of PMP22-associated neuropathies using fluorescence in situ hybridization (FISH) on archival peripheral nerve tissue preparations. Acta Neuropathol (Berl) 94:266–271

594. Lincoln J, Milner P, Appenzeller O, Burnstock G, Qualls C (1993) Innervation of normal human sural and optic nerves by noradrenaline- and peptide-containing nervi vasorum and nervorum: effect of diabetes and alcoholism. Brain Res 632:48–56

595. Lindberg C, Borg K, Edstrom L, Hedstrom A, Oldfors A (1991) Inclusion body myositis and Welander distal

myopathy: a clinical, neurophysiological and morphological comparison. J Neurol Sci 103:76–81

596. Linington C, Izumo S, Suzuki M, Uyemura K, Meyermann R, Wekerle H (1984) A permanent rat T cell line that mediates experimental allergic neuritis in the Lewis rat in vivo. J Immunol 133:1946–1950

597. Linington C, Wekerle H (1984) LiP2/A: A permanent P2 protein-specific T lymphozyte line mediating experimental allergic neuritis in the Lewis rat. Neurology (Minneap) 34:260

598. Linke RP (1999) Praktische Hinweise zur Diagnose und Therapie generalisierter Amyloidosen. Deutsches Ärzteblatt 96:B662–B663

599. Lippa CF, Chad DA, Smith TW, Kaplan MH, Hammer K (1986) Neuropathy associated with cryoglobulinemia. Muscle Nerve 9:626–631

600. Lisak RP, Bealmear B, Benjamins J, Skoff A (1998) Inflammatory cytokines inhibit upregulation of glycolipid expression by Schwann cells in vitro. Neurology 51:1661–1665

601. Livesey FJ, Fraher JP (1992) Experimental traction injuries of cervical spinal nerve roots: a scanning EM study of rupture patterns in fresh tissue. Neuropathol Appl Neurobiol 18:376–386

602. Liwnicz BH (1979) Bilateral trigeminal neurofibrosarcoma. Case report. J Neurosurg 50:253–256

603. Lorson CL, Strasswimmer J, Yao JM, Baleja JD, Hahnen E, Wirth B, Le T, Burghes AH, Androphy EJ (1998) SMN oligomerization defect correlates with spinal muscular atrophy severity. Nat Genet 19:63–66

604. Lossos A, Meiner Z, Barash V, Soffer D, Schlesinger I, Abramsky O, Argov Z, Shpitzen S, Meiner V (1998) Adult polyglucosan body disease in Ashkenazi Jewish patients carrying the Tyr329Ser mutation in the glycogen-branching enzyme gene. Ann Neurol 44:867–872

605. Lothe RA, Slettan A, Saeter G, Brogger A, Borresen AL, Nesland JM (1995) Alterations at chromosome 17 loci in peripheral nerve sheath tumors. J Neuropathol Exp Neurol 54:65–73

606. Louis MES, Peck SHS, Bowering D, Morgan GB, Blatherwick J, Banerjee S, Kettyls GDM, Black WA, Milling ME, Hauschild AHW, Tauxe RV, Blake PA (1988) Botulism from chopped garlic: delayed recognition of a major outbreak. Ann Int Med 108:363–368

607. Love S, Bateman DE, Hirschowitz L (1997) Bilateral lambda light chain amyloidomas of the trigeminal ganglia, nerves and roots. Neuropathol Appl Neurobiol 23:512–515

608. Love S, Hilton DA, Coakham HB (1998) Central demyelination of the Vth nerve root in trigeminal neuralgia associated with vascular compression. (discussion 11–2) Brain Pathol 8:1–11

609. Luke RA, Stern BJ, Krumholz A, Johns CJ (1987) Neurosarcoidosis: the long-term clinical course. Neurology 37:461–463

610. Lundberg PO, Wranne I, Brun A (1987) Family with optic atrophy and neurological symptoms. Acta Neurol Scand 43:87–105

611. Lundborg G, Gelberman RH, Longo FM, Powell HC, Varon S (1982) In vivo regeneration of cut nerves encased in silicone tubes: growth across a six-millimeter gap. J Neuropathol Exp Neurol 41:412–422

612. Lundborg G, Myers R, Powell H (1983) Nerve compression injury and increased endoneurial fluid pressure:

613. a "miniature compartment syndrome". J Neurol Neurosurg Psychiatry 46:1119–1124

613. Lundborg G, Zhao Q, Kanje M, Danielsen N, Kerns JM (1994) Can sensory and motor collateral sprouting be induced from intact peripheral nerve by end-to-side anastomosis? J Hand Surg [Br] 19:277–282

614. Lunn ER, Perry VH, Brown MC, Rosen H, Gordon S (1989) Absence of Wallerian degeneration does not hinder regeneration in peripheral nerve. Eur J Neurosci 1:27–33

615. Lunn MPT, Muir P, Brown LJ, MacMahon EME, Gregson NA, Hughes RAC (1999) Cytomegalovirus is not associated with IgM anti-myelin-associated glycoprotein/sulphate-2-glucuronyl paragloboside antibody-associated neuropathy. Ann Neurol 46:267–270

616. Lupski JR (2000) Recessive Charcot-Marie-Tooth disease. Ann Neurol 47:6–8

617. Luster AD (1998) Chemokines – chemotactic cytokines that mediate inflammation. N Engl J Med 338:436–445

618. Lutchman M, Rouleau GA (1996) Neurofibromatosis type 2: a new mechanism of tumor suppression. Trends Neurosci 19:373–377

619. Ma JJ, Nishimura M, Mine H, Kuroki S, Nukina M, Ohta M, Saji H, Obayashi H, Kawakami H, Saida T, Uchiyama T (1998) Genetic contribution of the tumor necrosis factor region in Guillain-Barré syndrome. Ann Neurol 44:815–818

620. Maas JJ, Beersma MF, Haan J, Jonkers GJ, Kroes AC (1996) Bilateral brachial plexus neuritis following parvovirus B19 and cytomegalovirus infection. Ann Neurol 40:928–932

621. MacCollin M, Braverman N, Viskochil D, Ruttledge M, Davis K, Ojemann R, Gusella J, Parry DM (1996) A point mutation associated with a severe phenotype of neurofibromatosis 2. Ann Neurol 40:440–445

622. MacDonald BK, Cockerell OC, Sander JW, Shorvon SD (2000) The incidence and lifetime prevalence of neurological disorders in a prospective community-based study in the UK. Brain 123:665–676

623. Mackinnon SE, Dellon AL, Hudson AR, Hunter DA (1986) Chronic human nerve compression – a histological assessment. Neuropathol Appl Neurobiol 12:547–565

624. Madrid R, Bradley WG (1975) The pathology of neuropathies with focal thickening of the myelin sheath (tomaculous neuropathy). Studies on the formation of the abnormal myelin sheath. J Neurol Sci 25:415–448

625. Maeda Y, Maeda R, Prineas JW, Ledeen RW (1994) Phosphatidylserine suppresses myelin-induced experimental allergic neuritis (EAN) in Lewis rats. J Neuropathol Exp Neurol 53:672–677

626. Magyar JP, Martini R, Ruelicke T, Aguzzi A, Adlkofer K, Dembic Z, Zielasek J, Toyka KV, Suter U (1996) Impaired differentiation of Schwann cells in transgenic mice with increased PMP22 gene dosage. J Neurosci 16:5351–5360

627. Makonkawkeyoon S, Limson-Pobre RN, Moreira AL, Schauf V, Kaplan G (1993) Thalidomide inhibits the replication of human immunodeficiency virus type 1. Proc Natl Acad Sci USA 90:5974–5978

628. Malandrini A, Guazzi GC, Alessandrini C, Federico A (1990) Peripheral nerve involvement in ataxia telangiectasia: histological and ultrastructural studies of peroneal nerve biopsy in two cases. Clin Neuropathol 9:109–114

629. Malandrini A, Palmeri S, Fabrizi GM, Villanova M, Berti G, Salvadori C, Gardini G, Motti L, Solime F, Guazzi GC

(1998) Juvenile Leigh syndrome with protracted course presenting as chronic sensory motor neuropathy, ataxia, deafness and retinitis pigmentosa: a clinicopathological report. J Neurol Sci 155:218–221

630. Malandrini A, Villanova M, Sabatelli P, Squarzoni S, Six J, Toti P, Guazzi G, Maraldi NM (1997) Localization of the laminin alpha 2 chain in normal human skeletal muscle and peripheral nerve: an ultrastructural immunolabeling study. Acta Neuropathol (Berl) 93:166–172

631. Malinow K, Yannakakis GD, Glusman SM, Edlow DW, Griffin J, Pestronk A, Powell DL, Ramsey-Goldman R, Eidelman BH, Medsger TA, Jr et al. (1986) Subacute sensory neuronopathy secondary to dorsal root ganglionitis in primary Sjögren's syndrome. Ann Neurol 20: 535–537

632. Mancardi GL, Di Rocco M, Schenone A, Veneselli E, Doria M, Abbruzzese M, Tabaton M, Borrone C (1992) Hereditary motor and sensory neuropathy with deafness, mental retardation and absence of large myelinated fibers. J Neurol Sci 110:121–130

633. March PA, Thrall MA, Brown DE, Mitchell TW, Löwenthal AC, Walkley SU (1997) GABAergic neuroaxonal dystrophy and other cytopathological alterations in feline Niemann-Pick disease type C. Acta Neuropathol (Berl) 94:164–172

634. Marchuk DA, Saulino AM, Tavakkol R, Swaroop M, Wallace MR, Andersen LB, Mitchell AL, Gutmann DH, Boguski M, Collins FS (1991) cDna cloning of the type 1 neurofibromatosis gene: complete sequence of the Nf1 gene product. Genomics 11:931–940

635. Mariman EC, Gabreels-Festen AA, van Beersum SE, Jongen PJ, van de Looij E, Baas F, Bolhuis PA, Ropers HH, Gabreels FJ (1994) Evidence for genetic heterogeneity underlying hereditary neuropathy with liability to pressure palsies. Hum Genet 93:151–156

636. Marrosu MG, Vaccargiu S, Marrosu G, Vannelli A, Cianchetti C, Muntoni F (1997) A novel point mutation in the peripheral myelin protein 22 (PMP22) gene associated with Charcot-Marie-Tooth disease type 1 A. Neurology 48:489–493

637. Martin JJ, Cras P, De Schutter E (1987) Spinal neuroaxonal dystrophy and angioneuromatosis. Acta Neuropathol (Berl) 73:19–24

638. Martin JJ, Lowenthal A, Ceuterick C, Vanier MT (1984) Juvenile dystonic lipidosis (variant of Niemann-Pick disease type C). J Neurol Sci 66:33–45

639. Martin JR (1984) Intra-axonal virus in demyelinative lesions of experimental herpes simplex type 2 infection. J Neurol Sci 63:63–74

640. Martini R, Zielasek J, Toyka KV, Giese KP, Schachner M (1995) Protein zero (P0)-deficient mice show myelin degeneration in peripheral nerves characteristic of inherited human neuropathies. Nat Genet 11:281–286

641. Maruff P, Tyler P, Burt T, Currie B, Burns C, Currie J (1996) Cognitive deficits in Machado-Joseph disease. Ann Neurol 40:421–427

642. Maruyama H, Kawakami H, Kohriyama T, Sakai T, Doyu M, Sobue G, Seto M, Tsujihata M, Oh-i T, Nishio T, Sunohara N, Takahashi R, Ohtake T, Hayashi M, Nishimura M, Saida T, Abe K, Itoyama Y, Matsumoto H, Nakamura S (1997) CAG repeat length and disease duration in Machado-Joseph disease: a new clinical classification. J Neurol Sci 152:166–171

643. Masini A, Scotti C, Calligaro A, Cazzalini O, Stivala LA, Bianchi L, Giovannini F, Ceccarelli D, Muscatello U, Tomasi A, Vannini V (1999) Zidovudine-induced experimental myopathy: dual mechanism of mitochondrial damage. J Neurol Sci 166:131–140

644. Mather K, Martin JE, Swash M, Vowles G, Brown A, Leigh PN (1993) Histochemical and immunocytochemical study of ubiquitinated neuronal inclusions in amyotrophic lateral sclerosis. Neuropathol Appl Neurobiol 19: 141–145

645. Matsuda M, Ikeda S, Sakurai S, Nezu A, Yanagisawa N, Inuzuka T (1996) Hypertrophic neuritis due to chronic inflammatory demyelinating polyradiculoneuropathy (CIDP): a postmortem pathological study. Muscle Nerve 19:163–169

646. Matsumoto S, Goto S, Kusaka H, Imai T, Murakami N, Hashizume Y, Okazaki H, Hirano A (1993) Ubiquitin-positive inclusion in anterior horn cells in subgroups of motor neuron diseases: a comparative study of adult-onset amyotrophic lateral sclerosis, juvenile amyotrophic lateral sclerosis and Werdnig-Hoffmann disease. J Neurol Sci 115:208–213

647. Matsumoto S, Goto S, Kusaka H, Ito H, Imai T (1994) Synaptic pathology of spinal anterior horn cells in amyotrophic lateral sclerosis: an immunohistochemical study. J Neurol Sci 125:180–185

648. Matsumura K, Chiba A, Yamada H, Fukuta-Ohi H, Fujita S, Endo T, Kobata A, Anderson LV, Kanazawa I, Campbell KP, Shimizu T (1997) A role of dystroglycan in Schwannoma cell adhesion to laminin. J Biol Chem 272: 13904–13910

649. Matsumura K, Nakasu S, Nioka H, Handa J (1993) Lectin histochemistry of normal and neoplastic peripheral nerve sheath. 2. Lectin binding patterns of Schwannoma and neurofibroma. Acta Neuropathol (Berl) 86:559–566

650. Matsumura K, Yamada H, Saito F, Sunada Y, Shimizu T (1997) Peripheral nerve involvement in merosin-deficient congenital muscular dystrophy and dy mouse. Neuromuscul Disord 7:7–12

651. Mattio TG, Nishida T, Minieka MM (1992) Lotus neuropathy: report of a case. Neurology 42:1636

652. Mazzeo A, Rodolico C, Monici MC, Migliorato A, Aguennouz M, Vita G (1997) Perineurium talin immunoreactivity decreases in diabetic neuropathy. J Neurol Sci 146:7–11

653. McCarthy BG, Hsieh ST, Stocks A, Hauer P, Macko C, Cornblath DR, Griffin JW, McArthur JC (1995) Cutaneous innervation in sensory neuropathies: evaluation by skin biopsy. Neurology 45:1848–1855

654. McCombe PA, van der Kreek SA, Pender MP (1992) Neuropathological findings in chronic relapsing experimental allergic neuritis induced in the Lewis rat by inoculation with intradural root myelin and treatment with low dose cyclosporin A. Neuropathol Appl Neurobiol 18:171–187

655. McEneaney D, Hawkins S, Trimble E, Smye M (1993) Porphyric neuropathy – a rare and often neglected differential diagnosis of Guillain-Barré syndrome (letter). J Neurol Sci 114:231–232

656. McLeod JG, Tuck RR, Pollard JD, Cameron J, Walsh JC (1984) Chronic polyneuropathy of undetermined cause. J Neurol Neurosurg Psychiatry 47:530–535

657. McLoughlin DM, Spargo E, Wassif WS, Newham DJ, Peters TJ, Lantos PL, Russell GF (1998) Structural and

functional changes in skeletal muscle in anorexia nervosa. Acta Neuropathol (Berl) 95:632–640

658. Medori R, Autilio-Gambetti L, Jenich H, Gambetti P (1988) Changes in axon size and slow axonal transport are related in experimental diabetic neuropathy. Neurology 38:597–601

659. Meier C, Grahmann F, Engelhardt A, Dumas M (1989) Peripheral nerve disorders in Lyme-Borreliosis. Nerve biopsy studies from eight cases. Acta Neuropathol (Berl) 79:271–278

660. Meier C, Vandevelde M, Steck A, Zurbriggen A (1984) Demyelinating polyneuropathy associated with monoclonal IgM-paraproteinaemia. Histological, ultrastructural and immunocytochemical studies. J Neurol Sci 63:353–367

661. Meijerink PH, Hoogendijk JE, Gabreels-Festen AA, Zorn I, Veldman H, Baas F, de Visser M, Bolhuis PA (1996) Clinically distinct codon 69 mutations in major myelin protein zero in demyelinating neuropathies. Ann Neurol 40:672–675

662. Mendell JR, Sahenk Z, Whitaker JN, Trapp BD, Yates AJ, Griggs RC, Quarles RH (1985) Polyneuropathy and IgM monoclonal gammopathy: studies on the pathogenetic role of anti-myelin-associated glycoprotein antibody. Ann Neurol 17:243–254

663. Menken M (1989) The 1985 National Ambulatory Medical Care Survey of neurologists. A clinician's perspective. Arch Neurol 46:1346–1348

664. Mercelis R, Hassoun A, Verstraeten L, De Bock R, Martin JJ (1990) Porphyric neuropathy and hereditary delta-aminolevulinic acid dehydratase deficiency in an adult. J Neurol Sci 95:39–47

665. Merlini L, Villanova M, Sabatelli P, Trogu A, Malandrini A, Yanakiev P, Maraldi NM, Kalaydjieva L (1998) Hereditary motor and sensory neuropathy Lom type in an Italian Gypsy family. Neuromuscul Disord 8:182–185

666. Messier G, Meyrier A, Robineau M, Kemeny JL (1986) Recurrent transient paralysis of a common oculomotor nerve in essential mixed cryoglobulinemia. Presse Med 15:579–580

667. Meucci N, Baldini L, Cappellari A, Di Troia A, Allaria S, Scarlato G, Nobile-Orazio E (1999) Anti-myelin-associated glycoprotein antibodies predict the development of neuropathy in asymptomatic patients with IgM monoclonal gammopathy. Ann Neurol 46:119–122

668. Midha R, Mackinnon SE, Becker LE (1994) The fate of Schwann cells in peripheral nerve allografts. J Neuropathol Exp Neurol 53:316–322

669. Midroni G, Bilbao JM (1995) Biopsy diagnosis of peripheral neuropathy. Butterworth-Heinemann, Boston Oxford Melbourne

670. Migheli A, Attanasio A, Schiffer D (1994) Ubiquitin and neurofilament expression in anterior horn cells in amyotrophic lateral sclerosis: possible clues to the pathogenesis. Neuropathol Appl Neurobiol 20:282–289

671. Miller R, Bartolo DC, Cervero F, Mortensen NJ (1989) Differences in anal sensation in continent and incontinent patients with perineal descent. Int J Colorectal Dis 4:45–49

672. Miller RG, Parry GJ, Pfaeffl W, Lang W, Lippert R, Kiprov D (1988) The spectrum of peripheral neuropathy associated with ARC and AIDS. Muscle Nerve 11:857–863

673. Millesi H (1968) Zum Problem der Überbrückung von Defekten peripherer Nerven. Wien Med Wochenschr 118:182–187

674. Mimura Y, Kuriyama M, Tokimura Y, Fujiyama J, Osame M, Takesako K, Tanaka N (1993) Treatment of cerebrotendinous xanthomatosis with low-density lipoprotein (LDL)-apheresis (see comments). J Neurol Sci 114:227–230

675. Misra VP, King RH, Harding AE, Muddle JR, Thomas PK (1991) Peripheral neuropathy in the Chediak-Higashi syndrome. Acta Neuropathol (Berl) 81:354–358

676. Misu K-i, Hattori N, Nagamatsu M, Ikeda S-i, Ando Y, Nakazato M, Takei Y-i, Hanyu N, Usui Y, Tanaka F, Harada T, Inukai A, Hashizume Y, Sobue G (1999) Late-onset familial amyloid polyneuropathy type I (transthyretin Met30-associated familial amyloid polyneuropathy) unrelated to endemic focus in Japan – clinicopathological and genetic features. Brain 122:1951–1962

677. Mito T, Takada K, Akaboshi S, Takashima S, Takeshita K, Origuchi Y (1989) A pathological study of a peripheral nerve in a case of neonatal adrenoleukodystrophy. Acta Neuropathol (Berl) 77:437–440

678. Mitsui Y, Kusunoki S, Hiruma S, Akamatsu M, Kihara M, Hashimoto S, Takahashi M (1999) Sensorimotor polyneuropathy associated with chronic lymphocytic leukemia, IgM antigangliosides antibody and human T-cell leukemia virus I infection. Muscle Nerve 22:1461–1465

679. Mitsuishi K, Takahashi A, Mizutani M, Ochiai K, Itakura C (1993) beta,beta'-Iminodipropionitrile toxicity in normal and congenitally neurofilament-deficient Japanese quails. Acta Neuropathol (Berl) 86:578–581

680. Mitsumoto H, Estes ML, Wilbourn AJ, Culver JE Jr (1992) Perineurial cell hypertrophic mononeuropathy manifesting as carpal tunnel syndrome. Muscle Nerve 15:1364–1368

681. Mitsumoto H, Ikeda K, Wong V, Cedarbaum JM, Lindsay RM (1993) Ciliary neurotrophic factor (CNTF) and brain-derived neurotrophic factor (BDNF) co-administration arrests loss of motor function in wobbler mice. Soc Neurosci Abst 19:199

682. Mitsumoto H, Wilbourn AJ, Goren H (1980) Perineurioma as the cause of localized hypertrophic neuropathy. Muscle Nerve 3:403–412

683. Miyata Y, Kashihara Y, Homma S, Kuno M (1986) Effects of nerve growth factor on the survival and synaptic function of Ia sensory neurons axotomized in neonatal rats. J Neurosci 6:2012–2018

684. Mizisin AP, Shelton GD, Wagner S, Rusbridge C, Powell HC (1998) Myelin splitting, Schwann cell injury and demyelination in feline diabetic neuropathy. Acta Neuropathol (Berl) 95:171–174

685. Mizusawa H, Matsumoto S, Yen SH, Hirano A, Rojas-Corona RR, Donnenfeld H (1989) Focal accumulation of phosphorylated neurofilaments within anterior horn cell in familial amyotrophic lateral sclerosis. Acta Neuropathol (Berl) 79:37–43

686. Mizusawa H, Watanabe M, Kanazawa I, Nakanishi T, Kobayashi M, Tanaka M, Suzuki H, Nishikimi M, Ozawa T (1988) Familial mitochondrial myopathy associated with peripheral neuropathy: partial deficiencies of complex I and complex IV. J Neurol Sci 86:171–184

687. Mogyoros I, Kiernan MC, Burke D, Bostock H (1997) Excitability changes in human sensory and motor axons

during hyperventilation and ischaemia. Brain 120:
317–325

688. Mohseni S, Hildebrand C (1988) Hypoglycaemic neuro-pathy in BB/Wor rats treated with insulin implants. Electron microscopic observations. Acta Neuropathol 96:151–156

689. Moll JWB, Antoine JC, Brashear HR, Delattre J, Drlicek M, Dropcho EJ, Giometto B, Graus F, Greelee J, Honnorat J, Jaeckle KA, Tanaka K, Vecht CJ (1995) Guidelines on the detection of paraneoplastic anti-neuronal-spedific antibodies: report from the Workshop to the Fourth Meeting of the International Society of Neuro-Immu-nology on paraneoplastic neurological disease, held October 22–23, 1994, in Rotterdam, The Netherlands. Neurology 45:1937–1941

690. Molnar M, Neudecker S, Schröder JM (1995) Increase of mitochondria in vasa nervorum of cases with mito-chondrial myopathy, Kearns-Sayre syndrome, progres-sive external ophthalmoplegia and MELAS. Neuro-pathol Appl Neurobiol 21:432–439

691. Molnár M, Zanssen S, Buse G, Schröder JM (1996) A lar-ge-scale deletion of mitochondrial DNA in a case with pure mitochondrial myopathy and neuropathy. Acta Neuropathol (Berl) 91:654–658

692. Monaco S, Bonetti B, Ferrari S, Moretto G, Nardelli E, Tedesco F, Mollnes TE, Nobile-Orazio E, Manfredini E, Bonazzi L et al. (1990) Complement-mediated demyelin-ation in patients with IgM monoclonal gammopathy and polyneuropathy. N Engl J Med 322:649–652

693. Monforte R, Estruch R, Valls-Solé J, Nicolas J, Villalta J, Urbano-Marquez A (1995) Autonomic and peripheral neuropathies in patients with chronic alcoholism. A dose-related toxic effect of alcohol. Arch Neurol 52: 45–51

694. Monton F, Coria F (1991) Reversible Schwann cell hyper-trophy in lead neuropathy. Neuropathol Appl Neurobiol 17:231–236

695. Montpetit VJ, Clapin DF, Tryphonas L, Dancea S (1988) Alteration of neuronal cytoskeletal organization in dor-sal root ganglia associated with pyridoxine neurotoxici-ty. Acta Neuropathol (Berl) 76:71–81

696. Moorhouse DF, Fox RI, Powell HC (1992) Immunotac-toid-like endoneurial deposits in a patient with mono-clonal gammopathy of undetermined significance and neuropathy (see comments). Acta Neuropathol (Berl) 84:484–494

697. Moosa A, Dubowitz V (1970) Peripheral neuropathy in Cockayne's syndrome. Arch Dis Child 45:674–677

698. Morris JL, Gibbins IL, Campbell G, Murphy R, Furness JB, Costa M (1986) Innervation of the large arteries and heart of the toad (Bufo marinus) by adrenergic and peptide-containing neurons. Cell Tissue Res 243:171–184

699. Mortier W, Görke W, Schröder JM (1997) Riesenaxon-Neuropathie – prognostische Aspekte. In: Jahrbuch der neuromuskulären Erkrankungen. Arcis München, pp 279–283

700. Moser AB, Borel J, Odone A, Naidu S, Cornblath D, San-ders DB, Moser HW (1987) A new dietary therapy for adrenoleukodystrophy: biochemical and preliminary clinical results in 36 patients. Ann Neurol 21:240–249

701. Moser HW (1993) Lorenzo oil therapy for adrenoleuko-dystrophy: a prematurely amplified hope (editorial; comment). Ann Neurol 34:121–122

702. Moser HW (1995) Clinical and therapeutic aspects of adrenoleukodystrophy and adrenomyeloneuropathy. J Neuropathol Exp Neurol 54:740–745

703. Mostacciuolo ML, Müller E, Fardin P, Micaglio GF, Bar-doni B, Guioli S, Camerino G, Danieli GA (1991) X-link-ed Charcot-Marie-Tooth disease. A linkage study in a large family by using 12 probes of the pericentromeric region. Hum Genet 87:23–27

704. Moulignier A, Authier FJ, Baudrimont M, Pialoux G, Bel-ec L, Polivka M, Clair B, Gray F, Mikol J, Gherardi RK (1997) Peripheral neuropathy in human immunodefi-ciency virus-infected patients with the diffuse infiltra-tive lymphocytosis syndrome. Ann Neurol 41:438–445

705. Moulin DE, Hagen N, Feasby TE, Amireh R, Hahn A (1997) Pain in Guillain-Barré syndrome (see com-ments). Neurology 48:328–331

706. Mourelatos Z, Yachnis A, Rorke L, Mikol J, Gonatas NK (1993) The Golgi apparatus of motor neurons in amyotrophic lateral sclerosis. Ann Neurol 33:608–615

707. Müller HD, Mugler M, Ramaekers VT, Schröder JM (2000) Hereditary motor and sensory neuropathy with absence of large myelinated fibers due to absence of lar-ge neurons in dorsal root ganglia and anterior horns, clinically associated with deafness, mental retardation, and epilepsy (HMSN-ADM). J Periph Nerv Sys 5:1–11

708. Müller HD, Mugler M, Schröder JM (1999) No molecu-lar genetic alterations identified so far in congenital absence of large myelinated nerve fibers, deafness and mental retardation (abstract). J Periph Nerv Sys 4: 297–298

709. Mumenthaler M, Schliack H, Stöhr M (1998) Läsionen peripherer Nerven. Diagnostik und Therapie, 7. Auflage. Thieme, Stuttgart New York

710. Munoz DG, Greene C, Perl DP, Selkoe DJ (1988) Accu-mulation of phosphorylated neurofilaments in anterior horn motoneurons of amyotrophic lateral sclerosis patients. J Neuropathol Exp Neurol 47:9–18

711. Murakami K, Sobue G, Iwase S, Mitsuma T, Mano T (1993) Skin sympathetic nerve activity in acquired idio-pathic generalized anhidrosis. Neurology 43:1137–1140

712. Murakami S, Mizobuchi M, Nakashiro Y, Doi T, Hato N, Yanagihara N (1996) Bell palsy and herpes simplex virus: identification of viral DNA in endoneurial fluid and muscle (see comments). Ann Intern Med 124:27–30

713. Murayama S, Mori H, Ihara Y, Bouldin TW, Suzuki K, Tomonaga M (1990) Immunocytochemical and ultra-structural studies of lower motor neurons in amyotro-phic lateral sclerosis. Ann Neurol 27:137–148

714. Murayama S, Ookawa Y, Mori H, Nakano I, Ihara Y, Kuzuhara S, Tomonaga M (1989) Immunocytochemical and ultrastructural study of Lewy body-like hyaline inclusions in familial amyotrophic lateral sclerosis. Acta Neuropathol (Berl) 78:143–152

715. Murphy JR, Ringel SP (1990) Survival prediction in amyotrophic lateral sclerosis (letter; comment). Muscle Nerve 13:657–658

716. Mutoh T, Senda Y, Sugimura K, Koike Y, Matsuoka Y, Sobue I, Takahashi A, Naoi M (1988) Severe orthostatic hypotension in a female carrier of Fabry's disease. Arch Neurol 45:468–472

717. Nacimiento W, Podoll K, Graeber MB, Topper R, Möbius E, Ostermann H, Noth J, Kreutzberg GW (1992) Con-tralateral early blink reflex in patients with facial nerve palsy: indication for synaptic reorganization in the

facial nucleus during regeneration. J Neurol Sci 109: 148–155

718. Nadkarni N, Lisak RP (1993) Guillain-Barré syndrome (GBS) with bilateral optic neuritis and central white matter disease. Neurology 43:842–843

719. Nagao M, Oka N, Akiguchi I, Kimura J (1995) Lectin binding to Renaut bodies. Acta Neurol Scand 92:344–347

720. Nagaoka U, Kato T, Kurita K, Arawaka S, Hosoya T, Yuki N, Shikama Y, Yamaguchi K, Sasaki H (1996) Cranial nerve enhancement on three-dimensional MRI in Miller Fisher syndrome. Neurology 47:1601–1602

721. Nagashima T, Seko K, Hirose K, Mannen T, Yoshimura S, Arima R, Nagashima K, Morimatsu Y (1988) Familial bulbo-spinal muscular atrophy associated with testicular atrophy and sensory neuropathy (Kennedy-Alter-Sung syndrome). Autopsy case report of two brothers. J Neurol Sci 87:141–152

722. Nakagawa M, Suehara M, Saito A, Takashima H, Umehara F, Saito M, Kanzato N, Matsuzaki T, Takenaga S, Sakoda S, Izumo S, Osame M (1999) A novel MPZ gene mutation in dominantly inherited neuropathy with focally folded myelin sheaths. Neurology 52:1271–1275

723. Nakanishi T, Sobue I, Toyokura Y, Nishitani H, Kuroiwa Y, Satoyoshi E, Tsubaki T, Igata A, Ozaki Y (1984) The Crow-Fukase syndrome: a study of 102 cases in Japan. Neurology 34:712–720

724. Nardelli E, Anzini P, Moretto G, Rizzuto N, Steck AJ (1994) Pattern of nervous tissue immunostaining by human anti-glycolipid antibodies. J Neurol Sci 122: 220–227

725. Nardelli E, Steck AJ, Barkas T, Schluep M, Jerusalem F (1988) Motor neuron syndrome and monoclonal IgM with antibody activity against gangliosides GM1 and GD1b. Ann Neurol 23:524–528

726. Navarro X, Kennedy WR, Fries TJ (1989) Small nerve fiber dysfunction in diabetic neuropathy. Muscle Nerve 12:498–507

727. Navon R, Khosravi R, Melki J, Drucker L, Fontaine B, Turpin JC, N'guyen B, Fardeau M, Rondot P, Baumann N (1997) Juvenile-onset spinal muscular atrophy caused by compound heterozygosity for mutations in the HEXA gene. Ann Neurol 41:631–638

728. Navon R, Seifried B, Gal-On NS, Sadeh M (1996) A new point mutation affecting the fourth transmembrane domain of PMP22 results in severe de novo Charcot-Marie-Tooth disease. Hum Genet 97:685–687

729. Neff NT, Prevette D, Houenou LJ, Lewis ME, Glicksman MA, Yin QW, Oppenheim RW (1993) Insulin-like growth factors: putative muscle-derived trophic agents that promote motoneuron survival. J Neurobiol 24:1578–1588

730. Nelis E, Haites N, Van Broeckhoven C (1999) Mutations in the peripheral myelin genes and associated genes in inherited peripheral neuropathies. Hum Mutat 13:11–28

731. Nelis E, Holmberg B, Adolfsson R, Holmgren G, van Broeckhoven C (1997) PMP22 Thr(118)Met: recessive CMT1 mutation or polymorphism? (letter). Nat Genet 15:13–14

732. Nelis E, Timmerman V, De Jonghe P, Vandenberghe A, Pham-Dinh D, Dautigny A, Martin JJ, Van Broeckhoven C (1994) Rapid screening of myelin genes in CMT1 patients by SSCP analysis: identification of new mutations and polymorphisms in the P0 gene. Hum Genet 94: 653–657

733. Nemni R, Fazio R, Corbo M, Sessa M, Comi G, Canal N (1987) Peripheral neuropathy associated with Crohn's disease. Neurology 37:1414–1417

734. Nemni R, Feltri ML, Fazio R, Quattrini A, Lorenzetti I, Corbo M, Canal N (1990) Axonal neuropathy with monoclonal IgG kappa that binds to a neurofilament protein. Ann Neurol 28:361–364

735. Nemni R, Mamoli A, Fazio R, Camerlingo M, Quattrini A, Lorenzetti I, Comola M, Galardi G, Canal N (1991) Polyneuropathy associated with IgA monoclonal gammopathy: a hypothesis of its pathogenesis. Acta Neuropathol (Berl) 81:371–376

736. Neufeld MY, Josiphov J, Korczyn AD (1992) Demyelinating peripheral neuropathy in Creutzfeldt-Jakob disease. Muscle Nerve 15:1234–1239

737. Neuhaus IM, Bone L, Wang S, Ionasescu V, Werner R (1996) The human connexin32 gene is transcribed from two tissue-specific promoters. Biosci Rep 16:239–248

738. Neundörfer B (1987) Polyneuritiden und Polyneuropathien. In: Neundörfer B, Schimrigk K, Soyka D (eds) Praktische Neurologie (vol 2) Edition Medizin VCH, Weinheim

739. Neundörfer B, Grahmann F, Engelhardt A, Harte U (1990) Postoperative effects and value of sural nerve biopsies: a retrospective study. Eur Neurol 30:350–352

740. Newman NJ (1993) Leber's hereditary optic neuropathy. New genetic considerations. Arch Neurol 50:540–548

741. Nicholson GA (1991) Penetrance of the hereditary motor and sensory neuropathy Ia mutation: assessment by nerve conduction studies. Neurology 41:547–552

742. Nicholson GA, Dawkins JL, Blair IP, Kennerson ML, Gordon MJ, Cherryson AK, Nash J, Bananis T (1996) The gene for hereditary sensory neuropathy type I (HSN-I) maps to chromosome 9q22.1-q22.3. Nat Genet 13:101–104

743. Nicholson GA, Valentijn LJ, Cherryson AK, Kennerson ML, Bragg TL, DeKroon RM, Ross DA, Pollard JD, McLeod JG, Bolhuis PA et al. (1994) A frame shift mutation in the PMP22 gene in hereditary neuropathy with liability to pressure palsies (published erratum appears in Nat Genet 1994 May;7(1):113). Nat Genet 6:263–266

744. Nicolas JM, Estruch R, Salamero M, Orteu N, Fernandez-Sola J, Sacanella E, Urbano-Marquez A (1997) Brain impairment in well-nourished chronic alcoholics is related to ethanol intake. Ann Neurol 41:590–598

745. Niehrs C (1996) Growth factors. Mad connection to the nucleus (news; comment). Nature 381:561–562

746. Nishizawa M, Sutherland WH, Nukada H (1995) Goshajinki-gan (herbal medicine) in streptozocin-induced diabetic neuropathy. J Neurol Sci 132:177–181

747. Nobile-Orazio E, Carpo M, Meucci N, Grassi MP, Capitani E, Sciacco M, Mangoni A, Scarlato G (1992) Guillain-Barré syndrome associated with high titers of anti-GM1 antibodies. J Neurol Sci 109:200–206

748. Nobile-Orazio E, Manfredini E, Carpo M, Meucci N, Monaco S, Ferrari S, Bonetti B, Cavaletti G, Gemignani F, Durelli L et al. (1994) Frequency and clinical correlates of anti-neural IgM antibodies in neuropathy associated with IgM monoclonal gammopathy. Ann Neurol 36: 416–424

749. Nobile-Orazio E, Meucci N, Baldini L, Di Troia A, Scarlato G (2000) Long-term prognosis of neuropathy associated with anti-MAG IgM M- proteins and its relationship to immune therapies. Brain 123:710–717

750. Nozaki K, Moskowitz MA, Maynard KI, Koketsu N, Dawson TM, Bredt DS, Snyder SH (1993) Possible origins and distribution of immunoreactive nitric oxide synthase-containing nerve fibers in cerebral arteries. J Cereb Blood Flow Metab 13:70–79

751. Nukada H, Anderson GM, McMorran PD (1997) Reperfusion nerve injury: pathology due to reflow and prolonged ischaemia. J Periph Nerv Sys 1:60–69

752. Nukada H, Dyck PJ (1987) Acute ischemia causes axonal stasis, swelling, attenuation, and secondary demyelination. Ann Neurol 22:311–318

753. Nukada H, McMorran PD (1994) Perivascular demyelination and intramyelinic oedema in reperfusion nerve injury. J Anat 185:259–266

754. Nukada H, McMorran PD, Shimizu J (2000) Acute inflammatory demyelination in reperfusion nerve injury. Ann Neurol 47:71–79

755. Nukada H, Pollock M, Haas LF (1982) The clinical spectrum and morphology of type II hereditary sensory neuropathy. Brain 105:647–665

756. Nukada H, Pollock M, Haas LF (1989) Is ischemia implicated in chronic multifocal demyelinating neuropathy? (see comments). Neurology 39:106–110

757. Nukada H, Powell HC, Myers RR (1992) Perineurial window: demyelination in nonherniated endoneurium with reduced nerve blood flow. J Neuropathol Exp Neurol 51:523–530

758. Nukada H, Powell HC, Myers RR (1993) Spatial distribution of nerve injury after occlusion of individual major vessels in rat sciatic nerves. J Neuropathol Exp Neurol 52:452–459

759. Nukada H, van Rij AM, Packer SG, McMorran PD (1996) Pathology of acute and chronic ischaemic neuropathy in atherosclerotic peripheral vascular disease. Brain 119:1449–1460

760. O' Leary C, Mann AC, Lough J, Willison HJ (1997) Muscle hypertrophy in multifocal motor neuropathy is associated with continuous motor unit activity. Muscle Nerve 20:479–485

761. Ochoa J, Fowler TJ, Gilliatt RW (1972) Anatomical changes in peripheral nerves compressed by a pneumatic tourniquet. J Anat 113:433–455

762. Ochoa JL (1993) Essence, investigation, and management of "neuropathic" pains: hopes from acknowledgment of chaos (editorial; see comments). Muscle Nerve 16:997–1008

763. Oda K, Fukushima N, Shibasaki H, Ohnishi A (1989) Hypoxia-sensitive hyperexcitability of the intramuscular nerve axons in Isaacs' syndrome. Ann Neurol 25:140–145

764. Odaka M, Yuki N, Yoshino H, Kasama T, Handa S, Irie F, Hirabayashi Y, Suzuki A, Hirata K (1998) N-glycolylneuraminic acid-containing GM1 is a new molecule for serum antibody in Guillain-Barré syndrome. Ann Neurol 43:829–834

765. Odergren T, Iwasaki N, Borg J, Forssberg H (1996) Impaired sensory-motor integration during grasping in writer's cramp. Brain 119:569–583

766. Ogawa-Goto K, Funamoto N, Abe T, Nagashima K (1990) Different ceramide compositions of gangliosides between human motor and sensory nerves. J Neurochem 55:1486–1493

767. Ogier H, Roels F, Cornelis A, Poll The BT, Scotto JM, Odievre M, Sandubray JM (1985) Absence of hepatic peroxisomes in a case of infantile Refsum's disease (letter). Scand J Clin Lab Invest 45:767–768

768. Ogino M, Orazio N, Latov N (1995) IgG anti-GM1 antibodies from patients with acute motor neuropathy are predominantly of the IgG1 and IgG3 subclasses. J Neuroimmunol 58:77–80

769. Ogleznev KY, Grigorian JA, Stange LA, Slavin KG (1992) Microsurgical treatment of spasmodic torticollis and hemifacial spasm. Neurology, International Symposium, Moscow

770. Oh SJ, Claussen GC, Kim DS (1997) Motor and sensory demyelinating mononeuropathy multiplex (multifocal motor and sensory demyelinating neuropathy): a separate entity of a variant of chronic inflammatory demyelinating polyneuropathy? J Periph Nerv Sys 2/4:363–369

771. Oh SJ, Claussen GC, Odabasi Z, Palmer CP (1995) Multifocal demyelinating motor neuropathy: pathologic evidence of 'inflammatory demyelinating polyradiculoneuropathy'. Neurology 45:1828–1832

772. Oh SJ, Slaughter R, Harrell L (1991) Paraneoplastic vasculitic neuropathy: a treatable neuropathy. Muscle Nerve 14:152–156

773. Ohnishi A, Dyck PJ (1974) Loss of small peripheral sensory neurons in Fabry's disease. Archiv Neurol 31:120–127

774. Ohnishi A, Inoue N, Yamamoto T, Murai Y, Hori H, Tanaka I, Koga M, Akiyama T (1986) Ethylene oxide neuropathy in rats. Exposure to 250 ppm. J Neurol Sci 74:215–221

775. Ohnishi A, Mitsudome A, Murai Y (1987) Primary segmental demyelination in the sural nerve in Cockayne's syndrome. Muscle Nerve 10:163–167

776. Ohnishi A, Murai Y, Ikeda M, Fujita T, Furuya H, Kuroiwa Y (1989) Autosomal recessive motor and sensory neuropathy with excessive myelin outfolding. Muscle Nerve 12:568–575

777. Ohnishi A, Yamashita Y, Goto I, Kuroiwa Y, Murakami S, Ikeda M (1979) De- and remyelination and onion bulb in cerebrotendinous xanthomatosis. Acta Neuropathol (Berl) 45:43–45

778. Ohnishi M, Tanaka Y, Tutui T, Bann S (1992) Extensive malignant Schwannoma of the mandibular nerve. Case report. Int J Oral Maxillofac Surg 21:280–281

779. Ohta M, Ellefson RD, Lambert EH, Dyck PJ (1973) Hereditary sensory neuropathy, type II. Clinical, electrophysiologic, histologic, and biochemical studies of a Quebec kinship. Arch Neurol 29:23–37

780. Okamoto K, Hirai S, Amari M, Iizuka T, Watanabe M, Murakami N, Takatama M (1993) Oculomotor nuclear pathology in amyotrophic lateral sclerosis. Acta Neuropathol (Berl) 85:458–462

781. Oksanen V (1986) Neurosarcoidosis: clinical presentations and course in 50 patients. Acta Neurol Scand 73:283–290

782. O-Kusky, Norman MG (1992) Sudden infant death syndrome: postnatal changes in the numerical density and total number of neurons in the hypoglossal nucleus. J Neuropathol Exp Neurol 51:577–584

783. Olney RK, Aminoff MJ, Gelb DJ, Lowenstein DH (1988) Neuromuscular effects distant from the site of botulinum neurotoxin injection. Neurology 38:1780–1783

784. Olsson Y (1990) Microenvironment of the peripheral nervous system under normal and pathological conditions. Crit Rev Neurobiol 5:265–311

785. Olsson Y, Reese TS (1971) Permeability of vasa nervorum and perineurium in mouse sciatic nerve studied by fluorescence and electron microscopy. J Neuropathol Exp Neurol 30:105–119

786. Ono S, Hashimoto K, Shimizu T, Mannen T, Toyokura Y (1989) Amyotrophic lateral sclerosis: electrophoretic study of amorphous material of skin (see comments). J Neurol Sci 92:159–167

787. Ono S, Mannen T, Toyokura Y (1989) Differential diagnosis between amyotrophic lateral sclerosis and spinal muscular atrophy by skin involvement. J Neurol Sci 91:301–310

788. Ono S, Yamauchi M (1993) Collagen fibril diameter and its relation to cross-linking of collagen in the skin of patients with amyotrophic lateral sclerosis. J Neurol Sci 119:74–78

789. Oomes PG, Jacobs BC, Hazenberg MP, Banffer JR, van der Meché FG (1995) Anti-GM1 IgG antibodies and Campylobacter bacteria in Guillain-Barré syndrome: evidence of molecular mimicry. Ann Neurol 38:170–175

790. Oomes PG, van der Meché FG, Markus-Silvis L, Meulstee J, Kleyweg RP (1991) In vivo effects of sera from Guillain-Barré subgroups: an electrophysiological and histological study on rat nerves. Muscle Nerve 14:1013–1020

791. Oppenheim RW, Prevette D, Haverkamp LJ, Houenou L, Yin QW, McManaman J (1993) Biological studies of a putative avian muscle-derived neurotrophic factor that prevents naturally occurring motoneuron death in vivo. J Neurobiol 24:1065–1079

792. Orrell RW (2000) Amyotrophic lateral sclerosis: copper/zinc superoxide dismutase (SOD1) gene mutations. Neuromuscul Disord 10:63–68

793. Orrell RW, King AW, Lane RJ, de Belleroche JS (1995) Investigation of a null mutation of the CNTF gene in familial amyotrophic lateral sclerosis. J Neurol Sci 132:126–128

794. Orso E, Broccardo C, Kaminski WE, Bottcher A, Liebisch G, Drobnik W, Gotz A, Chambenoit O, Diederich W, Langmann T, Spruss T, Luciani MF, Rothe G, Lackner KJ, Chimini G, Schmitz G (2000) Transport of lipids from golgi to plasma membrane is defective in Tangier disease patients and Abc1-deficient mice. Nat Genet 24:192–196

795. Owmann E, Lindvall-Axelsson M (1986) Cerebrovascular nerves and effetcts of amine transmitters and peptides on the brain circulation. Acta Physiol Scand 127, Suppl 552:95

796. Oyanagi K, Ikuta F, Horikawa Y (1989) Evidence for sequential degeneration of the neurons in the intermediate zone of the spinal cord in amyotrophic lateral sclerosis: a topographic and quantitative investigation. Acta Neuropathol (Berl) 77:343–349

797. Page RW, Moskowitz RW, Nash RE, Roessmann U (1977) Lower motor neuron disease with spinocerebellar degeneration. Ann Neurol 2:524–527

798. Palix C, Coignet J (1978) Un cas de polyneuropathie péripherique néo-natale par amyélinisation. Pédiatrie 33:201–207

799. Pamphlett R (1988) Axonal sprouting after botulinum toxin does not elicit a histological axon reaction. J Neurol Sci 87:175–185

800. Pamphlett R (1989) Early terminal and nodal sprouting of motor axons after botulinum toxin. J Neurol Sci 92:181–192

801. Pamphlett R, Bayliss A (1992) Lead uptake in motor axons. Muscle Nerve 15:620–625

802. Pamphlett R, Walsh J (1989) Infective endocarditis with inflammatory lesions in the peripheral nervous system. Acta Neuropathol (Berl) 78:101–104

803. Panegyres PK, Blumbergs PC, Leong AS, Bourne AJ (1990) Vasculitis of peripheral nerve and skeletal muscle: clinicopathological correlation and immunopathic mechanisms. J Neurol Sci 100:193–202

804. Panegyres PK, Mastaglia FL (1989) Guillain-Barré syndrome with involvement of the central and autonomic nervous systems (clinical conference). Med J Aust 150:655–659

805. Papadimitriou A, Comi GP, Hadjigeorgiou GM, Bordoni A, Sciacco M, Napoli L, Prelle A, Moggio M, Fagiolari G, Bresolin N, Salani S, Anastasopoulos I, Giassakis G, Divari R, Scarlato G (1998) Partial depletion and multiple deletions of muscle mtDNA in familial MNGIE syndrome. Neurology 51:1086–1092

806. Pareyson D (1999) Charcot-Mmarie-Tooth disease and related neuropathies: molecular basis for distinction and diagnosis. Muscle Nerve 22:1498–1509

807. Pareyson D, Taroni F, Botti S, Morbin M, Baratta S, Lauria G, Ciano C, Sghirlanzoni A (2000) Cranial neve involvement in CMT disease type 1 due to early growth response 2 gene mutation. Neurology 54:1696–1698

808. Parhad IM, Oishi R, Clark AW (1992) GAP-43 gene expression is increased in anterior horn cells of amyotrophic lateral sclerosis. Ann Neurol 31:593–597

809. Parman Y, Plante-Bordeneuve V, Guiochon-Mantel A, Eraksoy M, Said G (1999) Recessive inheritance of a new point mutation of the PMP22 gene in Dejerine-Sottas disease. Ann Neurol 45:518–522

810. Parry GJ (1993) Guillain-Barré Syndrome. Thieme, Stuttgart New York

811. Parry GJ, Clarke S (1988) Multifocal acquired demyelinating neuropathy masquerading as motor neuron disease. Muscle Nerve 11:103–107

812. Passafaro M, Clementi F, Pollo A, Carbone E, Sher E (1994) Omega-Conotoxin and Cd2+ stimulate the recruitment to the plasmamembrane of an intracellular pool of voltage-operated Ca2+ channels. Neuron 12:317–326

813. Paulson HL, Perez MK, Trottier Y, Trojanowski JQ, Subramony SH, Das SS, Vig P, Mandel JL, Fischbeck KH, Pittman RN (1997) Intranuclear inclusions of expanded polyglutamine protein in spinocerebellar ataxia type 3. Neuron 19:333–344

814. Paulus W, Jellinger K, Perneczky G (1991) Intraspinal neurothekeoma (nerve sheath myxoma). A report of two cases. Am J Clin Pathol 95:511–516

815. Payan H, Levine S (1965) Focal axonal proliferation in pons (central neurinoma). Arch Pathol 79:501–504

816. Payan MJ, Gambarelli D, Keller P, Lachard A, Garcin M, Vigouroux C, Toga M (1986) Melanotic neurofibroma: a case report with ultrastructural study. Acta Neuropathol (Berl) 69:148–152

817. Pearn J, Hudgson P (1979) Distal spinal muscular atrophy. A clinical and genetic study of 8 kindreds. J Neurol Sci 43:183–191

818. Pearson J, Pytel B (1978) Quantitative studies of ciliary and sphenopalatine ganglia in familial dysautonomia. J Neurol Sci 39:123–130

819. Pearson J, Pytel BA (1978) Quantitative studies of sympathetic ganglia and spinal cord intermedio-lateral gray columns in familial dysautonomia. J Neurol Sci 39: 47–59

820. Peiffer J, Kustermann-Kuhn B, Mortier W, Poremba M, Roggendorf W, Scholte HR, Schröder JM, Wendtland B, Wessel K, Zimmermann C (1988) Mitochondrial myopathies with necrotizing encephalopathy of the Leigh type. Pathol Res Pract 183:706–716

821. Peiffer J, Schlote W, Bischoff A, Boltshauser E, Müller G (1977) Generalized giant axonal neuropathy: a filament-forming disease of neuronal, endothelial, glial, Schwann cells in a patient without kinky hair. Acta Neuropathol (Berl) 40:213–218

822. Perentes E, Nakagawa Y, Ross GW, Stanton C, Rubinstein LJ (1987) Expression of epithelial membrane antigen in perineurial cells and their derivatives. An immunohistochemical study with multiple markers. Acta Neuropathol (Berl) 75:160–165

823. Perentes E, Rubinstein LJ (1986) Non-specific binding of mouse myeloma IgM immunoglobulins by human myelin sheaths and astrocytes. A potential complication of nervous system immunoperoxidase histochemistry. Acta Neuropathol (Berl) 70:284–288

824. Perry VH, Brown MC, Lunn ER, Tree P, Gordon S (1990) Evidence that very slow Wallerian degeneration in C57BL/Ola mice is an intrinsic property of the peripheral nerve. Eur J Neurosci 2:802–808

825. Peter HH (1991) Vaskulitiden. In: Gerok W, Hartmann F, Schustger HP (eds) Klinische Immunologie. (Innere Medizin der Gegenwart, vol 9). Urban & Schwarzenberg; München, Wien, Baltimore p 401–414

826. Peters A, Palay SL, Webster HD (1991) The fine structure of the nervous system, 3rd edn. WB Saunders, London

827. Pettersson CA (1993) Drainage of molecules from subarachnoid space to spinal nerve roots and peripheral nerve of the rat. A study based on Evans blue-albumin and lanthanum as tracers. Acta Neuropathol (Berl) 86: 636–644

828. Petty BG, Cornblath DR, Adornato BT, Chaudhry V, Flexner C, Wachsman M, Sinicropi D, Burton LE, Peroutka SJ (1994) The effect of systemically administered recombinant human nerve growth factor in healthy human subjects. Ann Neurol 36:244–246

829. Phillips DD, Hibbs RG, Ellison JP, Shapiro H (1972) An electron microscopic study of central and peripheral nodes of Ranvier. J Anat 111:229–238

830. Pickett JBD (1988) AAEE case report 16: Botulism. Muscle Nerve 11:1201–1205

831. Pingault V, Bondurand N, Kuhlbrodt K, Goerich DE, Préhu MO, Puliti A, Herbarth B, Hermans-Borgmeyer I, Legius E, Matthijs G, Amiel J, Lyonnet S, Ceccherini I, Romeo G, Smith JC, Read AP, Wegner M, Goossens M (1998) SOX10 mutations in patients with Waardenburg-Hirschsprung disease. Nat Genet 18:171–173

832. Plant GT, Mtanda AT, Arden GB, Johnson GJ (1997) An epidemic of optic neuropathy in Tanzania: characterization of the visual disorder and associated peripheral neuropathy. J Neurol Sci 145:127–140

833. Podvinec M (1984) Facial nerve disorders: anatomical, histological and clinical aspects. Adv Oto-Rhino-Laryng 32:124–193

834. Pollard JD, Baverstock J, McLeod JG (1987) Class II antigen expression and inflammatory cells in the Guillain-Barré syndrome. Ann Neurol 21:337–341

835. Pollard JD, McLeod JG, Honnibal TG, Verheijden MA (1982) Hypothyroid polyneuropathy. Clinical, electrophysiological and nerve biopsy findings in two cases. J Neurol Sci 53:461–471

836. Pollin MM, Griffiths IR (1987) Feline dysautonomia: an ultrastructural study of neurones in the XII nucleus. Acta Neuropathol (Berl) 73:275–280

837. Pollock M, Nicholson GI, Nukada H, Cameron S, Frankish P (1988) Neuropathy in multiple symmetric lipomatosis. Madelung's disease. Brain 111:1157–1171

838. Pollock M, Nukada H, Frith RW, Simcock JP, Allpress S (1983) Peripheral neuropathy in Tangier disease. Brain 106:911–928

839. Poll-The BT, Poulos A, Sharp P, Boue J, Ogier H, Odievre M, Saudubray JM (1985) Antenatal diagnosis of infantile Refsum's disease (letter). Clin Genet 27:524–526

840. Ponzin D, Menegus AM, Kirschner G, Nunzi MG, Fiori MG, Raine CS (1991) Effects of gangliosides on the expression of autoimmune demyelination in the peripheral nervous system. Ann Neurol 30:678–685

841. Pop PH, Joosten E, van Spreeken A, Gabreels-Festen A, Jaspar H, ter Laak H, Vos A (1984) Neuroaxonal pathology of central and peripheral nervous systems in cerebrotendinous xanthomatosis (CTX). Acta Neuropathol (Berl) 64:259–264

842. Poser CM (1987) The peripheral nervous system in multiple sclerosis. A review and pathogenetic hypothesis. J Neurol Sci 79:83–90

843. Powell HC, Myers RR (1984) Axonopathy and microangiopathy in chronic alloxan diabetes. Acta Neuropathol (Berl) 65:128–137

844. Powell HC, Myers RR (1996) The axon in Guillain-Barré syndrome: immune target or innocent bystander? (editorial; comment). Ann Neurol 39:4–5

845. Powell HC, Myers RR, Lampert PW (1982) Changes in Schwann cells and vessels in lead neuropathy. Am J Pathol 109:193–205

846. Powell HC, Myers RR, Mizisin AP, Olee T, Brostoff SW (1991) Response of the axon and barrier endothelium to experimental allergic neuritis induced by autoreactive T cell lines. Acta Neuropathol (Berl) 82:364–377

847. Powell HC, Rosoff J, Myers RR (1985) Microangiopathy in human diabetic neuropathy. Acta Neuropathol (Berl) 68:295–305

848. Preston DC, Kelly JJ Jr (1991) "Pseudospasticity" in Guillain-Barré syndrome. Neurology 41:131–134

849. Previtali SC, Archelos JJ, Hartung HP (1998) Expression of integrins in experimental autoimmune neuritis and Guillain-Barré syndrome. Ann Neurol 44:611–621

850. Priest JM, Fischbeck KH, Nouri N, Keats BJ (1995) A locus for axonal motor-sensory neuropathy with deafness and mental retardation maps to Xq24-q26. Genomics 29:409–412

851. Prior R, Schober R, Scharffetter K, Wechsler W (1992) Occlusive microangiopathy by immunoglobulin (IgM-kappa) precipitation: pathogenetic relevance in paraneoplastic cryoglobulinemic neuropathy. Acta Neuropathol (Berl) 83:423–426

852. Probst A, Ulrich J, Bischoff A, Boltshauser E (1981) Sensory ganglioneuropathy in infantile spinal muscular atrophy. Light and electronmicroscopic findings in two cases. Neuropediatrics 12:215–231

853. Pullen AH (1992) Presynaptic terminal loss from alpha-motoneurones following the retrograde axonal trans-

port of diphtheria toxin. Acta Neuropathol (Berl) 83:488-498

854. Pullen AH (1994) Neurofilament reorganisation and neurofilament antigen redistribution in spinal motoneurones following retrograde axonal transport of diphtheria toxin. Acta Neuropathol (Berl) 87:32-46

855. Pullen AH, Martin JE (1995) Ultrastructural abnormalities with inclusions in Onuf's nucleus in motor neuron disease (amyotrophic lateral sclerosis). Neuropathol Appl Neurobiol 21:327-340

856. Quarles RH, Weiss MD (1999) Autoantibodies associated with peripheral neuropathy. Muscle Nerve 22:800-822

857. Quasthoff S (1998) The role of axonal ion conductances in diabetic neuropathy: a review. Muscle Nerve 21:1246-1255

858. Quattrini A, Comi G, Nemni R, Martinelli V, Villa A, Caimi M, Wrabetz L, Canal N (1997) Axonal neuropathy associated with interferon-alpha treatment for hepatitis C: HLA-DR immunoreactivity in Schwann cells. Acta Neuropathol (Berl) 94:504-508

859. Quattrone A, Gambardella A, Bono F, Aguglia U, Bolino A, Bruni AC, Montesi MP, Oliveri RL, Sabatelli M, Tamburrini O, Valentino P, Van Broeckhoven C, Zappia M (1996) Autosomal recessive hereditary motor and sensory neuropathy with focally folded myelin sheaths: clinical, electrophysiologic, and genetic aspects of a large family. Neurology 46:1318-1324

860. Quinlivan R, Robb S, Hughes RA, Hall SM, Calver D (1993) Congenital sensory neuropathy in association with ichthyosis and anterior chamber cleavage syndrome. Neuromuscul Disord 3:217-221

861. Raivich G, Hellweg R, Graeber MB, Kreutzberg GW (1990) The expression of growth factor receptors during nerve regeneration. Restor Neurol Neurosci 1:217-223

862. Ram Z, Sadeh M, Walden R, Adar R (1991) Vascular insufficiency quantitatively aggravates diabetic neuropathy. Arch Neurol 48:1239-1242

863. Ramaekers VT, Lake BD, Harding B, Boyd S, Harden A, Brett EM, Wilson J (1987) Diagnostic difficulties in infantile neuroaxonal dystrophy. A clinicopathological study of eight cases. Neuropediatrics 18:170-175

864. Rance NE, McArthur JC, Cornblath DR, Landstrom DL, Griffin JW, Price DL (1988) Gracile tract degeneration in patients with sensory neuropathy and AIDS. Neurology 38:265-271

865. Raphael EA (1992) Plasma exchange in Guillain-Barré-Syndrome: one-year follow-up. Ann Neurol 32:94-97

866. Ratner N, Lieberman MA, Riccardi VM, Hong DM (1990) Mitogen accumulation in von Recklinghausen neurofibromatosis. Ann Neurol 27:298-303

867. Rebai T, Mhiri C, Heine P, Charfi H, Meyrignac C, Gherardi R (1989) Focal myelin thickenings in a peripheral neuropathy associated with IgM monoclonal gammopathy. Acta Neuropathol (Berl) 79:226-232

868. Rees JH, Gregson NA, Hughes RA (1995) Anti-ganglioside GM1 antibodies in Guillain-Barré syndrome and their relationship to Campylobacter jejuni infection. Ann Neurol 38:809-816

869. Ressot C, Latour P, Blanquet-Grossard F, Sturtz F, Duthel S, Battin J, Corbillon E, Ollagnon E, Serville F, Vandenberghe A, Dautigny A, Pham-Dinh D (1996) X-linked dominant Charcot-Marie-Tooth neuropathy (CMTX): new mutations in the connexin32 gene. Hum Genet 98:172-175

870. Riordan-Eva P, Sanders MD, Govan GG, Sweeney MG, Da Costa J, Harding AE (1995) The clinical features of Leber's hereditary optic neuropathy defined by the presence of a pathogenic mitochondrial DNA mutation. Brain 118:319-337

871. Ritz M-F, Erne B, Ferracin F, Vital A, Vital C, Steck AJ (1999) Anti-MAG IgM penetration into myelinated fibers correlates with the extent of myelin widening. Muscle Nerve 22:1030-1037

872. Rizzo WB, Phillips MW, Dammann AL, Leshner RT, Jennings SS, Avigan J, Proud VK (1987) Adrenoleukodystrophy: dietary oleic acid lowers hexacosanoate levels. Ann Neurol 21:232-239

873. Roa BB, Dyck PJ, Marks HG, Chance PF, Lupski JR (1993) Dejerine-Sottas syndrome associated with point mutation in the peripheral myelin protein 22 (PMP22) gene. Nat Genet 5:269-273

874. Roa BB, Garcia CA, Pentao L, Killian JM, Trask BJ, Suter U, Snipes GJ, Ortiz-Lopez R, Shooter EM, Patel PI et al. (1993) Evidence for a recessive PMP22 point mutation in Charcot-Marie-Tooth disease type 1A. Nat Genet 5:189-194

875. Roa BB, Garcia CA, Suter U, Kulpa DA, Wise CA, Mueller J, Welcher AA, Snipes GJ, Shooter EM, Patel PI et al. (1993) Charcot-Marie-Tooth disease type 1A. Association with a spontaneous point mutation in the PMP22 gene. N Engl J Med 329:96-101

876. Robert ME, Geraghty JJd, Miles SA, Cornford ME, Vinters HV (1989) Severe neuropathy in a patient with acquired immune deficiency syndrome (AIDS). Evidence for widespread cytomegalovirus infection of peripheral nerve and human immunodeficiency virus-like immunoreactivity of anterior horn cells. Acta Neuropathol (Berl) 79:255-261

877. Romics I, Bach D, Beutler W (1992) Malignant Schwannoma of kidney capsule. Urology 40:453-455

878. Ropert A, Metral S (1990) Conduction block in neuropathies with necrotizing vasculitis. Muscle Nerve 13:102-105

879. Ropper AH (1993) Accelerated neuropathy of renal failure. Arch Neurol 50:536-539

880. Ropper AH, Adelman L (1992) Early Guillain-Barré syndrome without inflammation. Arch Neurol 49:979-981

881. Rosales RL, Osame M, Madriaga EP, Navarro JC, Igata A (1988) Morphometry of intramuscular nerves in amyotrophic lateral sclerosis. Muscle Nerve 11:223-226

882. Rosen JL, Brown MJ, Hickey WF, Rostami A (1990) Early myelin lesions in experimental allergic neuritis. Muscle Nerve 13:629-636

883. Rosen SA, Wang H, Cornblath DR, Uematsu S, Hurko O (1989) Compression syndromes due to hypertrophic nerve roots in hereditary motor sensory neuropathy type I. Neurology 39:1173-1177

884. Rosenberg RN, Chutorian A (1967) Familial optico-acoustic nerve degeneration and polyneuropathy. Neurology 17:827-832

885. Ross AH, Grob P, Bothwell M, Elder DE, Ernst CS, Marano N, Ghrist BF, Slemp CC, Herlyn M, Atkinson B et al. (1984) Characterization of nerve growth factor receptor in neural crest tumors using monoclonal antibodies. Proc Natl Acad Sci USA 81:6681-6685

886. Rossiter JP, Anderson LL, Yang F, Cole GM (2000) Caspase-cleaved actin (fractin) immunolabelling of hirano bodies. Neuropathol Appl Neurobiol 26:342-346

887. Rothwell NJ, Hopkins SJ (1995) Cytokines and the nervous system II: actions and mechanisms of action. Trends Neurosci 18:130–136

888. Rouanet-Larriviere M, Vital C, Arne P, Favarel-Garrigues JC, Gin H, Vital A (2000) Guillain-Barré syndrome occurring in two women after ketoacidosic comatose state disclosing an insulin-dependent diabetes mellitus. J Peripher Nerv Syst 5:27–31

889. Rouleau GA, Clark AW, Rooke K, Pramatarova A, Krizus A, Suchowersky O, Julien JP, Figlewicz D (1996) SOD1 mutation is associated with accumulation of neurofilaments in amyotrophic lateral sclerosis. Ann Neurol 39:128–131

890. Rubin M, Karpati G, Wolfe LS, Carpenter S, Klavins MH, Mahuran DJ (1988) Adult onset motor neuronopathy in the juvenile type of hexosaminidase A and B deficiency. J Neurol Sci 87:103–119

891. Ruchoux MM, Maurage CA (1997) CADASIL: cerebral autosomal dominant arteriopathy with subcortical infarcts and leukoencephalopathy. J Neuropathol Exp Neurol 56:947–964

892. Rust S, Rosier M, Funke H, Real J, Amoura Z, Piette JC, Deleuze JF, Brewer HB, Duverger N, Denefle P, Assmann G (1999) Tangier disease is caused by mutations in the gene encoding ATP-binding cassette transporter 1. Nat Genet 22:352–355

893. Rust S, Walter M, Funke H, von Eckardstein A, Cullen P, Kroes HY, Hordijk R, Geisel J, Kastelein J, Molhuizen HO, Schreiner M, Mischke A, Hahmann HW, Assmann G (1998) Assignment of Tangier disease to chromosome 9q31 by a graphical. Nat Genet 20:96–98

894. Ruttledge MH, Narod SA, Dumanski JP, Parry DM, Eldridge R, Wertelecki W, Parboosingh J, Faucher MC, Lenoir GM, Collins VP et al. (1993) Presymptomatic diagnosis for neurofibromatosis 2 with chromosome 22 markers. Neurology 43:1753–1760

895. Ryberg B, Hindfelt B, Nilsson B, Olsson JE (1984) Antineural antibodies in Guillain-Barré syndrome and lymphocytic meningoradiculitis (Bannwarth's syndrome). Arch Neurol 41:1277–1281

896. Sabatelli M, Bertini E, Servidei S, Fernandez E, Magi S, Tonali P (1992) Giant axonal neuropathy: report on a case with focal fiber loss. Acta Neuropathol (Berl) 83:543–546

897. Sabatelli M, Mignogna T, Lippi G, Servidei S, Manfredi G, Ricci E, Bertini E, Lo Monaco M, Tonali P (1994) Autosomal recessive hypermyelinating neuropathy. Acta Neuropathol (Berl) 87:337–342

898. Sabatelli M, Mignogna T, Lippi G, Servidei S, Zollino M, Padua L, Lo Monaco M, De Armas L, Mereu ML, Tonali P (1998) Hereditary motor and sensory neuropathy with deafness, mental retardation, and absence of sensory large myelinated fibers: confirmation of a new entity. Am J Med Genet 75:309–313

899. Sadeh M, Martinovits G, Goldhammer Y (1989) Occurrence of both neurofibromatoses 1 and 2 in the same individual with a rapidly progressive course. Neurology 39:282–283

900. Said G (1990) Studies in the mechanisms of nerve lesions in leprous neuropathy. N Neurosci 2:85–94

901. Said G (1993) Asymptomatic nerve hypertrophy in lepromatous leprosy (editorial). Acta Leprol 8:119–120

902. Said G, Goulon-Goeau C, Lacroix C, Moulonguet A (1994) Nerve biopsy findings in different patterns of proximal diabetic neuropathy. Ann Neurol 35:559–569

903. Said G, Lacroix-Ciaudo C, Fujimura H, Blas C, Faux N (1988) The peripheral neuropathy of necrotizing arteritis: a clinicopathological study. Ann Neurol 23:461–465

904. Said G, Marion MH, Selva J, Jamet C (1986) Hypotrophic and dying-back nerve fibers in Friedreich's ataxia. Neurology 36:1292–1299

905. Saida K, Kawakami H, Ohta M, Iwamura K (1997) Coagulation and vascular abnormalities in Crow-Fukase syndrome. Muscle Nerve 20:486–492

906. Sakai T, Oda K (1993) Abundant reinnervation in peripheral nerves in Joseph disease. Neurology 43:428–430

907. Salazar-Grueso EF, Routbort MJ, Martin J, Dawson G, Roos RP (1990) Polyclonal IgM anti-GM1 ganglioside antibody in patients with motor neuron disease and variants. Ann Neurol 27:558–563

908. Salih MA, Maisonobe T, Kabiraj M, Rayess MA, al-Turaiki MH, Akbar M, Tahan A, Urtizberea JA, Grid D, Hamadouche T, Guilbot A, Brice A, Leguern E (2000) Autosomal recessive hereditary neuropathy with focally folded myelin sheaths and linked to chromosome 11q23: a distinct and homogeneous entity. Neuromuscul Disord 10:10–15

909. Samii M (1981) Centrocentral anastomosis of peripheral nerves: A neurosurgical treatment of amputation neuromas. In: Siegfried J, Zimmermann M (eds) Phantom and stump pain. Springer, Berlin Heidelberg New York, pp 123–125

910. Sancho S, Magyar JP, Aguzzi A, Suter U (1999) Distal axonopathy in peripheral nerves of PMP22-mutant mice. Brain 122:1563–1577

911. Sander D, Scholz CW, Eiben P, Klingelhofer J (1994) Postvaccinal plexus neuropathy following vaccination against tick-borne encephalitis and tetanus in a competitive athlete. Clin Investig 72:399

912. Sander S, Nicholson GA, Ouvrier RA, McLeod JG, Pollard JD (1998) Charcot-Marie-Tooth disease: histopathological features of the peripheral myelin protein (PMP22) duplication (CMT1A) and connexin32 mutations (CMTX1). Muscle Nerve 21:217–225

913. Sanders KA, Rowland LP, Murphy PL, Younger DS, Latov N, Sherman WH, Pesce M, Lange DJ (1993) Motor neuron diseases and amyotrophic lateral sclerosis: GM1 antibodies and paraproteinemia. Neurology 43:418–420

914. Santoro L, Perretti A, Crisci C, Ragno M, Massini R, Filla A, De Michele G, Caruso G (1990) Electrophysiological and histological follow-up study in 15 Friedreich's ataxia patients. Muscle Nerve 13:536–540

915. Santoro L, Perretti A, Filla A, De Michele G, Lanzillo B, Barbieri F, Crisci C, Rippa PG, Caruso G (1992) Is early onset cerebellar ataxia with retained tendon reflexes identifiable by electrophysiologic and histologic profile? A comparison with Friedreich's ataxia. J Neurol Sci 113:43–49

916. Santoro M, Thomas FP, Fink ME, Lange DJ, Uncini A, Wadia NH, Latov N, Hays AP (1990) IgM deposits at nodes of Ranvier in a patient with amyotrophic lateral sclerosis, anti-GM1 antibodies, and multifocal motor conduction block. Ann Neurol 28:373–377

917. Sasaki H, Kihara M, Zollman PJ, Nickander KK, Smithson IL, Schmelzer JD, Willner CL, Benarroch EE, Low PA (1997) Chronic constriction model of rat sciatic nerve:

nerve blood flow, morphologic and biochemical alterations. Acta Neuropathol (Berl) 93:62–70

918. Satchell PM, Hersch MI (1988) Firing rate may be a
determinant of nerve fibre vulnerability in axonopa-
thies. J Neurol Sci 87:289–297

919. Satsangi J, Donaghy M (1992) Multifocal peripheral neuropathy in eosinophilic fasciitis. J Neurol 239:91–92

920. Sawant-Mane S, Clark MB, Koski CL (1991) In vitro
demyelination by serum antibody from patients with
Guillain-Barré syndrome requires terminal complement complexes. Ann Neurol 29:397–404

921. Sayed AK, Bernhardt B, Perez-Atayde AR, Bannerman
RM (1987) Malignant Schwannoma in siblings with neurofibromatosis. Cancer 59:829–835

922. Scarpini E, Conti G, Chianese L, Baron P, Pizzul S, Basel-
lini A, Livraghi S, Scarlato G (1996) Induction of
p75NGFR in human diabetic neuropathy. J Neurol Sci
135:55–62

923. Schady W, Ochoa J (1984) Ehlers-Danlos in association
with tomaculous neuropathy (letter). Neurology 34:
1270–1271

924. Schaller E, Lassner F, Becker M, Walter GF, Berger A
(1991) Regeneration of autologous and allogenic nerve
grafts in a rat genetic model: preliminary report. J
Reconstr Microsurg 7:9–12

925. Schalow G, Zäch GA (1998) Neuronal reorganization
through oscillator formation training in patients with
CNS lesions. J Periph Nerv Sys 3:165–188

926. Schaumburg HH, Berger AR, Thomas PK (1992) Disorders of peripheral nerves, 2nd ed. FA Davis Company,
Philadelphia

927. Scheithauer BW, Woodruff JM, Erlandson RA (1999)
Tumors of the Peripheral Nervous System. Armed
Forces Institute of Pathology, Washington

928. Schenone A, Primavera A, De Martini I, Bianchini D,
Mancardi GL (1989) Amyloid neuropathy in light chain
multiple myeloma. Clin Neuropathol 8:156–157

929. Scherer SS (1996) Molecular specializations at nodes
and paranodes in peripheral nerve. Microsc Res Tech
34:452–461

930. Scherer SS, Chance PF (1995) Myelin genes: getting the
dosage right (news). Nat Genet 11:226–228

931. Schliack H (1968) Problems of surgical decompression
in idiopathic facial paralysis. Dtsch Med J 19:310–314

932. Schmalbruch H, Stender S, Boysen G (1987) Abnormalities in spinal neurons and dorsal root ganglion cells in
Tangier disease presenting with a syringomyelia-like
syndrome. J Neuropathol Exp Neurol 46:533–543

933. Schneider M, Obringer AC, Zackai E, Meadows AT
(1986) Childhood neurofibromatosis: risk factors for
malignant disease. Cancer Genet Cytogenet 21:347–354

934. Schnitzler A, Witte OW, Kunesch E, Freund HJ, Benecke
R (1998) Early-onset multisystem degeneration with
central motor, autonomic and optic nerve disturbances:
unusual Riley-Day syndrome or new clinical entity? J
Neurol Sci 154:205–208

935. Schober R, Reifenberger G, Kremer G, Urich H (1993)
Symmetrical neurofibroma with Schwann cell predomi-
nance and focal formation of microneurinomas. Acta
Neuropathol (Berl) 85:227–232

936. Schöls L, Amoiridis G, Przuntek H, Frank G, Epplen JT,
Epplen C (1997) Friedreich's ataxia. Revision of the phenotype according to molecular genetics. Brain 120:
2131–2140

937. Schonberger LB, Hurwitz ES, Katona P, Holman RC,
Bregman DJ (1981) Guillain-Barré syndrome: its epide-
miology and associations with influenza vaccination.
Ann Neurol 9:31–38

938. Schorr M, Zhou L, Schwechheimer K (1996) Expression
of ciliary neurotrophic factor is maintained in spinal
motor neurons of amyotrophic lateral sclerosis. J Neurol
Sci 140:117–122

939. Schröder J, Bohl J (1978) Altered ratio between axon
caliber and myelin thickness in sural nerves of children.
In: Canal N (ed) Peripheral neuropathies. Elsevier,
Amsterdam, pp 49–62

940. Schröder JM (1967) The role of Schwann cells in the formation of onion bulbs found in chronic neuropathies. J
Neuropathol Exp Neurol 26:135–136

941. Schröder JM (1968) Die Hyperneurotisationn Büngner-
scher Bänder bei der experimentellen Isoniazid-Neuro-
pathie: Phasenkontrast- und elektronenmikroskopische
Untersuchungen. Virch Arch Abt B Zellpath 1:131–156

942. Schröder JM (1968) Überzählige Schwannzellen bei der
Remyelinisation regenerierter und segmental demyeli-
nisierter Axone im peripheren Nerven. Verh Dtsch Ges
Pathol 52:222–228

943. Schröder JM. (1970) Zur Feinstruktur und quantitativen
Auswertung regenerierter peripherer Nervenfasern,
Proceedings of the VIth International Congress of Neu-
ropathology, Paris, pp 628–646

944. Schröder JM (1970) Zur Pathogenese der Isoniazid-
Neuropathie. I. Eine feinstrukturelle Differenzierung
gegenüber der Wallerschen Degeneration. Acta Neuropathol 16:301–323

945. Schröder JM (1970) Zur Pathogenese der Isoniazid-
Neuropathie. II. Phasenkontrast- und elektronenmikroskopische Untersuchungen am Rückenmark, an den
Spinalganglien und Muskelspindeln. Acta Neuropathol
16:324–341

946. Schröder JM (1972) Altered ratio between axon diameter and myelin sheath thickness in regenerated nerve
fibers. Brain Res 45:49–65

947. Schröder JM (1972) Das Perineurium als transitorische
Immunbarriere bei heterologer Nerventransplantation.
Vol. 46 Heft 116 B. Braun Melsungen AG, pp 317–323

948. Schröder JM (1974) Optic-electronic methods for evaluating peripheral nerve fibers quantitatively. Proceedings of the VIIth Internat. Congr. of Neuropath. Sept.
1–7, Budapest, pp 235–239

949. Schröder JM (1975) Degeneration and regeneration of
myelinated nerve fibers in experimental neuropathies.
In: Dyck PJ, Thomas PK, Lambert EH (eds) Periperal
Neuropathy. Saunders, Philadelphia London Toronto, pp
337–362

950. Schröder JM (1978) Die Feinstruktur markloser (Re-
makscher) Nervenfasern bei der Isoniazid-Neuropa-
thie. Acta Neuropathol 15:156–175

951. Schröder JM (1978) Zur Morphologie der Erkrankungen und Schädigungen peripherer Nerven. Therapie-
woche 28:4730–4747

952. Schröder JM (1982). Pathologie der Muskulatur. (Spezi-
elle pathologische Anatomie series, vol. 15) In: Doerr W,
Uehlinger E, Seifert G (eds) Springer, Berlin Heidelberg
New York, pp 1–813

953. Schröder JM (1982) Feinstrukturell-morphometrische
Analyse anaboler Myelinisationsstörungen im peripheren Nerven. Verh Dtsch Ges Pathol 66:272–275

954. Schröder JM (1984) Zur Morphologie hereditärer Polyneuropathien. In: Mortier W (ed) Moderne Diagnostik und Therapie bei Kindern. Grosse, Berlin, pp 14–22

955. Schröder JM (1984) Zur Pathologie der Polyneuropathien. Internist (Berl) 25:589–598

956. Schröder JM (1985) Degeneration und Regeneration nach Plexus-brachialis-Verletzung. In: Hase U, Reulen H-J (eds) Läsionen des Plexus brachialis. De Gruyter, Berlin New York, pp 65–70

957. Schröder JM (1986) Proliferation of epineurial capillaries and smooth muscle cells in angiopathic peripheral neuropathy. Acta Neuropathol (Berl) 72:29–37

958. Schröder JM (1987) Pathomorphologie der peripheren Nerven. In: Neundörfer B, Schimrigk K, Soyka D (eds) Praktische Neurologie, vol 2. Edition Medizin VCH, Weinheim, pp 11–104

959. Schröder JM (1987) Pathomorphologie der peripheren Nerven. In: Neundörfer B, Schimrigk K, Soyka D (eds) Polyneuritiden und Polyneuropathien. (Praktische Neurologie series, vol 2) Edition Medizin VCH, Weinheim, pp 11–104

960. Schröder JM (1988) Muskel- und Nervenbiopsien. In: Schliack H, Hopf JC (eds) Diagnostik in der Neurologie. Thieme, Stuttgart New York, pp 147–188

961. Schröder JM (1992) Nervenbiopsien. In: Pongratz D (ed) Klinische Neurologie. Urban & Schwarzenberg, München, pp 247–254

962. Schröder JM (1993) Neuropathy associated with mitochondrial disorders. Brain Pathol 3:177–190

963. Schröder JM (1993) Pathomorphologie peripherer Neuropathien. Nervenheilkunde 12:388–394

964. Schröder JM (1994) Veränderungen bei Verletzungen peripherer Nerven, Heilungsvorgänge und Neurombildung. In: Bundesärztekammer (ed) Fortschritt und Fortbildung in der Medizin (vol 18). Deutscher Ärzte-Verlag, Cologne, pp 197–202

965. Schröder JM (1995) Pathologie des peripheren Nervensystems. In: Remmele W, Peiffer J, Schröder JM (eds) Neuropathologie. Springer, Berlin Heidelberg New York, pp 347–402

966. Schröder JM (1996) Developmental and pathological changes at the node and paranode in human sural nerves. Microsc Res Tech 34:422–435

967. Schröder JM (1997) Peripheral neuropathies. Correlation between molecular genetic and fine structural diagnosis of inherited peripheral neuropathies. Brain Pathol 7:1299–1302

968. Schröder JM (1998) Recommendations for the examination of peripheral nerve biopsies. Virchows Arch 432: 199–205

969. Schröder JM (1999) Pathologie peripherer Nerven, Springer, Berlin Heidelberg New York, pp 1–862

970. Schröder JM (2000) Isoniazid. In: Schaumburg HH, Spencer PS (eds) Experimental and clinical neurotoxicology. Oxford University Press, New York Oxford

971. Schröder JM (2000) Cadmium. In: Spencer PS, Schaumburg HH (eds) Experimental and clinical neurotoxicology. Oxford University Press, New York Oxford, pp 276–280

972. Schröder JM (2000) Isoniazid. In: Spencer PS, Schaumburg HH (eds) Experimental and clinical neurotoxicology. Oxford University Press, New York, Oxford, pp 690–697

973. Schröder JM, Bertram M, Schnabel R, Pfaff U (1992) Nuclear and mitochondrial changes of muscle fibers in AIDS after treatment with high doses of zidovudine. Acta Neuropathol (Berl) 85:39–47

974. Schröder JM, Bohl J (1978) Altered ratio between axon caliber and myelin thickness in sural nerves of children. In: Canal N (ed) Peripheral Neuropathies. Elsevier, Amsterdam, pp 49–62

975. Schröder JM, Bohl J, von Bardeleben U (1988) Changes of the ratio between myelin thickness and axon diameter in human developing sural, femoral, ulnar, facial, and trochlear nerves. Acta Neuropathol (Berl) 76:471–483

976. Schröder JM, Dieler R, Skopnik H, Steinau G (1992) Immunohistochemical reactivity of neuropeptides in plastic-embedded semithin sections of the myenteric plexus in infantile hypertrophic pylorus stenosis. Acta Histochem Suppl 42:341–344

977. Schröder JM, Dodel R, Weis J, Stefanidis I, Reichmann H (1996) Mitochondrial changes in muscle phosphoglycerate kinase deficiency. Clin Neuropathol 15:34–40

978. Schröder JM, Gibbels E (1977) Marklose Nervenfasern im Senium und im Spätstadium der Thalidomid-Polyneuropathie: quantitativ-elektronenmikroskopische Untersuchungen. Acta Neuropathol (Berl) 39:271–280

979. Schröder JM, Heide G, Ramaekers V, Mortier W (1993) Subtotal aplasia of myelinated nerve fibers in the sural nerve. Neuropediatrics 24:286–291

980. Schröder JM, Himmelmann F (1992) Fine structural evaluation of altered Schmidt-Lanterman incisures in human sural nerve biopsies. Acta Neuropathol (Berl) 83:120–133

981. Schröder JM, Hoheneck M, Weis J, Deist H (1985) Ethylene oxide polyneuropathy: clinical follow-up study with morphometric and electron microscopic findings in a sural nerve biopsy. J Neurol 232:83–90

982. Schröder JM, Huffmann B, Braun V, Richter HP (1992) Spasmodic torticollis: severe compression neuropathy in rami dorsales of cervical nerves C1–6. Acta Neuropathol (Berl) 84:416–424

983. Schröder JM, Kaldenbach T, Piroth W (1996) Nuclear and mitochondrial changes of co-cultivated spinal cord, spinal ganglia and muscle fibers following treatment with various doses of zidovudine. Acta Neuropathol (Berl) 92:138–149

984. Schröder JM, Krabbe B, Weis J (1995) Oculopharyngeal muscular dystrophy: clinical and morphological follow-up study reveals mitochondrial alterations and unique nuclear inclusions in a severe autosomal recessive type. Neuropathol Appl Neurobiol 21:68–73

985. Schröder JM, Krämer KG, Hopf HC (1985) Granular nuclear inclusion body disease: fine structure of tibial muscle and sural nerve. Muscle Nerve 8:52–59

986. Schröder JM, Krücke W (1970) Zur Feinstruktur der experimentell-allergischen Neuritis beim Kaninchen. Acta Neuropathol (Berl) 14:261–283

987. Schröder JM, Matthiesen T (1985) Experimental thalidomide neuropathy: the morphological correlate of reduced conduction velocity. Acta Neuropathol (Berl) 65: 285–292

988. Schröder JM, May R, Shin YS, Sigmund M, Nase-Hüppmeier S (1993) Juvenile hereditary polyglucosan body disease with complete branching enzyme deficiency (type IV glycogenosis). Acta Neuropathol (Berl) 85: 419–430

989. Schröder JM, May R, Weis J (1993) Perineurial cells are the first to traverse gaps of peripheral nerves in silicone tubes. Clin Neurol Neurosurg 95(suppl):S78–S83

990. Schröder JM, Mayer M, Weis J (1996) Mitochondrial abnormalities and intrafamilial variability of sural nerve biopsy findings in adrenomyeloneuropathy. Acta Neuropathol (Berl) 92:64–69

991. Schröder JM, Molnár M (1997) Mitochondrial abnormalities and peripheral neuropathy in inflammatory myopathy, especially inclusion body myositis. Mol Cell Biochem 174:277–281

992. Schröder JM, Rollnik JD, Schubert M, Dengler R (1999) Demyelinating sensorimotor neuropathy with congenital cataract, mental retardation, and unique, dysplastic perineurial cells within the endoneurium. Acta Neuropathol 98:421–426

993. Schröder JM, Seiffert KE (1970) Die Feinstruktur der neuromatösen Neurotisation von Nerventransplanten. Virchows Arch B Cell Pathol 5:219–235

994. Schröder JM, Seiffert KE (1972) Untersuchungen zur homologen Nerventransplantation. Morphologische Ergebnisse. Zentralbl Neurochir 33:103–118

995. Schröder JM, Sellhaus B, Jörg J (1995) Identification of the characteristic vascular changes in a sural nerve biopsy of a case with cerebral autosomal dominant arteriopathy with subcortical infarcts and leukoencephalopathy (CADASIL). Acta Neuropathol (Berl) 89:116–121

996. Schröder JM, Sellhaus B, Wöhrmann T, Kögel B, Zwingenberger K (1995) Inhibitory effects of thalidomide on cellular proliferation, endoneurial edema and myelin phagocytosis during early wallerian degeneration. Acta Neuropathol (Berl) 89:415–419

997. Schröder JM, Senderek J, Bergmann C, Hermanns B (1999) Identification of DNA mutations in archival sural nerve biopsies confirmed by blood samples in HMSN X: occasional association with Becker's muscular dystrophy and color blindness (abstract). J Neurol Sci 166:166–167

998. Schröder JM, Senderek J, Bergmann C, Hermanns B, Ramaekers V, Quasthoff S (1998) Identification of CX32 mutations in paraffin-embedded sural nerve biopsies of 5 unrelated families with X-linked CMT (HMSN X), in one male associated with X-linked (Becker's) muscular dystrophy. J Periph Nerv Sys 3:302–303

999. Schröder JM, Senderek J, Hartmann C (2000) Identification of myelin protein zero (MPZ, Po) point mutations in sural nerve biopsies (abstract). Alzheimer's Reports 3:S32

1000. Schröder JM, Sommer C (1991) Mitochondrial abnormalities in human sural nerves: fine structural evaluation of cases with mitochondrial myopathy, hereditary and non-hereditary neuropathies, and review of the literature. Acta Neuropathol (Berl) 82:471–482

1001. Schröder JM, Thiex R, Senderek J, Bergmann C (1999) Molecular genetic identification of mutations in paraffin embedded, archival sural nerve biopsies of cases with HMSN Ia, Ib, X, and HNPP (abstract). Neuropathol Appl Neurobiol 25:30–31

1002. Schröder JM, Wang JF, Sindern E, Malin JP (1999) Polyneuropathy with osmiophilic membrane-bound, cytoplasmic inclusions in Schwann cells (POMCIS). Acta Neuropathol 98:427–432

1003. Schubert W, Schwan H (1995) Detection by 4-parameter microscopic imaging and increase of rare mononuclear blood leukocyte types expressing the Fc gamma RIII receptor (CD16) for immunoglobulin G in human sporadic amyotrophic lateral sclerosis (ALS). Neurosci Lett 198:29–32

1004. Schuelke M, Cervós-navarro J (1998) Degenerative changes in unmyelinated nerve fibers in late-infantile neuronal ceroidlipofuscinosis. A morphometric study of conjunctival biopsy specimens. Acta Neuropathol (Berl) 95:175–183

1005. Schuler U, Ehninger G (1995) Thalidomide: rationale for renewed use in immunological disorders. Drug Saf 12:364–369

1006. Schütz G, Schröder JM (1997) Number and size of epineurial blood vessels in normal and diseased human sural nerves. Cell Tissue Res 290:31–37

1007. Schwab ME, Thoenen H (1985) Dissociated neurons regenerate into sciatic but not optic nerve explants in culture irrespective of neurotrophic factors. J Neurosci 5:2415–2423

1008. Schwartzman RJ, Liu JE, Smullens SN, Hyslop T, Tahmoush AJ (1997) Long-term outcome following sympathectomy for complex regional pain syndrome type 1 (RSD). J Neurol Sci 150:149–152

1009. Schwendemann G, Arendt G, Noth J, Lange HW, Strauss W (1987) Diagnosis of juvenile-adult form of neuroaxonal dystrophy by electron microscopy of rectum and skin biopsy (letter). J Neurol Neurosurg Psychiatry 50:818–821

1010. Scoles DR, Baser ME, Pulst SM (1996) A missense mutation in the neurofibromatosis 2 gene occurs in patients with mild and severe phenotypes. Neurology 47:544–546

1011. Scoles DR, Huynh DP, Morcos PA, Coulsell ER, Robinson NG, Tamanoi F, Pulst SM (1998) Neurofibromatosis 2 tumour suppressor Schwannomin interacts with betaII-spectrin. Nat Genet 18:354–359

1012. Scott TF (1993) Neurosarcoidosis: progress and clinical aspects. Neurology 43:8–12

1013. Seiffert KE, Schindler P, Thomas E, Schröder JM, Hufschmidt F (1968) Experimentelle Technik und Ergebnisse der homologen Nerventransplantation. Langenbecks Arch Chir 322:598–601

1014. Seiler N, Schröder JM (1970) Beziehungen zwischen Polyaminen und Nucleinsäuren. II. Biochemische und feinstrukturelle Untersuchungen am peripheren Nerven während der Wallerschen Degeneration. Brain Res 22:81–103

1015. Senderek J, Bergmann C, Quasthoff S, Ramaekers VT, Schröder JM (1998) X-linked dominant Charcot-Marie-Tooth disease: nerve biopsies allow morphological evaluation and detection of connexin32 mutations (Arg15Trp, Arg22Gln). Acta Neuropathol (Berl) 95:443–449

1016. Senderek J, Hermanns B, Bergmann C, Boroojerdi B, Bajbouj M, Hungs M, Ramaekers VT, Quasthoff S, Karch D, Schröder JM (1999) X-linked dominant Charcot-Marie-Tooth neuropathy: clinical, electrophysiological, and morphological phenotype in four families with different connexin32 mutations. J Neurol Sci 167:90–101

1017. Senderek J, Hermanns B, Bergmann C, Boroojerdi B, Bajbouj M, Hungs M, Ramaekers VT, Quasthoff S, Karch D, Schröder JM (1999) X-linked dominant Charcot-Marie-Tooth neuropathy: clinical, electrophysiological, and morphological phenotype in four families with different connexin32 mutations. J Neurol Sci 167:90

1018. Senderek J, Hermanns B, Lehmann U, Bergmann C, Marx G, Kabus C, Timmermann V, Stoltenburg-Didinger G, Schröder JM (2000) Charcot-Marie-Tooth neuropathy type 2 and P0 point mutations: Two novel amino acid substitutions (Asp61Gly; Tyr119Cys) and a possible "hotspot" on Thr1214Met. Brain Pathology 10:235–248

1019. Sendtner M, Dittrich F, Hughes RA, Thoenen H (1994) Actions of CNTF and neurotrophins on degenerating motoneurons: preclinical studies and clinical implications. J Neurol Sci 124(suppl):77–83

1020. Sendtner M, Kreutzberg GW, Thoenen H (1990) Ciliary neurotrophic factor prevents the degeneration of motor neurons after axotomy. Nature 345:440–441

1021. Sendtner M, Schmalbruch H, Stöckli KA, Carroll P, Kreutzberg GW, Thoenen H (1992) Ciliary neurotrophic factor prevents degeneration of motor neurons in mouse mutant progressive motor neuronopathy. Nature 358:502–504

1022. Shapiro EG, Lipton ME, Krivit W (1992) White matter dysfunction and its neuropsychological correlates: a longitudinal study of a case of metachromatic leukodystrophy treated with bone marrow transplant. J Clin Exp Neuropsychol 14:610–624

1023. Shapiro L, Doyle JP, Hensley P, Colman DR, Hendrickson WA (1996) Crystal structure of the extracellular domain from P0, the major structural protein of peripheral nerve myelin. Neuron 17:435–449

1024. Sharief MK, McLean B, Thompson EJ (1993) Elevated serum levels of tumor necrosis factor-alpha in Guillain-Barré syndrome. Ann Neurol 33:591–596

1025. Sheth RD, Riggs JE, Hobbs GR, Gutmann L (1996) Age and Guillain-Barré syndrome severity. Muscle Nerve 19:375–377

1026. Shetty VP, Uplekar MW, Antia NH (1994) Immunohistological localization of mycobacterial antigens within the peripheral nerves of treated leprosy patients and their significance to nerve damage in leprosy. Acta Neuropathol (Berl) 88:300–306

1027. Shian WJ, Chi CC, Mak SC, Tzeng GY (1992) Late infantile form metachromatic leukodystrophy: report of one case. Chung Hua Min Kuo Hsiao Erh Ko I Hsueh Hui Tsa Chih 33:286–293

1028. Shillito P, Molenaar PC, Vincent A, Leys K, Zheng W, van den Berg RJ, Plomp JJ, van Kempen GT, Chauplannaz G, Wintzen AR et al. (1995) Acquired neuromyotonia: evidence for autoantibodies directed against K+ channels of peripheral nerves. Ann Neurol 38:714–722

1029. Shimada H, Chatten J, Newton WA Jr, Sachs N, Hamoudi AB, Chiba T, Marsden HB, Misugi K (1984) Histopathologic prognostic factors in neuroblastic tumors: definition. J Natl Cancer Inst 73:405–416

1030. Shoffner JM, Brown MD, Stugard C, Jun AS, Pollock S, Haas RH, Kaufman A, Koontz D, Kim Y, Graham JR et al. (1995) Leber's hereditary optic neuropathy plus dystonia is caused by a mitochondrial DNA point mutation. Ann Neurol 38:163–169

1031. Shupeck M, Ward KK, Schmelzer JD, Low PA (1989) Comparison of nerve regeneration in vascularized and conventional grafts: nerve electrophysiology, norepinephrine, prostacyclin, malondialdehyde, and the blood-nerve barrier. Brain Res 493:225–230

1032. Shy ME, Evans VA, Lublin FD, Knobler RL, Heiman-Patterson T, Tahmoush AJ, Parry G, Schick P, DeRyk TG (1989) Antibodies to GM1 and GD1b in patients with motor neuron disease without plasma cell dyscrasia. Ann Neurol 25:511–513

1033. Shy ME, Heiman-Patterson T, Parry GJ, Tahmoush A, Evans VA, Schick PK (1990) Lower motor neuron disease in a patient with autoantibodies against Gal(beta 1-3)GalNAc in gangliosides GM1 and GD1b: improvement following immunotherapy. Neurology 40:842–844

1034. Sieb JP, Breul P, Jerusalem F (1990) Neurofibromatose. Akt Neurol 17:173–178

1035. Sieb JP, Mattle H, Pirovino M (1989) Neurofibrosarkome bei Neurofibromatose 1. Dtsch Med Wochenschr 114:417–419

1036. Sigal LH, Tatum AH (1988) Lyme disease patients' serum contains IgM antibodies to Borrelia burgdorferi that cross-react with neuronal antigens. Neurology 38:1439–1442

1037. Sillevis Smitt PA, de Jong JM (1989) Animal models of amyotrophic lateral sclerosis and the spinal muscular atrophies. J Neurol Sci 91:231–258

1038. Silvestri G, Mongini T, Odoardi F, Modoni A, deRosa G, Doriguzzi C, Palmucci L, Tonali P, Servidei S (2000) A new mtDNA mutation associated with a progressive encephalopathy and cytochrome c oxidase deficiency. Neurology 54:1693–1696

1039. Simmons Z, Albers JW, Bromberg MB, Feldman EL (1993) Presentation and initial clinical course in patients with chronic inflammatory demyelinating polyradiculoneuropathy: comparison of patients without and with monoclonal gammopathy. Neurology 43:2202–2209

1040. Simmons Z, Albers JW, Sima AA (1992) Case-of-the-month: perineuritis presenting as mononeuritis multiplex. Muscle Nerve 15:630–635

1041. Simon LT, Horoupian DS, Dorfman LJ, Marks M, Herrick MK, Wasserstein P, Smith ME (1990) Polyneuropathy, ophthalmoplegia, leukoencephalopathy, and intestinal pseudo-obstruction: POLIP syndrome. Ann Neurol 28:349–360

1042. Simon LT, Ricaurte GA, Forno LS (1989) Chronic idiopathic ataxic neuropathy: neuropathology of a case. Acta Neuropathol (Berl) 79:104–107

1043. Simon R, Thier M, Kruttgen A, Rose-John S, Weiergraber O, Heinrich PC, Schröder JM, Weis J (1995) Human CNTF and related cytokines: effects on DRG neurone survival. Neuroreport 7:153–157

1044. Simone IL, Annunziata P, Maimone D, Liguori M, Leante R, Livrea P (1993) Serum and CSF anti-GM1 antibodies in patients with Guillain-Barré syndrome and chronic inflammatory demyelinating polyneuropathy. J Neurologic Sci 114:49–55

1045. Simpson LO (1988) Altered blood rheology in the pathogenesis of diabetic and other neuropathies. Muscle Nerve 11:725–744

1046. Sindern E, Patzold T, Vorgerd M, Shin YS, Podskarbi T, Schröder JM, Malin JP (1999) Adulte Polyglukosankörperkrankheit. Der Nervenarzt 8:745–749

1047. Singh G, Lott MT, Wallace DC (1989) A mitochondrial DNA mutation as a cause of Leber's hereditary optic neuropathy. N Engl J Med 320:1300–1305

1048. Sirdofsky MD, Hawley RJ, Manz H (1991) Progressive motor neuron disease associated with electrical injury. Muscle Nerve 14:977–980

1049. Sivieri S, Ferrarini AM, Lolli F, Matà S, Pinto F, Tavolato B, Gallo P (1997) Cytokine pattern in the cerebrospinal fluid from patients with GBS and CIDP. J Neurol Sci 147:93–95

1050. Sluga E (1970) Über eine Entmarkungsneuropathie bei G-Paraproteinämie. Wien Klin Wochenschr 82:667

1051. Small JR, Scadding JW, Landon DN (1990) A fluorescence study of changes in noradrenergic sympathetic fibres in experimental peripheral nerve neuromas. J Neurol Sci 100:98–107

1052. Smith B (1967) The myenteric plexus in Chagas' disease. J Pathol Bacteriol 94:462–463

1053. Smith IS (1994) The natural history of chronic demyelinating neuropathy associated with benign IgM paraproteinaemia. A clinical and neurophysiological study. Brain 117:949–957

1054. Smith TW, Bhawan J (1980) Tactile-like structures in neurofibromas. An ultrastructural study. Acta Neuropathol (Berl) 50:233–236

1055. Snider WD (1994) Functions of the neurotrophins during nervous system development: what the knockouts are teaching us. Cell 77:627–638

1056. Snooks SJ, Barnes PR, Swash M, Henry MM (1985) Damage to the innervation of the pelvic floor musculature in chronic constipation. Gastroenterology 89:977–981

1057. Sobel RA (1993) Vestibular (acoustic) Schwannomas: histologic features in neurofibromatosis 2 and in unilateral cases. J Neuropathol Exp Neurol 52:106–113

1058. Sobue G, Hashizume Y, Mitsuma T, Takahashi A (1987) Size-dependent myelinated fiber loss in the corticospinal tract in Shy-Drager syndrome and amyotrophic lateral sclerosis. Neurology 37:529–532

1059. Sobue G, Hashizume Y, Yasuda T, Mukai E, Kumagai T, Mitsuma T, Trojanowski JQ (1990) Phosphorylated high molecular weight neurofilament protein in lower motor neurons in amyotrophic lateral sclerosis and other neurodegenerative diseases involving ventral horn cells. Acta Neuropathol (Berl) 79:402–408

1060. Sobue G, Li M, Terao S, Aoki S, Ichimura M, Ieda T, Doyu M, Yasuda T, Hashizume Y, Mitsuma T (1997) Axonal pathology in Japanese Guillain-Barré syndrome: a study of 15 autopsied cases. Neurology 48:1694–1700

1061. Sobue G, Sonnenfeld K, Rubenstein AE, Pleasure D (1985) Tissue culture studies of neurofibromatosis: effects of axolemmal fragments and cyclic adenosine 3′,5′-monophosphate analogues on proliferation of Schwann-like and fibroblast-like neurofibroma cells. Ann Neurol 18:68–73

1062. Sobue G, Terao S, Hayashi F, Yamamoto K, Mitsuma T (1992) Involvement of the ventral horn cells in Guillain-Barré syndrome and chronic inflammatory demyelinating polyradiculoneuritis (in Japanese). Rinsho Shinkeigaku 32:447–450

1063. Soffer D, Benharroch D, Berginer V (1995) The neuropathology of cerebrotendinous xanthomatosis revisited: a case report and review of the literature. Acta Neuropathol (Berl) 90:213–220

1064. Solders G (1988) Discomfort after fascicular sural nerve biopsy. Acta Neurol Scand 77:503–504

1065. Solders G, Nennesmo I, Ernerudh J, Cruz M, Vrethem M (1999) Lymphocytes in sural nerve biopsies from patients with plasma cell dyscrasia and polyneuropathy. J Peripher Nerv Syst 4:91–98

1066. Somer H, Mäki T, Härkönen M (1992) Beta-adrenergic system in myotonic dystrophy. J Neurol Sci 111:214–217

1067. Sommer C, Schröder JM (1988) Binding of swine IgM immunoglobulins to peripheral nerve myelin sheaths in electron microscopic immunocytochemistry. Acta Neuropathol (Berl) 77:100–103

1068. Sommer C, Schröder JM (1989) Amyloid neuropathy: immunocytochemical localization of intra- and extracellular immunoglobulin light chains. Acta Neuropathol (Berl) 79:190–199

1069. Sommer C, Schröder JM (1989) Hereditary motor and sensory neuropathy with optic atrophy. Ultrastructural and morphometric observations on nerve fibers, mitochondria, and dense-cored vesicles. Arch Neurol 46:973–977

1070. Sommer C, Schröder JM (1992) Immune-mediated neuropathy and myopathy in post-streptococcal disease: electron-microscopical, morphometrical and immunohistochemical studies. Clin Neuropathol 11:77–86

1071. Sonneland P, Scheithauer B, LeChago J, Crawford B, Onofrio B (1986) Paraganglioma of the cauda equina region. Clinicopathologic study of 31 cases with special reference to immunocytology and ultrastructure. Cancer 58:1720–1723

1072. Sonnenfeld KH, Bernd P, Sobue G, Lebwohl M, Rubenstein AE (1986) Nerve growth factor receptors on dissociated neurofibroma Schwann-like cells. Cancer Res 46:1446–1452

1073. Sorenson EJ, Sima AA, Blaivas M, Sawchuk K, Wald JJ (1997) Clinical features of perineuritis. Muscle Nerve 20:1153–1157

1074. Sorenson EJ, Windebank AJ (1993) Relative importance of basement membrane and soluble growth factors in delayed and immediate regeneration of rat sciatic nerve. J Neuropathol Exp Neurol 52:216–222

1075. Southam E, Thomas PK, King RH, Goss-Sampson MA, Muller DP (1991) Experimental vitamin E deficiency in rats. Morphological and functional evidence of abnormal axonal transport secondary to free radical damage. Brain 114:915–936

1076. Spencer PS, Schaumburg HH (2000) Experimental and clinical neurotoxicology. Oxford University Press, New York, Oxford

1077. Spüler M, Dimpfel W, Tüllner HU (1987) Effect of gangliosides on nerve conduction velocity during diabetic neuropathy in the rat. Arch Int Pharmacodyn Ther 287:211–223

1078. St. Louis ME, Peck SH, Bowering D, Morgan GB, Blatherwick J, Banerjee S, Kettyls GD, Black WA, Milling ME, Hauschild AH et al. (1988) Botulism from chopped garlic: delayed recognition of a major outbreak. Ann Intern Med 108:363–368

1079. Steck AJ, Erne B, Gabriel JM, Schaeren-Wiemers N (1999) Paraproteinaemic neuropathies. Brain Pathol 9:361–368

1080. Steck AJ, Murray N, Dellagi K, Brouet JC, Seligmann M (1987) Peripheral neuropathy associated with monoclonal IgM autoantibody. Ann Neurol 22:764–767

1081. Stemmer-Rachamimov AO, Ino Y, Lim ZY, Jacoby LB, MacCollin M, Gusella JF, Ramesh V, Louis DN (1998) Loss of the NF2 gene and merlin occur by the tumorlet stage of Schwannoma development in neurofibromatosis 2. J Neuropathol Exp Neurol 57:1164–1167

1082. Stennert ER (1994) The facial nerve. An update on clinical and basic neuroscience research. AORL CG Suppl: 1–564

1083. Sterman AB, Schaumburg HH, Asbury AK (1980) The acute sensory neuronopathy syndrome: a distinct clinical entity. Ann Neurol 7:354–358

1084. Stevens A, Schabet M, Schott K, Wiethölter H (1989) Role of endoneural cells in experimental allergic neuritis and characterisation of a resident phagocytic cell. Acta Neuropathol (Berl) 77:412–419

1085. Stevens JC, Löfgren EP, Dyck PJ (1973) Histometric evaluation of branches of peroneal nerve: technique for combined biopsy of muscle nerve and cutaneous nerve. Brain Res 52:37–59

1086. Stewart JD, McKelvey R, Durcan L, Carpenter S, Karpati G (1996) Chronic inflammatory demyelinating polyneuropathy (CIDP) in diabetics. J Neurol Sci 142:59–64

1087. Stober T, Schimrigk K, Ganten D, Sherman DG (1986) Central nervous system control of the heart. Martinus Nijhoff Publishing, Boston Dordrecht Lancaster

1088. Stoebner P, Mezin P, Vila A, Grosse R, Kopp N, Paramelle B (1989) Microangiopathy of endoneurial vessels in hypoxemic chronic obstructive pulmonary disease (COPD). A quantitative ultrastructural study. Acta Neuropathol (Berl) 78:388–395

1089. Stögbauer F, Young P, Kuhlenbäumer G, Kiefer R, Timmermann V, Ringelstein EB, Wang JF, Schröder JM, Van Broeckhoven C, Weis J (1999) Autosomal dominant burning feet syndrome. J Neurol Neurosurg Psych 67:78–81

1090. Stoll G, Griffin JW, Li CY, Trapp BD (1989) Wallerian degeneration in the peripheral nervous system: participation of both Schwann cells and macrophages in myelin degradation. J Neurocytol 18:671–683

1091. Stoll G, Mueller HW, Trapp BD, Griffin JW (1989) Oligodendrocytes but not astrocytes express apolipoprotein E after injury of rat optic nerve. Glia 2:170–176

1092. Straub V, Wehnert M, Schröder JM, Voit T (2000) X-linked Emery-Dreifuss muscular dystrophy presenting with distal myopathy and peripheral nerve hypomyelination (abstract). Neuromusc Disord 10:362

1093. Stumpf DA, Sokol R, Bettis D, Neville H, Ringel S, Angelini C, Bell R (1987) Friedreich's disease: V. Variant form with vitamin E deficiency and normal fat absorption. Neurology 37: 68–74

1094. Suarez GA, Kelly JJ Jr (1993) Polyneuropathy associated with monoclonal gammopathy of undetermined significance: further evidence that IgM-MGUS neuropathies are different than IgG-MGUS. Neurology 43: 1304–1308

1095. Sunderland S (1978) Nerves and nerve injuries. Churchill Livingstone, Edinburgh London New York

1096. Sung JH, Hayano M, Desnick RJ (1977) Mannosidosis: Pathology of the nervous system. J Neuropathol Exp Neurol 35:807

1097. Swanson A (1963) Congenital insensitivity to pain with anhidrosis. Arch Neurol 8:299–306

1098. Tabaraud F, Lagrange E, Sindou P, Vandenberghe A, Levy N, Vallat JM (1999) Demyelinating X-linked Charcot-Marie-Tooth disease: unusual electrophysiological findings. Muscle Nerve 22:1442–1447

1099. Tabaraud F, Vallat JM, Hugon J, Ramiandrisoa H, Dumas M, Signoret JL (1990) Acute or subacute alcoholic neuropathy mimicking Guillain-Barré syndrome. J Neurol Sci 97:195–205

1100. Tachi N, Kasai K, Chiba S, Naganuma M, Uyemura K, Hayasaka K (1994) Expression of Po protein in sural nerve of a patient with hereditary motor and sensory neuropathy type III. J Neurol Sci 124:67–70

1101. Tachi N, Kozuka N, Ohya K, Chiba S, Sasaki K (1997) Tomaculous neuropathy in Charcot-Marie-Tooth disease with myelin protein zero gene mutation. J Neurol Sci 153:106–109

1102. Tackmann W, Porst H, van Ahlen H (1988) Bulbocavernosus reflex latencies and somatosensory evoked potentials after pudendal nerve stimulation in the diagnosis of impotence. J Neurol 235:219–225

1103. Tackmann W, Vogel P (1988) Fibre density, amplitudes of macro-EMG motor unit potentials and conventional EMG recordings from the anterior tibial muscle in patients with amyotrophic lateral sclerosis. A study on 51 cases. J Neurol 235:149–154

1104. Tagawa Y, Yuki N, Hirata K (1999) The 301 to 314 amino acid residue of beta-tubulin is not a target epitope for serum IgM antibodies in chronic inflammatory demyelinating polyneuropathy. J Neurol Sci 163:44–46

1105. Takahashi A, Mizutani M, Itakura C (1995) Acrylamide-induced peripheral neuropathy in normal and neurofilament-deficient Japanese quails. Acta Neuropathol (Berl) 89:17–22

1106. Takahashi H, Makifuchi T, Nakano R, Sato S, Inuzuka T, Sakimura K, Mishina M, Honma Y, Tsuji S, Ikuta F (1994) Familial amyotrophic lateral sclerosis with a mutation in the Cu/Zn superoxide dismutase gene. Acta Neuropathol (Berl) 88:185–188

1107. Takebe Y, Koide N, Takahashi G (1981) Giant axonal neuropathy: report of two siblings with endocrinological and histological studies. Neuropediatrics 12:392–404

1108. Tali ET, Yuh WT, Nguyen HD, Feng G, Koci TM, Jinkins JR, Robinson RA, Hasso AN (1993) Cystic acoustic Schwannomas: MR characteristics. AJNR Am J Neuroradiol 14:1241–1247

1109. Tallan EM, Harner SG, Beatty CW, Scheithauer BW, Parisi JE (1993) Does the distribution of Schwann cells correlate with the observed occurrence of acoustic neuromas? (published erratum appears in Am J Otol 1994 Mar;15(2):287). Am J Otol 14:131–134

1110. Tamas LB, Howe JF (1984) Physiological evaluation of the effect of fascicular ligation on neuromas in the rat. Neurosurgery 14:664–669

1111. Tanaka F, Sobue G, Doyu M, Ito Y, Yamamoto M, Shimada N, Yamamoto K, Riku S, Hshizume Y, Mitsuma T (1996) Differential pattern in tissue-specific somatic mosaicism of expanded CAG trinucleotide repeats in dentatorubral-pallidoluysian atrophy, Machado-Joseph disease, and X-linked recessive spinal and bulbar muscular atrophy. J Neurol Sci 135:43–50

1112. Tandan R, Bradley WG, Fillyaw MJ (1990) Giant axonal neuropathy: studies with sulfhydryl donor compounds. J Neurol Sci 95:153–162

1113. Tandan R, Little BW, Emery ES, Good PS, Pendlebury WW, Bradley WG (1987) Childhood giant axonal neuropathy. Case report and review of the literature. J Neurol Sci 82:205–228

1114. Tannier C, Hamidou M, Morlock G, Pages M (1988) Syndromes de Lambert-Eaton et de Schwartz-Bartter et neuropathie périphérique associés à un carcinome bronchique: à propos d'un cas. Neurophysiol Clin 18:285–290

1115. Taratuto AL, Sevlever G, Saccoliti M, Caceres L, Schultz M (1990) Giant axonal neuropathy (GAN): an immunohistochemical and ultrastructural study report of a Latin American case. Acta Neuropathol (Berl) 80: 680-683

1116. Tegner R, Tomé FM, Godeau P, Lhermitte F, Fardeau M (1988) Morphological study of peripheral nerve changes induced by chloroquine treatment. Acta Neuropathol (Berl) 75:253-260

1117. Tembl JI, Ferrer JM, Sevilla MT, Lago A, Mayordomo F, Vilchez JJ (1999) Neurologic complications associated with hepatitis C virus infection. Neurology 53:861-864

1118. Terao S, Sobue G, Hashizume Y, Mitsuma T, Takahashi A (1994) Disease-specific patterns of neuronal loss in the spinal ventral horn in amyotrophic lateral sclerosis, multiple system atrophy and X-linked recessive bulbospinal neuronopathy, with special reference to the loss of small neurons in the intermediate zone. J Neurol 241:196-203

1119. Theriault M, Dort J, Sutherland G, Zochodne DW (1998) A prospective quantitative study of sensory deficits after whole sural nerve biopsies in diabetic and nondiabetic patients. Surgical approach and the role of collateral sprouting. Neurology 50:480-484

1120. Thier M, Hall M, Heath JK, Pennica D, Weis J (1999) Trophic effects of cardiotrophin-1 and interleukin-11 on rat dorsal root ganglion neurons in vitro. Brain Res Mol Brain Res 64:80-84

1121. Thiex R, Schröder J (1998) PMP-22 gene duplications and deletions identified in archival, paraffin-embedded sural nerve biopsy specimens: correlation to structural changes. Acta Neuropathol (Berl) 96:13-21

1122. Thomas C, Love S, Powell HC, Schultz P, Lampert PW (1987) Giant axonal neuropathy: correlation of clinical findings with postmortem neuropathology. Ann Neurol 22:79-84

1123. Thomas FP, Lovelace RE, Ding XS, Sadiq SA, Petty GW, Sherman WH, Latov N, Hays AP (1992) Vasculitic neuropathy in a patient with cryoglobulinemia and anti-MAG IGM monoclonal gammopathy. Muscle Nerve 15: 891-898

1124. Thomas FP, Vallejos U, Foitl DR, Miller JR, Barrett R, Fetell MR, Knowles DM, Latov N, Hays AP (1990) B cell small lymphocytic lymphoma and chronic lymphocytic leukemia with peripheral neuropathy: two cases with neuropathological findings and lymphocyte marker analysis. Acta Neuropathol (Berl) 80:198-203

1125. Thomas PK (1995) Biopsy of peripheral nerve tissue. In: Asbury AK, Thomas PK (eds) Peripheral nerve disorders 2. Blue books of practical neurology. Butterworth-Heinemann, Oxford, pp 281-300

1126. Thomas PK, Claus D, Jaspert A, Workman JM, King RH, Larner AJ, Anderson M, Emerson JA, Ferguson IT (1996) Focal upper limb demyelinating neuropathy. Brain 119:765-774

1127. Thomas PK, Hollinrake K, Lascelles RG, DJ OS, Baillod RA, Moorhead JF, Mackenzie JC (1971) The polyneuropathy of chronic renal failure. Brain 94:761-780

1128. Thomas PK, King RH, Bradley JL (1997) Hypertrophic neuropathy: atypical appearances resulting from the combination of type I hereditary motor and sensory neuropathy and diabetes mellitus. Neuropathol Appl Neurobiol 23:348-351

1129. Thomas PK, King RH, Chiang TR, Scaravilli F, Sharma AK, Downie AW (1990) Neurofibromatous neuropathy. Muscle Nerve 13:93-101

1130. Thomas PK, King RHM, Workman JM, Schröder JM (2000) Hypertrophic perineurial dysplasia in multifocal and generalized peripheral neuropathies. Neuropathol Appl Neurobiol 26:536-543

1131. Thomas PK, Marques W Jr., Davis MB, Sweeney MG, King RH, Bradley JL, Muddle JR, Tyson J, Malcolm S, Harding AE (1997) The phenotypic manifestations of chromosome 17p11.2 duplication. Brain 120:465-478

1132. Thomas PK, Misra VP, King RH, Muddle JR, Wroe S, Bhatia KP, Anderson M, Cabello A, Vilchez J, Wadia NH (1994) Autosomal recessive hereditary sensory neuropathy with spastic paraplegia. Brain 117:651-659

1133. Thomas PK, Walker JG (1965) Xanthomatous neuropathy in primary biliary cirrhosis. Brain 88:1079-1088

1134. Thomas TD, Donofrio PD, Angelo J (1991) Peripheral neuropathy in cold agglutinin disease. Muscle Nerve 14:331-334

1135. Thrush DC, Holti G, Bradley WG, Campbell MJ, Walton JN (1974) Neurological manifestations of xeroderma pigmentosum in two siblings. J Neurol Sci 22: 91-104

1136. Timmerman V, De Jonghe P, Simokovic S, Löfgren A, Beuten J, Nelis E, Ceuterick C, Martin JJ, Van Broeckhoven C (1996) Distal hereditary motor neuropathy type II (distal HMN II): mapping of a locus to chromosome 12q24. Hum Mol Genet 5:1065-1069

1137. Timmerman V, Raeymaekers P, Nelis E, De Jonghe P, Muylle L, Ceuterick C, Martin JJ, Van Broeckhoven C (1992) Linkage analysis of distal hereditary motor neuropathy type II (distal HMN II) in a single pedigree. J Neurol Sci 109:41-48

1138. Tischner KH, Schröder JM (1972) The effects of cadmium chloride on organotypic cultures of rat sensory ganglia. A light and electron microscope study. J Neurol Sci 16:383-399

1139. Togashi S, Watanabe H, Nagasaka T, Shindo K, Shiozawa Z, Maeda S, Tawata M, Onaya T (1999) An aggressive familial amyloidotic polyneuropathy caused by a new variant transthyretin Lys 54. Neurology 53:637-639

1140. Torvik A, Torp S, Kase BF, Ek J, Skjeldal O, Stokke O (1988) Infantile Refsum's disease: a generalized peroxisomal disorder. Case report with postmortem examination. J Neurol Sci 85:39-53

1141. Tournev I, King RHM, Workman J, Nourallah M, Muddle JR, Kalaydjieva L, Romanski K, Thomas PK (1999) Peripheral nerve abnormalities in the congenital cataracts facial dysmorphism neuropathy (CCFDN) syndrome. Acta Neuropathol 98:165-170

1142. Tourtellotte WG, Milbrandt J (1998) Sensory ataxia and muscle spindle agenesis in mice lacking the. Nat Genet 20:87-91

1143. Tredici G, Petruccioli MG, Cavaletti G, Marmiroli P, Crespi V, Pioltelli P (1992) Sural nerve bioptic findings in essential cryoglobulinemic patients with and without peripheral neuropathy. Clin Neuropathol 11:121-127

1144. Treiber-Held S, Budjarjo-Welim H, Reimann D, Richter J, Kretzschmar HA, Hanefeld F (1994) Giant axonal neuropathy: a generalized disorder of intermediate filaments with longitudinal grooves in the hair. Neuropediatrics 25:89-93

1145. Trockel U, Schröder JM, Reiners KH, Toyka KV, Goerz G, Freund HJ (1983) Multiple exercise-related mononeuropathy with abdominal colic. J Neurol Sci 60:431–442

1146. Trojanowski JQ, Molenaar WM, Baker DL, Pleasure D, Lee VM (1991) Neural and neuroendocrine phenotype of neuroblastomas. Prog Clin Biol Res 366:335–341

1147. Troost D, Claessen N, van den Oord JJ, Swaab DF, de Jong JM (1993) Neuronophagia in the motor cortex in amyotrophic lateral sclerosis. Neuropathol Appl Neurobiol 19:390–397

1148. Troost D, Louwerse ES, de Jong JM, van Leersum GS, van Raalte JA (1989) Aberrant myelinated neurites in the anterior horns of a patient with amyotrophic lateral sclerosis. Clin Neuropathol 8:152–155

1149. Trotti D, Rolfs A, Danbolt NC, Brown RH Jr, Hediger MA (1999) SOD1 mutants linked to amyotrophic lateral sclerosis selectively inactivate a glial glutamate transporter. Nat Neurosci 2:427–433

1150. Tsang WY, Chan JK, Chow LT, Tse CC (1992) Perineurioma: an uncommon soft tissue neoplasm distinct from localized hypertrophic neuropathy and neurofibroma. Am J Surg Pathol 16:756–763

1151. Tsui JK, Bhatt M, Calne S, Calne DB (1993) Botulinum toxin in the treatment of writer's cramp: a double-blind study. Neurology 43:183–185

1152. Tsukada N, Koh CS, Inoue A, Yanagisawa N (1987) Demyelinating neuropathy associated with hepatitis B virus infection. Detection of immune complexes composed of hepatitis B virus surface antigen. J Neurol Sci 77:203–216

1153. Ueki A, Namba Y, Otsuka M, Okuno M, Nishimura M, Oda M, Ikeda K (1993) GAP-43 immunoreactivity is detected in the nerve terminals of patients with amyotrophic lateral sclerosis (letter). Ann Neurol 33:226–227

1154. Ulenkate HJ, Kaal EC, Gispen WH, Jennekens FG (1994) Ciliary neurotrophic factor improves muscle fibre reinnervation after facial nerve crush in young rats. Acta Neuropathol (Berl) 88:558–564

1155. Umehara F, Izumo S, Zyounosono M, Osame M (1990) An autopsied case of the Crow-Fukase syndrome: a neuropathological study with emphasis on spinal roots. Acta Neuropathol (Berl) 80:563–567

1156. Uncini A, Di Guglielmo G, Di Muzio A, Gambi D, Sabatelli M, Mignogna T, Tonali P, Marzella R, Finelli P, Archidiacono N et al. (1995) Differential electrophysiological features of neuropathies associated with 17p11.2 deletion and duplication. Muscle Nerve 18:628–635

1157. Uncini A, Di Muzio A, Chiavaroli F, Gambi D, Sabatelli M, Archidiacono N, Antonacci R, Marzella R, Rocchi M (1994) Hereditary motor and sensory neuropathy with calf hypertrophy is associated with 17p11.2 duplication. Ann Neurol 35:552–558

1158. Uncini A, Sabatelli M, Mignogna T, Lugaresi A, Liguori R, Montagna P (1996) Chronic progressive steroid responsive axonal polyneuropathy: a CIDP variant or a primary axonal disorder? Muscle Nerve 19:365–371

1159. Uncini A, Santoro M, Corbo M, Lugaresi A, Latov N (1993) Conduction abnormalities induced by sera of patients with multifocal motor neuropathy and anti-GM1 antibodies. Muscle Nerve 16:610–615

1160. Uncini A, Servidei S, Silvestri G, Manfredi G, Sabatelli M, Di Muzio A, Ricci E, Mirabella M, Di Mauro S, Tonali P (1994) Ophthalmoplegia, demyelinating neuropathy, leukoencephalopathy, myopathy, and gastrointestinal dysfunction with multiple deletions of mitochondrial DNA: a mitochondrial multisystem disorder in search of a name. Muscle Nerve 17:667–674

1161. Urschel BA, Hulsebosch CE (1990) Schwann cell-neuronal interactions in the rat involve nerve growth factor. J Comp Neurol 296:114–122

1162. Valenstein E, Watson RT, Parker JL (1978) Myokymia, muscle hypertrophy and percussion "myotonia" in chronic recurrent polyneuropathy. Neurology 28:1130–1134

1163. Valentijn LJ, Ouvrier RA, van den Bosch NH, Bolhuis PA, Baas F, Nicholson GA (1995) Dejerine-Sottas neuropathy is associated with a de novo PMP22 mutation. Hum Mutat 5:76–80

1164. Vallat JM, Gil R, Leboutet MJ, Hugon J, Moulies D (1987) Congenital hypo- and hypermyelination neuropathy. Two cases. Acta Neuropathol (Berl) 74:197–201

1165. Vallat JM, Jauberteau MO, Bordessoule D, Yardin C, Preux PM, Couratier P (1996) Link between peripheral neuropathy and monoclonal dysglobulinemia: a study of 66 cases. J Neurol Sci 137:124–130

1166. Vallat JM, Leboutet MJ, Braund KG, Grimaud J (1993) Immunotactoid-like endoneurial deposits in a patient with monoclonal gammopathy of undetermined significance and neuropathy (letter; comment). Acta Neuropathol (Berl) 86:212–214

1167. Vallat JM, Leboutet MJ, Henry P, Millan J, Dumas M (1991) Endoneurial proliferation of perineurial cells in leprosy. Acta Neuropathol (Berl) 81:336–338

1168. Vallat JM, Leboutet MJ, Jauberteau MO, Tabaraud F, Couratier P, Akani F (1994) Widenings of the myelin lamellae in a typical Guillain-Barré syndrome. Muscle Nerve 17:378–380

1169. Vallat JM, Sindou P, Preux PM, Tabaraud F, Milor AM, Couratier P, LeGuern E, Brice A (1996) Ultrastructural PMP22 expression in inherited demyelinating neuropathies. Ann Neurol 39:813–817

1170. Valls-Solé J, Graus F, Font J, Pou A, Tolosa ES (1990) Normal proprioceptive trigeminal afferents in patients with Sjögren's syndrome and sensory neuronopathy. Ann Neurol 28:786–790

1171. Valmier J, Mallie S, Baldy-Moulinier M (1993) Skeletal muscle extract and nerve growth factor have developmentally regulated survival promoting effects on distinct populations of mammalian sensory neurons. Muscle Nerve 16:397–403

1172. van Alfen N, van Engelen BG, Reinders JW, Kremer H, Gabreels FJ (2000) The natural history of hereditary neuralgic amyotrophy in the Dutch population: two distinct types? Brain 123:718–723

1173. van der Pol WL, van den Berg LH, Scheepers RH, van der Bom JG, van Doorn PA, van Koningsveld R, van den Broek MC, Wokke JH, van de Winkel JG (2000) IgG receptor IIa alleles determine susceptibility and severity of Guillain-Barré syndrome. Neurology 54:1661–1665

1174. van der Wey LP, Polder TW, Stegeman DF, Gabreels-Festen AA, Spauwen PH, Gabreels FJ (1996) Peripheral nerve elongation by laser Doppler flowmetry-monitored expansion: an experimental basis for future application in the management of peripheral nerve defects. Plast Reconstr Surg 97:568–576

1175. van Dijk GW, Wokke JH, Oey PL, Franssen H, Ippel PF, Veldman H (1995) A new variant of sensory ataxic neuropathy with autosomal dominant inheritance. Brain 118:1557–1563

1176. van Domburg PH, Gabreels-Festen AA, Gabreels FJ, de Coo R, Ruitenbeek W, Wesseling P, ter Laak H (1996) Mitochondrial cytopathy presenting as hereditary sensory neuropathy with progressive external ophthalmoplegia, ataxia and fatal myoclonic epileptic status. Brain 119:997–1010

1177. van Heyningen V (1994) Genetics. One gene – four syndromes (news; comment). Nature 367:319–320

1178. van Meeteren NLU, Brakkee JH, Helders PJM, Gispen WH (1998) The effect of exercise training on functional recovery after sciatic nerve crush in the rat. J Periph Nerv Sys 3:277–282

1179. Vanier MT, Suzuki K (1998) Recent advances in elucidating Niemann-Pick C disease. Brain Pathol 8:163–174

1180. Verma A, Berger JR, Snodgrass S, Petito C (1996) Motor neuron disease: a paraneoplastic process associated with anti-hu antibody and small-cell lung carcinoma. Ann Neurol 40:112–116

1181. Villanova M, Ceuterick C, Dotti MT, Santorelli FM, Casali C, Malandrini A, De Stefano N, Lubke U, Martin JJ, Guazzi GC, Federico A (1999) Detection of beta-A4 amyloid and its precursor protein in the muscle of a patient with juvenile neuronal ceroid lipofuscinosis (Spielmeyer-Vogt- Sjögren). Acta Neuropathol (Berl) 98:78–84

1182. Visser LH, Schmitz PI, Meulstee J, van Doorn PA, van der Meche FG (1999) Prognostic factors of Guillain-Barré syndrome after intravenous immunoglobulin or plasma exchange. Dutch Guillain-Barré Study Group. Neurology 53:598–604

1183. Vital A, Fontan D, Julien J, Talon P, Héron B, Routon M, G. P, Vital C (1998) Congenital insensitivity to pain with anhydrosis. Report of two unrelated cases. J Periph Nerv Sys 3:125–132

1184. Vital A, Lagueny A, Julien J, Ferrer X, Barat M, Hermosilla E, Rouanet-Larrivière M, Henry P, Bredin A, Louiset P, Herbelleau T, Boisseau C, Guiraud-Chaumeil B, Steck A, Vital C (2000) Chronic inflammatory demyelinating polyneuropathy associated with dysglobulinemia: a peripheral nerve biopsy study in 18 cases. Acta Neuropathol (Berl) 100:63–68

1185. Vital A, Latinville D, Aupy M, Dumas P, Vital C (1991) Inflammatory demyelinating lesions in two patients with IgM monoclonal gammopathy and polyneuropathy. Neuropathol Appl Neurobiol 17:415–420

1186. Vital A, Vital C (1985) Polyarteritis nodosa and peripheral neuropathy. Ultrastructural study of 13 cases. Acta Neuropathol (Berl) 67:136–141

1187. Vital A, Vital C (1993) Immunoelectron identification of endoneurial IgM deposits in four patients with Waldenstrom's macroglobulinemia: a specific ultrastructural pattern related to the presence of cryoglobulin in one case. Clin Neuropathol 12:49–52

1188. Vital A, Vital C, Ellie E, Ferrer X, Lagueny A, Ferrer AM, Broustet A, Gbikpi-Benissan G (1993) Malignant infiltration of peripheral nerves in the course of acute myelomonoblastic leukaemia: neuropathological study of two cases. Neuropathol Appl Neurobiol 19:159–163

1189. Vital A, Vital C, Julien J, Baquey A, Steck AJ (1989) Polyneuropathy associated with IgM monoclonal gammopathy. Immunological and pathological study in 31 patients. Acta Neuropathol (Berl) 79:160–167

1190. Vital A, Vital C, Rigal B, Decamps A, Emeriau JP, Galley P (1990) Morphological study of the aging human peripheral nerve. Clin Neuropathol 9:10–15

1191. Vital C, Deminière C, Lagueny A, Bergouignan FX, Pellegrin JL, Doutre MS, Clement A, Beylot J (1988) Peripheral neuropathy with essential mixed cryoglobulinemia: biopsies from 5 cases. Acta Neuropathol (Berl) 75:605–610

1192. Vital C, Gherardi R, Vital A, Kopp N, Pellissier JF, Soubrier M, Clavelou P, Bellance R, Delisle MB, Ruchoux MM et al. (1994) Uncompacted myelin lamellae in polyneuropathy, organomegaly, endocrinopathy, M-protein and skin changes syndrome. Ultrastructural study of peripheral nerve biopsy from 22 patients. Acta Neuropathol (Berl) 87:302–307

1193. Vital C, Heraud A, Vital A, Coquet M, Julien M, Maupetit J (1989) Acute mononeuropathy with angiotropic lymphoma. Acta Neuropathol (Berl) 78:105–107

1194. Vogel H, Halpert D, Horoupian DS (1990) Hypoplasia of posterior spinal roots and dorsal spinal tracts with arthrogryposis multiplex congenita (published erratum appears in Acta Neuropathol (Berl) 1991;81(4):474). Acta Neuropathol (Berl) 79:692–696

1195. Voiculescu V, Alexianu M, Popescu-Tismana G, Pastia M, Petrovici A, Dan A (1987) Polyneuropathy with lipid deposits in Schwann cells and axonal degeneration in cerebrotendinous xanthomatosis. J Neurol Sci 82:89–99

1196. von Deimling A, Krone W, Menon AG (1995) Neurofibromatosis type 1: pathology, clinical features and molecular genetics. Brain Pathol 5:153–162

1197. von Giesen HJ, Stoll G, Koch MC, Beneck R (1994) Mixed axonal-demyelinating polyneuropathy as predominant manifestation of myotonic dystrophy. Muscle Nerve 17:701–703

1198. Vrethem M, Cruz M, Wen-Xin H, Malm C, Holmgren H, Ernerudh J (1993) Clinical, neurophysiological and immunological evidence of polyneuropathy in patients with monoclonal gammopathies. J Neurol Sci 114:193–199

1199. Vriesendorp FJ, Flynn RE, Malone MR, Pappolla MA (1998) Systemic complement depletion reduces inflammation and demyelination in adoptive transfer experimental allergic neuritis. Acta Neuropathol (Berl) 95:297–301

1200. Vriesendorp FJ, Mishu B, Blaser MJ, Koski CL (1993) Serum antibodies to GM1, GD1b, peripheral nerve myelin, and Campylobacter jejuni in patients with Guillain-Barré syndrome and controls: correlation and prognosis. Ann Neurol 34:130–135

1201. Vujaskovic Z (1997) Structural and physiological properties of peripheral nerves after intraoperative irradiation. J Periph Nerv Sys 2:343–349

1202. Wallace DC, Singh G, Lott MT, Hodge JA, Schurr TG, Lezza AM, Elsas LJd, Nikoskelainen EK (1988) Mitochondrial DNA mutation associated with Leber's hereditary optic neuropathy. Science 242:1427–1430

1203. Waller A (1850) Experiments on the section of the glossopharyngeal and hypoglossal nerves of the frog, and observations of the alterations produced thereby in the structure of their primitive fibres. Phil Trans R Soc Lond (Biol):423–429

1204. Walton J, Rowland LP, McLeod JG (1994) World Federation of Neurology Research Group on Neuromuscular Disorders. J Neurol Sci 124(suppl):109–130

1205. Wanders RJ, Heymans HS, Schutgens RB, Poll-The BT, Saudubray JM, Tager JM, Schrakamp G, van den Bosch H (1988) Peroxisomal functions in classical Refsum's disease: comparison with the infantile form of Refsum's disease. J Neurol Sci 84:147–155

1206. Wang CH, Carter TA, Das K, Xu J, Ross BM, Penchaszadeh GK, Gilliam TC (1997) Extensive DNA deletion associated with severe disease alleles on spinal muscular atrophy homologues. Ann Neurol 42:41–49

1207. Wang J, Schröder J (1998) Morphometric evaluation of paraneoplastic neuropathies associated with carcinomas, lymphomas, and dysproteinemias. J Periph Nerv Sys 3:259–266

1208. Wang ZH, Walter GF, Gerhard L (1996) The expression of nerve growth factor receptor on Schwann cells and the effect of these cells on the regeneration of axons in traumatically injured human spinal cord. Acta Neuropathol (Berl) 91:180–184

1209. Warner LE, Hilz MJ, Appel SH, Killian JM, Kolodry EH, Karpati G, Carpenter S, Watters GV, Wheeler C, Witt D, Bodell A, Nelis E, Van Broeckhoven C, Lupski JR (1996) Clinical phenotypes of different MPZ (P0) mutations may include Charcot- Marie-Tooth type 1B, Dejerine-Sottas, and congenital hypomyelination. Neuron 17: 451–460

1210. Warner LE, Mancias P, Butler IJ, McDonald CM, Keppen L, Gene Koob K, Lupski JR (1998) Mutations in the early growth response 2 (EGR2) gene are associated with hereditary myelinopathies. Nat Genet 18:382–384

1211. Watabe K, Kumanishi T, Ikuta F, Oyake Y (1983) Tactile-like corpuscles in neurofibromas: immunohistochemical demonstration of S-100 protein. Acta Neuropathol (Berl) 61:173–177

1212. Watanabe M, Sugai Y, Concannon P, Koenig M, Schmitt M, Sato M, Shizuka M, Mizushima K, Ikeda Y, Tomidokoro Y, Okamoto K, Shoji M (1998) Familial spinocerebellar ataxia with cerebellar atrophy, peripheral neuropathy, and elevated level of serum creatine kinase, gamma-globulin, and alpha-fetoprotein. Ann Neurol 44: 265–269

1213. Wattchow DA, Cass DT, Furness JB, Costa M, O'Brion PE, Little KE, Pitkin J (1987) Abnormalities of peptide-containing nerve fibers in infantile hypertrophic pyloric stenosis. Gastroenterology 92:443–448

1214. Weber JR, Angstwurm K, Bove GM, Bürger W, Einhäupl KM, Dirnagl U, Moskowitz MA (1996) The trigeminal nerve and augmentation of regional cerebral blood flow during experimental bacterial meningitis. J Cereb Blood Flow Metab 16:1319–1324

1215. Webster HD (1962) Schwann cell alterations in metachromatic leukodystrophy: preliminary phase and electron microscopic abservations. J Neuropathol Exp Neurol:534–554

1216. Webster HD (1993) Development of peripheral nerve fibers. In: Dyck PJ, Thomas PK (eds) Peripheral neuropathy, vol 1. Saunders, Philadelphia London Toronto Montreal Sydney Tokyo, pp 243–266

1217. Webster HD, Schröder J, Asbury A, Adams R (1967) The role of Schwann cells in the formation of "onion bulbs" found in chronic neuropathies. J Neuropathol Exp Neurol 26:276–299

1218. Webster HD, Spiro D (1960) Phase and electron microscopic studies of experimental demyelination. I. Variations in myelin sheath contour in normal guinea pig sciatic nerve. J Neuropath Exp Neurol 19:42–68

1219. Webster HD, Spiro D, Waksman B, Adams RD (1961) Phase and electron microscopic studies of experimental demyelination. II. Schwann cell changes in guinea pig sciatic nerves during experimental diphtheritic neuritis. J Neuropath Exp Neurol:5–34

1220. Weiner NC, Newman NJ, Lessell S, Johns DR, Lott MT, Wallace DC (1993) Atypical Leber's hereditary optic neuropathy with molecular confirmation. Arch Neurol 50:470–473

1221. Weis J, Alexianu ME, Heide G, Schröder JM (1993) Renaut bodies contain elastic fiber components. J Neuropathol Exp Neurol 52:444–451

1222. Weis J, Dimpfel W, Schröder JM (1995) Nerve conduction changes and fine structural alterations of extra- and intrafusal muscle and nerve fibers in streptozotocin diabetic rats. Muscle Nerve 18:175–184

1223. Weis J, Lie DC, Ragoss U, Züchner SL, Schröder JM, Karpati G, Farruggella T, Stahl N, Yancopoulos GD, DiStefano PS (1998) Increased expression of CNTF receptor alpha in denervated human skeletal muscle. J Neuropathol Exp Neurol 57:850–857

1224. Weis J, May R, Schröder JM (1994) Fine structural and immunohistochemical identification of perineurial cells connecting proximal and distal stumps of transected peripheral nerves at early stages of regeneration in silicone tubes. Acta Neuropathol 88:159–165

1225. Weis J, Schröder JM (1989) Differential effects of nerve, muscle, and fat tissue on regenerating nerve fibers in vivo. Muscle Nerve 12:723–734

1226. Weis J, Schröder JM (1989) The influence of fat tissue on neuroma formation. J Neurosurg 71:588–593

1227. Weis J, Weber U, Schröder JM, Lemke R, Althoff H (1998) Phrenic nerves and diaphragms in sudden infant death syndrome. Forensic Sci Int 91:133–146

1228. Weissman JD, Constantinitis I, Hudgins P, Wallace DC (1992) 31P magnetic resonance spectroscopy suggests impaired mitochondrial function in AZT-treated HIV-infected patients. Neurology 42:619–623

1229. Werner RA, Albers JW, Franzblau A, Armstrong TJ (1994) The relationship between body mass index and the diagnosis of carpal tunnel syndrome. Muscle Nerve 17:632–636

1230. Westarp ME, Westphal KP, Kolde G, Wollinsky KH, Westarp MP, Dickob M, Kornhuber HH (1992) Dermal, serological and CSF changes in amyotrophic lateral sclerosis with and without intrathecal interferon beta treatment. Int J Clin Pharmacol Ther Toxicol 30: 81–93

1231. White W, Shiu MH, Rosenblum MK, Erlandson RA, Woodruff JM (1990) Cellular Schwannoma. A clinicopathologic study of 57 patients and 58 tumors. Cancer 66: 1266–1275

1232. Wicklein EM, Orth U, Gal A, Kunze K (1997) Missense mutation (R15 W) of the connexin32 gene in a family with X chromosomal Charcot-Marie-Tooth neuropathy with only female family members affected. J Neurol Neurosurg Psychiatry 63:379–381

1233. Wijdicks EF, Ropper AH (1990) Acute relapsing Guillain-Barré syndrome after long asymptomatic intervals. Arch Neurol 47:82–84

1234. Wiley RG, Stirpe F (1987) Neuronotoxicity of axonally transported toxic lectins, abrin, modeccin and volkensin in rat peripheral nervous system. Neuropathol Appl Neurobiol 13:39–53

1235. Wilichowski E, Ohlenbusch A, Korenke GC, Hunneman DH, Hanefeld F (1998) Identical mitochondrial DNA in monozygotic twins with discordant adrenoleukody-strophy phenotype (letter). Ann Neurol 43:835–836

1236. Willems PJ, Vits L, Wanders RJ, Coucke PJ, Van der Auwera BJ, Van Elsen AF, Raeymaekers P, Van Broeck-hoven C, Schutgens RB, Dacremont G et al. (1990) Link-age of DNA markers at Xq28 to adrenoleukodystrophy and adrenomyeloneuropathy present within the same family. Arch Neurol 47:665–669

1237. Williams HB (1984) The painful stump neuroma and its treatment. Clin Plast Surg 11:79–84

1238. Willison HJ, Chancellor AM, Paterson G, Veitch J, Singh S, Whitelaw J, Kennedy PG, Warlow CP (1993) Antiglyco-lipid antibodies, immunoglobulins and paraproteins in motor neuron disease: a population based case-control study. J Neurol Sci 114:209–215

1239. Windebank A (1993) Polyneuropathy due to nutritio-nal deficiency and alcoholism. In: Dyck P, Thomas P, Griffin J, Low P, Poduslo J (eds) Peripheral neuropa-thy. WB Saunders Company, Philadelphia, pp 1310– 1321

1240. Windebank AJ, Blexrud MD, Dyck PJ, Daube JR, Karnes JL (1990) The syndrome of acute sensory neuropathy: clinical features and electrophysiologic and pathologic changes. Neurology 40:584–591

1241. Windebank AJ, Smith AG, Russell JW (1994) The effect of nerve growth factor, ciliary neurotrophic factor, and ACTH analogs on cisplatin neurotoxicity in vitro. Neu-rology 44:488–494

1242. Winek RR, Scheithauer BW, Wick MR (1989) Meningio-ma, meningeal hemangiopericytoma (angioblastic meningioma), peripheral hemangiopericytoma, and acoustic Schwannoma. A comparative immunohisto-chemical study. Am J Surg Pathol 13:251–261

1243. Winkler J, Ramirez GA, Kuhn HG, Peterson DA, Day-Lollini PA, Stewart GR, Tuszynski MH, Gage FH, Thal LJ (1997) Reversible Schwann cell hyperplasia and sprout-ing of sensory and sympathetic neurites after intraven-tricular administration of nerve growth factor. Ann Neurol 41:82–93

1244. Wirnsberger GH, Becker H, Ziervogel K, Hofler H (1992) Diagnostic immunohistochemistry of neuroblastic tumors. Am J Surg Pathol 16:49–57

1245. Witt FA (1993) Alkoholische Polyneuropathie: Experi-mentelle Untersuchungen über frühe und späte Stadien der direkten Alkoholwirkung auf Axone, Markscheiden und Blutgefäße. Universitätsklinikum, Institut für Neu-ropathologie. Rheinisch-Westfälische Technische Hoch-schule, Aachen

1246. Wokke JH, Jennekens FG, van den Oord CJ, Veldman H, van Gijn J (1988) Histological investigations of muscle atrophy and end plates in two critically ill patients with generalized weakness. J Neurol Sci 88:95–106

1247. Wolfe DE, Schindler D, Desnick RJ (1995) Neuroaxonal dystrophy in infantile alpha-N-acetylgalactosaminidase deficiency. J Neurol Sci 132:44–56

1248. Woodruff JM, Chernik NL, Smith MC, Millett WB, Foote FW, Jr. (1973) Peripheral nerve tumors with rhab-domyosarcomatous differentiation (malignant "Triton" tumors). Cancer 32:426–439

1249. Woodruff JM, Godwin TA, Erlandson RA, Susin M, Mar-tini N (1981) Cellular Schwannoma: a variety of Schwan-noma sometimes mistaken for a malignant tumor. Am J Surg Pathol 5:733–744

1250. Woodruff M (1960) The transplantation of tissue and organ. CC Thomas, Springfield Illinois

1251. Wright A, Dyck PJ (1995) Hereditary sensory neuro-pathy with sensorineural deafness and early-onset dementia. Neurology 45:560–562

1252. Wright GD, Patel MK, Mikel J (1988) An adult onset metachromatic leukodystrophy with dominant inheri-tance and normal arylsulphatase A levels. J Neurol Sci 87:153–166

1253. Xu D, Pollock M (1994) Experimental nerve thermal injury. Brain 117:375–384

1254. Yagihashi S (1995) Pathology and pathogenetic mecha-nisms of diabetic neuropathy. Diabetes Metab Rev 11:193–225

1255. Yagihashi S (1997) Pathogenetic mechanisms of diabetic neuropathy: lessons from animal models. J Periph Nerv Syst 2:113–132

1256. Yamamoto M, Sobue G, Mukoyama M, Matsuoka Y, Mitsuma T (1996) Demonstration of slow acetylator genotype of N-acetyltransferase in isoniazid neuro-pathy using an archival hematoxylin and eosin section of a sural nerve biopsy specimen. J Neurol Sci 135:51–54

1257. Yamamoto T, Vincent A, Ciulla TA, Lang B, Johnston I, Newsom-Davis J (1991) Seronegative myasthenia gravis: a plasma factor inhibiting agonist-induced acetylcholi-ne receptor function copurifies with IgM. Ann Neurol 30:550–557

1258. Yamasaki H, Itakura C, Mizutani M (1991) Hereditary hypotrophic axonopathy with neurofilament deficiency in a mutant strain of the Japanese quail. Acta Neuro-pathol (Berl) 82:427–434

1259. Yasaki S, Dyck PJ (1991) Spatial distribution of fiber degeneration in acute hypoglycemic neuropathy in rat. J Neuropathol Exp Neurol 50:681–692

1260. Yasuda H, Dyck PJ (1987) Abnormalities of endoneurial microvessels and sural nerve pathology in diabetic neu-ropathy. Neurology 37:20–28

1261. Yasuda T, Sobue G, Mitsuma T (1987) Nerve growth fac-tor receptors on dissociated dermal and plexiform neu-rofibroma Schwann-like cells (in Japanese). Rinsho Shinkeigaku 27:923–930

1262. Yasuda T, Sobue G, Mitsuma T, Takahashi A, Hashizume Y (1989) Nerve growth factor receptor immunoreactivi-ty in human benign peripheral nerve sheath tumor. Acta Neuropathol (Berl) 77:591–598

1263. Yiannikas C, McLeod JG, Walsh JC (1983) Peripheral neuropathy associated with polycythemia vera. Neuro-logy 33:139–143

1264. Yokota T, Wada Y, Furukawa T, Tsukagoshi H, Uchihara T, Watabiki S (1987) Adult-onset spinocerebellar syn-drome with idiopathic vitamin E deficiency. Ann Neurol 22:84–87

1265. Yomishi N, Tanaka T, Hara A, Bunai Y, Kato K, Mori H (1992) Extra-adrenal pheochromocytoma-ganglioneu-roma. A case report. Pathol Res Pract Dec;188:1098–1113

1266. Yoshida S, Mitani K, Wakayama I, Kihira T, Yase Y (1995) Bunina body formation in amyotrophic lateral sclerosis: a morphometric-statistical and trace element study fea-turing aluminum. J Neurol Sci 130:88–94

1267. Younes-Chennoufi AB, Léger JM, Hauw JJ, Preud'hom-me JL, Bouche P, Aucouturier P, Ratinahirana H, Lubetz-ki C, Lyon-Caen O, Baumann N (1992) Ganglioside GD1b is the target antigen for a biclonal IgM in a case of sen-sory-motor axonal polyneuropathy: involvement of N-acetylneuraminic acid in the epitope. Ann Neurol 32:18–23

1268. Young P, Wiebusch H, Stögbauer F, Ringelstein B, Assmann G, Funke H (1997) A novel frameshift mutation in PMP22 accounts for hereditary neuropathy with liability to pressure palsies. Neurology 48:450–452

1269. Younger DS, Dalmau J, Inghirami G, Sherman WH, Hays AP (1994) Anti-Hu-associated peripheral nerve and muscle microvasculitis. Neurology 44:181–183

1270. Yuki N (1994) Pathogenesis of axonal Guillain-Barré syndrome: hypothesis. Muscle Nerve 17:680–682

1271. Yuki N, Handa S, Tai T, Takahashi M, Saito K, Tsujino Y, Taki T (1995) Ganglioside-like epitopes of lipopolysaccharides from Campylobacter jejuni (PEN 19) in three isolates from patients with Guillain-Barré syndrome. J Neurol Sci 130:112–116

1272. Yuki N, Miyatani N, Sato S, Hirabayashi Y, Yamazaki M, Yoshimura N, Hayashi Y, Miyatake T (1992) Acute relapsing sensory neuropathy associated with IgM antibody against B-series gangliosides containing a GalNAc beta 1–4(Gal3–2 alpha NeuAc8–2 alpha NeuAc)beta 1 configuration. Neurology 42:686–689

1273. Yuki N, Takahashi M, Tagawa Y, Kashiwase K, Tadokoro K, Saito K (1997) Association of Campylobacter jejuni serotype with antiganglioside antibody in Guillain-Barré syndrome and Fisher's syndrome. Ann Neurol 42:28–33

1274. Yuki N, Wakabayashi K, Yamada M, Seki K (1997) Overlap of Guillain-Barré syndrome and Bickerstaff's brainstem encephalitis. J Neurol Sci 145:119–121

1275. Yuki N, Yamada M, Sato S, Ohama E, Kawase Y, Ikuta F, Miyatake T (1993) Association of IgG anti-GD1a antibody with severe Guillain-Barré syndrome. Muscle Nerve 16:642–647

1276. Yuki N, Yoshino H, Sato S, Shinozawa K, Miyatake T (1992) Severe acute axonal form of Guillain-Barré syndrome associated with IgG anti-GD1a antibodies. Muscle Nerve 15:899–903

1277. Yundt KD, Grubb RL Jr, Diringer MN, Powers WJ (1998) Autoregulatory vasodilation of parenchymal vessels is impaired during cerebral vasospasm. J Cereb Blood Flow Metab 18:419–424

1278. Zanssen S, Molnar M, Buse G, Schröder JM (2000) Novel cluster of tRNALeu(UUR) mutations in a sporadic case of infantile myopathy restricted to muscle tissue. Neuropediatrics 31:93–96

1279. Zanssen S, Molnar M, Buse G, Schröder JM (1998) Mitochondrial cytochrome b-gene deletion in Kearns Sayre syndrome associated with a mild type of peripheral neuropathy. Clin Neuropathol 17:291–296

1280. Zanssen S, Molnar M, Schröder JM, Buse G (1997) Multiple mitochondrial tRNA(Leu[UUR]) mutations associated with infantile myopathy. Mol Cell Biochem 174:231–236

1281. Zeng L, Worseg A, Redl H, Schlag G (1994) Peripheral nerve repair with nerve growth factor and fibrin matrix. Eur J Plast Surg 17:228–232

1282. Zerres K, Rudnik-Schöneborn S, Forrest E, Lusakowska A, Borkowska J, Hausmanowa-Petrusewicz I (1997) A collaborative study on the natural history of childhood and juvenile onset proximal spinal muscular atrophy (type II and III SMA): 569 patients. J Neurol Sci 146:67–72

1283. Zerres K, Wirth B, Rudnik-Schöneborn S (1997) Spinal muscular atrophy - clinical and genetic correlations. Neuromuscul Disord 7:202–207

1284. Zettl UK, Gold R, Toyka KV, Hartung HP (1995) Intravenous glucocorticosteroid treatment augments apoptosis of inflammatory T cells in experimental autoimmune neuritis (EAN) of the Lewis rat. J Neuropathol Exp Neurol 54:540–547

1285. Zhao J, Yoshioka K, Miike T, Kageshita T, Arao T (1991) Nerve growth factor receptor immunoreactivity on the tunica adventitia of intramuscular blood vessels in childhood muscular dystrophies. Neuromuscul Disord 1:135–141

1286. Zhao JX, Ohnishi A, Itakura C, Mizutani M, Yamamoto T, Hayashi H, Murai Y (1993) Smaller number of large myelinated fibers and focal myelin thickening in mutant quails deficient in neurofilaments. Acta Neuropathol (Berl) 86:242–248

1287. Zhao JX, Ohnishi A, Itakura C, Mizutani M, Yamamoto T, Hayashi H, Murai Y (1994) Greater number of microtubules per axon of unmyelinated fibers of mutant quails deficient in neurofilaments: possible compensation for the absence of neurofilaments. Acta Neuropathol (Berl) 87:332–336

1288. Zhao JX, Ohnishi A, Itakura C, Mizutani M, Yamamoto T, Hojo T, Murai Y (1995) Smaller axon and unaltered numbers of microtubules per axon in relation to number of myelin lamellae of myelinated fibers in the mutant quail deficient in neurofilaments. Acta Neuropathol (Berl) 89:305–312

1289. Zhu J, Link H, Weerth S, Linington C, Mix E, Qiao J (1994) The B cell repertoire in experimental allergic neuritis involves multiple myelin proteins and GM1. J Neurol Sci 125:132–137

1290. Zielasek J, Martini R, Suter U, Toyka KV (2000) Neuromyotonia in mice with hereditary myelinopathies. Muscle Nerve 23:696–701

1291. Zielasek J, Martini R, Toyka KV (1996) Functional abnormalities in Po-deficient mice resemble human hereditary neuropathies linked to Po gene mutations. Muscle Nerve 19:946–952

1292. Ziemssen F, Sindern E, Schröder JM, Shin YS, Zange J, Kilimann MW, Malin JP, Vorgerd M (2000) Novel missense mutations in the glycogen-branching enzyme gene in adult polyglucosan body disease. Ann Neurol 47:536–540

1293. Zifko U, Hahn A (1997) Migrant sensory neuropathy:Report of 5 cases and review of the literature. J Periph Nerve System 2:244–249

1294. Zimmer C, Gosztonyi G, Cervós-Navarro J, von Moers A, Schröder JM (1992) Neuropathy with lysosomal changes in Marinesco-Sjögren syndrome: fine structural findings in skeletal muscle and conjunctiva. Neuropediatrics 23:329–335

1295. Zochodne D (1996) Is early diabetic neuropathy a disorder of thedorsal root ganglion? J Periph Nerv Sys 2:119–130

1296. Zochodne DW (1994) Autonomic involvement in Guillain-Barré syndrome: a review. Muscle Nerve 17:1145–1155

1297. Zochodne DW (1999) Diabetic neuropathies: features and mechanisms. Brain Pathol 9:369–391

1298. Zochodne DW, Bolton CF, Wells GA, Gilbert JJ, Hahn AF, Brown JD, Sibbald WA (1987) Critical illness polyneuropathy. A complication of sepsis and multiple organ failure. Brain 110:819–841

1299. Zochodne DW, Nguyen C (1999) Increased peripheral nerve microvessels in early experimental diabetic neuropathy: quantitative studies of nerve and dorsal root ganglia. J Neurol Sci 166:40–46

1300. Zuber M, Sebald M, Bathien N, de Recondo J, Rondot P (1993) Botulinum antibodies in dystonic patients treated with type A botulinum toxin: frequency and significance. Neurology 43:1715–1718

References added in proof:

1301. Böker DK, Schönberg F, Gullotta F (1984) Localized hypertrophic neuropathy – a rare, clinically almost unknown syndrome. Clin Neuropathol 3:228-230

1302. Mersiyanova IV, Perepelov AV, Polyakov AV, Sitnikov VF, Dadali EL, Oparin RB, Petrin AN, Evgrafov OV (2000) A new variant of Charcot-Marie-Tooth disease type 2 is probably the result of a mutation in the neurofilament-light gene (see comments). Am J Hum Genet 67:37–46

1303. Ring HZ, Chang H, Guilbot A, Brice A, LeGuern E, Francke U (1999) The human neuregulin-2 (NRG2) gene: cloning, mapping and evaluation as a candidate for the autosomal recessive form of Charcot-Marie-Tooth disease linked to 5q. Hum Genet 104:326–332

1304. Sommer C, Schröder JM (1995) HLA-DR expression in peripheral neuropathies: the role of Schwann cells, resident and hematogenous macrophages, and endoneurial fibroblasts. Acta Neuropathol (Berl) 89:63–71

Subject Index

The manufacturer's authorised representative in the EU is Springer
Nature Customer Service Centre GmbH, Europaplatz 3, 69115 Heidelberg,
Germany. If you have any concerns regarding our products, please
contact ProductSafety@springernature.com

Printed and bound by CPI Group (UK) Ltd, Croydon, CR0 4YY
29/04/2026
02099553-0005